BRAIN–COMPUTER INTERFACES

BRAIN–COMPUTER INTERFACES

PRINCIPLES AND PRACTICE

EDITED BY Jonathan R. Wolpaw, MD

WADSWORTH CENTER

NEW YORK STATE DEPARTMENT OF HEALTH

ALBANY, NY

Elizabeth Winter Wolpaw, PhD

EMERITA PROFESSOR OF CHEMISTRY

SIENA COLLEGE

LOUDONVILLE, NY

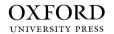

UNIVERSITY PRESS

OXFORD
UNIVERSITY PRESS

Oxford University Press, Inc., publishes works that further
Oxford University's objective of excellence
in research, scholarship, and education.

Oxford New York
Auckland   Cape Town   Dar es Salaam   Hong Kong   Karachi
Kuala Lumpur   Madrid   Melbourne   Mexico City   Nairobi
New Delhi   Shanghai   Taipei   Toronto

With offices in
Argentina   Austria   Brazil   Chile   Czech Republic   France   Greece
Guatemala   Hungary   Italy   Japan   Poland   Portugal   Singapore
South Korea   Switzerland   Thailand   Turkey   Ukraine   Vietnam

Published by Oxford University Press, Inc.
198 Madison Avenue, New York, New York 10016
www.oup.com

Oxford is a registered trademark of Oxford University Press

Library of Congress Cataloging-in-Publication Data

Brain–computer interfaces : principles and practice / [edited by] Jonathan R. Wolpaw, Elizabeth Winter Wolpaw.
    p. ; cm.
Includes bibliographical references and index.
ISBN 978-0-19-538885-5 (hardcover)
1. Brain mapping. 2. Pattern recognition systems. 3. Signal processing—Digital techniques. I. Wolpaw, Jonathan R.
II. Wolpaw, Elizabeth Winter.
[DNLM: 1. Brain Mapping. 2. Brain—physiology. 3. Pattern Recognition, Automated. 4. Self-Help Devices.
5. Signal Processing, Computer-Assisted. 6. User-Computer Interface. WL 335]
RC386.6.B7B624 2012
616.800285—dc23   2011018572

This material is not intended to be, and should not be considered, a substitute for medical or other professional advice.
Treatment for the conditions described in this material is highly dependent on the individual circumstances. And,
although this material is designed to offer accurate information with respect to the subject matter covered and to be
current as of the time it was written, research and knowledge about medical and health issues are constantly evolving,
and dose schedules for medications are being revised continually, with new side effects recognized and accounted
for regularly. Readers must therefore always check the product information and clinical procedures with the most
up-to-date published product information and data sheets provided by the manufacturers and the most recent codes of
conduct and safety regulation. The publisher and the authors make no representations or warranties to readers, express
or implied, as to the accuracy or completeness of this material. Without limiting the foregoing, the publisher and the
authors make no representations or warranties as to the accuracy or efficacy of the drug dosages mentioned in the
material. The authors and the publisher do not accept, and expressly disclaim, any responsibility for any liability, loss,
or risk that may be claimed or incurred as a consequence of the use and/or application of any of the contents of this
material.

9 8 7 6 5 4 3 2

Printed in China
on acid-free paper

Dedicated to
Michael, Sarah, Eliana, Vered, Maya, and Gabriella,
children of the 21st century

PREFACE

The possibility that signals recorded from the brain might be used for communication and control has engaged popular and scientific interest for many decades. However, it is only in the last 25 years that sustained research has begun, and it is only in the last 15 that a recognizable field of brain–computer interface (BCI) research and development has emerged. This new field is now populated by some hundreds of research groups around the world, and new groups are appearing continually. The explosive growth of this field is evident in the fact that a majority of all the BCI research articles ever published have appeared in the past five years.

This surge in scientific interest and activity arises from a combination of three factors. First and most obvious is the recent appearance of powerful inexpensive computer hardware and software that can support the complex high-speed analyses of brain activity essential to real-time BCI operation. Until quite recently, much of the rapid online signal processing used in current and contemplated BCIs was either impossible or extremely expensive. Now, hardware and software are no longer limiting factors: given the appropriate expertise, almost any promising BCI design can be implemented quickly and inexpensively.

The second factor is the greater understanding of the central nervous system (CNS) that has emerged from animal and human research over the past 50 years, particularly the voluminous new information about the nature and functional correlates of brain signals such as EEG activity and neuronal action potentials. Along with this new understanding have come improved methods for recording these signals, in both the short-term and the long-term. The continuing increases in basic knowledge and improvements in technology are enabling and guiding steadily more sophisticated and productive BCI research. Particularly important is the veritable revolution in the appreciation of the brain's remarkable capacity for adaptation, both in normal life and in response to trauma or disease. This new appreciation is a stunning change from the conception of the hardwired CNS that prevailed only 20 or 30 years ago. It generates enormous excitement about the possibilities for using these adaptive capacities to create novel interactions between the brain and computer-based devices, interactions that can replace, restore, enhance, supplement, or improve the brain's natural interactions with its external and internal environments.

The third factor is new recognition of the needs and abilities of people disabled by disorders such as cerebral palsy, spinal cord injury, stroke, amyotrophic lateral sclerosis (ALS), multiple sclerosis, and muscular dystrophies. Home ventilators and other life-support technology now enable even the most severely disabled people to live for many years. Furthermore, it is now understood that people who have very little voluntary muscle control can lead enjoyable and productive lives if they can be given even the most basic means of communication and control. BCIs, even in their currently limited state of development, can serve this need.

The distinctive property of BCI research and development, beyond its remarkable recent growth, is that it is inherently and necessarily multidisciplinary. The sequence of operations that lead from the user's brain to the BCI's action indicates this clearly. Appropriate selection of the brain signals that a BCI uses depends on our understanding of neuroscience, both basic and applied. Recording these signals properly depends on the physical sciences as well as on electrical and materials engineering and sometimes on neurosurgery and tissue biology as well. Appropriate, efficient, and timely processing of the recorded signals requires computer science and applied mathematics. The design and operation of the algorithms that translate signal features into device commands that achieve the user's intent depend on systems engineering as well as on understanding of spontaneous and adaptive changes in brain function. The selection of appropriate user populations and the implementation of appropriate applications require clinical neurology and rehabilitation engineering and depend on expertise in assistive technology. Finally, management of the complex ongoing interaction between the user and the application device requires understanding of behavioral psychology and human factors engineering. All these disparate disciplines, and effective cooperation among them, are essential if BCI research and development are to be successful in their primary goal, to provide important new communication and control options to people with severe disabilities.

The multidisciplinary nature of BCI research was a major impetus for this book and is the first principle of its structure and content. The book is intended to provide an introduction to and summary of essentially all major aspects of BCI research and development. Its goal is to be a comprehensive, balanced, and coordinated presentation of the field's key principles, current practice, and future prospects. It is aimed at scientists, engineers, and clinicians at all levels, and it is designed to be accessible to people with a basic undergraduate-level background in biology, physics, and mathematics. In response to the inherently multidisciplinary nature of the field, it seeks to introduce people from the many different relevant disciplines to all aspects of BCI research and thereby enable them to interact most productively. Attention has been paid to ensuring that the chapters mesh into a reasonably coordinated and logical whole, while at the same time preserving the sometimes differing views of the individual authors.

Each chapter tries to present its topic in a didactic format so that the reader can acquire the basic knowledge needed to work effectively with researchers and clinicians from the wide range of disciplines engaged in BCI research. For example, the chapters on signal processing (chapters 7 and 8) do more than simply review the various signal analysis methods that have been used in BCIs. They try to provide an accessible introduction to the broad range of signal analysis methods that might conceivably be applied to BCI use, and they outline the comparative advantages and disadvantages of these methods for specific BCI purposes. The goal is to enable the reader to participate actively in choosing from among alternative methods.

The book has six major parts. The Introduction stakes out the book's territory by carefully defining what is and what is not a brain–computer interface and it identifies six important themes that appear throughout the book. Part II introduces the different kinds of electrical and metabolic brain signals that BCIs might use; these chapters are necessarily long and challenging because they present many fundamental principles that underlie the subjects of all of the subsequent chapters. Part III proceeds through each of the components that constitute a BCI system, from signal acquisition to output commands, and discusses the applications that these commands control. Part IV reviews the principal kinds of BCIs developed to date and describes the current state of the art. Part V addresses the issues involved in the realization, validation, and dissemination of BCI systems useful to people with severe disabilities. Success in these difficult tasks is critical for the future of BCI technology. Part V also considers the possibilities for BCI uses that go beyond the assistive communication and control applications that have engaged the most attention up to the present; these further possibilities include BCI applications that could serve people with or without disabilities. In addition, Part V includes a chapter discussing the ethical issues associated with BCI research and development. Part VI, the Conclusion, considers the key problems that must be solved if BCIs are to fulfill the high expectations that so many people have for them.

Many people have contributed to this book. Each chapter is a unique and essential part of the whole. We hope that together they tell a coherent and exciting story and that therefore the whole is even greater than the sum of its parts.

Jonathan R. Wolpaw
Elizabeth Winter Wolpaw
Albany, New York
September 2011

ACKNOWLEDGMENTS

Brain–computer interface research and development is a team sport and so has been the realization of this book. No single author could have written it. The contribution of every one of the chapter authors was essential to our goal of presenting a comprehensive view of this complex new field. Coming from a wide variety of disciplines, they are brought together here by their knowledge of and commitment to research in areas important to BCI research and development. In this volume, they share their expertise and the fruits of their own work and that of other researchers and clinicians all over the world. Some of the authors have been engaged in BCI research since its beginnings, others have joined the ranks more recently, and still others work in related fields. All of them have generously contributed to make this book possible. We thank them all for this generosity and for their patience through the numerous steps of the process.

We are indebted to the many experts who served as external reviewers. Their names are listed on pages xvii–xviii of this volume. They represent many different disciplines and hail from many different places. Their insightful comments and suggestions have made the chapters substantially better. We also thank our colleagues at the Wadsworth Center for their numerous helpful comments and suggestions; we are particularly grateful to Chadwick Boulay, Peter Brunner, Natalie Dowell-Mesfin, Markus Neuper, Jeremy Hill, and Stuart Lehrman for their excellent technical advice and assistance.

People disabled by neuromuscular disorders have been and remain the primary impetus for BCI development. Their courage in facing the difficult challenges of their lives is an inspiration to all of us. We thank them all for this inspiration and especially want to thank those who have participated in many of the studies reported here. They are truly partners in this work.

Many institutions, both public and private, located in many countries around the world, have supported the research that is the substance of these chapters. Without their generous and enthusiastic support, virtually none of the work reported in this book would have been possible.

Finally, we would like to thank our editors at Oxford University Press. It has been a pleasure to get to know and work with Craig Allen Panner, Associate Editorial Director for Neuroscience, Neurology, and Psychiatry, who encouraged us to embark on this project in the first place. We thank him heartily for giving us this opportunity and for his wise guidance and unfaltering patience throughout the process. We thank Assistant Editor Kathryn Winder for her enthusiasm and for her unerring attention to detail in seeing this project through to completion. We also thank Production Editor Karen Kwak, and Viswanath Prasanna, Elissa Schiff, and the rest of Oxford's production team for their extraordinary care in turning the manuscript into a polished product.

It has been a privilege to work with all of these remarkable people, and we are grateful to have had the chance to do so. We hope that this volume provides a valuable foundation, framework, and resource for those engaged, or involved in any other way, in BCI research and development.

CONTENTS

PART SIX
CONCLUSION

CONTRIBUTORS

Brendan Z. Allison, PhD
Laboratory of Brain-Computer Interfaces
Institute for Knowledge Discovery
Graz University of Technology
Graz, Austria

Kim D. Anderson, PhD
Miami Project to Cure Paralysis
University of Miami
Miami, Florida, USA

Yael Arbel, PhD, CCC-SLP
Department of Communication Sciences
    and Disorders
University of South Florida
Tampa, Florida, USA

Niels Birbaumer, PhD
Institute of Medical Psychology and
    Behavioral Neurobiology
Eberhard-Karls-University of Tübingen
Tübingen, Germany, and
IRCCS Ospedale San Camillo
Istituto di Ricovero e Cura a Carattere Scientifico
Venezia Lido, Italy

Benjamin Blankertz, PhD
Department of Computer Science
Berlin Institute of Technology
Berlin, Germany

Janis J. Daly, PhD
Departments of Neurology
Louis B. Stokes Cleveland Veterans Affairs
    Medical Center, and
Case Western Reserve University School of Medicine
Cleveland, Ohio, USA

Emanuel Donchin, PhD
Department of Psychology
University of South Florida
Tampa, Florida, USA

John P. Donoghue, PhD
Department of Neuroscience
Brown University
Providence, Rhode Island, USA

Josef Faller, MSc
Laboratory of Brain-Computer Interfaces
Institute for Knowledge Discovery
Graz University of Technology
Graz, Austria

Joseph J. Fins, MD, FACP
Division of Medical Ethics
Weill Cornell Medical College
New York, New York, USA

Christoph Guger, PhD
g. tec Guger Technologies OG
Schiedlberg, Austria

Nicholas Hatsopoulos, PhD
Department of Organismal Biology and Anatomy
Committee on Computational Neuroscience
University of Chicago
Chicago, Illinois, USA

Leigh R. Hochberg, MD, PhD
Rehabilitation R&D Service
Department of Veterans Affairs Medical Center, and
School of Engineering
Brown University
Providence, Rhode Island, USA, and
Department of Neurology
Massachusetts General Hospital, and
Harvard Medical School
Boston, Massachusetts, USA

Jane E. Huggins, PhD
Department of Physical Medicine and Rehabilitation
Department of Biomedical Engineering
University of Michigan
Ann Arbor, Michigan, USA

Daryl R. Kipke, PhD
Department of Biomedical Engineering
University of Michigan
Ann Arbor, Michigan, USA

Dean J. Krusienski, PhD
Department of Electrical and Computer Engineering
Old Dominion University
Norfolk, Virginia, USA

Sangkyun Lee, MSc, Dr rer nat
Max-Planck Institute for Biological Cybernetics
Eberhard-Karls-University of Tübingen
Tübingen, Germany

Gerald E. Loeb, MD
Department of Biomedical Engineering
University of Southern California
Los Angeles, California, USA

Kip A. Ludwig, PhD
CVRx˚, Inc.
Minneapolis, Minnesota, USA

Steven G. Mason, PhD
Left Coast Biometrics Inc.
Vancouver, British Columbia, Canada

Dennis J. McFarland, PhD
Laboratory of Neural Injury and Repair
Wadsworth Center
New York State Department of Health
Albany, New York, USA

Lee E. Miller, PhD
Department of Physiology
Department of Physical Medicine and Rehabilitation
Department of Biomedical Engineering
Northwestern University
Chicago, Illinois, USA

Klaus-Robert Müller, PhD
Department of Computer Science
Berlin Institute of Technology
Berlin, Germany

Christa Neuper, PhD
Department of Psychology
University of Graz, and
Institute for Knowledge Discovery
Graz University of Technology
Graz, Austria

Paul L. Nunez, PhD
Emeritus Professor of Biomedical Engineering
Tulane University, and
Cognitive Dissonance, LLC
New Orleans, Louisiana, USA

Kevin J. Otto, PhD
Department of Biological
Sciences and Weldon School of Biomedical Engineering
Purdue University
West Lafayette, Indiana, USA

Gert Pfurtscheller, MSc, PhD
Emeritus Professor
Institute for Knowledge Discovery
Graz University of Technology
Graz, Austria

José C. Principe, PhD
Computational NeuroEngineering Laboratory
University of Florida
Gainesville, Florida, USA

Nick F. Ramsey, PhD
Department of Neurology and Neurosurgery
Division of Neuroscience
Rudolf Magnus Institute of Neuroscience
University Medical Center Utrecht
Utrecht, The Netherlands

Frances J. R. Richmond, PhD
School of Pharmacy
University of Southern California
Los Angeles, California, USA

Gerwin Schalk, MS, MS, PhD
Wadsworth Center
New York State Department of Health, and
Department of Biomedical Sciences
University at Albany, SUNY, and
Department of Neurology
Albany Medical College
Albany, New York, USA

Hansjörg Scherberger, MD
German Primate Center
Department of Biology
University of Göttingen
Göttingen, Germany

Mary-Jane Schneider, PhD
Department of Health Policy Management
   and Behavior
School of Public Health
University at Albany, SUNY, and
Laboratory of Neural Injury and Repair
Wadsworth Center
New York State Department of Health
Albany, New York, USA

Eric W. Sellers, PhD
Department of Psychology
East Tennessee State University
Johnson City, Tennessee, USA

Ranganatha Sitaram, MEng, PhD
Institute of Medical Psychology and
    Behavioral Neurobiology
Eberhard-Karls-University of Tübingen
Tübingen, Germany

Ramesh Srinivasan, PhD
Department of Cognitive Sciences
University of California
Irvine, California, USA

Michael Tangermann, Dr rer nat
Department of Computer Science
Berlin Institute of Technology
Berlin, Germany

Theresa M. Vaughan, BA
Laboratory of Neural Injury and Repair
Wadsworth Center
New York State Department of Health
Albany, New York, USA

J. Adam Wilson, PhD
Department of Neurosurgery
University of Cincinnati
Cincinnati, Ohio, USA

Elizabeth Winter Wolpaw, PhD
Professor Emerita of Chemistry
Siena College, and
Wadsworth Center
New York State Department of Health
Albany, New York, USA

Jonathan R. Wolpaw, MD
Wadsworth Center
New York State Department of Health, and
Department of Biomedical Sciences
University at Albany, SUNY
Albany, New York, USA

Debra Zeitlin, MA, CCC-SLP, ATP
Center For Rehabilitation Technology
Helen Hayes Hospital
New York State Department of Health
West Haverstraw, New York, USA

CHAPTER REVIEWERS

Brendan Z. Allison, PhD
Laboratory of Brain-Computer Interfaces
Institute for Knowledge Discovery
Graz University of Technology
Graz, Austria

Charles W. Anderson, PhD
Department of Computer Science
Colorado State University
Fort Collins, Colorado, USA

Tracy Cameron, PhD
St. Jude Medical
Neuromodulation Division
Plano, Texas, USA

Jose M. Carmena, PhD
Department of Electrical Engineering and
    Computer Sciences
Helen Wills Neuroscience Institute
University of California, Berkeley
Berkeley, California, USA

Bruce H. Dobkin, MD
Department of Neurology
Geffen/UCLA School of Medicine
Reed Neurologic Research Center
University of California Los Angeles
Los Angeles, California, USA

Richard P. Dum, PhD
Department of Neurobiology
University of Pittsburgh School of Medicine
Pittsburgh, Pennsylvania, USA

Thomas C. Ferree, PhD
Department of Radiology and Program in Biomedical
    Engineering
University of Texas Southwestern Medical Center
Dallas, Texas, USA

Jeremy Hill, DPhil
Laboratory of Neural Injury and Repair
Wadsworth Center
New York State Department of Health
Albany, New York, USA

Meltem Izzetoglu, PhD
School of Biomedical Engineering
Drexel University
Philadelphia, Pennsylvania, USA

Albert Kok, PhD
Emeritus Professor of Physiological Psychology
University of Amsterdam
Amsterdam, The Netherlands

Robert Leeb, PhD
Chair in Non-Invasive Brain-Machine Interface
École Polytechnique Fédérale de Lausanne
Lausanne, Switzerland

David M. LeMaster, PhD
Wadsworth Center
New York State Department of Health and
University at Albany, SUNY
Albany, New York, USA

Lee E. Miller, PhD
Department of Physiology
Department of Physical Medicine and Rehabilitation
Department of Biomedical Engineering
Northwestern University
Chicago, Illinois, USA

Fernando H. Lopes da Silva, MD, PhD
Emeritus Professor, Swammerdam Institute
    for Life Sciences
Center of NeuroSciences
University of Amsterdam
Amsterdam, The Netherlands

Dennis J. McFarland, PhD
Laboratory of Neural Injury and Repair
Wadsworth Center
New York State Department of Health
Albany, New York, USA

Michael C. Morton, MA
Global Regulatory Affairs Department
Medtronic, Inc.
Minneapolis, Minnesota, USA

Richard Normann, PhD
Department of Bioengineering
University of Utah
Salt Lake City, Utah, USA

Robert Oostenveld, PhD
Donders Institute for Brain, Cognition and Behaviour
Centre for Cognitive Neuroimaging
Radboud University Nijmegen
Nijmegen, The Netherlands

Nick F. Ramsey, PhD
Department of Neurology and Neurosurgery
Division of Neuroscience
Rudolf Magnus Institute of Neuroscience
University Medical Center Utrecht
Utrecht, The Netherlands

Robert L. Ruff, MD, PhD
Departments of Neurology
Louis B. Stokes Cleveland Veterans Affairs Medical Center
Case Western Reserve University School of Medicine
Cleveland, Ohio, USA

William Zev Rymer, MD, PhD
Rehabilitation Institute of Chicago
Department of Physiology
Department of Biomedical Engineering
Department of Physical Medicine and Rehabilitation
Northwestern University
Chicago, Illinois, USA

Krishna V. Shenoy, PhD
Department of Electrical Engineering
Department of Bioengineering
Department of Neurobiology
Stanford University
Stanford, California, USA

Karen L. Smith, MSc
Laboratory of Neural Injury and Repair
Wadsworth Center
New York State Department of Health
Albany, New York, USA

Aiko K. Thompson, PhD
Helen Hayes Hospital
West Haverstraw, New York, USA, and
Wadsworth Center
New York State Department of Health
Albany, New York, USA

Wei Wang, MD, PhD
Department of Physical Medicine and Rehabilitation
School of Medicine
Department of Bioengineering
Swanson School of Engineering
University of Pittsburgh
Pittsburgh, Pennsylvania, USA

Katryna Warren, BSc
St. Jude Medical
Neuromodulation Division
Plano, Texas, USA

Nikolaus Weiskopf, Dr rer nat
Wellcome Trust Centre for Neuroimaging
UCL Institute of Neurology
University College London
London, UK

Carolee Winstein, PhD, PT, FAPTA
Division Biokinesiology and Physical Therapy
Herman Ostrow School of Dentistry
Department of Neurology
Keck School of Medicine
University of Southern California
Los Angeles, California, USA

Steven L. Wolf, PhD, PT, FAPTA, FAHA
Department of Rehabilitation Medicine
Department of Medicine
Department of Cell Biology
Emory University School of Medicine
Atlanta, Georgia, USA

PART I. | INTRODUCTION

1 | BRAIN–COMPUTER INTERFACES: SOMETHING NEW UNDER THE SUN

JONATHAN R. WOLPAW AND ELIZABETH WINTER WOLPAW

In 1924, Hans Berger, Professor of Psychiatry at the University of Jena in Germany, discovered that electrical signals produced by the human brain could be recorded from the scalp. After five years of further study, Berger published the first of 14 articles that established electroencephalography (EEG) as a basic tool for clinical diagnosis and brain research (Berger, 1929). In 1938, just as his work had begun to receive international recognition, the German government closed his laboratory and forced him into retirement. The year was momentarily brightened for him by a holiday greeting from Herbert Jasper, a young North American neuroscientist at the start of a stellar career. Jasper sent to Berger the drawing shown in figure 1.1. It implies, albeit in a fanciful way, that EEG signals could also be used for communication.

This possibility—that people could act through brain signals rather than muscles—has fascinated scientists and nonscientists alike for many years. Now, nearly a century after Berger's epochal discovery, possibility is becoming reality. Although the reality is new and tentative and very modest, its excitement and potential are driving the burgeoning field of brain–computer interface research (fig. 1.2). This book is about that field—the principles that underlie it, its achievements so far, the problems that confront it, and its prospects for the future.

WHAT IS A BRAIN–COMPUTER INTERFACE?

As currently understood, the function of the central nervous system (CNS) is to respond to events in the outside world or the body by producing outputs that serve the needs of the organism. All the natural outputs of the CNS are neuromuscular or hormonal. A brain–computer interface (BCI) provides the CNS with new output that is neither neuromuscular nor hormonal. *A BCI is a system that measures CNS activity and converts it into artificial output that replaces, restores, enhances, supplements, or improves natural CNS output and thereby changes the ongoing interactions between the CNS and its external or internal environment.*

Understanding this definition requires an understanding of each of its key terms, beginning with *CNS*. The CNS is comprised of the brain and the spinal cord and is distinguished from the peripheral nervous system (PNS), which is comprised of the peripheral nerves and ganglia and the sensory receptors. The structures of the CNS are distinguished by their location within the meningeal coverings (or meninges), by their unique cell types and histology, and by their function in integrating the many different sensory inputs to produce appropriate motor outputs. In contrast, the PNS is not within the meninges, lacks the unique CNS histology, and serves mainly to convey sensory inputs to the CNS and to convey motor outputs from it.

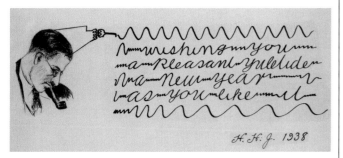

Figure 1.1 *This drawing was included in a holiday greeting that Herbert Jasper sent to Hans Berger in 1938. It is an early rendering of what is now called a brain-computer interface. (© Photo Deutsches Museum, Munich.)*

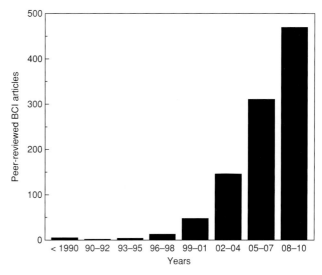

Figure 1.2 *BCI articles in the peer-reviewed scientific literature. In the past 15 years, BCI research, which was initially limited to a few isolated laboratories, has emerged as a very active and rapidly growing scientific field. The majority of research articles have appeared in the past five years. (Updated from Vaughan and Wolpaw, 2006.)*

CNS activity consists of the electrophysiological, neuro-chemical, and metabolic phenomena (e.g., neuronal action potentials, synaptic potentials, neurotransmitter releases, oxygen consumption) that occur continually in the CNS. These phenomena can be quantified by monitoring electric or magnetic fields, hemoglobin oxygenation, or other parameters using sensors on the scalp, on the surface of the brain, or within the brain (fig. 1.3). A BCI records these *brain signals*, extracts specific measures (or *features*) from them, and converts (or *translates*) these features into *artificial outputs* that act on the outside world or on the body itself. Figure 1.3 illustrates the five types of applications that a BCI output might control. For each of these five application types, it shows one of many possible examples.

A BCI output might *replace* natural output that has been lost as a result of injury or disease. For example, a person who can no longer speak might use a BCI to type words that are then spoken by a speech synthesizer. Or a person who has lost limb control might use a BCI to operate a motorized wheelchair. In these examples the BCI outputs *replace* lost natural outputs.

A BCI output might *restore* lost natural output. For example, a person with spinal cord injury whose arms and hands are paralyzed might use a BCI to stimulate the paralyzed muscles via implanted electrodes so that the muscles move the limbs. Or a person who has lost bladder function due to multiple sclerosis might use a BCI to stimulate the peripheral nerves that control the bladder, thus enabling urination. In these examples, the BCI outputs *restore* the natural outputs.

A BCI output might *enhance* natural CNS output. For example, a person performing a task that requires continuous attention over a prolonged period (e.g., driving a vehicle or serving as a sentry) might use a BCI that detects the brain activity preceding lapses in attention and then provides an output (e.g., a sound) that alerts the person and restores attention. By preventing the attentional lapses that periodically impair natural CNS output (and might cause traffic accidents), the BCI *enhances* the natural output.

A BCI output might *supplement* natural CNS output. For example, a person who is controlling the position of a computer cursor with a hand-operated joystick might use a BCI to select items that the cursor reaches. Or a person might use a BCI to control a third (i.e., robotic) arm and hand. In these cases, the BCI *supplements* natural neuromuscular output with an additional, artificial output.

Finally, a BCI output might conceivably *improve* natural CNS output. For example, a person whose arm movements have been impaired by a stroke involving the sensorimotor

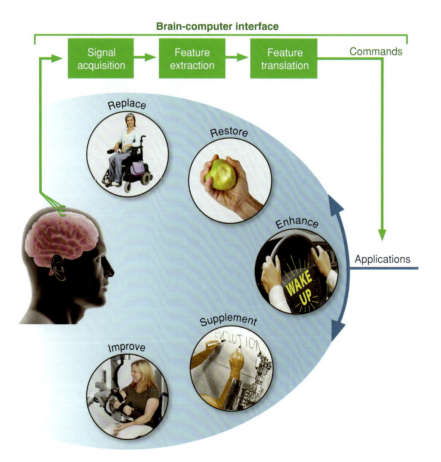

Figure 1.3 *The basic design and operation of a brain-computer interface (BCI) system. In this illustration, the BCI is shown in green. Electrical signals reflecting brain activity are acquired from the scalp, from the cortical surface, or from within the brain. The signals are analyzed to measure signal features (such as amplitudes of EEG rhythms or firing rates of single neurons) that reflect the user's intent. These features are translated into commands that operate application devices that replace, restore, enhance, supplement, or improve natural CNS outputs. (Modified from Wolpaw et al., 2002.) (Supplement image © Stelarc, http://stelarc.org; Improve image © Hocoma AG, www.hocoma.com.)*

cortex might use a BCI that measures signals from the damaged cortical areas and then stimulates muscles or controls an orthotic device so as to improve arm movements. Because this BCI application enables more normal movements, its repeated use may induce activity-dependent CNS plasticity that *improves* the natural CNS output and thereby helps the person to regain more normal arm control.

The first two types of BCI application, replacement or restoration of lost natural outputs, are the goals of most current BCI research and development, and examples of them appear many times throughout this book. At the same time, the other three kinds of BCI applications are also possible and are drawing increasing attention (chapters 22 and 23).

The last part of the definition states that a BCI *changes the ongoing interactions between the CNS and its external or internal environment.* The CNS interacts continuously with the outside world and with the body. These interactions consist of its motor outputs to the environment together with its sensory inputs from the environment. By measuring CNS activity and converting it into artificial outputs that affect the environment, BCIs change not only the CNS outputs but also the sensory inputs coming from the environment. These changes in sensory input are commonly referred to as *feedback*. Devices that simply monitor brain activity and do not use it to *change* the ongoing interactions between the CNS and its environment are not BCIs.

BCI TERMINOLOGY

PROVENANCE OF THE TERM BCI AND ITS PRESENT DEFINITION

Although an EEG-based BCI was demonstrated by Grey Walter in 1964 (Graimann et al., 2010a), the term *brain-computer interface* was apparently first used by Jacques Vidal in the 1970s. He applied the term very broadly, using it to describe any computer-based system that produced detailed information on brain function. Nevertheless, in the course of his work, Vidal developed a system that satisfies the narrower present-day meaning (Vidal, 1973, 1977). Vidal's system used the visual evoked potential (VEP) recorded from the scalp over the visual cortex to determine the direction of eye gaze (i.e., the visual fixation point) and thus to determine the direction in which the user wanted to move a cursor. Several years earlier, in the first neuron-based BCI, Eberhard Fetz and his collaborators had shown that monkeys could learn to use a single cortical neuron to control a meter needle to gain food rewards (Fetz, 1969; Fetz and Finocchio, 1971).

The BCI definition presented at the beginning of this chapter is based on the definitions and discussions in a number of reviews over the past decade (Donoghue, 2002; Wolpaw et al., 2002; Schwartz, 2004; Kübler and Müller, 2007; Daly and Wolpaw, 2008; Graimann et al., 2010a). It is intended to be comprehensive and definitive and, at the same time, to relate BCIs to the *sensorimotor hypothesis* (Young, 1990; Wolpaw, 2002), which is the theoretical foundation of modern neuroscience. The sensorimotor hypothesis is that the whole function of the CNS is to respond to external and internal events with appropriate outputs. In accord with this hypothesis, BCIs are defined as systems that translate brain signals into new kinds of outputs.

SYNONYMOUS OR SUBSIDIARY TERMS

The term *brain-machine interface* (BMI) was used as early as 1985 to describe implanted devices that stimulate the brain (Joseph, 1985) but was not applied specifically to devices that provide new outputs until more recently (e.g., Donoghue, 2002). In practice the term BMI has been applied mainly to systems that use cortical neuronal activity recorded by implanted microelectrodes. At present, BCI and BMI are synonymous terms, and the choice between them is largely a matter of personal preference. One reason for preferring BCI to BMI is that the word "machine" in BMI suggests an inflexible conversion of brain signals into output commands and thus does not reflect the reality that a computer and the brain are partners in the interactive adaptive control needed for effective BCI (or BMI) operation.

The terms *dependent BCI* and *independent BCI* were introduced in 2002 (Wolpaw et al., 2002). In accord with the basic BCI definition, both use brain signals to control their applications, but they differ in their dependence on natural CNS output. A dependent BCI uses brain signals that depend on muscle activity. For example, the BCI described by Vidal (1973, 1977) used the amplitude of a VEP that depended on gaze direction and thus on the muscles that controlled gaze. A dependent BCI is essentially an alternative method for detecting messages carried in natural CNS outputs. Although it does not give the brain a new output that is independent of natural outputs, it may still be useful (e.g., Sutter, 1992) (chapter 14).

In contrast, an *independent BCI* does not depend on natural CNS output; in independent BCIs, muscle activity is not essential for generating the brain signals that the BCI uses. For example, in BCIs based on EEG sensorimotor rhythms (SMRs) (chapter 13), the user may employ mental imagery to modify SMRs so as to control the BCI output. For people with severe neuromuscular disabilities, independent BCIs are likely to be more useful. At the same time it is important to recognize that most actual BCIs are neither purely dependent nor purely independent. The output of a steady-state VEP-based BCI may reflect the user's degree of attention (in addition to the user's gaze direction) (chapter 14). Conversely, most SMR-based BCIs rely on the user having sufficient visual function (and thus gaze control) to watch the results of the BCI's output commands (e.g., cursor movements).

The recent term *hybrid BCI* is applied in two different ways (Graimann et al., 2010b). It can describe a BCI that uses two different kinds of brain signals (e.g., VEPs and SMRs) to produce its outputs. Alternatively, it can describe a system that combines a BCI output with a natural muscle-based output (chapter 23). In the latter usage, the BCI output supplements a natural CNS output (e.g., as illustrated in fig. 1.3).

Another recent term, *passive BCI*, is applied to BCI applications that use brain signals that are correlated with aspects of the user's current state, such as level of attention (Zander and Kothe, 2011). For example, a BCI might detect EEG features preceding lapses in attention and produce an output (e.g., a sound) that alerts the user and restores attention (Chapter 23). The term *passive* is meant to distinguish these BCI applications from those that provide communication and control (i.e., *active* BCIs). However, *passive* and *active* are subjective terms that lack clear neuroscientific definitions. Furthermore, continued use of a passive BCI might well induce CNS adaptations that improve its performance, so that the term *passive* becomes no longer applicable. Thus, it seems preferable to categorize BCI applications simply as shown in figure 1.3, in which case passive BCIs will generally fit into the *enhance* or *supplement* category.

RELATED NEUROTECHNOLOGY

The recent explosion of BCI research is part of a surge of interest in a broad spectrum of new technologies and therapies that promise unprecedented understanding of and access to the brain and its disorders. These include structural and functional imaging methods of high resolution and specificity, chronically implanted devices for stimulating specific structures, molecules and particles that can encourage and guide neuronal regeneration and reconnection, cells that can replace lost tissues, and rehabilitation regimens that can restore useful function. A number of these new methods *act directly on the brain*, and thus contrast with BCIs, which, as defined here, allow the brain to *act directly on the world*. At the same time, some of these methods (e.g., direct stimulation of cortical or subcortical sensory areas) are likely to be incorporated into future BCI systems to improve their performance (chapters 5 and 16).

Direct input methods, together with BCIs (which provide direct outputs), fit into the general class of brain interfaces. Whether direct input methods will someday acquire their own designation (e.g., computer-brain interfaces [CBIs]) remains to be seen. The BCI definition described here recognizes the novel nature of devices that provide new CNS *outputs*.

SIX IMPORTANT THEMES

The rest of this chapter introduces six themes that we believe are important for understanding BCI research and development. These themes arise explicitly or implicitly many times in this book, and they are introduced here to emphasize and clarify their importance.

BCIs CREATE NEW CNS OUTPUTS THAT ARE FUNDAMENTALLY DIFFERENT FROM NATURAL OUTPUTS

The natural function of the CNS is to produce muscular and hormonal outputs that serve the needs of the organism by acting on the outside world or on the body. BCIs provide the CNS with *additional artificial outputs* derived from brain signals. Thus, they require the CNS, which has evolved to produce muscular and hormonal outputs, to now produce entirely new kinds of outputs. For example, the sensorimotor cortical areas, which normally interact with subcortical and spinal areas to control muscles, are now asked instead to control certain brain

signals (e.g., neuronal firing patterns or EEG rhythms). The profound implications of this requirement become apparent when BCI use is considered in terms of how the CNS normally operates. The research of the past 200 years, and especially of recent decades, has revealed two basic principles that govern how the CNS produces its natural outputs.

The first principle is that *the task of creating natural outputs is distributed throughout the CNS, from the cerebral cortex to the spinal cord.* No single area is wholly responsible for a natural output. As illustrated in an extremely simplified form in figure 1.4A, the selection, formulation, and execution of actions such as walking, speaking, or playing the piano are achieved through collaboration among cortical areas, basal ganglia, thalamic nuclei, cerebellum, brainstem nuclei, and spinal-cord interneurons and motoneurons. For example, while cortical areas initiate walking and oversee its progression, the rhythmic high-speed sensorimotor interactions needed to ensure effective locomotion are handled largely by spinal-cord circuitry (McCrea and Rybak, 2008; Ijspeert, 2008; Guertin and Steuer, 2009). The end product of this widely distributed CNS activity is the appropriate excitation of the spinal (or brainstem) motoneurons that activate muscles and thereby produce actions. Furthermore, although activity in the various CNS areas involved often correlates with motor action, the activity in any one area may vary substantially from one trial (i.e., one performance of a particular action) to the next. Nevertheless, the coordinated activations of all the areas ensure that the action itself is very stable across trials.

The second principle is that *normal CNS outputs (whether they be walking across a room, speaking specific words, or playing a particular piece on the piano) are mastered and maintained by initial and continuing adaptive changes in all the CNS areas involved.* In early development and throughout later life, neurons and synapses throughout the CNS change continually to acquire new actions (i.e., new skills) and to preserve those already acquired (e.g., Carroll and Zukin, 2002; Gaiarsa et al., 2002; Vaynman and Gomez-Pinilla, 2005; Saneyoshi et al., 2010; Wolpaw, 2010). This activity-dependent plasticity is responsible for acquiring and maintaining standard skills such as walking and talking as well as specialized skills such as dancing and singing, and it is guided by the results that are produced. For example, as muscle strength, limb length, and body weight change with growth and aging, CNS areas change so as to maintain these skills. Furthermore, the basic characteristics of the CNS (i.e., its anatomy, physiology, and mechanisms of plasticity) on which this continuing adaptation operates are the products of evolution guided by the need to produce appropriate actions, that is, to appropriately control the spinal motoneurons that activate the muscles. In figure 1.4A, to emphasize that this adaptation occurs and that it is directed at optimizing the natural CNS outputs (i.e., muscle activations), all of the CNS areas are shown in the same color as the muscles.

In light of these two principles—the many areas that contribute to natural CNS outputs and the continual adaptive plasticity in these areas—BCI use is a unique challenge for a CNS that has evolved and is continually adapting to produce the natural CNS outputs. Unlike natural CNS outputs, which are produced by spinal motoneurons, a BCI output is produced

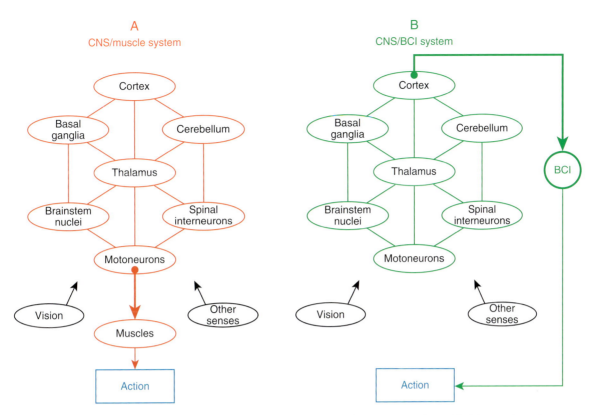

Figure 1.4 *CNS production of a muscle-based action versus CNS production of a BCI-based action. (A) This greatly simplified diagram shows the production of a normal motor action by the many CNS areas that collaborate to control spinal (or brainstem) motoneurons and thereby activate muscles. The red color indicates that all the CNS areas adapt to optimize muscle control. (B) This diagram shows the production of a BCI-mediated action by the same CNS areas, which now collaborate to optimize the control by the cortical area that produces the brain signals that the BCI translates into its output commands. The BCI assigns to the cortex the output role normally performed by spinal motoneurons and thereby asks that the CNS areas adapt to optimize an entirely new kind of output. This change in the target of CNS adaptation is indicated in this illustration by the fact that the color of all these areas (green) now matches the color of the BCI. (Modified from Wolpaw, 2007.)*

not by motoneuron activity but, rather, by signals that reflect activity in another CNS area (e.g., motor cortex). Normally the activity in this other area (e.g., motor cortex) is simply one of many contributors to natural CNS output. However, when its signals control a BCI, this activity actually *becomes* the CNS output. Figure 1.4B illustrates this fundamental change. The area that produces the signals that the BCI uses (i.e., the cortex in this illustration) takes on the role normally performed by spinal motoneurons. That is, the cortex produces the final product—the output—of the CNS. How well the cortex can perform this new role depends in part on how well the many CNS areas that normally adapt to control spinal motoneurons (which are downstream in natural CNS function) can instead adapt to control the relevant cortical neurons and synapses (which are largely upstream in natural CNS function). Figure 1.4B indicates this change in the goal of adaptation by now showing the CNS areas in the same color as the BCI, which, instead of the muscles, now produces the action.

For example, a BCI asks the cerebellum (which normally helps to ensure that motoneurons activate muscles so that movement is smooth, rapid, and accurate) to change its role to that of helping to ensure that the set of cortical neurons recorded by a microelectrode array produces patterns of action potentials that move a cursor (or a prosthetic limb) smoothly, rapidly, and accurately. The degrees to which the cerebellum

and other key areas can adapt to this new purpose remain uncertain. The ultimate capacities and practical usefulness of BCIs depend in large measure on the answers to this question.

The evidence to date shows that the adaptation necessary to control activity in the CNS areas responsible for the signals used by BCIs is certainly possible but that it is as yet imperfect. BCI outputs are in general far less smooth, rapid, and accurate than natural CNS outputs, and their trial-to-trial, day-to-day, and week-to-week variability is disconcertingly high. These problems (particularly the problem of poor reliability) and the various approaches to addressing them, are major concerns in BCI research, and they are discussed often in this book.

BCI OPERATION DEPENDS ON THE INTERACTION OF TWO ADAPTIVE CONTROLLERS

Natural CNS outputs are optimized for the goals of the organism, and the adaptation that achieves this optimization occurs primarily in the CNS. In contrast, BCI outputs can be optimized by adaptations that occur not only in the CNS but also in the BCI itself. In addition to adapting to the amplitudes, frequencies, and other basic characteristics of the user's brain signals, a BCI may also adapt to improve the fidelity with which its outputs match the user's intentions, to improve the effectiveness of adaptations in the CNS, and perhaps to guide the adaptive processes in the CNS.

Thus, BCIs introduce a second adaptive controller that can also change to ensure that the organism's goals are realized. BCI usage therefore depends on the effective interaction of *two adaptive controllers: the user's CNS and the BCI.* The management of this complex interaction between the adaptations of the CNS and the concurrent adaptations of the BCI is among the most difficult problems in BCI research. The challenges it poses arise at many points throughout this book.

CHOOSING SIGNAL TYPES AND BRAIN AREAS

Brain signals recorded by a variety of different electrophysiological and metabolic methods can serve as BCI inputs (chapters 12–18). These signals differ considerably in topographical resolution, frequency content, area of origin, and technical requirements. Figure 1.5 shows the range of electrophysiological methods from EEG to electrocorticography (ECoG) to intracortical recording and indicates the multiple scales of the brain signals available for BCIs, from the centimeter scale of EEG through the millimeter scale of ECoG to the tens-of-microns scale of neuronal action potentials. All of these electrophysiological methods have been used for BCIs and warrant continued evaluation, as do the metabolic methods discussed in chapters 4 and 18. Each has its own advantages and disadvantages. Which methods will prove most useful for which purposes is as yet unknown, and the answers will depend on a host of scientific, technical, clinical, and commercial factors.

On the one hand, the role of neuronal action potentials (spikes) as basic units of communication between neurons suggests that spikes recorded from many neurons could provide numerous degrees of freedom and might thus be the best signals for BCIs to use. Furthermore, the strong relationships between cortical neuronal activity and normal motor control

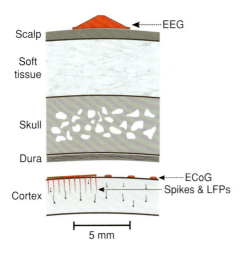

Figure 1.5 *Recording sites for electrophysiological signals used by BCI systems. EEG is recorded by electrodes on the scalp. ECoG is recorded by electrodes on the cortical surface. Neuronal action potentials (spikes) or local field potentials (LFPs) are recorded by microelectrode arrays inserted into the cortex (or other brain areas). A few representative cortical pyramidal neurons are indicated. (Modified from Wolpaw and Birbaumer, 2006.)*

(chapter 2) provide logical starting points for development of BCI-based control of devices such as robotic arms (chapter 16). On the other hand, the fundamental importance of CNS adaptation for all BCIs, and the evidence that adaptive methods can elicit multiple degrees of freedom even from EEG signals (chapter 13), suggest that the difference between the BCI performance provided by single neurons and by EEG may not be nearly as great as the difference in their topographical resolutions.

Questions about signal selection are empirical issues that can be resolved only by experiment, not by a priori assumptions about the inherent superiority of one signal type or another. For BCIs, the critical issue is which signals can provide the best measure of the user's intent, that is, which signals constitute the best language for communicating to the BCI the output desired by the user. This question can be conclusively answered only by experimental results.

Selection of the best brain areas from which to record the signals is also an empirical question. Studies to date have focused mainly on signals from sensorimotor (and visual) cortical areas. The usefulness of signals from other cortical or subcortical areas is also being explored (e.g., chapter 17). This is an important question, especially because the sensorimotor cortices of many prospective BCI users have been damaged by injury or disease and/or their visual function may be compromised. Different brain areas may well differ in their adaptive capacities and in other factors that may affect their ability to serve as the sources of new CNS outputs.

RECOGNIZING AND AVOIDING ARTIFACTS

Like most communication and control systems, BCIs face the problems of artifacts that obscure the signals that convey output commands. For BCIs, artifacts may come from the environment (e.g., electromagnetic noise from power lines or appliances), from the body (e.g., muscle (electromyographic [EMG]) activity, eye movement (electrooculographic [EOG]) activity, cardiac (electrocardiographic [EKG]) activity, bodily movements) or from the BCI hardware (e.g., electrode instability, amplifier noise). The different varieties of artifacts and the measures for eliminating them or reducing their impact are addressed in chapters 6 and 7. Particularly for BCIs that record brain signals noninvasively, artifacts present a danger that warrants some discussion even in this introductory chapter.

The first requirement for any BCI study or demonstration is to ensure that it is, in fact, using a BCI (i.e., that *brain signals,* not other types of signals, control its output). Systems that use other kinds of biological signals, such as EMG activity, may be valuable in their own right, but they are not BCIs. Unfortunately, nonbrain signals such as EMG activity may readily masquerade as brain signals. Electrodes placed anywhere on the scalp can record EMG activity from cranial muscles or EOG activity that equals or exceeds EEG activity in amplitude and that overlaps with it in frequency range. Because people can readily control cranial EMG or EOG activity and may not even be aware that they are doing so, such nonbrain activity may contaminate or even dominate the signals recorded by a BCI and may thereby ensure that the BCI outputs are produced in part, or even entirely, by nonbrain signals. Clearly, effective BCI research and development are not possible in such circumstances. (Indeed, even in the scientific literature there are examples of putative BCI studies in which EMG signals masquerade as EEG signals, so that the results reflect cranial-muscle control rather than brain-signal control.) Commercial devices (e.g., for gaming) that are currently marketed as BCIs often do not differentiate EEG from EMG or other nonbrain signals. Only if it is certain that the control signals arise from brain activity and not from other activity can the results of BCI studies be useful to people whose severe disabilities have eliminated their control of nonbrain signals.

To avoid the danger of contamination by nonbrain signals, EEG-based BCI studies need to incorporate topographical and frequency analyses that are sufficiently comprehensive to distinguish between brain and nonbrain signals. Noninvasive metabolic BCI studies may need to incorporate analogous precautions. EEG studies that simply record from a single site, or that focus on a single narrow frequency band, cannot reliably discriminate between EEG and EMG, and thus, their results may be misleading. These issues are addressed in greater detail in chapters 6 and 7.

BCI OUTPUT COMMANDS: GOAL SELECTION OR PROCESS CONTROL

A BCI can produce two kinds of output commands: a command that *selects a goal* or a command that *controls a process*. Figure 1.6 illustrates these two options applied to the movement of a motorized wheelchair.

In the *goal-selection* protocol shown at the top, the user and the BCI simply communicate the goal (i.e., the user's intent) to software in the application, and it is the application that then manages the process that accomplishes that intent. For example, the BCI might communicate the goal of moving to a location facing the television. The application device (i.e., the wheelchair) then produces the several concurrent sequences of actions (e.g., movements in x and y directions, turning,

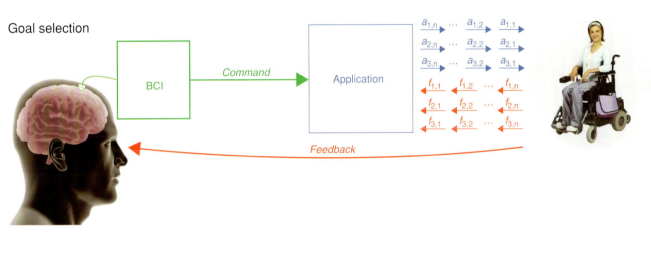

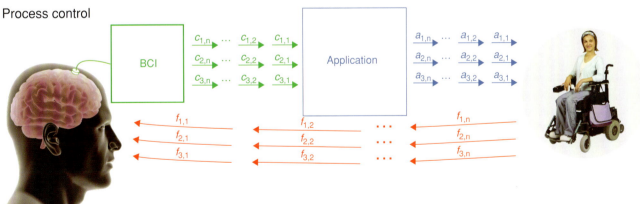

Figure 1.6 *BCI outputs: goal selection versus process control. BCI output commands can either select goals or control processes. In goal selection the BCI command specifies only the user's intent; the process that achieves this intent is accomplished by the application (i.e., the motorized wheelchair), which produces several concurrent sequences of actions (e.g., $a_{1,t=1}$, $a_{1,t=2}$ . . . $a_{1,t=n}$; $a_{2,t=1}$, $a_{2,t=2}$ . . . $a_{2,t=n}$; etc.) that control its movement and also manage the ongoing interactions between these actions and the resulting sequences of feedback (e.g., $f_{1,t=1}$, $f_{1,t=2}$ . . . $f_{1,t=n}$; $f_{2,t=1}$, $f_{2,t=2}$ . . . $f_{2,t=n}$; etc.). The feedback to the user is mainly the end result. In process control the brain and the BCI provide several concurrent sequences of commands (e.g., $c_{1,t=1}$, $c_{1,t=2}$ . . . $c_{1,t=n}$; $c_{2,t=1}$, $c_{2,t=2}$ . . . $c_{2,t=n}$; etc.) that correspond to the sequences of actions that the application produces; and the brain and the BCI continue to manage the ongoing interactions between these actions and the resulting feedback. The most successful BCIs are likely to combine goal selection and process control appropriately for each purpose and to thereby emulate the distributed control characteristic of natural muscle-based CNS outputs. (Modified from Wolpaw, 2007.)*

braking) (denoted by a's in fig. 1.6[top]) that move the wheelchair to the desired location at a safe speed. The wheelchair application also receives concurrent detailed feedback (denoted by f's) that allows it to adjust its actions as needed to avoid dangers such as staircases and obstacles such as walls, furniture, and other people. As the figure illustrates, the goal-selection protocol places most of the burden (i.e., for complex high-speed interactive control) on the application. The BCI simply communicates the goal, and the user simply views, and benefits from, the overall result. This example is analogous to using a global positioning system (GPS) to select a destination and then putting your vehicle on automatic pilot (assuming of course that it is equipped with this option!).

In contrast, in the *process-control* protocol shown at the bottom of figure 1.6, the user and the BCI control all the details of the process that accomplishes the user's intent. The user and BCI produce sequences of commands (denoted by c's), which the wheelchair simply converts into actions (e.g., movements in x and y directions, turning, braking). The user processes the concurrent sequences of feedback to adjust the BCI's commands appropriately. The user and the BCI manage all the details of the process that puts the user in front of the television. The wheelchair simply does exactly what it is told to do. If goal selection is like using a GPS and an automatic pilot, process control is like driving the vehicle yourself and making all the decisions on which way to turn, how fast to go, when to stop, and so forth.

A simple summary of the difference between these two kinds of BCI output commands is that in goal selection the BCI tells the application what to do, whereas in process control it tells it how to do it. As chapters 12–18 illustrate, goal-selection and process-control protocols have both been used in a variety of BCIs, noninvasive as well as invasive.

From the point of view of the CNS and the BCI, goal selection is relatively easy. It requires only that the BCI provide the goal (i.e., the user's intent), which is the one part of the desired action that the application alone cannot provide. Once the goal is communicated, the application software and hardware are expected to achieve the goal rapidly and reliably. Goal selection is generally most appropriate for simpler BCI applications in which the set of possible commands is relatively small and fully defined (e.g., word-processing or wheelchair navigation in a specific environment with limited destinations). For more demanding applications, in which the set of possible goals may be large and not fully defined, or in which unexpected complications can occur (e.g., multidimensional control of a robotic arm or wheelchair navigation in different environments with many possible destinations), it may be necessary to use process control, which generally places greater demands on the CNS and the BCI.

As illustrated in figure 1.4A, natural CNS outputs are the product of the combined activity of many areas from the cortex to the spinal cord. Furthermore, the distribution of control varies appropriately from action to action. For example, a lengthy clinical and experimental literature indicates that the cortex plays a much greater role in fine finger control than it does in gross movements such as hand grasp (Porter and Lemon, 1993). In accord with the terminology used here, the cortex sometimes functions in a process-control manner in which it controls every detail of an action, and at other times it functions in a goal-selection manner in which it delegates the details to subcortical areas.

The most effective and desirable BCIs are likely to be those that imitate to the greatest extent possible the action-appropriate distribution of control that characterizes natural CNS function. To do this, BCIs might combine the two approaches of goal selection and process control. For example, in reaching to and grasping an object with a robotic arm, the cortex and the BCI might command the three-dimensional movement of the hand, the hand orientation, and the grasp while the application device might handle the details of the movements of the individual limb segments and the details of wrist rotation and finger flexion. Such distributed designs, which place fewer demands on the user and the BCI, may also be more realistic in the present state of BCI development. As progress continues, and as BCIs incorporate more elaborate and timely feedback from the evolving action to the CNS, goal selection and process control might be combined so that BCIs can emulate with steadily growing fidelity the speed, reliability, and ease of the brain's natural outputs.

VALIDATING AND DISSEMINATING USEFUL BCI APPLICATIONS

Because of the complexity and multidisciplinary requirements of BCI development, most research groups focus on a single aspect, such as recording hardware, signal processing, or application design. This focus is both understandable and important for making substantive contributions. At the same time, the continuation and ultimate success of BCI development depend on realizing systems that are useful to the people with severe disabilities who are the principal reason for the existence of the field and for the substantial attention and support it currently receives. Thus, it is essential to develop systems that are clinically useful.

This task is an extremely demanding endeavor. It requires effective interdisciplinary collaborations and management of the complicated clinical and administrative requirements of human research (chapter 20) as well as attention to the more or less unique ethical issues associated with BCI research (chapter 24). Clinically useful BCI systems must function effectively and reliably in complex and often changing environments. They must be usable by nonexperts without excessive technical support and must provide applications that improve the lives of their users. These requirements constitute a hard and unforgiving test for systems first developed in the laboratory. At the same time, satisfying them validates the entire field of BCI research and development.

Even when BCI systems are clinically validated, their wider dissemination to the people who need them most faces several practical challenges. The dissemination of new medical technologies is typically a commercial endeavor and thus requires a reasonable expectation of profitability. However, the number of people who need the relatively modest capabilities of current BCIs, or of the BCIs likely to be available in the near future, is relatively small by typical marketing standards.

Thus, the immediate user population may not be large enough to attract and reward the commercial entities that could manufacture, market, and support current BCIs for those who need them most. Effective approaches to this problem may lie in therapeutic BCI applications (chapter 22) that can serve larger populations (e.g., people who have had strokes) and in well-structured commercial initiatives that target both the core group of people with severe disabilities and the much larger numbers of people in the general population who might use BCIs for other purposes (chapter 23). These difficult issues and their potential solutions are discussed in chapters 21 and 24.

SUMMARY

The CNS interacts continuously with the outside world and the body through its natural neuromuscular and hormonal outputs. *BCIs measure CNS activity and convert it into artificial outputs that replace, restore, enhance, supplement, or improve the natural CNS outputs.* Thus, BCIs change the interactions between the CNS and its environment. The *new CNS outputs* that the BCI creates are fundamentally different from natural CNS outputs, which come from spinal motoneurons. BCI outputs come from brain signals that reflect activity elsewhere in the CNS (e.g., motor cortex). Effective BCI operation requires that the CNS control that activity nearly as accurately and reliably as it normally controls motoneurons. The achievement of such accuracy and reliability is a major challenge for BCI research.

The adaptations that optimize natural CNS outputs occur mainly in the CNS. In contrast, the adaptations that optimize BCI outputs can also occur in the BCI. Thus, BCI operation relies on the interaction between, and the adaptive capacities of, *two adaptive controllers*: the CNS and the BCI. The design of this additional adaptive controller (i.e., the BCI) and the management of its interactions with the adaptations of the CNS constitute a particularly challenging aspect of BCI research.

BCIs might use any of a variety of *different kinds of brain signals* recorded in a variety of different ways from a variety of different brain areas. Questions of which signals from which brain areas are best for which applications are empirical issues that need to be answered by experiment.

Like other communication and control interfaces, BCIs can encounter *artifacts* that obscure or imitate their critical signals. EEG-based BCIs must exercise particular care to avoid mistaking nonbrain signals recorded from the head (e.g., cranial EMG activity) for brain signals. This entails appropriately comprehensive topographical and spectral analyses.

BCI outputs can either *select a goal* or *control a process*. Ultimately, BCIs are likely to be most successful by combining goal selection and process control, that is, by distributing control between the BCI and the application in a manner appropriate to the current action. By such distribution, they could most closely emulate natural CNS function.

The continuation and ultimate success of BCI development depend on realizing systems that are useful to people with severe disabilities. The *clinical evaluation and validation* of BCIs are demanding endeavors requiring interdisciplinary collaboration and satisfaction of the complicated requirements of clinical research.

BCI research, which occupied only a handful of laboratories 15 years ago, is now an explosively growing field involving hundreds of research groups throughout the world. Its excitement and potential are drawing many young scientists and engineers into a vibrant research community that is engaging the numerous issues and pursuing the great promise of BCI technology. The intent of this book is to contribute to the further growth and success of this community by providing a solid grounding in fundamental principles and methods, by summarizing the current state of the art, and by raising and discussing critical issues.

REFERENCES

Berger, H. Uber das electrenkephalogramm des menchen. Arch Psychiatr Nervenkr 87:527–570, 1929.t

Carroll, R.C., and Zukin, R.S. NMDA-receptor trafficking and targeting: implications for synaptic transmission and plasticity. Trends Neurosci 25(11):571–577, 2002.

Daly, J.J., and Wolpaw, J.R. Brain-computer interfaces in neurological rehabilitation. Lancet Neurol 7:1032–1043, 2008.

Donoghue, J.P. Connecting cortex to machines: recent advances in brain interfaces. Nature Neurosci 5(Suppl):1085–1088, 2002.

Fetz, E.E. Operant conditioning of cortical unit activity. Science 163:955–958, 1969.

Fetz, E.E., and Finocchio, D.V. Operant conditioning of specific patterns of neural and muscular activity. Science 174:431–435, 1971.

Gaiarsa, J.L., Caillard, O., and Ben-Ari, Y. Long-term plasticity at GABA-ergic and glycinergic synapses: mechanisms and functional significance. Trends Neurosci 25(11):564–570, 2002.

Graimann, B., Allison, B., and Pfurtscheller, G. Brain-computer interfaces: a gentle introduction. In: Brain-Computer Interfaces (B. Graimann, B. Allison, G. Pfurtscheller, eds.), Berlin: Springer, 2010a, pp. 1–27.

Graimann, B., Allison, B., and Pfurtscheller, G. (eds.), Brain-Computer Interfaces, Berlin: Springer, 2010b, p. 21 et passim.

Guertin, P.A., and Steuer, I. Key central pattern generators of the spinal cord. J Neurosci Res 87:2399–2405, 2009.

Ijspeert, A.J. Central pattern generators for locomotion control in animals and robots: a review. Neural Netw 21:642–653, 2008.

Joseph, A.B. Design considerations for the brain-machine interface. Med Hypoth 17:191–195, 1985.

Kübler, A., and Müller, K.R. An introduction to brain-computer interfacing. In: Toward Brain-Computer Interfacing (G. Dornbhege, J.d.R. Millán, T. Hinterberger, D.J. McFarland, K.-R. Müller, eds.). Cambridge, MA: MIT Press, 2007, pp. 1–26.

McCrea, D.A., and Ryback, I.A. Organization of mammalian locomotor rhythm and pattern generation. Brain Res Rev 57:134–146, 2008.

Porter, R., and Lemon, R. Corticospinal Function and Voluntary Movement. Oxford: Clarendon Press, 1993.

Saneyoshi, T., Fortin, D.A., and Soderling, T.R. Regulation of spine and synapse formation by activity-dependent intracellular signaling pathways. Curr Opin Neurobiol 20(1):108–115, 2010.

Schwartz, A.B. Cortical neural prosthetics. Annu Rev Neurosci 27:487–507, 2004.

Sutter EE. The brain response interface: communication through visually induced electrical brain responses. J Microcomput Appl 15:31–45, 1992.

Vaughan, T.M., and Wolpaw, J.R. The Third International Meeting on Brain-Computer Interface Technology: Making a Difference (Editorial). IEEE Trans Neural Syst Rehab Eng 14:126–127, 2006.

Vaynman, S., and Gomez-Pinilla, F. License to run: exercise impacts functional plasticity in the intact and injured central nervous system by using neurotrophins. Neurorehabil Neural Repair 19(4): 283–295, 2005.

Vidal, J.J. Towards direct brain–computer communication. Annu Rev Biophys Bioeng 2:157–180, 1973.

Vidal, J.J. Real-time detection of brain events in EEG. IEEE Proc 65:633–664 [Special issue on Biological Signal Processing and Analysis], 1977.

Wolpaw, J.R. Memory in neuroscience: rhetoric versus reality. Behav Cognit Neurosci Rev 1:130–163, 2002.

Wolpaw, J.R. Brain-computer interfaces as new brain output pathways. J Physiol 579:613–619, 2007.

Wolpaw, J.R. What can the spinal cord teach us about learning and memory? Neuroscientist 16(5):532–549, 2010.

Wolpaw, J.R., and Birbaumer, N. Brain-computer interfaces for communication and control. In: Textbook of Neural Repair and Rehabilitation; Neural Repair and Plasticity (M.E. Selzer, S. Clarke, L.G. Cohen, P. Duncan, F.H. Gage, eds.), Cambridge: Cambridge University Press, 2006, pp. 602–614.

Wolpaw, J.R., Birbaumer, N., McFarland, D.J., Pfurtscheller, G., and Vaughan TM. Brain-computer interfaces for communication and control. Clin Neurophysiol 113:767–791, 2002.

Young, R.M. Mind, Brain and Adaptation in the Nineteenth Century. Oxford: Oxford University Press, 1990.

Zander, T.O. and Kothe, C. Towards passive brain-computer interfaces: applying brain-computer interface technology to human-machine systems in general. J Neur Engin 8:025005(5pp), 2011.

PART II. | BRAIN SIGNALS FOR BCIs

2 | NEURONAL ACTIVITY IN MOTOR CORTEX AND RELATED AREAS

LEE E. MILLER AND NICHOLAS HATSOPOULOS

In 1870, Eduard Hitzig and Gustav Fritsch applied electrical stimuli to a region on the surface of a dog's brain that caused the limb on the opposite side of its body to move. This observation was critical in a number of respects. It demonstrated that, like muscles, the brain is electrically excitable. By finding limb movement represented in a particular area, it also addressed the larger issue of whether different parts of the brain, and of the cerebral cortex in particular, were devoted to different functions. In the middle of the 19th century opinions on this point ranged from that of the minute cortical specialization held by the phrenologists (Gall and Spurzheim 1809), to that of Pierre Flourens, who held that the cerebral cortex was largely unspecialized (Flourens 1824). Based on their experiments, Hitzig and Fritsch ultimately described the area of the brain that we now know as the *primary motor cortex* (Fritsch and Hitzig 1870). Also in the 1870s, David Ferrier conducted experiments similar to those of Hitzig and Fritsch using monkeys as subjects (Ferrier 1873).

Today, neurosurgeons routinely use electrical stimulation to map the brains of awake human patients undergoing surgical procedures for treatment of severe epilepsy or tumor resection. The goal is to identify *eloquent cortex*, (i.e., areas where damage will result in paralysis or in loss of sensation or linguistic ability). These methods were pioneered by the Canadian neurosurgeon Wilder Penfield, whose work led to the now familiar map of the *motor homunculus* that is reproduced in different versions in nearly every textbook dealing with neuroscience (Penfield and Boldrey 1937; Penfield 1958) (fig. 2.1). This map depicts the areas of motor cortex associated with distinct motor functions. It is a distorted image of the body in which parts that require more finely graded control (e.g., the hand) have disproportionately large representations.

Beyond the primary motor cortex, Penfield identified the areas that we now refer to as the premotor cortex and the supplementary motor area (Penfield and Welch 1951). These names (and the names of several other premotor areas) reflect their connections into primary motor cortex and their relatively sparse projections into the spinal cord. Other investigators working in the same period included Woolsey and colleagues (Woolsey et al. 1952), who used a variety of techniques in experimental animals to map not only the motor cortex but also the sensory areas of cortex that are part of a larger network of sensory, association, and motor areas that function together to produce normal movement.

At about the time of Woolsey's experiments, the first recordings of electrical activity from single neurons in the brains of either awake or lightly anesthetized animals were conducted in the laboratories of Vernon Mountcastle, David Hubel, Herbert Jasper, and Edward Evarts (Mountcastle 1957; Hubel 1957; Jasper et al. 1958; Evarts 1966). By inserting microelectrodes into the cortex so that their exposed tips were close to individual cortical neurons, they were able to record single *action potentials*, or *spikes*, from these neurons.

An *action potential* is a brief (about 1 msec) and highly stereotyped fluctuation in neuronal membrane potential that occurs when excitatory synaptic input to the neuron triggers an abrupt, transient opening of channels in the cell's membrane, through which specific ions can flow. These action potentials are actively regenerated as they travel down a neuron's axon to provide synaptic input to other neurons. Action potentials are

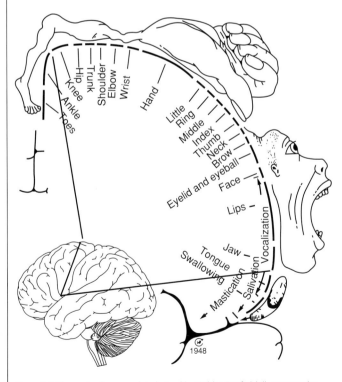

Figure 2.1 *The motor homunculus derived by Wilder Penfield illustrating the effects of electrical stimulation of the cortex of human neurosurgical patients. Adapted from Nolte (2002).*

viewed as the basic units of interneuronal communication and information transfer in the nervous system. A detailed description of this fundamental phenomenon may be found in any basic neurophysiology textbook.

These seminal neuronal-recording experiments began to reveal the relationships between neuronal discharge (i.e., spikes) in motor and sensory areas of cortex and movements or external sensory events. In the decades since these first studies, tremendous improvements have been made in microelectrode and electronics technology so that it is now possible to record the activity of many tens or hundreds of neurons simultaneously. This new technology has helped give rise to the brain-computer interface (BCI), whereby such recordings can be interpreted by a computer and used as a source of control signals, ultimately to provide movement or communication to a paralyzed person.

This chapter has six sections. The first four discuss the anatomy and functional roles of the brain areas that are most relevant to the development of BCI technology. This coverage is intended to provide a basic background for those readers who are not familiar with these topics and a succinct review for those readers who are. The final two sections discuss the information content of neuronal discharge recorded from these areas and review current methods for recording and analyzing spikes from many cortical neurons simultaneously (these two topics are discussed further in chapters 5 and 16).

OVERVIEW OF BRAIN ANATOMY

In humans, most of the brain consists of the two paired *cerebral hemispheres* (fig. 2.2). Each hemisphere is covered with *cortex*, a structure that varies in thickness in different regions from about 1.5 to 4.0 mm. The cortex is known colloquially as *gray matter* because of the color imparted by its large number of neurons. Beneath the cortex are a number of other deeper gray-matter structures, the *subcortical* areas including the basal ganglia, cerebellum, brainstem, and thalamus. The brain's *white matter* (so-called because of its lighter color) consists of the many nerve fibers that interconnect the various cortical areas and that connect the cortex to subcortical areas (and visa versa).

The left panel of figure 2.3 shows the trajectory of a single corticospinal fiber (i.e., one that extends from the cortex to the spinal cord). This fiber starts in motor cortex, goes through the cerebral peduncle, the pons, and into the medulla, where it crosses to the other side of the body and enters the spinal cord. It ultimately projects to interneurons and motoneurons in the ventral horn of the spinal cord on that side. Thus, in general, corticospinal fibers from neurons on one side of the brain activate muscles on the other side of the body.

Because the cerebral cortex is responsible for movement planning and because it is relatively accessible experimentally, it is the brain area of primary focus in most BCI research. Accordingly, this section of the chapter will focus mainly on the cortex, with brief additional discussion of the subcortical areas with which it is interconnected and that affect and modulate its activity.

TERMINOLOGY FOR DIRECTIONS IN THE CNS

Several different coordinate axes are used to describe directions within the body in general and the CNS in particular (fig. 2.2). The *mediolateral axis is perpendicular to the midline,* and the body is bilaterally symmetrical along this axis. That is, the zero point of the mediolateral axis is at the midline, and the value rises as distance to the left or right increases. The *rostral* (or *cranial*) to *caudal* axis (also called the *rostrocaudal* axis) goes from the head (or more precisely, the face or mouth) to the tail. Thus, the most rostral part of the CNS is the front of the frontal lobe, and the most caudal is the end of the spinal cord. The third axis is the *dorsoventral* axis; it is perpendicular to both the mediolateral and rostrocaudal axes, and goes from the back (or *dorsum*) to the front (or *ventrum*). In a quadruped, these definitions remain consistent for the spinal cord and brain. In a biped, the rostrocaudal and dorsoventral axes rotate forward, such that the dorsoventral axis becomes parallel to the gravity vector (fig. 2.2, lower).

Axis terminology is further complicated by the anterior-posterior axis. In general, *anterior* refers to the direction toward the front of the head or body (i.e., the face or abdomen), and *posterior* refers to the opposite direction. However, when applied to the brain, the anterior-posterior axis is the same as the rostrocaudal axis. Thus, the front edge of the frontal lobe is the most rostral, or anterior part, of the cerebrum, and the tip of the occipital lobe is the most caudal or posterior. In contrast, when applied to the spinal cord, the anterior-posterior axis is the same as the dorsoventral axis. Finally, the terms used for specifying location along the main axis of a limb are *proximal* and *distal*: *proximal* means close to the body, whereas *distal* means far from the body (e.g., the hand or foot).

THE CEREBRAL CORTEX

The cerebral cortex has four major parts, or *lobes*:

- *frontal*
- *parietal*
- *occipital*
- *temporal*

Whereas the cerebral cortex of lower mammals (e.g., rodents, rabbits, and some primates) is a relatively smooth sheet, the cerebral cortex of higher mammals is highly convoluted by a set of gyri (ridges) and sulci (grooves) that divide the cortex into distinct anatomical regions. The convolutions have presumably evolved to increase cortical volume while maintaining an unchanged thickness. The sulci and gyri define the four main lobes of the cerebral cortex, as well as other cortical subdivisions (fig. 2.2). The *frontal and parietal lobes* are separated by the *central sulcus (CS),* which is a deep groove between the cortical folds (called *gyri*) (fig. 2.2). The *frontal lobe* lies on the anterior side of the CS and the *parietal lobe* lies on its posterior side. The gyrus on the anterior side of the CS is the *precentral gyrus*, that on the posterior side is the

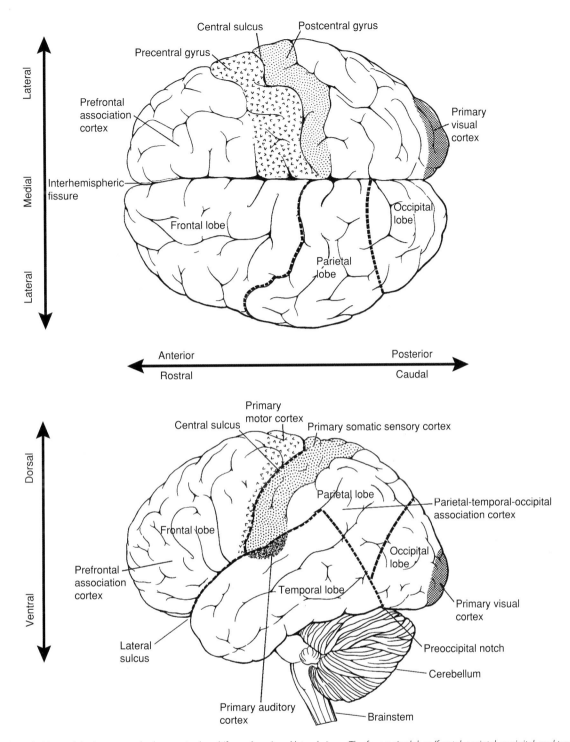

Figure 2.2 Major divisions of the human cerebral cortex in dorsal (from above) and lateral views. The four major lobes (frontal, parietal, occipital, and temporal) are indicated, as well as several of the functionally defined cortical areas. Adapted from Kandel et al. (1991).

postcentral gyrus. Primary motor cortex (M1) lies along the anterior wall of CS and continues into the precentral gyrus. Primary somatosensory cortex (S1) lies along the posterior wall of the CS and continues into the postcentral gyrus.

The frontal lobe is dramatically expanded in humans, even compared to our closest primate relatives. Much of this expansion is within the most anterior, *prefrontal area* (fig. 2.2), which is involved in higher-order executive function, including complex cognitive behaviors, personality, and decision making.

Posterior (or caudal) to the CS are the *parietal lobe* and then the *occipital lobe.* Primary somatosensory cortex (S1) is within the most anterior part of the parietal lobe. Farther posterior, in what is referred to as the *posterior parietal cortex* (PPC), is a region of *multimodal association cortex,* that receives input from the somatosensory, visual, and auditory sensory areas that surround it.

The *occipital lobe,* at the posterior pole of the brain, consists primarily of visual areas. The *temporal lobes* are located ventrally

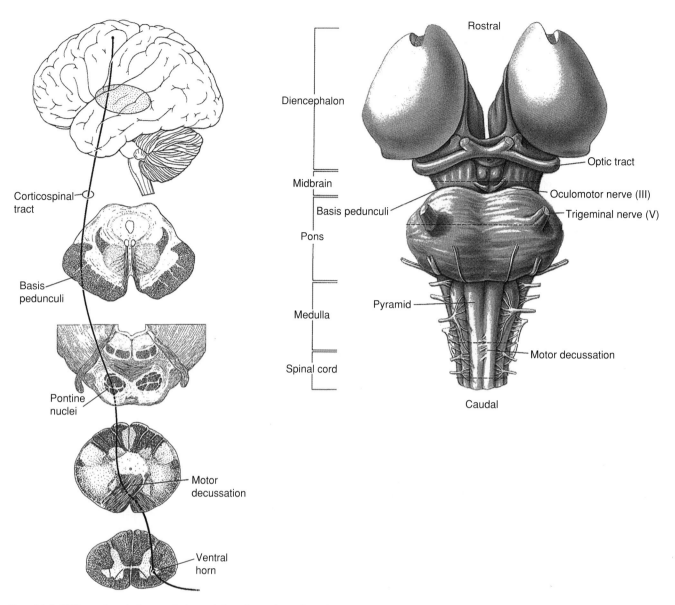

Figure 2.3 (Left) The corticospinal tract as it descends from the cerebrum through the brainstem to the spinal cord. (Right) Ventral view of the midbrain, pons, medulla, and spinal cord; the cerebellum (not shown) is behind (i.e., dorsal to) the pons and medulla. Adapted from Kandel et al. (1991).

along the sides of the brain. They are critical for auditory signal processing, higher-level visual processing, and memory.

The cerebral cortex has three histologically distinguishable parts: the neocortex; the paleocortex; and the archicortex. The *neocortex* comprises most of the cortex in mammals and is discussed in detail in this chapter. The paleocortex and archicortex are evolutionarily older forms of cortex. The paleocortex comprises a region at the bottom (i.e., the ventral side) of the cerebrum that includes, but is not limited to, the olfactory cortex. The archicortex (largely synonymous with the *hippocampus*) is a structure located deep within the temporal lobes that plays a critical role in the formation of new memories and in spatial navigation.

In the early 1900s, Korbinian Brodmann differentiated approximately 50 areas within the cerebral cortex, based largely on the distribution, density, and types of cells within each area (Brodmann 1909). His published cytoarchitectonic map provided the framework for many subsequent investigations into the functional differentiation of the cerebral cortex. This map is shown in figure 2.4, and some of the important areas are noted in table 2.1. With the advent of modern anatomical and physiological techniques, many of the Brodmann areas have been further subdivided. The overlap between the anatomically defined maps and functional maps determined later by physiological methods is rather remarkable.

THE SIX LAYERS OF NEOCORTEX

Neocortex is composed of six morphologically distinct layers (labeled I–VI), distinguishable mainly by the types of cells they contain. *Pyramidal cells* (named for their pyramidal shape) are projection neurons (i.e., their axons extend to other cortical regions and/or to subcortical regions as far away as the spinal cord). Of the nonpyramidal neurons, *stellate* cells (also called *granule* cells) are the most numerous; stellate cells have extensive

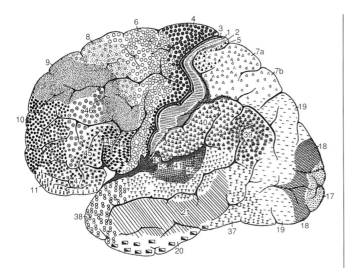

Figure 2.4 Lateral view of the cerebral cortex from the work of Korbinian Brodmann. Each of the different symbols represents an area Brodmann considered to be anatomically distinct. He identified and numbered a total of more than 50 such areas. His numbering is best understood in terms of his sectioning methodology. Unlike modern brain sectioning, which usually proceeds along the rostrocaudal axis, Brodmann sectioned along the dorsoventral axis, so that his areal numbering begins at the top of the brain (i.e., the central sulcus) and often alternates anteriorly and posteriorly as it proceeds ventrally. From Nolte (2002).

TABLE 2.1 Common names and abbreviations of the major cortical motor areas together with their Brodmann and Matelli designations*

COMMON NAME	COMMON ABBREVIATION	BRODMANN (Vogt 1919)	MATELLI
Primary motor cortex	M1	4	F1
Premotor cortex (Dorsal, rostral division)	PMdr	6 (6aβ)	F7
Premotor cortex (Dorsal, caudal division)	PMdc	6 (6aα)	F2
Premotor cortex (Ventral, rostral division)	PMvr	6 (6aα)	F5
Premotor cortex (Ventral, caudal division)	PMvc	6 (4c)	F4
Supplementary motor area	SMA	6 (6aα)	F3
Presupplementary motor area	pre-SMA	6 (6aβ)	F6
Cingulate motor area (rostal division)	CMAr	24	24c
Cingulate motor area (caudal division)	CMAc	23	24d
Anterior intraparietal area	AIP	7	
Ventral intraparietal area	VIP	5/7	
Medial intraparietal area	MIP	5	
Parietal reach region	PRR	5	
Primary somatosensory cortex	S1	1, 2, 3	
Prefrontal cortex	PFC	9	

*Matelli et al. (1985, 1991).

dendrites that arise from the cell body and that terminate, along with the axon, within a restricted region of the cortex. Stellate cells are primarily involved in processing information locally.

Layer I, the outermost layer of the neocortex, is called the molecular layer. It contains very few neurons and is composed mostly of the dendrites arising from pyramidal neurons in deeper layers and horizontally running axons. Layer II is called the external granular layer and contains mostly stellate cells and small pyramidal cells. Layer III is called the external pyramidal layer and contains both small and medium-sized pyramidal cells. It is the primary source of fibers that interconnect the different areas of cortex. Layer IV is the internal granular layer. It contains many nonpyramidal neurons and receives much of the input coming to the cortex. These fibers that come *to* the cortex (and are therefore called *afferent* fibers) originate in the thalamus and carry signals from each of the primary senses. Layer V is the internal pyramidal layer. It contains the largest pyramidal cells, the source of the long axons that project *out* of the cerebrum (and are therefore called *efferent* fibers). The largest of these Layer V pyramidal cells are located in the primary motor cortex and are referred to as Betz cells (Betz 1874). Finally, Layer VI, called the multiform layer, contains the greatest variety of cell types. It is the source of most fibers from the cortex (i.e., efferent fibers) to the thalamus.

In different cortical regions, the amount of cortex devoted to a given layer varies depending on the function of the area. For example, the primary visual and somatic sensory cortices have an input layer IV that is much thicker than that in the primary motor cortex; in contrast, the output layer V predominates in primary motor cortex. In sensory regions of cortex, layer IV contains a large number of granule cells. These regions are therefore often referred to as *granular cortex*. In contrast, motor areas of cortex lack a prominent layer IV and are termed *agranular*.

Intracortical efferents arising in layer III project ipsilaterally within a given gyrus and interconnect cortical regions in different lobes of the ipsilateral side. The longest fibers travel in association bundles. For example, the superior longitudinal fasciculus contains the fibers that interconnect the frontal and parietal lobes. Fibers projecting between the hemispheres travel primarily through the corpus callosum, which contains some 300 million fibers.

SUBCORTICAL AREAS

The major subcortical areas of the brain that interact with cortex and are intimately involved in motor and sensory function include the:

- *thalamus*
- *brainstem*

- *basal ganglia*
- *cerebellum*

The *thalamus* is located below the cortex and deep within the cerebrum. It serves as the main gateway to the cerebral cortex for sensory inputs from the spinal cord and from other subcortical structures including the basal ganglia and cerebellum. It also receives input from the cerebral cortex, which suggests that the thalamus plays a complex regulatory function.

The *brainstem* is at the base of brain (just visible in fig. 2.2, lower panel). The brainstem, consisting of the *midbrain, pons,* and *medulla oblongata,* can be seen in greater detail in figure 2.3. The medulla oblongata connects to the spinal cord. The brainstem contains nerve fibers descending to and ascending from the spinal cord; it also contains a number of motor and sensory nuclei, collections of neurons that further process these signals. The most numerous of these are within the pons (and are known collectively as the *pontine nuclei*).

The *basal ganglia* are a collection of interconnected nuclei located deep within the cerebrum. They are strongly connected with the cerebral cortex and play a critical role in movement. Both Parkinson's disease and Huntington's chorea are associated with pathology in the basal ganglia.

The *cerebellum* (derived from the Latin for *little brain*) is nestled under the posterior part of the cerebral hemispheres (see fig. 2.2, lower panel). The cerebellum is involved in the production of smooth, coordinated movements as well as in motor learning and adaptation. Although it has no direct connections to the spinal cord, it influences movement indirectly by way of its connections to the cerebrum and brainstem. People with disorders of the cerebellum are still able to move, but their movements lack normal coordination; these characteristic deficits are known collectively as *ataxia*.

CORTICAL EFFERENT PROJECTIONS

Nerve fibers that leave the cortex are called *cortical efferent fibers*; fibers that enter the cortex are called *cortical afferent fibers*. The cortical efferent fibers converge to pass through the *internal capsule*, a very dense collection of cortical afferent and efferent fibers located just lateral to the thalamus. From the internal capsule, these and other descending fibers form the paired *cerebral peduncles* (*basis pedunculi* in fig. 2.3) each of which contains roughly 20 million fibers. Between 85% and 95% of these fibers terminate within the brainstem, the largest proportion within the pontine nuclei. This *corticopontine pathway* also provides a massive projection from many regions of the cerebral cortex to the cerebellum. Other efferent fibers from the cortex end in the caudate and putamen (collectively known as the *striatum*), the input nuclei of the basal ganglia (see below). Other cortical efferents, known collectively as *corticobulbar fibers*, terminate in the lower brainstem area and include projections to both motor and sensory brainstem nuclei.

The remaining one million cortical fibers form the *medullary pyramids* (which give the *pyramidal tract* its name) and continue to the spinal cord as the *corticospinal* (CST) tract. Eighty to ninety percent of these CST fibers cross the midline at the *pyramidal decussation* (as shown in fig. 2.3) within the caudal medulla and run in the lateral columns of the spinal cord in primates and cats. (In rats, the CST is at the base of the dorsal columns of the spinal cord.) The remaining fibers remain uncrossed until they terminate bilaterally in the spinal cord, and constitute the *ventromedial CST*. In primates particularly, some corticospinal fibers synapse directly on motoneurons within the ventral (or anterior) horn of the spinal gray matter, especially motoneurons supplying the distal extremities. Some CST fibers (those arising from S1) project into the dorsal (or posterior) horn of the spinal gray matter, which receives sensory afferents coming in from the peripheral nerves. However, the majority of CST fibers project to the intermediate zone and influence motoneurons (which are located in the ventral [anterior] horn of the spinal gray matter) indirectly, through spinal interneurons.

MOTOR AND SENSORY AREAS OF THE CEREBRAL CORTEX

The cerebral cortex is the area of greatest interest in BCI research because it is most accessible to electrode probes (as well as to scalp recording) and because it is highly involved in the executive function of motor and communication behaviors.

The cortical surface features provide convenient landmarks for the identification of particular regions of the brain. In monkeys, the small spur extending posteriorly from the arcuate sulcus (see fig. 2.5), is a useful mediolateral landmark approximating the region of the cortex that controls proximal arm movements (Georgopoulos et al. 1982). In humans, a distinctive portion of the precental gyrus known as the "hand knob" marks the region controlling hand movements (Yousry et al. 1997). These landmarks are often used to guide implantation of intracortical electrodes. However, although they are useful for localization during surgery to place electrodes, the deep sulci make experimental access to the cortex with multielectrode recording techniques more difficult.

Table 2.1 lists the main motor areas of the brain that have been identified by a number of different classification systems. The most widely used are shown in the table and include the common names (column 1); their common abbreviations (column 2); the cytoarchitectonic areas described for the monkey by Brodmann (1909) and by Vogt (1919) (column 3); and a later system based on cytochrome-oxidase staining in the monkey (column 4) (Matelli et al. 1985; Matelli et al. 1991). In this chapter, we use primarily the common names and abbreviations shown in columns 1 and 2 of table 2.1.

CORTICAL SPECIALIZATION

PRIMARY MOTOR CORTEX
Primary motor cortex (M1), located in the frontal lobe, is a brain region of great importance in BCI research because of its close relation to movement control. Fritsch and Hitzig (1870) and Ferrier (1873) were able to activate muscles with relatively weak electrical stimulation in this area because of the relatively

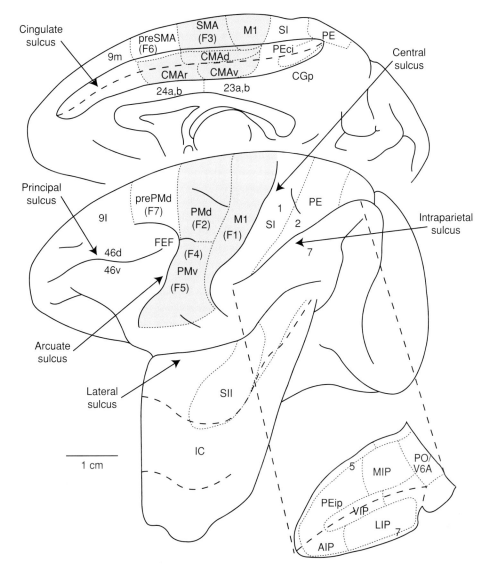

Figure 2.5 *Identification of cortical areas in the macaque monkey. Anterior is to the left and posterior is to the right. The cingulate and lateral sulci are unfolded, and each fundus (i.e., the deepest part of the sulcus) is indicated by a bold dashed line. The intraparietal sulcus is unfolded similarly and shown as an inset. The borders between cytoarchitectonic areas are delineated with dotted lines. M1 and the premotor areas are shaded. Abbreviations: AIP, LIP, MIP, VIP are anterior, lateral, medial, and ventral intraparietal areas, respectively; CMAd, CMAv, CMAr are dorsal, ventral, and rostral cingulate motor areas, respectively; F1 to F7 are cytoarchitectonic areas in the frontal lobe according to Matelli et al. (1985, 1991); IC is insular cortex; M1 is primary motor cortex; PMd is dorsal premotor area; PMv is ventral premotor area; prePMd is predorsal premotor area; preSMA is presupplementary motor area; SI is primary somatosensory cortex; SII is secondary somatosensory cortex; SMA is the supplementary motor area; PE and PEip are parietal areas (Pandya and Seltzer 1982); PO is the parietooccipital area or V6A (Wise et al. 1997); 9m, 9l, 46d, 46v are prefrontal areas (Walker 1940; Barbas and Pandya 1989). Adapted from Dum and Strick (2005).*

large density here of giant Betz cells whose axons form the CST. In primates particularly, these cells frequently project directly to spinal motoneurons, which probably contributes to their ability to activate small sets of muscles (Lemon 2008).

The primary motor cortex is organized somatotopically. That is, particular regions of M1 are devoted primarily to the control of particular body areas. This organization is reflected in Penfield's homunculus (fig. 2.1), in which an oddly shaped body is drawn along the central sulcus. Representations of the legs and feet are found within the medial wall of the cerebrum; the trunk, upper arm, and hand representations occur progressively more laterally in the hemisphere; and the face is most lateral. Although neighboring body parts are typically represented within neighboring areas of cortex, these body parts are spatially distorted because control of some body parts is more complex than that of others. For example, control of the many facial or hand muscles is much more complex than is control of the much larger biceps muscle that flexes the elbow. Consequently, a greater amount of cortical area is devoted to the control of the face or the hand than to the upper arm. These general principles of somatotopic organization apply to sensory as well as motor areas of cortex.

Despite the basic appeal of this textbook caricature of cerebral cortex motor representation, a true motor map probably bears a good bit less resemblance to the body (Schieber 2001). Figure 2.6, taken from work in Cheney's laboratory, contains a map that is analogous to Penfield's in that it shows the spatial distribution of motor areas that represent various body areas

(Park et al. 2001). The solid line in this figure represents the lip of the anterior bank of the precentral gyrus. The parallel dashed line indicates the fundus of the central sulcus and the posterior limit of M1. This study achieved much higher spatial resolution than those of Penfield, because it used *intracortical*, rather than surface stimulation and because the stimulating currents were almost 1000-fold smaller. Although the gross features of figure 2.6 are similar to those in figure 2.1 (i.e., the face most lateral, the legs most medial, and the hand and arms in between; see also Sessle and Wiesendanger 1982), it lacks the individual digits and simple linear mapping along the sulcus of the familiar homunculus.

Since Penfield and Woolsey identified the primary and premotor cortices, many additional motor cortical areas have been identified. Although not shown in figure 2.5, M1 can be subdivided into two regions: caudal M1 (M1c) (essentially that lying within the sulcus); and rostral M1 (M1r) (the portion on the cortical surface and extending rostrally—or anteriorly—nearly to the arcuate sulcus [ArS in fig. 2.5]). Neurons in M1c, nearest to the somatosensory cortex, are more strongly influenced by somatosensory inputs than are neurons in M1r (Strick and Preston 1978a; Strick and Preston 1978b). A variety of other motor areas have been identified that have projections into M1.

PREMOTOR CORTEX

Premotor cortex (PM), also located in the frontal lobe, is the area anterior (rostral) to the primary motor cortex (fig. 2.5). In monkeys, the border between the M1 and PM falls roughly midway between the central sulcus (CS) and the arcuate sulcus

(ArS) (see fig. 2.5). As noted in the figure, the PM is divided into dorsal (PMd) and ventral (PMv) areas. Each of these is sometimes further divided into rostral (PMdr and PMvr) and caudal (PMdc and PMvc) areas. These subdivisions are distinguished by differences in their parietal and prefrontal inputs, by their outputs to M1, and by whether or not they project to the spinal cord (Ghosh and Gattera 1995; Matelli et al. 1998; Fujii et al. 2000).

In addition to these premotor areas, there are several other limb-related premotor areas that have been identified within the frontal lobe of the monkey. These can be seen in the upper drawing in figure 2.5: the supplementary motor area (SMA) and the cingulate motor area (CMA). SMA is located medial to PMdc, and is primarily within the interhemispheric fissure. It extends slightly onto the exposed surface of the cortex. CMA is located entirely on the medial wall within the cingulate sulcus. As seen in figure 2.5, the CMA has been further subdivided into rostral (CMAr), dorsal (CMAd) and ventral (CMAv) areas.

Electrical stimulation applied to the premotor cortices can elicit movement as in M1. However, somewhat higher currents are required here than for M1, and the movements tend not to be isolated to individual parts of the hand or limbs as they are for M1. All of these premotor areas (except for PMdr) are characterized by fairly extensive spinal projections in parallel with those from M1 (Hutchins et al. 1988; Dum and Strick 1991).

SOMATOSENSORY CORTEX

The *primary somatosensory cortex* (S1), located in the parietal lobe, is important in movement because it conveys the sensations of touch, temperature, pain, and limb position that are important in guiding movement. S1 lies in the most anterior part of the parietal lobe. It starts along the posterior (caudal) wall of the CS and extends into the postcentral gyrus. It receives both tactile and proprioceptive (see below) input from the spinal cord by way of the thalamus.

The sense of touch originates from a combination of mechanoreceptors located either superficially or deep in the skin. Both the depth and the spacing of the receptors determine the spatial resolution of the signals they convey, from the exquisite sensitivity of the tips of the fingers, to the much less sensitive skin on the trunk. In addition, some of these receptors remain sensitive to maintained contact (slowly adapting receptors), whereas others are optimized to sense changes (rapidly adapting receptors).

S1 also conveys *proprioception*, the sense of both limb position and movement. Although less a part of our conscious awareness than either vision or somatosensory modalities, proprioception is, nevertheless, quite important for planning and guiding movement. Proprioceptive input is derived primarily from two types of receptors within the muscles: muscle spindles that are sensitive both to muscle length and to rate of stretch, and Golgi tendon organs that sense muscle force.

As is true of other senses, somatosensory input is relayed to the cerebral cortex by the *thalamus*. The thalamus is located deep within the brain and is subdivided into a number of regions, each of which processes input from a different sensory modality. Thalamic somatosensory inputs converge on several cerebral cortical areas, which together comprise S1. These include

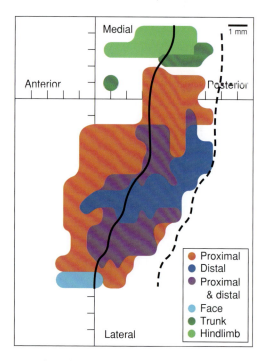

Figure 2.6 *Map of the effects of intracortical microstimulation within primary motor cortex of a monkey. The map indicates the body parts that were activated by stimulation at each point in cortex. The central sulcus has been unfolded. The dashed line indicates the fundus (i.e., bottom) of the central sulcus. The solid line is the crown of the precentral gyrus. Adapted from Park et al. (2001).*

Brodmann areas 3a, 3b, 1, and 2 (fig. 2.7). Area 3a receives primarily proprioceptive input, whereas 3b receives tactile input. The border between 3a and 3b lies within the central sulcus, but its location varies considerably among individuals (Krubitzer et al. 2004). Area 1 is similar to area 3b in that it responds mostly to tactile stimuli, receiving a combination of inputs from the thalamus and area 3b. On the other hand, area 2 is similar in many respects to 3a in that it is predominantly proprioceptive, receiving input both from the thalamus and from area 3a.

Perhaps unexpectedly, S1 also sends many axons to the spinal cord, but the axons terminate mainly in the dorsal part (i.e., the dorsal horn) of the spinal gray matter and are thought to regulate spinal reflexes and afferent input to the cerebrum (Liu and Chambers 1964; Coulter and Jones 1977; Yezierski et al. 1983; Ralston and Ralston 1985).

POSTERIOR PARIETAL CORTEX

The PPC (i.e., areas 5 and 7, including the regions within the intraparietal sulcus in fig. 2.5) is also involved in sensory function. It is an example of a multimodal *association cortex*, in that many of these neurons receive a combination of visual, auditory, and somatosensory inputs (Blatt et al. 1990; Andersen et al. 1997; Breveglieri et al. 2006). The PPC probably combines this sensory input to form an internal map of the limbs and their relation to the external world that is used to guide movement planning. Lesions within this part of the brain can cause a disorder called *hemispatial neglect*, in which a person becomes unable to recognize the limbs on the opposite side of the body.

Vision and proprioception are undoubtedly the most important of the sensory input modalities that guide movements. Visual signals from the occipital lobe follow two divergent paths, one extending into the PPC and the other into the

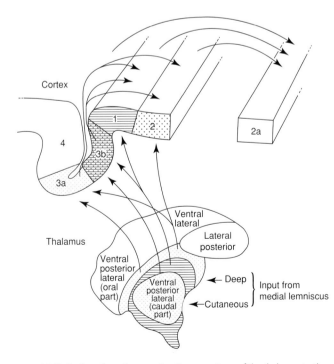

Figure 2.7 *Projections from the somatosensory portions of the thalamus to the primary somatosensory cortex. Adapted from Kandel et al. (1991).*

temporal lobe. These have been referred to, respectively, as the *dorsal and ventral visual streams* (Ungerleider and Mishkin 1982), and the function of these two streams has traditionally been divided into object-*location* (the "where" or dorsal stream), and object-*recognition* (the "what" or ventral stream). Another view is that these two streams might more properly be viewed as vision-for-action and vision-for-perception, respectively (Goodale and Milner 1992), a view that reflects the anatomy of the dorsal action stream, which passes from visual cortex into the PPC and then into the motor areas of the frontal lobe.

As with the visual system's division into object-recognition for perception and object-location for action, the somatosensory system may be similarly divided into representations for perception and action. The ventral stream (perception) analog projects from the secondary somatosensory cortex (SII in figure 2.5) to the insula and is thought to be involved in tactile learning and memory (Mishkin 1979; Friedman et al. 1986). The dorsal stream analog (action) enters the PPC together with visual input and then projects to the frontal lobe.

Within the PPC are several areas that play important roles in the control of movement. These lie near the intraparietal sulcus (IPS) (fig. 2.5). The lateral intraparietal area (LIP) (see fig. 2.5, inset showing detail of the IPS) is primarily involved in the control of saccadic (i.e., rapid) eye movements (Robinson et al. 1978). The ventral intraparietal area (VIP) (fig. 2.5, inset) is located in the groove at the bottom of the IPS and contains neurons with complex tactile/visual receptive fields. VIP is thought to be involved in the coding of space in egocentric, head-centered coordinates (Duhamel et al. 1997, 1998), a function that may be important for both head and limb movements.

The anterior and medial intraparietal areas (AIP and MIP) (fig. 2.5, inset) are both involved in arm and hand movements: MIP is devoted primarily to reaching movements; AIP is devoted to the control of grasping (Mountcastle et al. 1975; Taira et al. 1990; Cohen and Andersen 2002).

An area that has received considerable attention recently is the parietal reach region (PRR) which includes MIP as well as the dorsal aspect of the parietooccipital area (PO; also known as visual area, V6A). Many neurons in PRR encode the endpoint of limb movements in a gaze-centered coordinate system (Batista et al. 1999). These regions project to the PM area PMd, while the ventral and lateral areas (VIP, AIP) project to PMv (Wise et al. 1997; Dum and Strick 2005; Chang et al. 2008). VIP and AIP may specifically target PMvc and PMvr, respectively (Luppino et al. 1999).

PREFRONTAL CORTEX

The prefrontal cortex (PFC), located in the frontal lobe, surrounds the principal sulcus and includes Brodmann areas 9 and 46 (seen in fig. 2.5). It is usually not grouped with other cortical areas involved in motor control in the primate brain because of its differing anatomical connections and lack of stimulation-evoked movements. The PFC does not contribute to the CST as do primary motor and premotor cortices and parts of the parietal cortex (Lemon 2008); and, unlike premotor and PPC areas, the PFC does not directly project to or receive inputs from M1 (Picard and Strick 2001). The dorsal and ventral aspects of the PFC project to the dorsal and ventral premotor areas, respectively. In spite of these many differences from the other cortical motor areas, PFC is included here because it appears to have a major role in high-level executive functions relating to movement.

The most dramatic and famous example of the loss of function due to prefrontal damage is that of Phineas Gage. Gage sustained an injury in 1848 when a long, one-inch diameter iron rod was driven through his head while he was setting an explosive charge to level a railway roadbed, destroying a major portion of his frontal lobes (Damasio et al. 1994). Although he lived and functioned normally in many respects, his friends described dramatic changes in his personality. What little is known about the ensuing psychological changes derives largely from the comments of John Martyn Harlow, the physician who cared for Gage both in the immediate aftermath of the accident, and in the ensuing decade before he died. The formerly friendly and reliable Gage had become, quoting Harlow, "impulsive, unreliable, unable to carry out his plans, was profane and now lacked deference towards others. So marked was this change, that his friends said he 'was no longer Gage'" (Harlow 1868).

In addition to the PFC's apparent role in less well-defined executive functions, its role in short-term memory has been highlighted by a large number of well-controlled lesion experiments and clinical studies as well as electrophysiological recordings from animals. The maintenance of *spatial working memory* in particular appears to be a function of PFC (Jacobsen 1935; Funahashi et al. 1989; Goldman-Rakic 1995). It is experimentally difficult to separate this function from that of control of the spatial focus of attention, which may also be an important component of PFC function (Lebedev et al. 2004).

CEREBRAL CORTICAL AREAS AND MOTOR CONTROL

To understand how the brain controls the limbs, and particularly to understand the role of the cortex, the conceptual framework of a motor hierarchy is very helpful. In this conceptual framework, motor control is seen as a set of functions that are hierarchically organized and performed in series. Although it is not always possible to segregate particular functions within distinct cortical and subcortical structures, the concept of motor hierarchy serves as a useful aid in understanding the functional differences among various brain structures.

The concept of a motor hierarchy can be understood along at least four different dimensions:

- *time (planning vs. execution)*
- *encoding (abstract vs. concrete coding)*
- *complexity (simple vs. complex movements)*
- *source (external vs. internal movement initiation).*

Using these four dimensions as guidelines, we will consider six major cortical areas that have been described in this chapter: M1, PMd, PMv, SMA, PPC, and S1. We choose these cortical areas because they are particularly relevant for cortically controlled BCIs since they are intimately involved in the planning and execution of voluntary movements and because several have been the focus of past and current BCI development. Using the results of electrical stimulation and single-neuron recording studies, we will consider each of these cortical areas along each of the four dimensions. Finally, we will consider the roles of these areas in the motor hierarchy in the context of reaching to grasp an object, a natural behavior that traces its evolutionary roots to primate foraging and arboreal locomotion.

THE TIME DIMENSION: PLANNING VERSUS EXECUTION

Motor behavior can be viewed as a process of planning or preparation, followed in time by execution of that plan. Because planning precedes execution and is considered to provide more general, abstract information about the movement (see next section), it is viewed as a process that occurs higher in the motor hierarchy than execution. Planning includes several tasks: the identification of a goal (e.g., a target to be reached); the selection of the limb to be used (e.g., the right upper limb); and finally the specification of a path to the target (e.g., where the hand moves to reach the target). In complex, ethologically relevant behaviors, it is often impossible to temporally separate planning from execution since they overlap in time. An experimental approach to separate planning from execution is the *instructed-delay* paradigm. In this paradigm an instructional cue is first presented to inform the subject (human or animal) which of several possible movements should be performed. This cue is followed by an enforced-delay period (typically several hundred milliseconds) during which the cue is present and planning can occur, but movement execution is not allowed. At the end of the delay, a *go* cue instructs the subject to make the movement. In some experiments a period requiring a short-term memory process is incorporated by removing the instruction cue before the end of the delay period.

Using this paradigm, investigators have been able to determine which cortical and subcortical areas are involved in the planning process. This is accomplished by examining the modulation of neural activity during the delay period. Riehle (2005) proposed three criteria that must be met for neural activity to be considered planning-related: (1) modulation of spiking (i.e., neuronal action potential) frequency relative to baseline must occur during the planning period; (2) this modulation must be related to the movement to be made after the *go* cue; and (3) trial-by-trial variations in this modulation must predict trial-to-trial variations in the movement features (e.g., reaction time, success, or failure).

PRIMARY MOTOR AND DORSAL PREMOTOR CORTICES

Although there are strong reciprocal connections between PM and M1, electrophysiological data suggest that PM is more strongly engaged during planning, whereas M1 is more intimately involved in movement execution.

Modulation in M1 typically begins only 50–200 msec before movement onset, providing strong evidence that M1 is involved in the execution phase (Evarts 1968; Georgopoulos et al. 1982). As illustrated in figure 2.8, the modulation profiles of different M1 neurons are quite heterogeneous: they include both transient (*phasic*) and sustained (*tonic*) components, as well as various combinations of increasing or decreasing firing rates (Cheney and Fetz 1980; Kalaska et al. 1989). A number of studies have also observed that if an instructed-delay paradigm is used (enforcing a delay between the presentation of a movement target and the subsequent movement initiation cue), early planning-related activity can be observed prior to the initiation cue (Tanji and Evarts 1976). This activity has been used to predict the upcoming movement direction (Georgopoulos et al. 1989).

Premotor cortex also exhibits rate modulation locked to movement onset. Activity during the delay period is greater in PM than in M1 (Godschalk et al. 1981; Weinrich and Wise 1982; Riehle and Requin 1989; Riehle 1991; Crammond and Kalaska 2000). Moreover, several studies show that preparatory modulation typically occurs earlier in PM (in particular PMd) than in M1 (Riehle 1991; Kalaska and Crammond 1992) (fig. 2.9).

These findings support the conclusion that PM is more closely related to planning, whereas M1 is more closely involved in execution. It may therefore be said that PM resides higher in the motor hierarchy than M1 (Weinrich and Wise 1982). At the same time the data suggest that, although PM exhibits more robust and earlier preparatory activity, a gradient of preparatory-to-execution functions exists along the rostrocaudal dimension of the precentral gyrus (Johnson et al. 1996).

POSTERIOR PARIETAL CORTEX

For visually-guided movements, the PPC (including Brodmann areas 5 and 7), and regions within the intraparietal sulcus, may be viewed as even higher in the motor hierarchy than PM. PPC receives visual information related both to the movement goal and to the state of the limb (via direct inputs from extrastriate areas including V2, V3, V4, medial temporal area [MT], and medial superior temporal area [MST]). This visual information is retinotopic (i.e., in a coordinate system anchored to the retina) (Baizer et al. 1991). In fact, neurons in the PRR appear to code arm-movement direction in a retinotopic coordination system much like that of other visual cortical areas (Batista et al. 1999). Several studies have shown that area-5 neurons exhibit broad *directional tuning* like that of M1 (see below), such that single-neuron firing rates vary with target direction even during an instructed-delay period prior to movement (Kalaska et al. 1983; Crammond and Kalaska 1989).

However, Kalaska and colleagues report evidence that directional signals in M1 do not necessarily originate in parietal cortex (Kalaska et al. 1983). Using an identical center-out movement task, they directly compared neurons of M1 with those of area 5 and demonstrated that, on average, M1 neurons began modulating their firing-rates about 60 msec earlier than area-5 neurons. The earlier responses in M1 do not support the idea that the directional signals in M1 originate in parietal cortex. Because the earliest area-5 neurons began modulating before movement onset, the authors speculate that at least some of the directional responses in area 5 may represent an efference copy from M1 (i.e., a copy of the signal from M1 used to inform area 5 about the command being sent in parallel to the CST) rather than proprioceptive feedback. Given that PPC is not one homogeneous area, one way to reconcile these conflicting viewpoints is to consider that certain parts of PPC, such as PRR within the intraparietal sulcus, sit higher in the temporal hierarchy and send inputs to M1, whereas other parts, such as area 5 on the gyrus (where Kalaska et al. (1983) recorded), sit lower in the temporal hierarchy and receive efference copy information from M1.

PREFRONTAL CORTEX

Despite the relatively distant connection of lateral PFC to M1 and to the spinal cord, activity in lateral PFC does change during sensorimotor tasks (Tanji and Hoshi 2008). Di Pellegrino and Wise (1991) compared the activity of prefrontal and premotor cortical neurons during a modified instructed-delay task. They found that, like PM neurons, prefrontal neurons show direction-dependent discharges related to movement onset. However, prefrontal discharge was more phasic, more stimulus-related, and began 150 msec earlier on average than PM discharge. These observations place PFC higher on the motor control hierarchy than PM.

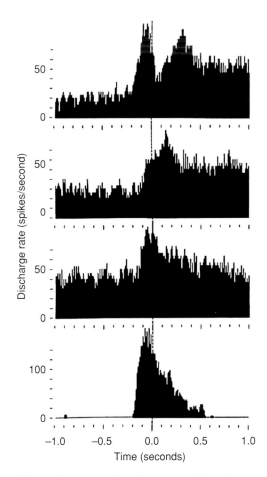

Figure 2.8 *Differing firing-rate profiles of four neurons in the primary motor cortex during a reaching task against a constant load. Each plot represents the average firing rate as a function of time. The onset of movement is at time 0. Redrawn from Kalaska et al. (1989).*

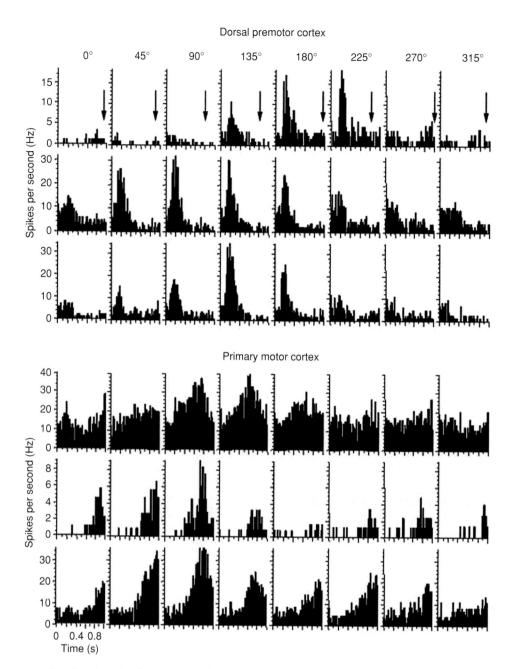

Figure 2.9 *Simultaneous recordings from three dorsal premotor cortical neurons (PMd) and three M1 neurons during an eight-direction, reaching task. (A) Perievent histograms for three PMd neurons (rows) aligned on the onset of an instructed-delay period for each movement direction (columns). Arrows point to the average movement onset time. (B) Perievent histograms from three M1 neurons. Time zero represents the onset of the instruction cue for both sets of figures. Notice that the PMd neurons exhibit modulation early in the instructed-delay period, whereas the M1 neurons do not. From Hatsopoulos et al. (2004).*

THE ENCODING DIMENSION: ABSTRACT VERSUS CONCRETE CODING

A movement can be described with different levels of abstraction. These range from the most abstract (e.g., the movement goal itself, represented by a target in space), to the somewhat less abstract (e.g., the hand movement necessary to reach the goal), to the most concrete (e.g., the temporal sequence of muscle contractions necessary to move the hand). Theories of biological motor control have borrowed concepts from robotics in an effort to elucidate these different levels of abstraction. In robotics, a goal and the desired trajectory plan for the

end-effector are specified in a coordinate system linked to a stationary part of the robot. Using this model for the nervous system, the movement goal or trajectory plan would be represented in an egocentric coordinate system (i.e., a coordinate system anchored to the body). The trajectory plan would be further transformed from body coordinates into joint coordinates using the so-called *inverse kinematics equations*, which dictate how the angular position of each of the joints evolves over time [i.e., $\theta(t)$] to execute the trajectory plan along each dimension:

$$F[x(t)] = \theta(t)$$

(2.1)

where $x(t)$ is a time-varying vector of end-effector positions, $\theta(t)$ is the vector of joint angular positions, and F is a nonlinear function.

Because movement is ultimately governed by forces obeying Newton's second law, the joint trajectories are realized using a set of torque trajectories $\tau(t)$ determined by the inverse dynamics equation:

$$G[\boldsymbol{\theta}(t), \dot{\boldsymbol{\theta}}(t), \ddot{\boldsymbol{\theta}}(t)] = \boldsymbol{\tau}(t) \tag{2.2}$$

where $\tau(t)$ is the vector of time-varying angular torques and G is a nonlinear function of the angular position, velocity, and acceleration of the joints.

Using this robotics perspective, a given brain area might represent (or *encode*) one of the different levels of movement abstraction. That is, it might encode an abstract goal in world or egocentric coordinates; it might encode the kinematics of the arm and hand in egocentric or joint-centered coordinates; or it might encode the forces or muscle activities required to realize the kinematics.

PRIMARY MOTOR CORTEX
Early Work

Beginning 40 years go with the work of Evarts (1968) and continuing to the present, research in behavioral electrophysiology has attempted to determine the motor variables encoded in the activity of single cells in M1. Despite much effort the results are still not entirely clear. Evarts's postulate was that M1 represented kinetic variables (e.g., joint torque or its derivatives) and thus corresponded to the final transformation on the right side of equation 2.2. This view was supported by the early data from his laboratory as well as by a number of succeeding studies (Smith et al. 1975; Hepp-Reymond et al. 1978; Cheney and Fetz 1980; Kalaska et al. 1989; Taira et al. 1996; Hepp-Reymond et al. 1999; Cabel et al. 2001), with further support coming from studies showing that the activity of a population of neurons (i.e., *population activity*) in M1 can be used to predict grip force, joint torque, or EMG activity (Carmena et al. 2003; Westwick et al. 2006; Pohlmeyer, Solla, et al. 2007; Fagg et al. 2009; Pohlmeyer et al. 2009).

Directional Tuning

There is now strong evidence that cells in M1 encode signals representing the movement of the hand in space (i.e., the input to eq. 2.1), including information about direction. Georgopoulos and colleagues (1982) performed the classic experiment testing this postulate. In this experiment monkeys were required to make hand movements from a central position to one of eight peripheral targets. About 75% of M1 neurons exhibited broad *directional tuning* during these movements. That is, each neuron displayed a preferential response to one direction, called the cell's *preferred direction* (PD). The peak discharge during movements made to other directions was a function of the cosine of the angle between the cell's PD and the actual direction of motion (fig. 2.10). The presence of directional tuning has been an extremely robust finding that has been replicated in many other studies of M1 for both two-dimensional and three-dimensional reaching (Schwartz et al.

1988; Kalaska et al. 1989; Maynard et al. 1999; Moran and Schwartz 1999).

Kinematic Information

Although movement direction has been the most extensively studied, there is also evidence that M1 neurons represent other kinematic features of movement, including velocity, position, and movement distance (Georgopoulos et al. 1984; Fu et al. 1993; Kurata 1993; Ashe and Georgopoulos 1994; Fu et al. 1995; Paninski et al. 2004). Over the past 25 years this model of M1 as a source of kinematic signals has emerged as the dominant viewpoint. With a few exceptions (Carmena et al. 2003; Pohlmeyer, Perreault, et al. 2007; Moritz et al. 2008; Fagg et al. 2009; Gupta and Ashe 2009; Pohlmeyer et al. 2009), it has served as the basis for all BCIs that use M1 neuronal activity to control movement.

Population Vectors

Georgopoulos showed that the PDs and discharge rates of a large population of neurons can be combined to predict movement direction (Georgopoulos et al. 1986). This is called the *population vector approach*. It simply takes the vector-sum of preferred directions among a population of directionally

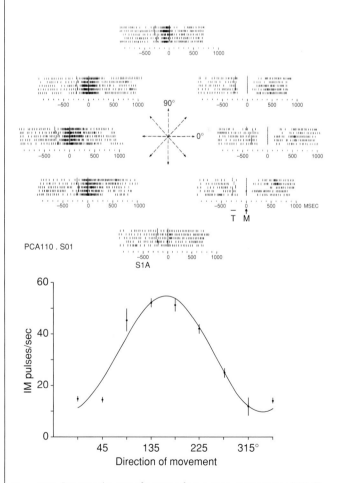

Figure 2.10 *Directional tuning of a neuron from primary motor cortex (M1). (Top panel) Raster plots (i.e., spikes) from one M1 neuron over repeated movements in each of eight movement directions. (Bottom panel) The average spike rate from the same neuron as a function of direction. A cosine function was used to fit the data. From Georgopoulos et al. (1982).*

tuned neurons after weighting each PD-vector by the firing rate of the corresponding neuron. Using the population-vector approach, Schwartz and colleagues demonstrated that more complex movement paths with time-varying directions can be decoded as well (Schwartz 1992; Schwartz and Moran 1999). This approach has been used in real-time BCIs to guide the movement of virtual and robotic devices in three dimensions (Taylor et al. 2002; Velliste et al. 2008).

Other Studies

Despite the numerous demonstrations supporting kinematic encoding of hand movement in M1, there have been a number of studies suggesting a more complex picture (e.g., studies of M1 discharges during isometric contraction [i.e., muscle contractions without movement]) (Taira et al. 1996; Boline and Ashe 2005; Sergio et al. 2005). The directional tuning of most (but not all) M1 neurons during movement is affected by changes in external load, initial hand position, and arm posture (Kalaska et al. 1989; Caminiti et al. 1990; Caminiti et al. 1991; Scott and Kalaska 1995). Furthermore, for individual M1 neurons, context-dependent effects can also alter the relationship between firing rate and force (Hepp-Reymond et al. 1999).

Strick's laboratory examined the postural dependence of M1 discharge with a behavioral paradigm in which monkeys were trained to perform wrist movements in one of four directions (flexion, extension, radial deviation, and ulnar deviation) with the forearm supinated, pronated, or midway between the two extremes (Kakei et al. 1999). Since forearm rotation changes the pulling direction of muscles (thereby changing the muscles' preferred directions computed in extrinsic, body-centered coordinates), they used measurement of the shifts of M1-neuron PDs in the different postures to show that individual M1 neurons represented movement in either a muscle-based (intrinsic) or body-centered (extrinsic) coordinate system (fig. 2.11). Forearm rotation did not affect discharge rate for 20% of the neurons, affected the magnitude but not the PD of discharge for 30%, and (much in the way it affected muscle discharge) affected the PD for 32%. These results suggest that both low-level muscle activations and higher-level hand movements are represented within M1.

There is also evidence that discharge in M1 may even represent target location, regardless of arm-movement direction. Alexander and colleagues developed a behavioral paradigm to distinguish activity related to spatial features of the target from activity related to arm movement (Shen and Alexander 1997a). Monkeys were trained to control a cursor with movements of a joystick using whole-arm movements similar to those in Georgopoulos's study (Georgopoulos et al. 1982). In one condition, the joystick and cursor movements were identical. However, in a second condition, they rotated the spatial mapping between the joystick and cursor motion by 90 degrees such that upward movement of the cursor now required a rightward movement of the joystick. During reaction time and movement time, the activity of roughly 40%–50% of neurons was exclusively related to the direction of arm movement, regardless of the target location or cursor movement. However, during the instruction, delay, and reaction time periods, the activity of 10%–15% of the neurons was related to the target

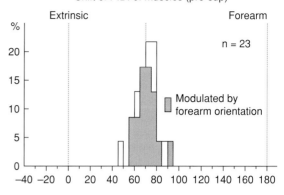

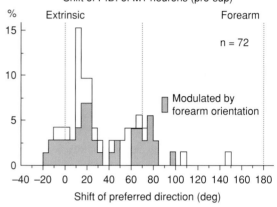

Figure 2.11 *Change in preferred direction (PD) of muscle activity (upper panel) and M1 neuronal activity (lower panel) as the forearm was rotated from the fully pronated to the fully supinated orientation. Shaded regions indicate cases in which the peak magnitude of activity changed by more than 30% with wrist orientation. The dashed vertical lines suggest three possible coordinate systems: extrinsic (i.e., world-fixed) coordinates; forearm-fixed coordinates; or intrinsic coordinates that reflect the average 70° rotation of muscle PDs. The PD rotation of many neurons behaved much like that of muscles, but another larger group did not rotate. Forearm orientation affected the magnitude of most muscles and neurons. n is the number of neurons studied. Adapted from Kakei et al. (1999).*

location or the direction of cursor movement independent of the required limb movement.

The strong correlations among the different movement-related signals have made it very difficult to address the question of what M1 actually encodes. Likewise, theoretical studies have taken opposing views on the question of the primacy of high- or low-level tuning within M1 (Mussa-Ivaldi 1988; Todorov 2000; Fagg et al. 2002). Given the currently contradictory state of the literature, a number of interpretations are possible. First, M1 might encode an as yet undiscovered feature of movement that may be partially correlated with the parameters of movement already examined. Second, M1 might not be a functionally homogeneous area, but, rather, may contain a heterogeneous set of neurons that together possess the full range of representations postulated from the robotics perspective. A third possibility, entirely consistent with the second, is that the motor cortex serves as a substrate for implementing the transformation from sensory to motor coordinate systems. In summary, there is at present no clear consensus as to M1's position along the abstract-to-concrete dimension.

PREMOTOR AND POSTERIOR PARIETAL CORTICES

In contrast to the ambiguity regarding M1, the picture appears to be clearer for PM and PPC. Using the rotated visual-display paradigm described above, Shen and Alexander (1977b) found that neurons representing target location were much more common in dorsal premotor (PMd) cortex than in M1. Likewise, Strick and colleagues found that most ventral premotor cortical (PMv) neurons encode wrist-movement direction in a body-centered coordinate system, with virtually none encoding it in muscle coordinates (Kakei et al. 2001).

Several studies have also described a spatial gradient of target selectivity in which more M1 neurons with higher-order, abstract properties were found rostrally, near the boundary between M1 and PMd (Alexander and Crutcher 1990; Johnson et al. 1996).

A recent study directly compared the ability of simultaneously recorded populations of M1 and PMd neurons to decode discrete target location versus continuous hand position in an instructed-delay, center-out task (Hatsopoulos et al. 2004). Although target location and movement direction were not explicitly dissociated, this study found that PMd populations could more accurately predict target direction prior to movement, whereas M1 populations could more faithfully reconstruct continuous hand position. These findings further support the notion that PM activity is related to an abstract goal.

Kalaska and colleagues compared the effects of a bias-load force imposed systematically in different directions during center-out hand movements in neurons in M1 and in area 5 of the PPC (Kalaska et al. 1989, 1990). M1 neurons exhibited a mixture of different load effects. In contrast, area-5 neurons were almost completely unaffected by the added load and thus appear to represent the kinematics of movement regardless of the force required to move.

THE COMPLEXITY DIMENSION: COMPLEX VERSUS SIMPLE MOVEMENTS

Many everyday movements are complex and can be viewed as either sequential or simultaneous recruitment of simpler movements. For example, typing on a keyboard or playing the piano requires a sequence of finger movements, and reaching to grasp an object requires coordination across proximal and distal segments of the upper limb. Moreover, bimanual movements require the coordination of both limbs. At a behavioral level, complex movements are typically not just the concatenation of simpler movements, since one movement element may affect the execution of another element. This is particularly evident in the language phenomenon of co-articulation, in which the production of one phoneme is influenced by the need to produce the next phoneme (Daniloff and Moll 1968; Benguerel and Cowan 1974). It is also evident in piano playing (Engel et al. 1997) and probably in many other complex movements. These behavioral phenomena suggest that there are specialized neural circuits that link and coordinate simple movements into more complex sequences.

SUPPLEMENTARY MOTOR CORTEX AND PRIMARY MOTOR CORTEX

Beginning with the classical stimulation studies of Penfield (Penfield and Welch 1951), it has been recognized that the *supplementary motor area* (SMA) of the cortex is an important area in the representation of complex movements involving multiple limb segments.

Single-neuron recordings have demonstrated that SMA neurons fire preferentially for complex movement sequences compared to simple movements. In a task using a series of push-pull movements of a handle, individual SMA neurons fired only for particular sequences of movements, but not for any single movement in isolation (Shima and Tanji 2000). For example, as illustrated in figure 2.12, one SMA neuron fired whenever a pull was followed by a push, but not when these movements were performed in other sequences or in combinations with other movements.

However, recent studies have called into question the view that movement-sequence representations reside within SMA but not within M1. Lu and Ashe demonstrated that M1 neurons preferentially encode specific memorized movement sequences (Lu and Ashe 2005). They also found that injections of muscimol (a drug that inhibits neuronal activity) into M1 increased errors during memorized sequences, without increasing errors in nonsequenced movements.

The electrical stimulation used in Penfield's experiments was of much greater intensity and longer duration than that typically used in the most recent intracortical-stimulation studies. However, using lengthy stimulation trains (500–1000 msec) and relatively high current intensity to stimulate frontal lobe (including M1) and parietal lobe, Graziano et al. (2002, 2004) elicited seemingly goal-directed movements that

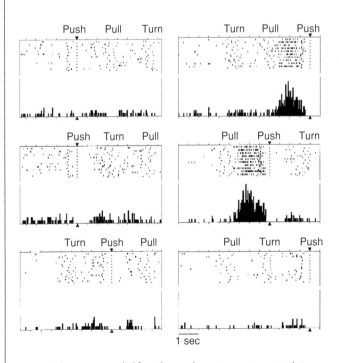

Figure 2.12 A neuron recorded from the supplementary motor cortex that responds during the combination of a pull movement followed by a push movement but that does not respond to individual movement elements. From Shima and Tanji (2000).

mimicked ethologically relevant behaviors involving complex movements of multiple limb segments. Although the interpretation of these observations is controversial given the large magnitude and long duration of electrical stimulation, they suggest that cortical control of movement sequences may be distributed beyond SMA.

THE SOURCE DIMENSION: EXTERNAL VERSUS INTERNAL MOVEMENT INITIATION

A movement can be triggered and initiated by an external stimulus, or it may be initiated internally by motivation. For example, one may reach for and grasp a cup among several other visually presented objects after instruction to do so (i.e., external initiation), or one may simply decide to reach out for the cup to satisfy a desire for the hot coffee it contains (i.e., internal initiation). The distinction between external and internal initiation is particularly evident in the generation of complex movements such as those involved in playing a musical instrument: a pianist can play from sheet music that provides visual instructions as to which keys to press, for how long, and in which order (i.e., external initiation); or, with repeated practice, the pianist can remember and generate (i.e, internal initiation) the proper sequence of key presses without the support of external stimuli.

The distinction between external and internal movement guidance can be seen rather dramatically in Parkinson's disease. Although severe akinesia can prevent some people with Parkinson's disease from initiating even a simple step on their own, they may be able to walk if visual cues are placed on the ground.

SUPPLEMENTARY MOTOR AND PREMOTOR CORTICES

Experimental evidence provides support for the existence of two separate neural circuits (in SMA and PM) that subserve internally guided versus externally guided movements, respectively. Electrophysiological experiments in behaving monkeys suggest that SMA is particularly important for internally generated movements. Mushiake and colleagues trained monkeys to press a set of buttons in various sequences (Mushiake et al. 1991). To train the animals to perform a particular button-press sequence, lights within the buttons were turned on in the proper sequence to cue each movement. After several repetitions the lights within the buttons were gradually dimmed until they were completely extinguished. A significant number of SMA neurons began to modulate only after the lights had been extinguished and stopped firing when the lights were restored. These SMA neurons were thus understood to be related to internal initiation of movement.

In contrast, a second neural circuit involving the PM (PMd and PMv) appears to be involved in externally-generated movements. In the same experiment (Mushiake et al. 1991), a large number of PMd and PMv neurons fired while the lights remained illuminated, but stopped firing once the lights were extinguished. In contrast, M1 neurons did not differentiate between the two conditions. This study suggests that area 6 (the area containing both SMA and PM cortices) has specialized circuits dedicated to internal and external movement generation. In contrast, M1, which is lower in the motor hierarchy, is not affected by this contextual difference.

VISUALLY GUIDED REACH-TO-GRASP (PREHENSION) BEHAVIOR

Thus far we have described a motor hierarchy understood on the basis of the four dimensions outlined above. These descriptions have been framed in general terms. We now look in detail at a concrete example, that of prehension, the act of reaching to grasp an object, to see how these hierarchical functions throughout the cortex lead to purposeful movement.

Prehension is a fundamental feature of human behavior. It traces its evolutionary roots to primates foraging for food in arboreal environments, and it has supported the development of more complex actions, such as tool use. Current BCI research is studying prehension in order to develop cortically controlled BCI systems capable of moving to locations and grasping objects.

TWO CORTICAL NETWORKS SUBSERVE PREHENSION

Prehension is interesting from the perspective of motor control because it is a complex behavior that requires the coordination of proximal and distal components of the arm. Electrophysiological data provide some evidence for two cortical networks, one supporting reach behavior and the other supporting grasp (fig. 2.13). The *dorsal* network—including area 5d (in the PPC), MIP (medial intraparietal area), PMdc (the caudal portion of dorsal PM), and M1—appears to be specialized for control of shoulder and elbow movements (i.e., for *reach* behaviors). Corticospinal projections from PMdc and rostral M1 (i.e., on the precentral gyrus) terminate predominantly in upper cervical (i.e., neck) segments of the spinal cord containing motoneuron pools innervating proximal musculature (He et al. 1993). A recent electrical-stimulation study suggests that there is a dorsal-to-ventral topography within PMd, such that stimulation above the arcuate spur elicits predominantly proximal arm movements (Raos et al. 2003). In contrast, the *ventral* network including the anterior intraparietal area (AIP), rostral portion of the ventral PM (PMvr), and M1 (particularly the caudal portion of M1 buried in the central sulcus) has been postulated to control distal movements such as *grasping* (Kurata and Tanji 1986; Rizzolatti et al. 1988; Jeannerod et al. 1995). The AIP and PMvr possess similar functional properties, including both visual and motor responses to grasped objects. Not surprisingly, given AIP's proximity to visual input, AIP's discharge appears to depend more on the shape of the grasped object and less on the actual details of the grasp (Jeannerod et al. 1995).

Unlike AIP neurons, many PMvr neurons appear to be more sensitive to different types of grasp (Taira et al. 1990; Sakata et al. 1995; Raos et al. 2006). There appear to be at least two functionally distinct groups of grasp-related neurons in PMvr. In monkeys, the first group (called *canonical neurons*) discharges not only for particular types of grasps but also when the monkey simply observes the grasped object (Rizzolatti et al. 1988; Rizzolatti and Fadiga 1998). A second group (called

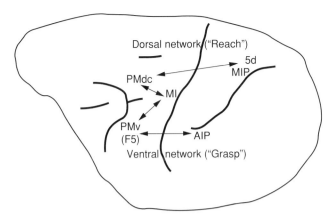

Figure 2.13 Two proposed neural networks in the macaque monkey cortex involved in control of proximal reaching movements and distal grasping movements, respectively. A dorsal reach network consists of the superior parietal cortex (area 5d and MIP), caudal dorsal premotor cortex (PMdc) and primary motor cortex (M1). A ventral grasp network includes the anterior intraparietal area (AIP), rostral ventral premotor cortex (PMv; F5), and M1.

mirror neurons) discharges even when a monkey watches another individual (either monkey or human) make a particular grasping movement (di Pellegrino et al. 1992; Gallese et al. 1996). Thus, AIP appears to represent more abstract information (i.e., higher in the motor hierarchy) than does PMvr, which itself is clearly at a higher level in the hierarchy than M1.

PRIMARY MOTOR CORTEX

The primary motor cortex (M1) is clearly involved in the control of distal as well as proximal components of arm movements. We have already described evidence that M1 neurons encode a variety of proximal reach movement parameters. Electrophysiological recordings in behaving monkeys have also shown that single neurons in M1 modulate their activity with many different aspects of distal limb function, including torque about the wrist (Evarts 1966; Murphy et al. 1979; Cheney and Fetz 1980; Kurata 1993; Kakei et al. 1999) and grip force (Hepp-Reymond et al. 1978; Muir and Lemon 1983; Wannier et al. 1991; Maier et al. 1993).

Lesions of M1 or the pyramidal tract in monkeys cause transient paresis or paralysis of the proximal limb and persistent loss of finely controlled wrist and finger movements (in particular, the loss of the ability to fractionate the movements of individual digits) (Denny-Brown 1950; Lawrence and Kuypers 1968a; Passingham et al. 1978). Intracortical microelectrode stimulation of M1 using short stimulation trains and low-current amplitudes can elicit muscle contractions and movements about the shoulder, elbow, wrist, and finger joints (Asanuma et al. 1976; Huntley and Jones 1991; Donoghue et al. 1992). Longer stimulation trains (lasting several hundred milliseconds) can elicit complex, apparently goal-directed movements involving proximal and distal joints that appear similar to natural reaching and grasping (Graziano et al. 2002, 2004). Consistent with these observations, a number of imaging and stimulation studies indicate that proximal and distal representations are intermingled and distributed throughout the arm area of M1 (Huntley and Jones 1991; Donoghue et al. 1992; Schieber and Hibbard 1993; Sanes et al. 1995).

Thus, despite extensive study, the existence of a strictly topographic organization within the arm area of M1 is still somewhat controversial. Modern stimulation studies argue for the existence of a *concentric* or *horse-shoe* organization, with distal representations mainly in the caudal portion of M1 (including the anterior bank of the central sulcus) that are surrounded by a zone of proximal-arm representations (see fig. 2.6) (Kwan et al. 1978a, 1978b; Park et al. 2001; Park et al. 2004). In between these two zones is a third zone in which low-current stimuli elicit activity in combinations of proximal and distal muscles (Park et al. 2001). There are two possible functional interpretations of this intermediate zone: that single neurons encoding either distal or proximal components are intermingled in close proximity to each other and can be excited concurrently with electrical stimulation; or, alternatively, that single neurons encode both proximal and distal components. Based on strong congruence between stimulus-triggered and spike-triggered averaging of EMG signals, Park et al. (2001, 2004) argue in favor of the second interpretation. As for the inner distal and outer proximal zones, coordination of reach and grasp might appear in the form of spatiotemporal patterning of the firing of these two populations of neurons.

Recent anatomical studies using retrograde transneuronal rabies-virus transport from individual muscles have demonstrated that direct projections from cortex to spinal motoneurons arise almost exclusively from the caudal portion of M1 in the anterior bank of the central sulcus (Rathelot and Strick 2006). Moreover, these studies demonstrate that motor neurons innervating proximal as well as distal muscles receive these monosynaptic projections and form a medial-to-lateral topography within caudal M1 such that proximal cells reside more medially and distal cells more laterally. Therefore, caudal M1 may be a particularly important area for producing coordinated reach-to-grasp behaviors.

SOMATOSENSORY FEEDBACK IN CONTROL OF MOVEMENT

PROPRIOCEPTION

At present, the user of a BCI that controls movement of a cursor or robotic limb must rely on relatively slow visual feedback to guide the movement and to correct errors. In contrast, in normal movements these functions are accomplished in large part by the proprioceptive system. People suffering loss of proprioceptive feedback can rely on watching their limbs, but their movements are typically slower and less coordinated than normal and require great concentration (Ghez et al. 1995; Sainburg et al. 1995). Thus, sensorimotor feedback in the form of proprioception is an important modulator of movement control.

Proprioceptive sense comes from a variety of muscle and joint sensory organs (e.g., muscle spindles, Golgi tendon organs, joint receptors, etc.). Their inputs converge onto cortical areas 3a and 2 of the primary somatosensory cortex (S1). Additional complexity arises because the position and velocity sensitivities of muscle spindles can be modulated by descending input from the brain (Burke et al. 1978; Loeb and Duysens 1979;

Prochazka 1981) and because both Golgi tendon organs (Houk and Henneman 1967; Crago et al. 1982) and joint receptors (Grigg 1975; Millar 1973) are differentially sensitive to actively and passively generated forces. As a result, cortical responses to perturbations during movement are likely to differ from those during rest. Indeed, studies that have compared the discharge of S1 neurons during active and passive movements find only partial correspondence (Soso and Fetz 1980; Prud'homme and Kalaska 1994). In this and in many other respects, the discharges of area 2 and 3a cells appear to be fairly similar.

NEURONAL ACTIVITY IN S1 AND RELATED AREAS

Movement-related neuronal activity in S1 is predominantly phasic (i.e., occurring during the movement itself), is often proportionate to movement speed, and in most cases is combined with lesser tonic, or position-related discharge (Soso and Fetz 1980; Gardner and Costanzo 1981; Wise and Tanji 1981). One study of planar, center-out reaching movements made in a variety of directions revealed sinusoidal-shaped tuning curves very much like those of neurons in M1 (Prud'homme and Kalaska 1994).

The earliest studies of the signals in S1 were those of Mountcastle in the late 1950s and focused largely on the sense of touch (Mountcastle 1957; Mountcastle et al. 1957). Mountcastle established that all the primary sensory and motor cortical areas are composed of distinct columns of neurons extending from the most superficial to the deepest layers of cortex. He further suggested that these *columns* might act as elemental computational units, each processing inputs from one part of the body and one type of receptor (Mountcastle 1957). As these inputs are transmitted through the cortex, from area 3b to area 1 and then into the secondary somatosensory cortex, they gradually combine inputs from different receptor types and cortical areas, thereby conveying more complex, multimodal representations of stimuli within larger receptive fields. This progression in receptive-field complexity and size continues as the somatosensory signals propagate into the PPC, where they are combined with visual and auditory inputs.

This progression of signal processing was recently analyzed in the context of a sensorimotor decision-making process (de Lafuente and Romo 2006). Monkeys were trained to discriminate the presence or absence of a vibratory stimulus applied to the fingertip. The monkeys indicated the presence or absence of the stimulus by making one of two different movements. This was an easy task unless the amplitude of the stimulus was quite small, in which case the monkeys made frequent mistakes. Recordings were made from a number of different cortical areas during the period in which the monkey was making its decision. The results showed that the correspondence between the monkey's final judgment and the neuronal discharge increased as the recordings shifted from the primary somatosensory cortex to the secondary somatosensory cortex, to the PMdc. Conversely, regardless of the monkey's ultimate decision, activity in the primary sensory areas corresponded with the properties of the mechanical stimulus.

CHANGES IN SOMATOTOPIC MAPS AFTER INJURY

If BCIs that use cortical neuronal activity are to be useful to people with severe disabilities, it will be important to take into account the dramatic changes in cortical somatotopic maps that occur after both peripheral and central injuries. A good example of this dramatic change is the phantom-limb sensation experienced by many amputees, in which sensory afferents from the remaining portion of the limb innervate the adjacent denervated cortex, causing them to sense the presence of the limb despite its absence (Flor et al. 2007).

Less dramatically, prolonged and selective use of particular digits causes their cortical representations to increase in size (Pascual-Leone and Torres 1993; Nudo et al. 1996; Xerri et al. 1996). Furthermore, mechanical coupling of two digits has been shown to cause their cortical maps to fuse (Clark et al. 1988; Jenkins et al. 1990). Similar changes have been demonstrated in response to either cortical or peripheral electrical stimulation (Nudo et al. 1990; Recanzone et al. 1990).

These observations have important implications for people with neurological disorders, for the possible use of BCIs that depend on signals originating in specific sensorimotor cortical areas, and for the incorporation of BCIs with sensory-feedback methods that depend on cortical stimulation.

SUBCORTICAL AREAS

Subcortical areas also make important contributions to motor behaviors. However, due to their less accessible locations, they are less pertinent to BCI technology, at least in its present state. Thus, we discuss these areas only briefly. In the future, as recording technology and scientific understanding continue to improve, these subcortical areas may assume greater importance in BCI research and development. The major subcortical areas that we discuss are the:

- *thalamus*
- *brainstem*
- *basal ganglia*
- *cerebellum*

THE THALAMUS

As previously noted, the thalamus provides the principal input to the cerebral cortex, conveying inputs from the spinal cord as well as from subcortical areas. It consists of a number of distinct nuclei divided into lateral, medial, anterior, intralaminar, midline, and reticular groups. The lateral group is further subdivided into ventral and dorsal tiers. Thalamic nuclei fall into two general classes: relay nuclei and diffuse-projection nuclei. The relay nuclei subserve a single sensory modality or motor area, and they interact reciprocally with fairly circumscribed regions of the cerebral cortex. In contrast, the diffuse-projection nuclei influence broad regions of cortex and have important connections to both the basal ganglia and the limbic system (Morgane et al. 2005). They are thought to be involved in the regulation of arousal, emotion, and cognitive state (Jones 1981; Van der Werf et al. 2002).

The ventral tier of the lateral group of thalamic nuclei contains the ventral anterior (VA) and ventral lateral (VL) nuclei. These are the main motor nuclei of the thalamus and convey inputs from the basal ganglia and cerebellum to specific areas of the cerebral cortex. In turn, these cortical areas project back to the basal ganglia and cerebellum. These interconnections appear to constitute well defined loops that originate and terminate in specific cortical areas. In addition to the traditional motor and premotor cortical areas that have been recognized for decades, it is also now evident that motor areas within the medial wall of the cerebrum, and even nonmotor areas in temporal lobe and PFC, are involved in similar loops (Middleton and Strick 2000).

THE BRAINSTEM

We have already described cerebral cortical projections that descend into subcortical areas and to the spinal cord. There are also brainstem areas that project to the spinal cord. These include the red nucleus, the brainstem reticular formation, the vestibular nuclei, and the superior colliculus. Their spinal projections have been divided into lateral and medial systems, based on the location of their terminations in the spinal cord, which largely overlap with the lateral (crossed) and ventromedial (uncrossed) corticospinal systems, respectively (Kuypers et al. 1962). Brainstem motor areas are most prominent in lower mammals and decline in prominence relative to the cerebral cortex as one ascends phylogenetically toward humans.

The main component of the lateral system is the red nucleus, which receives somatotopically organized projections from the cerebellum and, to a lesser extent, from the primary motor cortex. Its output, the rubrospinal tract crosses the midline within the brainstem and descends in the lateral column of the spinal cord. Like the crossed CST, it terminates in regions of the cord that influence motoneurons of limb and hand (or paw) muscles. The rubrospinal tract is involved in independent use of the limb, primarily reach and grasp movements (Lawrence and Kuypers 1968b).

The medial brainstem system includes primarily the reticular, vestibular, and tectal nuclei. Their outputs (the reticulospinal, vestibulospinal, and tectospinal tracts) descend in the ventral column of the spinal cord. Like the uncrossed CST, they target primarily interneurons and propriospinal neurons that control axial and proximal limb muscles on both sides of the body and appear to be principally involved in the control of whole-body posture, orienting, and locomotion (Lawrence and Kuypers 1968b).

THE BASAL GANGLIA

The basal ganglia are a group of nuclei located deep within the cerebrum (fig. 2.14). These highly interconnected nuclei are implicated in a range of motor disorders, including Parkinson's disease and Huntington's chorea. The earliest models of the basal ganglia viewed them as essentially a funnel, receiving inputs from disparate cortical areas and sending output exclusively to the motor cortex (Kemp and Powell 1971). More recently, it has been recognized that the output of the basal ganglia targets a much broader range of cortical areas, comprising (much like the corticocerebellar pathways [see below]) several parallel loops (Alexander et al. 1986). These include the motor, oculomotor, lateral orbitofrontal, dorsolateral prefrontal, and anterior cingulate, or limbic circuits. Although these loops are thought to be largely separate, there is likely to be some degree of convergence within their thalamic or cortical targets (Joel and Weiner 1994; Hoover and Strick 1999).

As shown in figure 2.14, the head of the caudate nucleus is adjacent to the putamen, with the two structures separated by fibers of the internal capsule. Functionally, they are considered to be one structure, the *striatum*, which serves as the primary input nucleus of the basal ganglia. The striatum receives inputs from throughout the cerebral cortex, the brainstem, and the thalamus. The basal ganglia also include the *globus pallidus* and the *substantia nigra*. These structures are the principal output nuclei. They send a large number of inhibitory fibers to the ventroanterior (VA) and ventrolateral (VL) nuclei of the thalamus. The thalamus in turn sends excitatory projections to various motor-related areas, including the primary motor cortex, the supplementary motor area, PM, and the PFC. Output from the basal ganglia also goes directly to the superior colliculus and is involved in eye and head movements.

The basal ganglia are thought to be involved in the expectation of reward, and the prediction of actions to optimize them, particularly within the prefrontal and limbic circuits (Kawagoe et al. 1998; Schultz et al. 2000). Evidence is also emerging of the important role of the basal ganglia in promoting the learning of actions (including sequences of movements) that optimize

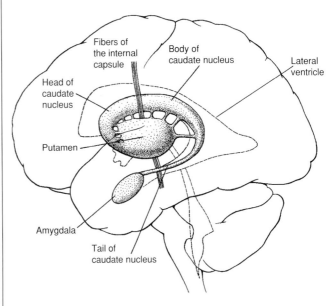

Figure 2.14 Location of the basal ganglia deep within the cerebral cortex, parallel to the lateral ventricle. The fibers of the internal capsule pass through the striatum, causing a separation between the caudate and the putamen. Although it is located in close proximity to the tail of the caudate nucleus, the amygdala is not considered part of the basal ganglia. The basal ganglia output nuclei, globus pallidus, and substantia nigra, are medial to the putamen and are not visible in this figure. From Kandel et al. (1991).

reward (Graybiel 1995, 2005). Degenerative changes within the basal ganglia are associated with a number of motor and cognitive disorders, most prominently Parkinson's and Huntington's diseases.

THE CEREBELLUM

LOCATION, ORGANIZATION, AND CONNECTIONS

The cerebellum sits on the dorsal surface of the brainstem caudal to the cerebrum. The cerebellar cortex is highly convoluted into many folds or *folia*, to a much greater extent than the gyri and sulci of the cerebral cortex, and is divided by a series of fissures running roughly mediolaterally. Figure 2.15 presents a dorsal view of the human cerebellum. The primary fissure divides the anterior lobe from the posterior lobe, and the posteriolateral fissure divides the posterior lobe from the flocculonodular lobe (not visible in this view). Although the cerebellum is symmetrical about the midline, it is not divided at the midline, as is the cerebrum.

The cerebellar cortex has only three layers, and unlike the cerebrum, there is little variation across different cortical regions. With few exceptions, the same neuronal types, in the same proportion, with the same well-defined interconnections, are found throughout the cerebellar cortex. The *Purkinje cells*, which are the cerebellar output neurons and are among the largest neurons in the CNS, are in the middle layer. Beneath the cerebellar cortex are the cerebellar nuclei, which receive the Purkinje cell axons from the cerebellar cortex, and are the main source of the cerebellar output fibers. Moving mediolaterally are found the fastigial, interpositus, and dentate nuclei, which receive the outputs from the most medial (i.e., the vermis), intermediate (i.e., paravermis), and most lateral (i.e., hemispheric) parts of the cerebellar cortex, respectively. The cerebellar hemispheres have become greatly enlarged in the phylogenetic transition from cats to monkeys to humans and are often called the neocerebellum, while the vermis and paravermis constitute the paleocerebellum. The flocculonodular lobe (also called the archicerebellum) is the most primitive part of the cerebellum, and it sends its axons directly to the vestibular nuclei in the brainstem.

Multiple maps of the body-surface representation in the cerebellar cortex have been made (e.g., Snider and Stowell 1944). Representation of the trunk is usually placed within the vermis, with the limbs in the hemispheres. The flocculonodular lobe receives mainly visual and vestibular input (Snider and Stowell 1944; Manni and Petrosini 2004) and is chiefly involved in balance and eye movements.

Cerebellar inputs and outputs pass through the anterior, middle, and posterior *cerebellar peduncles*. The inputs come from many different sources in the pontine nuclei and the spinal cord. Cerebellar outputs go to the cerebral cortex via the ventral lateral nucleus of the thalamus and to a variety of brainstem motor areas, including the red nucleus which gives rise to the rubrospinal tract.

The cerebellum and the cerebrum are closely interconnected. The leg, arm, and face regions of the primary motor cortex send separate, parallel projections to the cerebellum

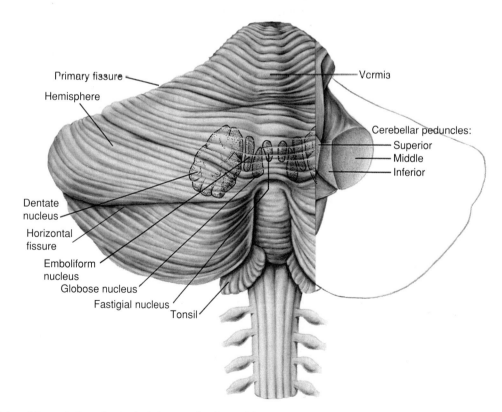

Figure 2.15 *Dorsal view of the cerebellum, showing both the cortical surface and the underlying paired nuclei. The right hemisphere has been removed to reveal the three cerebellar peduncles that connect the cerebellum to the brainstem. From Kandel et al. (1991).*

through the pons. The cerebellar nuclei, in turn, project back through the VL nucleus of the thalamus to the same cortical regions. Thus, closed loops connect the leg, arm, and face representations in the motor cortex to those in the cerebellum. Similar closed-loop circuits with the cerebellum appear to exist for each of the premotor areas in the frontal lobe (Dum and Strick 2003; Kelly and Strick 2003; Glickstein et al. 2009; Strick et al. 2009).

CEREBELLAR FUNCTION

Current understanding of cerebellar function began with Gordon Holmes, a neurologist who served with the British Forces in France during World War I. Holmes made repeated observations of the effects of gunshot wounds in the cerebellum and visual cortex (areas which, being relatively unprotected by the back of the helmet, were quite vulnerable to injury) (Pearce 2004). Holmes quoted one of his patients, who had a lesion of the right cerebellar hemisphere as saying, "the movements of my left arm are done subconsciously, but I have to think out each movement of the right arm. I come to a dead stop in turning, and have to think before I start again" (Holmes 1939). Based on such observations, Holmes wrote numerous papers giving classic descriptions of cerebellar disorders (Holmes 1939).

The effects of cerebellar lesions are unlike those resulting from injury to the cerebrum. In particular, motor deficits are ipsilateral to the side of the injury, and they do not result in paralysis. Damage to the cerebellar hemispheres is associated with a broad spectrum of disorders of limb movements. The term ataxia is used generally to describe the resulting incoordination, which may include: dysmetria (wrong-amplitude movements), intention tremor occurring particularly near the end of movement, disdiadochokinesia (inability to perform a rapidly alternating movement), or decomposition of complex movements into several components. Such findings indicate that the cerebellum is important in fine-tuning the details of movement, and in coordinating the limbs and limb segments so that complex movements occur smoothly and automatically. These findings have generated a variety of models for how the cerebellum performs these functions (e.g., Lacquaniti and Maioli 1989; Paulin 1989; Miall et al. 1993; Kawato 1999; Spoelstra et al. 2000; Kawato and Gomi 1992; Wolpert et al. 1998).

In addition, the cerebellum has long been known to play a role in motor learning, including the recalibration of eye/hand coordination during growth, as well as adaptive adjustments in the vestibular reflexes that control eye and head movements to stabilize vision (Gellman et al. 1985; Stone and Lisberger 1986; Kim et al. 1987; Wang et al. 1987; Lou and Bloedel 1992). Cerebellar injury is associated with a loss of the ability to adapt movements to changing conditions.

Although the cerebellum has traditionally been viewed as a motor structure, recent views suggest that it also helps to optimize the acquisition of sensory information (Gao et al. 1996; Blakemore et al. 2001) and to organize higher cognitive functions (Kim et al. 1994; Daum and Ackermann 1995; Thach 2007). Such higher-order functions are thought to be located within the hemispheres and dentate nucleus.

INFORMATION IN ACTION POTENTIALS (SPIKES)

Neuronal *action potentials* (or *spikes*) are believed to be the basic units of interneuronal communication and information transfer in the CNS. In accord with this understanding, the second section of this chapter discussed the functional correlates of various cortical areas largely in terms of the amount of activity (i.e., the numbers of spikes produced). In this section we consider exactly *how* spikes or series of spikes (*spike trains*) might *encode* the information important for motor control. There are several hypotheses about the way in which information might be encoded in spiking activity. This is important for BCI technology, which is based on the premise that brain signals can be decoded and used to control devices.

RATE-CODING HYPOTHESIS

The prevailing view today is referred to as the *rate-coding hypothesis*. It posits that information is transmitted by neurons through the *rate* at which they produce spikes. The notion of a rate code was first clearly articulated by Adrian and Zotterman (1926), who recorded action potentials from cutaneous nerve fibers in the leg of a cat as the pressure applied to the footpad was varied. While *spike amplitude* remained stable, the *number of spikes* counted over several seconds was proportional to the pressure applied. This observation suggested that spike *frequency*, or *rate*, is the fundamental mechanism of coding information. This is called the *rate-coding hypothesis*.

Since the seconds-long time interval used in this initial study appeared to be too long to encode the rapidly changing sensory, motor, and cognitive information associated with motor behaviors, later investigators refined the rate-coding hypothesis by considering much smaller time windows able to accommodate rapid variations (Richmond et al. 1987). Nevertheless, the preferred operational time scale of neurons and the appropriate time scale for measurement of spike rates remain unsettled.

In many BCI applications, spikes are counted in bins (i.e., time periods) of 20–100 msec (Serruya et al. 2002; Taylor et al. 2002; Carmena et al. 2003; Pohlmeyer et al. 2009). Counting spikes in bins is a common method for estimating firing rates. However, this method has certain problems. First, the temporal boundaries of the bins are chosen arbitrarily with respect to the occurrence of individual spikes (e.g., so that a given spike might span two adjacent bins). Second, when bin width (i.e., duration) is reduced to improve temporal resolution, the rate resolution decreases (because rate is computed in increments of 1/binwidth) (Dayan and Abbott 2001). An alternate method not extensively used in BCI applications is to convolve a spike train with a Gaussian or similar filter in order to translate the point process into a continuous rate signal (French and Holden 1971; Dayan and Abbott 2001). With this approach, the width of the Gaussian filter acts much like the bin width in standard binning, and it determines the temporal resolution at which the firing rate is measured.

TEMPORAL-CODING HYPOTHESIS

The *temporal-coding hypothesis* offers an alternative viewpoint. In this hypothesis information is encoded in the fine temporal patterns of spikes. That is, the precise temporal pattern of spike occurrences carries information beyond the total number of spikes. There is much debate as to what the essential distinction is between rate and temporal coding. Some researchers argue that by shrinking the bin width or Gaussian-filter width to some arbitrarily small value, a rate code becomes indistinguishable from a temporal code, and that, therefore, there is no fundamental difference between the two hypotheses. Others argue that if temporal patterns of action potentials measured on a millisecond (as opposed to tens or hundreds of milliseconds) time scale do carry behavioral information, then these patterns constitute proof of a temporal code. Theunissen and Miller (1995) have proposed a formal distinction between the two hypotheses by appealing not only to the temporal fluctuations of the neural response but also to the temporal variations in the stimulus or behavior that is encoded. They argue that if temporal patterns in a spike train are fluctuating faster than the stimulus or behavior and carry information about the stimulus or behavior, then this is evidence for a temporal code. For example, if we consider the original work of Adrian, who monitored action potentials in cutaneous nerve fibers under different levels of maintained pressure (Adrian and Zotterman 1926), any pattern of spike trains within the measurement period (beyond that of the mean spike rate) that correlated with the pressure level would constitute a temporal code.

Although some data support the idea of temporal coding in sensory systems (Richmond et al. 1987; Middlebrooks et al. 1994), there is less evidence of temporal coding in the motor system, at least at the single-neuron level. However, a number of studies suggest that precise temporal synchrony between neurons in the motor cortex may carry behavioral information. For example, Riehle and colleagues recorded simultaneously from multiple M1 neurons while monkeys performed a simple reaching task in which the cue to move could occur at one of several predictable time points. Significant synchronization between pairs of M1 neurons occurred at these expected cue times even when the firing rates of the constituent neurons did not change at these times (Riehle et al. 1997). The authors suggest that rate and temporal coding are not mutually exclusive, but, rather, provide complementary information, in which the firing rate of individual neurons encodes movement information, while the synchrony between neurons encodes expectation or enhanced attention (Middlebrooks et al. 1994). In another study (Hatsopoulos et al. 1998), M1 neurons appeared to synchronize transiently near the onset of a reaching movement, and the magnitude of synchrony changed with the direction of movement. A follow-up study suggested that this synchrony, while present in pairs of M1 neurons, carries directional information that is redundant with the simple rate coding of individual neurons (Oram et al. 2001).

SPIKE RECORDING AND PROCESSING

The spikes of cortical neurons are detected by microelectrodes that penetrate into cortex so that their tips (or other recording surfaces) are close to the neurons. This section discusses the techniques used to record and analyze spikes (see also chapters 5, 7, and 16). Recording of field potentials by electroencephalographic (EEG) methods is described in chapters 3 and 6.

MICROELECTRODES

The first reported use of penetrating electrodes to record spikes from individual cortical neurons was probably Renshaw's study in the late 1930s using an agar-filled micropipette and a vacuum-tube amplifier (Renshaw et al. 1940). It was not until the early 1950s that metal *microelectrodes* were used to record spikes from neurons in visual, somatosensory, and motor cortices (Hubel 1957; Mountcastle 1957; Jasper et al. 1958; Hubel 1959; Evarts 1966). These microelectrodes were essentially insulated wires with sharpened uninsulated tips.

Many different types of microelectrodes are now in use for intracortical recordings, including multielectrode arrays that can be chronically implanted in the brain for months or even years. Several commonly used variations are shown in figure 2.16. The simplest of these are *microwire* electrodes, arrays of thin wires soldered to a connector in two or more rows (fig. 2.16A). The diameter of the wires is typically 25–50 μm, and their composition may be steel, tungsten, or platinum-iridium. The tips of the wires are generally cut off at an angle to produce sufficient sharpness to penetrate the pia mater (the innermost and thinnest of the three meningeal layers surrounding the brain). Because of the high flexibility of these wires, they must be stiffened during insertion. A coating of polyethylene glycol is typically used to accomplish this and makes it possible to construct electrodes as long as 20 mm or more. The coating is dissolved with warm saline as the electrodes are inserted slowly into the cortex to the desired depth. The electrodes are stabilized in position by anchoring the connector directly to the skull with an adhesive such as methyl methacrylate.

If the tips of electrodes in an array are ≤50 μm apart, the spike of a given neuron may be detected at more than one electrode. This offers more than just redundancy. A single electrode often records spikes from several different neurons, and it may be difficult to identify the spikes produced by each individual neuron. Separation is usually accomplished on the basis of differences in spike shapes (see section on Spike Sorting in this chapter). The spike-sorting process can be more reliable if the spikes of an individual neuron are recorded by more than one electrode. This was the rationale behind the *stereotrode* (McNaughton et al. 1983), which was constructed by twisting together two 25-μm platinum/iridium wires and cutting the ends with a sharp scissors. Subsequently, four wires were used for the same purpose, giving rise to the *tetrode* (Gray et al. 1995). These have been further bundled into arrays of as many as 12 tetrodes, each adjustable in depth (Wilson and McNaughton 1993; Yamamoto and Wilson 2008; Kloosterman et al. 2009; Nguyen et al. 2009), providing the ability to record quite reliably from large numbers of neurons and to record spikes from a given neuron on several electrodes simultaneously (fig. 2.16B).

An alternative design that has recently become available commercially (Microprobes for Life Sciences, http://www.microprobes.com/; Plexon Neurotechnology Research Systems, http://www.plexon.com/) is the *floating microelectrode array* (fig. 2.16C). This array consists of as many as 36 electrodes mounted in a small ceramic substrate, and bonded to thin connecting wires (i.e., leads). The electrode tips are finely etched and generally have somewhat better recording properties than microwires, the tips of which are simply the cut ends of the wire. The array geometry is highly customizable, with electrodes as long as 10 mm. The array is inserted much like a microwire array, but the flexible leads run to a connector

mounted on the skull. This allows the electrode array to float on the surface of the cortex, thereby reducing movement relative to brain tissue.

A similar rationale was part of the motivation for the 100-electrode *Utah array*, invented nearly 20 years ago by Richard Normann at the University of Utah (Jones et al. 1992) and now available commercially through Blackrock Microsystems (http://www.blackrockmicro.com/) (fig. 2.16D). Many different laboratories have now adopted it for high-density cortical recordings. The array is constructed from a block of silicon, formed into 100 cone-shaped spikes separated by 0.4 mm and either 1.0 or 1.5 mm long. The tips are metalized with either platinum or iridium; the shank is insulated with silicon nitride. The electrodes are connected via very thin wires to a separate skull-mounted connector. Unlike other microelectrode arrays that are inserted relatively slowly into the cortex, the Utah array is inserted at very high speed (in <1 msec) to a calibrated distance using a pneumatic inserter. This approach is designed to reduce the mechanical dimpling of the surface that is otherwise typically associated with the insertion of such a large number of electrodes.

The use of a silicon substrate allows for the adoption of some of the technology developed for the fabrication of integrated circuits. An excellent example of this strategy is the *Michigan probe* originally developed at the University of Michigan and now available commercially from NeuroNexus Technologies (http://www.neuronexustech.com/) (fig. 2.16E). The basic electrode consists of a single shank approximately 15 μm thick, 150 μm wide, and up to 10 mm long, etched from silicon. Along the length of this shank are as many as 64 iridium, gold, or platinum contacts, each routed to a connector at the base of the shank. A variety of electrodes are available with different geometries and numbers of contacts. Moreover, several of these devices can be combined in a single package to form a more complex planar device. The design of the Michigan probes provides an opportunity to integrate electronic circuitry onto the same substrate as the electrode array itself.

The *U-Probe* (Plexon Neurotechnology Research Systems, http://www.plexon.com/) is another example of an electrode with multiple contact sites along its length (fig. 2.16F). Unlike the Michigan probe, its overall geometry is more like the traditional electrode, with a cylindrical cross section and a conical tip.

NOISE REDUCTION AND ELECTRODE SIGNAL CONDITIONING

The spikes recorded from these microelectrodes have amplitudes on the order of tens to several hundred microvolts, and the impedance of the electrodes ranges from several hundred kilohms to several megaohms. Consequently, the recordings are quite prone to noise from a variety of sources such as power lines, lights, and electrical equipment. In addition, simply bending the leads generates tiny microphonic currents that can be as large as the spikes if care is not taken to eliminate them. The process of eliminating noise from the recorded signals is

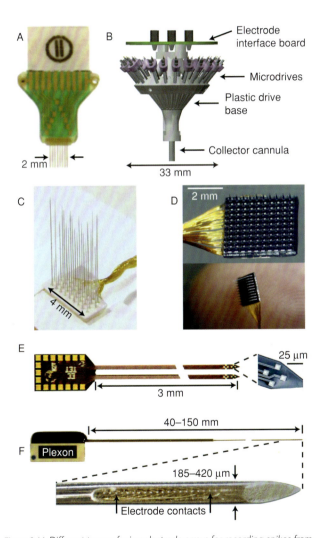

Figure 2.16 *Different types of microelectrode arrays for recording spikes from cortical neurons. (A) Microwires (Tucker Davis Technologies). (B) Multiple tetrode microdrive (Kloosterman et al. 2009; Nguyen et al. 2009). (C) Floating microelectrode array (Microprobe, Inc.) (D) Array of 100 silicon electrodes (Utah array) (Blackrock Microsystems). (E) Planar multisite silicon electrodes (Michigan electrodes) (Neuronexus Technologies). (F) Metal multisite electrode, the "U-Probe" (Plexon).*

called *conditioning*. Conditioning eliminates irrelevant aspects of the signals so that the spikes can be discerned. The most effective approach is to condition the signals as close to the electrodes as possible so that the subsequent transmission through longer leads is less prone to interference. This is accomplished in several steps.

The first step is amplification of the signal very close to the electrode by a *headstage*. Commercially available headstages range from very simple voltage followers constructed from discrete transistors to more sophisticated integrated-circuit devices with 10x or greater voltage gain and appropriate bandpass filtering (see chapter 7). Most of the companies offering electrode arrays also provide headstages configured for their particular arrays. Since substantial noise can arise from the wires connecting the headstage to the next stage of processing, recent interest has focused on using telemetry to eliminate the need for these wires. Several telemetered headstages with as many as 96 channels are available commercially (e.g., Triangle Biosystems, Inc., http://www.trianglebiosystems.com/; Biosignal Group Corp., http://www.biosignalgroup.com/).

After this initial step of signal conditioning is accomplished at the headstage, further filtering and amplification are typically required. These further steps are discussed in greater detail in chapters 7 and 9. Some degree of high-pass filtering (chapter 7) is usually necessary because of the high gain (10,000x) required and because of the DC offsets (i.e., abrupt voltage shifts) and low-frequency noise introduced by movement artifacts. Such filtering does not impair spike detection since most of the power in spikes is in frequencies of 300 Hz to 10 kHz. However, in addition to spikes it is often desirable to record local field potentials (LFPs) (see chapter 3), which have lower frequencies, so the high-pass filter should be kept below 10 Hz. In addition, an appropriate (i.e., 5–10 kHz) anti-aliasing low-pass filter (chapter 7) is typically applied, and then the signals are digitized at rates of 25–40 kHz. Further digital filtering may be helpful in subsequent stages to deal with particular noise sources or to help in identifying spikes from different neurons.

SPIKE SORTING

For most of the history of single-neuron behavioral electrophysiology, researchers relied on single, moveable microelectrodes, positioning their tips very near the cell body of one neuron in order to selectively capture its extracellular voltage waveform. More recently, however, with the advent of multielectrode technology, it is not always practical to isolate single neurons, either because it is too time-consuming to position each electrode close to a single neuron or because the electrodes are rigidly fixed in one position and may or may not be near a particular neuron. In response to this problem, over the past decade sophisticated algorithms for identifying the spikes of individual neurons have become prevalent in microelectrode electrophysiology. This process is called *spike sorting*, and a relatively large literature describing a number of different approaches has emerged (see (Lewicki 1998) for a review).

The assumption underlying all spike-sorting algorithms is that the size and shape of the spikes from a single neuron are highly stereotyped and differ from those coming from other neurons. Therefore, all algorithms begin by representing the spike waveform according to some feature set. The simplest is the fluctuation of the spike voltage over time. Sets of representative examples of these waveforms can be selected from several minutes of recorded data, and an average waveform can be computed and used as a template to sort subsequent spikes. Each spike that is subsequently collected can be compared to each of the template waveforms with any of a number of different similarity metrics. If the match is sufficiently close, it is assumed to have been generated from the corresponding template neuron (Tolias et al. 2007; Rebesco et al. 2010).

Another approach is to represent the spike waveform using an appropriate reduced-dimensionality basis set. For example, assuming that the action potential is sampled at 40 kHz for 1.5 msec, there are 60 voltage values per action potential. Given that the action potential is highly autocorrelated in time, the dimensionality of the signal can be reduced from 60 to perhaps two or three dimensions using an analysis technique called *principal components analysis* (PCA) (chapter 7), while still accounting for most of the variance across individual spikes. Alternatively, a small set of arbitrarily chosen features can be defined (e.g., spike width, peak-to-trough amplitude, or time-to-peak voltage). By thus projecting the action potential waveforms into a lower-dimensional space, distinct clusters often emerge, each potentially corresponding to a single neuron. In a process called *cluster-cutting*, boundaries separating the clusters can be manually defined so that it is often possible to isolate more than one neuron from a single microelectrode.

With the growing use of multielectrode methods that allow 100 or more neurons to be recorded simultaneously, manual spike-discrimination methods have become extremely tedious or entirely impractical. Automated methods have been developed to address this problem and to eliminate the subjectivity characteristic of manual methods (Wood et al. 2004). Nonparametric clustering algorithms (e.g., k-means or fuzzy clustering) can automatically discover partitions between naturally occurring clusters in the PCA or feature space. However, many of these methods have an inherent weakness in that they require prior knowledge of the expected number of clusters (Lewicki 1998). More powerful spike-sorting algorithms that can also estimate the number of distinct clusters in a data set have been developed (Lewicki 1994; Wood and Black 2008). By using Bayes's rule (see chapter 8), the probability that a given spike waveform belongs to a particular cluster can be used to sort spikes into distinct clusters.

SUMMARY

The ease with which we make arm and hand movements is due to the interaction of many different cortical and subcortical brain areas. This network is necessary to transform a high-level, abstract representation of a movement goal into the sequence of muscle activations necessary to effect the movement. The goal might be represented initially in visual coordinates, or it might be generated internally. Feedback to guide the movement is normally provided both by the somatosensory and visual systems. The cerebellum is thought to refine the dynamics of the movement through its interconnections with the cerebral cortex. The basal ganglia are important in initiating and optimizing actions.

In this chapter we review these anatomical connections and the neuronal activity that occurs throughout the network during movement. Although the cerebellum and basal ganglia play critical roles in the production of normal movements, their locations make them relatively inaccessible either to arrays of chronically implanted electrodes or to noninvasive electroencephalography. On the other hand, the exposed cerebral cortical surface is accessible to both EEG electrodes and to the various types of implanted multielectrode arrays now available for recording neuronal action potentials (spikes).

Among the exposed cortical areas, the primary motor cortex (M1) is so named because of its strong anatomical connections to the spinal cord and because its neuronal activity is closely related to that of the muscles that produce movements and to particular aspects of the movements, such as direction. As a result, M1 neurons have been the focus of most intracortical BCI development efforts up to the present. Just anterior to M1 within the frontal lobe are several premotor areas that represent more complex and abstract movement plans. Within the PPC are several different areas that appear to combine visual and somatosensory signals into an internal map of the body and its environment that is important in movement production. Many of the neurons in these higher-order motor areas represent limb movements in complex, gaze-dependent coordinates. In designing a BCI, its intended application might drive the choice of area from which neuronal activity will be recorded.

Although BCI research has focused on extracting motor-related information from cortical neurons, there is increasing interest in the possibility that somatosensory information comparable to that from skin and muscle receptors might be provided to the user during BCI operation by electrically *activating* appropriate brain areas. Realization of this possibility would be facilitated by increased understanding of the neuronal coding in these areas and by development of methods for activating individual neurons.

A variety of multielectrode arrays are currently available, and sophisticated algorithms have been developed for identifying the spikes of different neurons and for extracting the movement-related information each provides. However, several cortical areas most promising for BCI development, including parts of primary motor and sensory cortex and reach-related areas of PPC, are located deep within cortical sulci where they are not readily accessible to current recording technology. Thus, substantial technological challenges remain to be addressed.

REFERENCES

Adrian ED, Zotterman Y (1926) The impulses produced by sensory nerve endings: Part 3. Impulses set up by touch and pressure. J Physiol 61:465–483.

Alexander GE, Crutcher MD (1990) Neural representations of the target (goal) of visually guided arm movements in three motor areas of the monkey. J Neurophysiol 64:164–178.

Alexander GE, DeLong MR, Strick PL (1986) Parallel organization of functionally segregated circuits linking basal ganglia and cortex. Annu Rev Neurosci 9:357–381.

Andersen RA, Snyder LH, Bradley DC, Xing J (1997) Multimodal representation of space in the posterior parietal cortex and its use in planning movements. Annu Rev Neurosci 20:303–330.

Asanuma H, Arnold A, Zarzecki P (1976) Further study in the excitation of pyramidal tract cells by intracortical microstimulation. Exp Brain Res 26:443–461.

Ashe J, Georgopoulos AP (1994) Movement parameters and neural activity in motor cortex and area 5. Cereb Cortex 4:590–600.

Baizer JS, Ungerleider LG, Desimone R (1991) Organization of visual inputs to the inferior temporal and posterior parietal cortex in macaques. J Neurosci 11:168–190.

Barbas H, Pandya DN (1989) Architecture and intrinsic connections of the prefrontal cortex in the rhesus monkey. J Comp Neurol 286:353–375.

Batista AP, Buneo CA, Snyder LH, Andersen RA (1999) Reach plans in eye-centered coordinates. Science 285:257–260.

Benguerel AP, Cowan HA (1974) Coarticulation of upper lip protrusion in French. Phonetica 30:41–55.

Betz W (1874) Anatomischer Nachweis zweier Gehirncentra. Centralblatt Med Wissenschaft 12:578–580, 595–599.

Blakemore SJ, Frith CD, Wolpert DM (2001) The cerebellum is involved in predicting the sensory consequences of action. Neuroreport 12: 1879–1884.

Blatt GJ, Andersen RA, Stoner GR (1990) Visual receptive field organization and cortico-cortical connections of the lateral intraparietal area (area LIP) in the macaque. J Comp Neurol 299:421–445.

Boline J, Ashe J (2005) On the relations between single cell activity in the motor cortex and the direction and magnitude of three-dimensional dynamic isometric force. Exp Brain Res 167:148–159.

Breveglieri R, Galletti C, Gamberini M, Passarelli L, Fattori P (2006) Somatosensory cells in area PEc of macaque posterior parietal cortex. J Neurosci 26:3679–3684.

Brodmann K (1909) Comparative Localization Study of the Brain According to the Principles of Cellular Structures [in German]. Leipzig: JA Barth Verlag.

Burke D, Hagbarth KE, Lofstedt L (1978) Muscle spindle responses in man to changes in load during accurate position maintenance. J Physiol 276: 159–164.

Cabel DW, Cisek P, Scott SH (2001) Neural activity in primary motor cortex related to mechanical loads applied to the shoulder and elbow during a postural task. J Neurophysiol 86:2102–2108.

Caminiti R, Johnson PB, Galli C, Ferraina S, Burnod Y (1991) Making arm movements within different parts of space: The premotor and motor cortical representation of a coordinate system for reaching to visual targets. J Neurosci 11:1182–1197.

Caminiti R, Johnson PB, Urbano A (1990) Making arm movements within different parts of space: Dynamic aspects in the primate motor cortex. J Neurosci 10:2039–2058.

Carmena JM, Lebedev MA, Crist RE, O'Doherty JE, Santucci DM, Dimitrov D, Patil PG, Henriquez CS, Nicolelis MA (2003) Learning to control a brain-machine interface for reaching and grasping by primates. PLoS Biol 1:193–208.

Chang SW, Dickinson AR, Snyder LH (2008) Limb-specific representation for reaching in the posterior parietal cortex. J Neurosci 28:6128–6140.

Cheney PD, Fetz EE (1980) Functional classes of primate corticomotorneuronal cells and their relation to active force. J Neurophysiol 44:773–791.

Clark SA, Allard T, Jenkins WM, Merzenich MM (1988) Receptive fields in the body-surface map in adult cortex defined by temporally correlated inputs. Nature 332:444–445.

Cohen YE, Andersen RA (2002) A common reference frame for movement plans in the posterior parietal cortex. Nat Rev Neurosci 3:553–562.

Coulter JD, Jones EG (1977) Differential distribution of corticospinal projections from individual cytoarchitectonic fields in the monkey. Brain Res 129:335–340.

Crago PE, Houk JC, Rymer WZ (1982) Sampling of total muscle force by tendon organs. J Neurophysiol 47:1069–1083.

Crammond DJ, Kalaska JF (1989) Neuronal activity in primate parietal cortex area 5 varies with intended movement direction during an instructed-delay period. Exp Brain Res 76:458–462.

Crammond DJ, Kalaska JF (2000) Prior information in motor and premotor cortex: Activity during the delay period and effect on pre-movement activity. J Neurophysiol 84:986–1005.

Damasio H, Grabowski T, Frank R, Galaburda AM, Damasio AR (1994) The return of Phineas Gage: Clues about the brain from the skull of a famous patient. Science 264:1102–1105.

Daniloff R, Moll K (1968) Coarticulation of lip rounding. J Speech Hear Res 11:707–721.

Daum I, Ackermann H (1995) Cerebellar contributions to cognition. Behav Brain Res 67:201–210.

Dayan P, Abbott LF (2001) Theoretical Neuroscience: Computational and Mathematical Modeling of Neural Systems. Cambridge, MA: MIT Press.

de Lafuente V, Romo R (2006) Neural correlate of subjective sensory experience gradually builds up across cortical areas. Proc Natl Acad Sci USA 103:14266–14271.

Denny-Brown D (1950) Disintegration of motor function resulting from cerebral lesions. J Nerv Ment Dis 112:1–45.

di Pellegrino G, Fadiga L, Fogassi L, Gallese V, Rizzolatti G (1992) Understanding motor events: A neurophysiological study. Exp Brain Res 91:176–180.

di Pellegrino G, Wise SP (1991) A neurophysiological comparison of three distinct regions of the primate frontal lobe. Brain 114:951–978.

Donoghue JP, Leibovic S, Sanes JN (1992) Organization of the forelimb area in squirrel monkey motor cortex: Representation of digit, wrist, and elbow muscles. Exp Brain Res 89:1–19.

Duhamel JR, Bremmer F, BenHamed S, Graf W (1997) Spatial invariance of visual receptive fields in parietal cortex neurons. Nature 389:845–848.

Duhamel JR, Colby CL, Goldberg ME (1998) Ventral intraparietal area of the macaque: Congruent visual and somatic response properties. J Neurophysiol 79:126–136.

Dum RP, Strick PL (1991) The origin of corticospinal projections from the premotor areas in the frontal lobe. J Neurosci 11:667–689.

Dum RP, Strick PL (2003) An unfolded map of the cerebellar dentate nucleus and its projections to the cerebral cortex. J Neurophysiol 89:634–639.

Dum RP, Strick PL (2005) Motor areas of the frontal lobe: The anatomical substrate for the central control of movement. In: Riehle A, Vaadia E (eds.) Motor Cortex in Voluntary Movements. Boca Raton, FL: CRC Press, pp. 3–47.

Engel KC, Flanders M, Soechting JF (1997) Anticipatory and sequential motor control in piano playing. Exp Brain Res 113:189–199.

Evarts EV (1966) Pyramidal tract activity associated with a conditioned hand movement in the monkey. J Neurophysiol 29:1011–1027.

Evarts EV (1968) Relation of pyramidal tract activity to force exerted during voluntary movement. J Neurophysiol 31:14–27.

Fagg AH, Ojakangas GW, Miller LE, Hatsopoulos NG (2009) Kinetic trajectory decoding using motor cortical ensembles. IEEE Trans Neural Syst Rehabil Eng 17:487–496.

Fagg AH, Shah A, Barto AG (2002) A computational model of muscle recruitment for wrist movements. J Neurophysiol 88:3348–3358.

Ferrier D (1873) Experimental researches in cerebral physiology and pathology. West Riding Lunatic Asylum Med Rep 3:30–96.

Flor H, Nikolajsen L, Jensen TS (2007) Phantom limb pain: A case of maladaptive CNS plasticity? Nat Rev Neurosci 7:873–881.

Flourens P (1824) Recherches experimentales sur les propriétés et les fonctions du système nerveux dans les animaux vertebres. Paris: Crevot.

French AS, Holden AV (1971) Alias-free sampling of neuronal spike trains. Kybernetik 8:165–171.

Friedman DP, Murray EA, O'Neill JB, Mishkin M (1986) Cortical connections of the somatosensory fields of the lateral sulcus of macaques: Evidence for a corticolimbic pathway for touch. J Comp Neurol 252:323–347.

Fritsch G, Hitzig E (1870) Ueber dir elektrische Erregbarkeit des Grosshirns. Arch Anat Physiol Leipzig 37:330–332.

Fu QG, Flament D, Coltz JD, Ebner TJ (1995) Temporal encoding of movement kinematics in the discharge of primate primary motor and premotor neurons. J Neurophysiol 73:836–854.

Fu QG, Suarez JI, Ebner TJ (1993) Neuronal specification of direction and distance during reaching movements in the superior precentral premotor area and primary motor cortex of monkeys. J Neurophysiol 70:2097–2116.

Fujii N, Mushiake H, Tanji J (2000) Rostrocaudal distinction of the dorsal premotor area based on oculomotor involvement. J Neurophysiol 83:1764–1769.

Funahashi S, Bruce CJ, Goldman-Rakic PS (1989) Mnemonic coding of visual space in the monkey's dorsolateral prefrontal cortex. J Neurophysiol 61:331–349.

*Gall F, Spurzheim J (1809) Recherches sur le Système Nerveux en General, et Sur Celui du Cerveau en Particulier. Shoell, Paris.

Gallese V, Fadiga L, Fogassi L, Rizzolatti G (1996) Action recognition in the premotor cortex. Brain 119:593–609.

Gao JH, Parsons LM, Bower JM, Xiong JH, Li JQ, Fox PT (1996) Cerebellum implicated in sensory acquisition and discrimination rather than motor control. Science 272:545–547.

Gardner EP, Costanzo RM (1981) Properties of kinesthetic neurons in somatosensory cortex of awake monkeys. Brain Res 214:301–319.

Gellman R, Gibson AR, Houk JC (1985) Inferior olivary neurons in the awake cat: Detection of contact and passive body displacement. J Neurophysiol 54:40–60.

Georgopoulos AP, Caminiti R, Kalaska JF (1984) Static spatial effects in motor cortex and area 5: Quantitative relations in a two-dimensional space. Exp Brain Res 54:446–454.

Georgopoulos AP, Crutcher MD, Schwartz AB (1989) Cognitive spatial-motor processes. 3. Motor cortical prediction of movement direction during an instructed delay period. Exp Brain Res 75:183–194.

Georgopoulos AP, Kalaska JF, Caminiti R, Massey JT (1982) On the relations between the direction of two-dimensional arm movements and cell discharge in primate motor cortex. J Neurosci 2:1527–1537.

Georgopoulos AP, Schwartz AB, Kettner RE (1986) Neuronal population coding of movement direction. Science 233:1416–1419.

Ghez C, Gordon J, Ghilardi MF (1995) Impairments of reaching movements in patients without proprioception. II. Effects of visual information on accuracy. J Neurophysiol 73:361–372.

Ghosh S, Gattera R (1995) A comparison of the ipsilateral cortical projections to the dorsal and ventral subdivisions of the macaque premotor cortex. Somatosens Mot Res 12:359–378.

Glickstein M, Sultan F, Voogd J (2009) Functional localization in the cerebellum. Cortex 47:59–80.

Godschalk M, Lemon RN, Nijs HGT, Kuypers HGJM (1981) Behaviour of neurons in monkey periarcuate and precentral cortex before and during visually guided arm and hand movements. Exp Brain Res 44:113–116.

Goldman-Rakic PS (1995) Cellular basis of working memory. Neuron 14:477–485.

Goodale MA, Milner AD (1992) Separate visual pathways for perception and action. Trends Neurosci 15:20–25.

Gray CM, Maldonado PE, Wilson M, McNaughton B (1995) Tetrodes markedly improve the reliability and yield of multiple single-unit isolation from multi-unit recordings in cat striate cortex. J Neurosci Methods 63:43–54.

Graybiel AM (1995) Building action repertoires: Memory and learning functions of the basal ganglia. Curr Opin Neurobiol 5:733–741.

Graybiel AM (2005) The basal ganglia: Learning new tricks and loving it. Curr Opin Neurobiol 15:638–644.

Graziano MS, Cooke DF, Taylor CS, Moore T (2004) Distribution of hand location in monkeys during spontaneous behavior. Exp Brain Res 155:30–36.

Graziano M, Taylor C, Moore T (2002) Complex movements evoked by microstimulation of precentral cortex. Neuron 34:841–851.

Grigg P (1975) Mechanical factors influencing response of joint afferent neurons from cat knee. J Neurophysiol 38:1473–1484.

Gupta R, Ashe J (2009) Offline decoding of end-point forces using neural ensembles: Application to a brain-machine interface. IEEE Trans Neural Syst Rehabil Eng 17:254–262.

Harlow J (1868) Recovery from the passage of an iron bar through the head. Publ Mass Med Soc 2: 327.

Hatsopoulos N, Joshi J, O'Leary JG (2004) Decoding continuous and discrete motor behaviors using motor and premotor cortical ensembles. J Neurophysiol 92:1165–1174.

Hatsopoulos NG, Ojakangas CL, Paninski L, Donoghue JP (1998) Information about movement direction obtained from synchronous activity of motor cortical neurons. Proc Natl Acad Sci USA 95:15706–15711.

He SQ, Dum RP, Strick PL (1993) Topographic organization of corticospinal projections from the frontal lobe: Motor areas on the lateral surface of the hemisphere. J Neurosci 13:952–980.

Hepp-Reymond MC, Kirkpatrick-Tanner M, Gabernet L, Qi HX, Weber B (1999) Context-dependent force coding in motor and premotor cortical areas. Exp Brain Res 128:123–133.

Hepp-Reymond MC, Wyss UR, Anner R (1978) Neuronal coding of static force in the primate motor cortex. J Physiol [Paris] 74:287–291.

Holmes G (1939) The cerebellum of man. Brain 62:1–30.

Hoover JE, Strick PL (1999) The organization of cerebellar and basal ganglia outputs to primary motor cortex as revealed by retrograde transneuronal transport of herpes simplex virus type 1. J Neurosci 19:1446–1463.

Houk J, Henneman E (1967) Responses of Golgi tendon organs to active contractions of the soleus muscle of the cat. J Neurophysiol 30:466–481.

Hubel DH (1957) Single unit activity in visual cortex of the unanesthetized cat. Fed Proc 16:63.

Hubel DH (1959) Single unit activity in striate cortex of unrestrained cats. J Physiol 147:226–238.

Huntley GW, Jones EG (1991) Relationship of intrinsic connections to forelimb movement representations in monkey motor cortex: A correlative anatomic and physiological study. J Neurophysiol 66:390–413.

Hutchins KD, Martino AM, Strick PL (1988) Corticospinal projections from the medial wall of the hemisphere. Exp Brain Res 71:667–672.

Jacobsen CF (1935) Functions of the frontal association cortex in primates. Arch Neurol Psychiatry 33:558–569.

Jasper H, Ricci G, Doane B (1958) Patterns of cortical neurone discharge during conditioned motor responses in monkeys. In: Wolstenholme G, O'Connor C (eds.) Neurological Basis of Behaviour. Boston: Little, Brown, pp. 277–294.

Jeannerod M, Arbib MA, Rizzolatti G, Sakata H (1995) Grasping objects: The cortical mechanisms of visuomotor transformation. Trends Neurosci 18:314–320.

Jenkins WM, Merzenich MM, Ochs MT, Allard T, Guic-Robles E (1990) Functional reorganization of primary somatosensory cortex in adult owl monkeys after behaviorally controlled tactile stimulation. J Neurophysiol 63:82–104.

Joel D, Weiner I (1994) The organization of the basal ganglia-thalamocortical circuits: Open interconnected rather than closed segregated. Neuroscience 63:363–379.

Johnson PB, Ferraina S, Bianchi L, Caminiti R (1996) Cortical networks for visual reaching: Physiological and anatomical organization of frontal and parietal lobe arm regions. Cereb Cortex 6:102–119.

Jones EG (1981) Functional subdivision and synaptic organization of the mammalian thalamus. Intern Rev Physiol 25:173–245.

Jones KE, Campbell PK, Normann RA (1992) A glass/silicon composite intra-cortical electrode array. Ann Biomed Eng 20:423–437.

Kakei S, Hoffman DS, Strick PL (1999) Muscle and movement representations in the primary motor cortex. Science 285:2136–2139.

Kakei S, Hoffman DS, Strick PL (2001) Direction of action is represented in the ventral premotor cortex. Nat Neurosci 4:1020–1025.

Kalaska JF, Caminiti R, Georgopoulos AP (1983) Cortical mechanisms related to the direction of two-dimensional arm movements: Relations in parietal area 5 and comparison with motor cortex. Exp Brain Res 51:247–260.

Kalaska JF, Cohen DAD, Prud'homme M, Hyde ML (1990) Parietal area 5 neuronal activity encodes movement kinematics, not movement dynamics. Exp Brain Res 80:351–364.

Kalaska JF, Cohon DAD, Hyde ML, Prud'homme M (1989) A comparison of movement direction-related versus load direction-related activity in primate motor cortex, using a two-dimensional reaching task. J Neurosci 9:2080–2102.

Kalaska JF, Crammond DJ (1992) Cerebral cortical mechanisms of reaching movements. Science 255:1517–1523.

Kandel E, Schwartz J, Jessel T (1991) Principles of Neural Science. Norwalk, CT: Appleton & Lange.

Kawagoe R, Takikawa Y, Hikosaka O (1998) Expectation of reward modulates cognitive signals in the basal ganglia. Nat Neurosci 1:411–416.

Kawato M (1999) Internal models for motor control and trajectory planning. Curr Opin Neurobiol 9:718–727.

Kawato M. Gomi H (1992) A computational model of four regions of the cerebellum based on feedback-error learning. Biol Cybernet 68:95–103.

Kelly RM, Strick PL (2003) Cerebellar loops with motor cortex and prefrontal cortex of a nonhuman primate. J Neurosci 23:8432–8444.

Kemp JM, Powell TP (1971) The connexions of the striatum and globus pallidus: Synthesis and speculation. Philos Trans R Soc Lond B [Biol Sci] 262:441–457.

Kim JH, Wang JJ, Ebner TJ (1987) Climbing fiber afferent modulation during treadmill locomotion in the cat. J Neurophysiol 57:787–802.

Kim SG, Ugurbil K, Strick PL (1994) Activation of a cerebellar output nucleus during cognitive processing. Science 265:949–951.

Kloosterman F, Davidson TJ, Gomperts SN, Layton SP, Hale G, Nguyen DP, Wilson MA (2009) Micro-drive array for chronic in vivo recording: drive fabrication. J Vis Exp 16:1094–1097. http://www.jove.com/details.stp?id=1094.

Krubitzer L, Huffman KJ, Disbrow E, Recanzone G (2004) Organization of area 3a in macaque monkeys: Contributions to the cortical phenotype. J Comp Neurol 471:97–111.

Kurata K (1993) Premotor cortex of monkeys: Set- and movement-related activity reflecting amplitude and direction of wrist movements. J Neurophysiol 69:187–200.

Kurata K, Tanji J (1986) Premotor cortex neurons in macaques: Activity before distal and proximal forelimb movements. J Neuroscience 6:403–411.

Kuypers HGJM, Fleming WR, Farinholt JW (1962) Subcorticospinal projections in the rhesus monkey. J Comp Neurol 118:107–131.

Kwan H, MacKay W, Murphy J, Wong Y (1978a) An intracortical microstimulation study of output organization in precentral cortex of awake primates. J Phyisol [Paris] 74:231–233.

Kwan HC, MacKay WA, Murphy JT, Wong YC (1978b) Spatial organization of precentral cortex in awake primates. II. Motor outputs. J Neurophysiol 41:1120–1131.

Lacquaniti F, Maioli C (1989) Adaptation to suppression of visual information during catching. J Neurosci 9:149–159.

Lawrence DG, Kuypers HGJM (1968a) The functional organization of the motor system in the monkey. I. The effects of bilateral pyramidal lesions. Brain 91:1–14.

Lawrence DG, Kuypers HGJM (1968b) The functional organization of the motor system in the monkey. II. The effects of lesions of the descending brain-stem pathways. Brain 91:15–36.

Lebedev MA, Messinger A, Kralik JD, Wise SP (2004) Representation of attended versus remembered locations in prefrontal cortex. PLoS Biol 2:e365.

Lemon RN (2008) Descending pathways in motor control. Annu Rev Neurosci 31:195–218.

Lewicki MS (1994) Bayesian modeling and classification of neural signals. Neural Comput 6:1005–1030.

Lewicki MS (1998) A review of methods for spike sorting: The detection and classification of neural action potentials. Network: Comput Neural Syst 9:53–78.

Liu CN, Chambers WW (1964) An experimental study of the cortico-spinal system in the monkey (Macaca mulatta). The spinal pathways and preterminal distribution of degenerating fibers following discrete lesions of the pre- and postcentral gyri and bulbar pyramid. J Comp Neurol 123: 257–283.

Loeb GE, Duysens J (1979) Activity patterns in individual hindlimb primary and secondary muscle spindle afferents during normal movements in unrestrained cats. J Neurophysiol 42:420–440.

Lou JS, Bloedel JR (1992) Responses of sagittally aligned Purkinje cells during perturbed locomotion: Synchronous activation of climbing fiber inputs. J Neurophysiol 68:570–580.

Lu X, Ashe J (2005) Anticipatory activity in primary motor cortex codes memorized movement sequences. Neuron 45:967–973.

Luppino G, Murata A, Govoni P, Matelli M (1999) Largely segregated parietofrontal connections linking rostral intraparietal cortex (areas AIP and VIP) and the ventral premotor cortex (areas F5 and F4). Exp Brain Res 128:181–187.

Maier MA, Bennett KMB, Hepp-Reymond MC, Lemon RN (1993) Contribution of the monkey corticomotoneuronal system to the control of force in precision grip. J Neurophysiol 69:772–785.

Manni E, Petrosini L (2004) A century of cerebellar somatotopy: A debated representation. Nat Rev Neurosci 5:241–249.

Matelli M, Govoni P, Galletti C, Kutz DF, Luppino G (1998) Superior area 6 afferents from the superior parietal lobule in the macaque monkey. J Comp Neurol 402:327–352.

Matelli M, Luppino G, Rizzolatti G (1985) Patterns of cytochrome oxidase activity in the frontal agranular cortex of the macaque monkey. Behav Brain Res 18:125–136.

Matelli M, Luppino G, Rizzolatti G (1991) Architecture of superior and mesial area 6 and the adjacent cingulate cortex in the macaque monkey. J Comp Neurol 311:445–462.

Maynard EM, Hatsopoulos NG, Ojakangas CL, Acuna BD, Sanes JN, Normann RA, Donoghue JP (1999) Neuronal interactions improve cortical population coding of movement direction. J Neurosci 19:8083–8093.

McNaughton BL, O'Keefe J, Barnes CA (1983) The stereotrode: A new technique for simultaneous isolation of several single units in the central nervous system from multiple unit records. J Neurosci Methods 8: 391–397.

Miall RC, Weir DJ, Wolpert DM, Stein JF (1993) Is the cerebellum a Smith predictor? J Motor Behav 25:203–216.

Middlebrooks JC, Clock AE, Xu L, Green DM (1994) A panoramic code for sound location by cortical neurons. Science 264:842–844.

Middleton FA, Strick PL (2000) Basal ganglia and cerebellar loops: Motor and cognitive circuits. Brain Res Brain Res Rev 31:236–250.

Millar J (1973) Joint afferent fibres responding to muscle stretch, vibration and contraction. Brain Res 63:380–383.

Mishkin M (1979) Analogous neural models for tactual and visual learning. Neuropsychologia 17:139–151.

Moran DW, Schwartz AB (1999) Motor cortical representation of speed and direction during reaching. J Neurophysiol 82:2676–2692.

Morgane PJ, Galler JR, Mokler DJ (2005) A review of systems and networks of the limbic forebrain/limbic midbrain. Prog Neurobiol 75:143–160.

Moritz CT, Perlmutter SI, Fetz EE (2008) Direct control of paralysed muscles by cortical neurons. Nature 456:639–642.

Mountcastle VB (1957) Modality and topographic properties of single neurons of cat's somatic sensory cortex. J Neurophysiol 20:408–434.

Mountcastle VB, Davies PW, Berman AL (1957) Response properties of neurons of cat's somatic sensory cortex to peripheral stimuli. J Neurophysiol 20:374–407.

Mountcastle VB, Lynch JC, Georgopoulos A, Sakata H, Acuna C (1975) Posterior parietal association cortex of the monkey: Command functions for operations within extrapersonal space. J Neurophysiol 38:871–908.

Muir RB, Lemon RN (1983) Corticospinal neurons with a special role in precision grip. Brain Res 261:312–316.

Murphy J, Kwan H, Wong Y (1979) Differential effects of reciprocal wrist torques on responses of somatopically identified neurons of precentral cortex in awake primates. Brain Res 172:329–377.

Mushiake H, Inase M, Tanji J (1991) Neuronal activity in the primate premotor, supplementary, and precentral motor cortex during visually guided and internally determined sequential movements. J Neurophysiol 66:705–718.

Mussa-Ivaldi FA (1988) Do neurons in the motor cortex encode movement direction? An alternative hypothesis. Neurosci Lett 91:106–111.

Nguyen, D. P., Layton, S. P., Hale, G., Gomperts, S. N., Davidson, T. J., Kloosterman, F., Wilson, M. A. (2009) Micro-drive array for chronic in vivo recording: Tetrode assembly. J Vis Exp 26:1098–1100 http://www.jove.com/details.stp?id=1098.

Nolte J (2002) The Human Brain: An Introduction to Its Functional Anatomy. St. Louis: Mosby.

Nudo RJ, Jenkins WM, Merzenich MM (1990) Repetitive microstimulation alters the cortical representation of movements in adult rats. Somatosens Mot Res 7:463–483.

Nudo RJ, Milliken GW, Jenkins WM, Merzenich MM (1996) Use-dependent alterations of movement representations in primary motor cortex of adult squirrel monkeys. J Neurosci 16:785–807.

Oram MW, Hatsopoulos NG, Richmond BJ, Donoghue JP (2001) Excess synchrony in motor cortical neurons provides redundant direction information with that from coarse temporal measures. J Neurophysiol 86:1700–1716.

Pandya DN, Seltzer B (1982) Intrinsic connections and architectonics of posterior parietal cortex in the rhesus monkey. J Comp Neurol 204:196–210.

Paninski L, Fellows MR, Hatsopoulos NG, Donoghue JP (2004) Spatiotemporal tuning of motor cortical neurons for hand position and velocity. J Neurophysiol 91:515–532.

Park MC, Belhaj-Saïf A, Gordon M, Cheney PD (2001) Consistent features in the forelimb representation of primary motor cortex in rhesus macaques. J Neurosci 21:2784–2792.

Park MC, Belhaj-Saif A, Cheney PD (2004) Properties of primary motor cortex output to forelimb muscles in rhesus macaques. J Neurophysiol 92:2968–2984.

Pascual-Leone A, Torres F (1993) Plasticity of the sensorimotor cortex representation of the reading finger in Braille readers. Brain 116 (1):39–52.

Passingham R, Perry H, Wilkinson F (1978) Failure to develop a precision grip in monkeys with unilateral neocortical lesions made in infancy. Brain Res 145:410–414.

Paulin MG (1989) A Kalman-filter theory of the cerebellum. In: Arbib MA, Amari S (eds.) Dynamic Interactions in Neural Networks: Models and Data. New York: Springer-Verlag, pp. 241–259.

Pearce JM (2004) Sir Gordon Holmes (1876–1965). J Neurol Neurosurg Psychiatry 75:1502–1503.

Penfield W (1958) Some mechanisms of consciousness discovered during electrical stimulation of the brain. Proc Natl Acad Sci USA 44:51–66.

Penfield W, Boldrey E (1937) Somatic motor and sensory representation in the cerebral cortex of man as studied by electrical stimulation. Brain 60:389–443.

Penfield W, Welch K (1951) The supplementary motor area in the cerebral cortex. Arch Neurol Psychiatry 66:289–317.

Picard N, Strick PL (2001) Imaging the premotor areas. Curr Opin Neurobiol 11:663–672.

Pohlmeyer EA, Oby ER, Perreault EJ, Solla SA, Kilgore KL, Kirsch RF, Miller LE (2009) Toward the restoration of hand use to a paralyzed monkey: Brain-controlled functional electrical stimulation of forearm muscles. PLoS One 4:e5924.

Pohlmeyer EA, Perreault EJ, Slutzky MW, Kilgore KL, Kirsch RF, Taylor DM, Miller LE (2007) Real-Time Control of the Hand by Intracortically Controlled Functional Neuromuscular Stimulation. In: IEEE 10th international conference on rehab robotics, vol. 10, Noordwijk, The Netherlands, pp 454–458.

Pohlmeyer EA, Solla SA, Perreault EJ, Miller LE (2007) Prediction of upper limb muscle activity from motor cortical discharge during reaching. J Neural Eng 4:369–379.

Prochazka A (1981) Muscle spindle function during normal movement. Int Rev Physiol 25:47–90.

Prud'homme MJL, Kalaska JF (1994) Proprioceptive activity in primary somatosensory cortex during active arm reaching movements. J Neurophysiol 72:2280–2301.

Ralston DD, Ralston HJ, 3rd (1985) The terminations of corticospinal tract axons in the macaque monkey. J Comp Neurol 242:325–337.

Raos V, Franchi G, Gallese V, Fogassi L (2003) Somatotopic organization of the lateral part of area F2 (dorsal premotor cortex) of the macaque monkey. J Neurophysiol 89:1503–1518.

Raos V, Umilta MA, Murata A, Fogassi L, Gallese V (2006) Functional properties of grasping-related neurons in the ventral premotor area F5 of the macaque monkey. J Neurophysiol 95:709–729.

Rathelot JA, Strick PL (2006) Muscle representation in the macaque motor cortex: An anatomical perspective. Proc Natl Acad Sci USA 103: 8257–8262.

Rebesco JM, Stevenson IH, Koerding K, Solla SA, Miller LE (2010) Rewiring neural interactions by micro-stimulation. Front Systems Neurosci 4:39.

Recanzone GH, Allard TT, Jenkins WM, Merzenich MM (1990) Receptive-field changes induced by peripheral nerve stimulation in SI of adult cats. J Neurophysiol 63:1213–1225.

Renshaw B, Forbes A, Morison BR (1940) Activity of isocortex and hippocampus: Electrical studies with micro-electrodes J Neurophysiol 3:74–105.

Richmond BJ, Optican LM, Podell M, Spitzer H (1987) Temporal encoding of two-dimensional patterns by single units in primate inferior temporal cortex. I. Response characteristics. J Neurophysiol 57:132–146.

Riehle A (1991) Visually induced signal-locked neuronal activity changes in precentral motor areas of the monkey: Hierarchical progression of signal processing. Brain Res 540:131–137.

Riehle A (2005) Preparation for action: One of the key functions of the motor cortex. In: Riehle A, Vaadia E (eds.) Motor Cortex in Voluntary Movements. Boca Raton, FL: CRC Press.

Riehle A, Grun S, Diesmann M, Aertsen A (1997) Spike synchronization and rate modulation differentially involved in motor cortical function. Science 278:1950–1953.

Riehle A, Requin J (1989) Monkey primary motor and premotor cortex: single-cell activity related to prior information about direction and extent of an intended movement. J Neurophysiol 61:534–549.

Rizzolatti G, Camarda R, Fogassi L, Gentilucci M, Luppino G, Matelli M (1988) Functional organization of inferior area 6 in the macaque monkey. II. Area F5 and the control of distal movements. Exp Brain Res 71:491–507.

Rizzolatti G, Fadiga L (1998) Grasping objects and grasping action meanings: The dual role of monkey rostroventral premotor cortex (area F5). Novartis Found Symp 218:81–95; discussion 95–103.

Robinson DL, Goldberg ME, Stanton GB (1978) Parietal association cortex in the primate: Sensory mechanisms and behavioral modulations. J Neurophysiol 41:910–932.

Sainburg RL, Ghilardi MF, Poizner H, Ghez C (1995) Control of limb dynamics in normal subjects and patients without proprioception. J Neurophysiol 73:820–835.

Sakata H, Taira M, Murata A, Mine S (1995) Neural mechanisms of visual guidance of hand action in the parietal cortex of the monkey. Cereb Cortex 5:429–438.

Sanes JN, Donoghue JP, Thangaraj V, Edelman RR, Warach S (1995) Shared neural substrates controlling hand movements in human motor cortex. Science 268:1775–1777.

Schieber MH (2001) Constraints on somatotopic organization in the primary motor cortex. J Neurophysiol 86:2125–2143.

Schieber MH, Hibbard LS (1993) How somatotopic is the motor cortex hand area? Science 261:489–492.

Schultz W, Tremblay L, Hollerman JR (2000) Reward processing in primate orbitofrontal cortex and basal ganglia. Cereb Cortex 10:272–284.

Schwartz AB (1992) Motor cortical activity during drawing movements: Single-unit activity during sinusoid tracing. J Neurophysiol 68:528–541.

Schwartz AB, Kettner RE, Georgopoulos AP (1988) Primate motor cortex and free arm movements to visual targets in three-dimensional space. I. Relations between single cell discharge and direction of movement. J Neurosci 8:2913–2927.

Schwartz AB, Moran DW (1999) Motor cortical activity during drawing movements: Population representation during lemniscate tracing. J Neurophysiol 82:2705–2718.

Scott SH, Kalaska JF (1995) Changes in motor cortex activity during reaching movements with similar hand paths but different arm postures. J Neurophysiol 73:2563–2567.

Sergio LE, Hamel-Paquet C, Kalaska JF (2005) Motor cortex neural correlates of output kinematics and kinetics during isometric-force and arm-reaching tasks. J Neurophysiol 94:2353–2378.

Serruya MD, Hatsopoulos NG, Paninski L, Fellows MR, Donoghue JP (2002) Instant neural control of a movement signal. Nature 416:141–142.

Sessle B, Wiesendanger M (1982) Structural and functional definition of the motor cortex in the monkey (*Macaca fascicularis*). J Physiol 323:245.

Shen L, Alexander G (1997a) Neural correlates of a spatial sensory-to-motor transformation in primary motor cortex. J Neurophysiol 77:1171–1194.

Shen L, Alexander G (1997b) Preferential representation of instructed target location versus limb trajectory in Dorsal Premotor Area. J Neurophysiol 77:1195–1212.

Shima K, Tanji J (2000) Neuronal activity in the supplementary and presupplementary motor areas for temporal organization of multiple movements. J Neurophysiol 84:2148–2160.

Smith AM, Hepp-Reymond MC, Wyss UR (1975) Relation of activity in precentral cortical neurons to force and rate of force change during isometric contractions of finger muscles. Exp Brain Res 23:315–332.

Snider RS, Stowell A (1944) Receiving areas of the tactile, auditory, and visual systems in the cerebellum. J Neurophysiol 7:331–357.

Soso MJ, Fetz EE (1980) Responses of identified cells in postcentral cortex of awake monkeys during comparable active and passive joint movements. J Neurophysiol 43:1090–1110.

Spoelstra J, Schweighofer N, Arbib MA (2000) Cerebellar learning of accurate predictive control for fast-reaching movements. Biol Cybernet 82:321–333.

Stone LS, Lisberger SG (1986) Detection of tracking errors by visual climbing fiber inputs to monkey cerebellar flocculus during pursuit eye movements. Neurosci Lett 72:163–168.

Strick PL, Dum RP, Fiez JA (2009) Cerebellum and nonmotor function. Annu Rev Neurosci 32:413–434.

Strick PL, Preston JB (1978a) Multiple representation in the primate motor cortex. Brain Res 154:366–370.

Strick PL, Preston JB (1978b) Sorting of somatosensory afferent information in primate motor cortex. Brain Res 156:364–368.

Taira M, Boline J, Smyrnis N, Georgopoulos AP, Ashe J (1996) On the relations between single cell activity in the motor cortex and the direction and magnitude of three-dimensional static isometric force. Exp Brain Res 109:367–376.

Taira M, Mine S, Georgopoulos AP, Murata A, Sakata H (1990) Parietal cortex neurons of the monkey related to the visual guidance of hand movement. Exp Brain Res 83:29–36.

Tanji J, Evarts E (1976) Anticipatory activity of motor cortex neurons in relation to direction of an intended movement. J Neurophysiol 39:1062–1068.

Tanji J, Hoshi E (2008) Role of the lateral prefrontal cortex in executive behavioral control. Physiol Rev 88:37–57.

Taylor DM, Tillery SI, Schwartz AB (2002) Direct cortical control of 3D neuroprosthetic devices. Science 296:1829–1832.

Thach WT (2007) On the mechanism of cerebellar contributions to cognition. Cerebellum 6:163–167.

Theunissen F, Miller JP (1995) Temporal encoding in nervous systems: A rigorous definition. J Comput Neurosci 2:149–162.

Todorov E (2000) Direct cortical control of muscle activation in voluntary arm movements: A model. Nat Neurosci 3:391–398.

Tolias AS, Ecker AS, Siapas AG, Hoenselaar A, Keliris GA, Logothetis NK (2007) Recording chronically from the same neurons in awake, behaving primates. J Neurophysiol 98:3780–3790.

Ungerleider LG, Mishkin M (1982) Two cortical visual systems. In: Ingle DJ, Goodale MA, Mansfield RJW (eds) Analysis of Visual Behavior. Cambridge, MA: MIT Press.

Van der Werf YD, Witter MP, Groenewegen HJ (2002) The intralaminar and midline nuclei of the thalamus. Anatomical and functional evidence for participation in processes of arousal and awareness. Brain Res Brain Res Rev 39:107–140.

Velliste M, Perel S, Spalding MC, Whitford AS, Schwartz AB (2008) Cortical control of a prosthetic arm for self-feeding. Nature 453:1098–1101.

Vogt V (1919) Allgemeine Ergebnisse unserer Hirnforschung. Vierte Mitteilung: Die physiologische Bedeutung der architektonischen Rindenfelderung auf Grund neuer Rindenizungen. J Psych Neurol (Leipzig) 25:279–462.

Walker A (1940) A cytoarchitectural study of the prefrontal area of the macaque monkey. J Comp Neurol 73:59–86.

Wang JJ, Kim JH, Ebner TJ (1987) Climbing fiber afferent modulation during a visually guided, multi-joint arm movement in the monkey. Brain Res 410:323–329.

Wannier TM, Maier MA, Hepp-Reymond MC (1991) Contrasting properties of monkey somatosensory and motor cortex neurons activated during the control of force in precision grip. J Neurophysiol 65:572–589.

Weinrich M, Wise SP (1982) The premotor cortex of the monkey. J Neurosci 2:1329–1345.

Westwick DT, Pohlmeyer EA, Solla SA, Miller LE, Perreault EJ (2006) Identification of multiple-input systems with highly coupled inputs: Application to EMG prediction from multiple Intracortical electrodes. Neural Comput 18:329–355.

Wilson MA, McNaughton BL (1993) Dynamics of the hippocampal ensemble code for space. Science 261:1055–1058.

Wise SP, Boussaoud D, Johnson PB, Caminiti R (1997) Premotor and parietal cortex: Corticocortical connectivity and combinatorial computations. Annu Rev Neurosci 20:25–42.

Wise SP, Tanji J (1981) Neuronal responses in sensorimotor cortex to ramp displacements and maintained positions imposed on hindlimb of the unanesthetized monkey. J Neurophysiol 45:482–500.

Wolpert DM, Miall RC, Kawato M (1998) Internal models in the cerebellum. Trends Cog Sci 2:338–347.

Wood F, Black MJ (2008) A nonparametric Bayesian alternative to spike sorting. J Neurosci Methods 173:1–12.

Wood F, Black MJ, Vargas-Irwin C, Fellows M, Donoghue JP (2004) On the variability of manual spike sorting. IEEE Trans Biomed Eng 51:912–918.

Woolsey CN, Settlage PH, Meyer DR, Sencer W, Pinto Hamuy T, Travis AM (1952) Patterns of localization in precentral and "supplementary" motor areas and their relation to the concept of a premotor area. Res Publ Assoc Res Nerv Ment Dis 30:238–264.

Xerri C, Coq JO, Merzenich MM, Jenkins WM (1996) Experience-induced plasticity of cutaneous maps in the primary somatosensory cortex of adult monkeys and rats. J Physiol [Paris] 90:277–287.

Yamamoto J, Wilson MA (2008) Large-scale chronically implantable precision motorized microdrive array for freely behaving animals. J Neurophysiol 100:2430–2440.

Yezierski RP, Gerhart KD, Schrock BJ, Willis WD (1983) A further examination of effects of cortical stimulation on primate spinothalamic tract cells. J Neurophysiol 49:424–441.

Yousry TA, Schmid UD, Alkadhi H, Schmidt D, Peraud A, Buettner A, Winkler P (1997) Localization of the motor hand area to a knob on the precentral gyrus. A new landmark. Brain 120:141–157.

3 | ELECTRIC AND MAGNETIC FIELDS PRODUCED BY THE BRAIN

PAUL L. NUNEZ

In most present-day BCI systems electric or magnetic signals produced by brain activity are used to convey the user's intentions to the BCI system. This chapter focuses primarily on *electric* rather than *magnetic* recording because electric recording (particularly by electroencephalography [EEG]) is convenient, widely used, and inexpensive, whereas magnetic recording by magnetoencephalography (MEG) is expensive, cumbersome, and remains largely confined to research settings. For purposes of our discussion in this chapter, we may categorize brain electric fields as belonging to four classes according to the nature and spatial scale of the neural activity that produces them. Chapter 2 deals with the first of these (i.e., action potentials produced by individual neurons), and this chapter addresses the other three classes. These three classes encompass the electric fields produced by the activity of neurons and their synapses at three spatial scales of measurement. These three scales, measuring *micro-, meso-, and macroscale fields,* are determined by the size and location of their respective recording electrodes.

- *Microscale fields*, in practice, are the *local field potentials (LFPs)* that are recorded within brain (usually cortical) tissue and mostly reflect current sources related to synaptic activity occurring within perhaps 0.1–1.0 mm of the recording electrode, that is, within tissue volumes typically in the 10^{-3} to 1 mm^3 range.

- *Mesoscale fields* are mostly recorded from the surface of cortex. Such recordings are called the *electrocorticogram (ECoG)*. They are believed to reflect mainly synaptic and other source activity occurring over a substantial portion of the depth of local cortex (2–5 mm), that is, within tissue volumes of 1–20 mm^3.

- *Macroscale fields* are recorded as the *electroencephalogram (EEG)*. These are obtained from the scalp. Each electrode reflects synaptic source activity occurring within large parts of the underlying brain, perhaps 10–40 cm^2 of the cortical sheet, or cortical tissue volumes in the 10^3 to 10^4 mm^3 range. Thus, EEG represents the space-averaged source activity in tissue containing on the order of 100 million to a billion neurons.

TABLE 3.1 Approximate scales of cortical tissue

SPATIAL SCALE	SIGNAL TYPE	MEASUREMENT RANGE (mm)	EXAMPLES OF BRAIN STRUCTURES
Microscale	LFP	$< 10^{-1}$	Cell body, synaptic knob
Mesoscale	ECoG	10^{-1} to 10	Module to macrocolumn
Macroscale	EEG	> 10	Brodmann area, lobe, brain

Table 3.1 lists these three scales, their recording methods, and examples of the neuroanatomical structures at each scale. Note that each of today's methods for recording electric fields covers only one of the scale ranges. Table 3.2 lists cortical structures related to function and links them to these three scales.

A BCI usually focuses on the electric fields or potentials generated in a particular brain area, those associated with a particular motor or cognitive function, or both. Its goal is to enable a person to use these fields for communication and control, substituting BCI technology for the normal use of muscles. Thus, just as understanding muscle-based movement entails understanding how muscles generate force and the characteristics of that force, effective BCI research necessarily

TABLE 3.2 Spatial scales of cortical tissue structure related to function

STRUCTURE	DIAMETER (mm)	# NEURONS	ANATOMICAL DESCRIPTION
Minicolumn	0.03	10^2	Spatial extent of inhibitory connections
Module	0.3	10^4	Input scale for corticocortical fibers
Macrocolumn	3.0	10^6	Intracortical spread of pyramidal cell
Region	50	10^8	Brodmann area
Lobe	170	10^9	Areas bordered by major cortical folds
Hemisphere	400	10^{10}	Half of brain

begins with some basic information about brain physiology, anatomy, and physics: How are the brain's electric fields generated? How are they distributed through the head? What determines their spatial and temporal characteristics? How are they best distinguished from other fields of brain or nonbrain origin? These basic questions are the business of the present chapter. It is intended to be a concise and accessible summary of the physical principles important for understanding LFP, ECoG, and EEG signals and for employing these signals in BCI research and development. We begin with a brief treatment of electric field fundamentals and go on to address the principles that underlie the behavior of these fields within the brain and in other tissues of the head.

We first provide a short nontechnical overview. Synaptic and action potentials at neural membranes create current sources, the so-called *generators* of LFP, ECoG, and EEG signals. These same current sources also generate magnetic fields (those detected by MEG), but with different sensitivity to specific source characteristics. As we will see, MEG is partly independent of, and complementary, to EEG. At the low frequencies that are of interest in electrophysiology, the electric and magnetic fields are *uncoupled*; that is, each may be estimated without reference to the other. For this reason, we will avoid the label *electromagnetic* which implies a single (coupled) field and which generally exhibits much more complicated dynamic behaviors.

Much of the membrane current from source regions remains in the local tissue and forms small current loops that may pass through the intercellular, membrane, and extracellular media. Such local source activity may be recorded as LFP. In addition, some of the source current may reach the cortical surface to be recorded as ECoG, and a little even gets as far as the scalp to be recorded as EEG. The manner in which source current spreads through brain, CSF, skull, and scalp tissue is called *volume conduction* and is determined by the geometric (i.e., due to surface shapes) and electrical *resistivity* of these tissues. For example, skull tissue has a high resistivity, causing current generated in local cortical regions to spread widely. (This is one reason that the cortical region contributing to potentials recorded at each scalp electrode is much larger than the electrode itself.) The second contributor to this space-averaging effect is the physical separation (about 1 cm) between cortical sources and scalp. In EEG, this current-spreading also contributes to the knotty issue of choice of a reference electrode, to be discussed in more detail in chapter 6. Whereas large-scale measures like EEG provide the big picture but no local details, small-scale measures like LFPs provide local detail but only very sparse spatial coverage. Thus, these measures plus the intermediate-scale ECoG provide *complementary* and *largely independent* measures of brain source activity at different spatial scales and therefore with different levels of description.

Many physics and engineering books provide excellent treatments of electric field fundamentals. Why then is this chapter necessary? First, texts on electric circuits or electromagnetic fields focus on issues of minimal interest in electrophysiology and are not, by themselves, very useful in the current context. Introductory electrical engineering is concerned with one-dimensional current in wires, rather than volume current in three spatial dimensions. Elementary physics courses emphasize fields due to charges in *dielectrics* (i.e., insulators) rather than the membrane current sources generating fields. The practical problems in electrophysiology require a much different emphasis, one that treats current sources in conductive media.

The second reason for this chapter is the most obvious and most important. Electric currents and fields depend on the medium that contains them. Living tissue presents unique problems as a medium for these currents. In particular, spatial scale is a central issue in all of electrophysiology, specifically in the critical distinction among the *microscopic, mesoscopic,* and *macroscopic* fields. The nature of brain electric fields depends strongly on the scale under study. In a complex system with nontrivial relationships among dynamics at different spatial and temporal scales, it is important to appreciate that no one scale is intrinsically better than another (Nunez 2010). The usual elementary relations between charges and electric fields are of minimal use in electrophysiology. *Static membrane charge produces no electric field that can be recorded by an extracellular electrode.* This is because many charged particles (ions such as Na^+, Cl^-, etc.) in the extracellular fluid change position to shield membrane charge. Thus, the electric field due to the static charges in the extracellular space is essentially zero (i.e., it is electroneutral, except at atomic scales). In a conducting medium like living tissue, this charge shielding impels a focus not on charges (the usual focus in describing electric fields and potentials in insulators) but, rather, on current sources.

A third justification for this chapter is that electrophysiology is concerned exclusively with fields of *low frequency.* Although currents generally produce magnetic fields, it is only at field frequencies in the megahertz range or higher (i.e., frequencies far above those found in the brain) that they form nonnegligible *electromagnetic fields* and associated propagating waves. The fields generated in tissue are well below the megahertz range. This allows us to focus, instead, on *quasistatic electric* or *quasistatic magnetic fields.* We use the *quasistatic approximation*, in which electric fields (e.g., those measured by EEG) occur as if magnetic fields do not exist and in which magnetic fields (e.g., those measured by MEG) occur as if electric fields do not exist. It is important to note here that although some time intervals of EEG records may appear as waves traveling across the scalp (as revealed by progressive EEG phase shifts), these events are *not* due to electromagnetic waves. Rather, such "brain waves" owe their origins to some combination of synaptic delays, intrinsic cellular dynamics, and action-potential propagation delays, and they originate at least partly from the selectively nonlinear behavior of active cell membranes.

To begin our introduction to the physiological electric fields that can be measured and used for BCIs, we first give a short overview of electric circuits with emphasis on the ideas that carry over naturally to brain electric fields. The goal is to provide the electric-field novice with a robust bridge to the more advanced topic of multiscale brain electric fields. The basic physics and physiology supporting the ideas of this chapter are presented in more technical depth in (Nunez and Srinivasan 2006a) where a more extensive reference list may also be found.

CURRENTS AND POTENTIALS IN ELECTRIC CIRCUITS

OHM'S LAW IN ELECTRIC CIRCUITS

Electric current is defined as the directed motion of positive charge (coulombs) per unit time. It is measured in units of amperes (A), where one ampere equals one coulomb/second (C/sec). However, the positive current direction is an arbitrary definition. In metal wires the carriers of current are negatively charged electrons moving in directions opposite to positive current. By contrast, current carriers in living tissue are positive *and* negative ions moving in opposite directions, and *both* of these movements contribute to the total current in tissue volume conductors.

In a typical electric circuit, the small resistance contributed by the wire may be neglected so that opposition to current occurs only at discrete circuit elements with *resistance R*. Ohm's law (eq. 3.1) relates the potential difference ($V_1 - V_2$) across resistor terminals to the current I passing through the resistor

$$V_1 - V_2 = RI \qquad (3.1)$$

Current moves from higher to lower potentials, so that positive current in equation (3.1) is consistent with V_1 greater than V_2. The process is somewhat analogous to water flow down a pipe, with volume flow (liters per second) representing current, and the heights of the pipe ends representing the two voltages. According to this analogy, current, like water, flows "downhill" as indicated in figure 3.1. The pipe's resistance to water flow depends on its cross-sectional area and the frictional force applied to the water by the pipe wall. This metaphor emphasizes that *potential differences*, not potentials, cause current to flow. This distinction has long been a source of confusion in the EEG community when reference-electrode effects are evaluated. Although idealized electric circuits typically allow for a convenient reference location where the potential may be set to zero, actual human heads, which contain unknown sources of current, are not so cooperative. The important issue of reference selection is extensively discussed in chapter 6.

EQUIVALENCE OF VOLTAGE AND CURRENT SOURCES

Voltages and currents may be generated by several kinds of sources. Figure 3.2 shows two circuits: an *ideal independent voltage source* (an AC or alternating-current generator) (upper panel) and an *ideal independent current source* (lower panel) (typically a separate circuit containing transistors and voltage sources). *Ideal* here means that the magnitude of the voltage or current produced by an independent source is a fixed property and is not affected by other elements in the circuit. (Note that in all circuit images in this chapter, arbitrary combinations of circuit elements are represented by rectangles, as in the case of box *X*; their inner details are not relevant to this discussion.) Representation of sources as ideal and independent is not universally valid. For example, if a switch in series with the current source is opened, thereby disconnecting it from other parts of the circuit, the current must go to zero unless the source supplies enough power to cause electrons to jump the air gap in the switch, creating sparks. However, with proper circuit design, the ideal source assumption will be valid whenever box *X* contains normal circuit elements.

The ideal voltage source V_S (fig. 3.2, upper panel) in series with the resistor R is equivalent to the ideal current source I_S (fig. 3.2, lower panel) in parallel with the same resistor R in the following sense. In both cases, $V_s = RI_s$ and all the currents and voltages in the network represented by box *X* are identical, regardless of whether the terminals (*a*, *b*) of the box are connected to the voltage or current source network. This equivalence principle, closely associated with Thevenin's theorem of electrical engineering (see any introductory engineering text on electric circuits) is valid irrespective of the complexity of the network in box *X*, which might contain hundreds of nonlinear circuit elements. The equivalence of voltage and current sources also occurs in volume conductors such as the head. Whereas smaller-scale electrophysiology (LFP and single-neuron studies) may be concerned with membrane potentials measured by small electrodes (see chapters 2, 5), data from

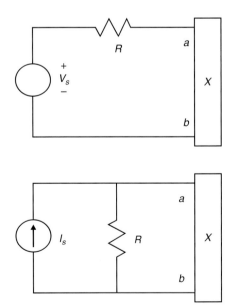

Figure 3.2 Circuit with ideal independent sources: voltage source (upper panel) and current source (lower panel). The equivalence of voltage and current sources is described in the text. All the currents and voltages in the electric network represented by X are unchanged when the voltage source (upper) is replaced by the current source (lower). The network X is arbitrary, perhaps containing thousands of nonlinear circuit elements.

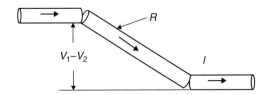

Figure 3.1 Fluid flow rate through the central pipe (liters/sec) depends on the height difference between its two ends V_1–V_2 and the pipe resistance R. The fluid flow is analogous to current flux through a resistor with a voltage difference across its terminals.

macroscale EEG are more conveniently related to the *multiple* synaptic current sources produced within mesoscale tissue volumes. Just as they are in electric circuits such as those shown in figure 3.2, these current and voltage source descriptions can be regarded as equivalent for electrical phenomena in the head.

The sources shown in figure 3.2 are *independent*: they are fixed regardless of what happens in box *X*. By contrast, figure 3.3 shows a circuit with an ideal *dependent* (i.e., controlled) current source, indicated by the diamond symbol. In this example, the current I_S is controlled by the voltage in some other part of the circuit according to some rule, $I_S = f(V_X)$. This control is provided by some influence not indicated in the figure, typically a separate circuit. Given the dense interconnectivity of cerebral cortex, dependent sources provide more realistic cortical analogs than independent sources.

IMPEDANCE IN ELECTRIC CIRCUITS

Fundamentally, circuit dynamics are governed by differential equations, which model resistive, capacitive, and inductive elements. However, for cases in which all sources produce sinusoidal voltages or currents and all circuit elements are linear, electrical engineers have devised a clever trick to bypass some of the mathematics. The trick is to employ complex circuit variables such as *impedance*, which have real and imaginary parts. Impedance (*Z*) is the AC equivalent of *resistance* and accounts for phase shifts due to capacitive and inductive properties of circuit elements. Ohm's law (eq. 3.1) remains valid, provided that resistance *R* is replaced by impedance *Z*. *Z* is a complex quantity providing for phase shifts between current and voltage. Resistors, capacitors, and inductors are often combined in circuit analysis to form equivalent impedance. The real and imaginary parts of *Z* are labeled the composite *resistance* and *reactance*, respectively, of the combined circuit elements.

At frequencies of interest in EEG, inductive effects (coupling of electric and magnetic fields) in macroscopic neural tissue masses are entirely negligible. Capacitive effects have also been found to be negligible in most studies, although small but measureable capacitive phase shifts were found in at least one study of live human skull (Akhtari et al. 2002) . Thus, in addressing macroscale tissue volume conduction, we usually use *impedance* and *resistance* interchangeably. However, even at macroscopic scales, capacitive effects may be important at electrode/tissue interfaces where the contact approximates a resistor and capacitor in parallel. This occurs because chemical reactions take place at the metal/tissue interface where tissue ion current induces tiny electron current in the amplifier circuit. Capacitive effects are, of course, quite important at the microscopic scale of individual cells. Indeed, membranes in states well below threshold for action-potential firing are modeled as chains of resistors in parallel with capacitors, similar to coaxial TV cables, but with zero inductance.

Tissue volume conduction adds several complications not present in electric circuits, but volume conduction is simpler in other ways. The first major simplification is the neglect of magnetic induction. As noted, brain currents can produce genuine *electromagnetic fields* (propagating waves or *far fields*) only at field frequencies in the megahertz range or higher, frequencies far above those found in the brain. It is thus reasonable to use the *quasistatic approximation*, in which electric fields (e.g., those measured by EEG) occur as if magnetic fields do not exist, and magnetic fields (e.g., those measured by MEG) occur as if electric fields do not exist. Thus, EEG wave propagation across the scalp is *not electromagnetic*; rather, its origins are some combination of axonal propagation and synaptic (i.e., postsynaptic potential) delays.

LINEAR SUPERPOSITION IN ELECTRIC CIRCUITS

A second major simplification in tissue volume conduction occurs because, for the weak electric fields detected by EEG, tissue appears to behave *linearly* at macroscopic scales. By this we mean that in this context, bulk neural tissue obeys Ohm's law. (By contrast, neural cell membranes become nonlinear near their thresholds for firing action potentials; this is a microscale phenomenon.) At the macroscale of bulk tissue that is relevant for EEG studies, and at frequencies below perhaps 10–100 kHz, current largely bypasses high-resistance membranes and thereby obeys Ohm's law.

For electric circuits, the analogous linearity is indicated in figure 3.4, in which the rectangular boxes stand for arbitrary combinations of linear resistors, capacitors, inductors, and/or any other linear elements, including independent sources. The current source I_1 in figure 3.4 (upper panel) generates numerous voltages and currents within networks represented by the rectangles; V_1 is any such voltage. Similarly, the current source I_2 (fig. 3.4, middle panel) generates the voltage V_2 at the same location as V_1. Figure 3.4 (lower panel) shows that when the two current sources are turned on simultaneously, the potential at this location is simply the sum $V_1 + V_2$. This simple outcome does not hold true if the boxes contain nonlinear elements.

About 10 billion synapses producing current sources occupy regions the size of a cortical macrocolumn (see section *Multiple Scales of Cortical Sources* below and table 3.2 in this chapter) with diameter of 1–3 mm and containing perhaps a 10^5 to 10^6 neurons. If I_1 and I_2 were to represent two cortical current sources, such as the net source current produced in two cortical columns, figure 3.4 correctly indicates that the resulting dural or scalp potential is simply the sum of

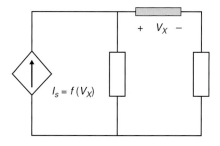

Figure 3.3 *Circuit with ideal dependent source. The diamond symbol represents a dependent current source with its output given by the function* $I_S = f(V_X)$, *that is, controlled by the voltage* V_X *across the terminals of the gray box (representing arbitrary circuit elements). This control occurs through processes not shown in the image, possibly a separate circuit. The white boxes also represent arbitrary circuit elements.*

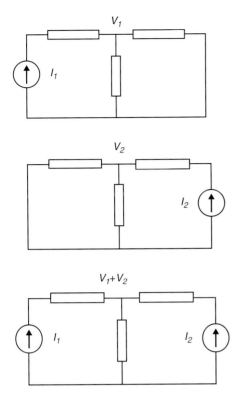

Figure 3.4 *Superposition in a linear electric network. In this figure only, rectangles represent linear circuit elements. In the upper and middle panels, current sources* I_1 *and* I_2 *produce voltages* V_1 *and* V_2, *respectively, when acting separately. When both sources are turned on together (lower panel), the resulting voltage at the same location is* $V_1 + V_2$. *This simple result does not hold true in nonlinear circuits.*

potentials generated by each column separately. This result does not require that the sources oscillate at equal frequencies or even produce sinusoidal oscillations at all; only the validity of Ohm's law is required. This linearity of the tissue volume conductor must not be confused with the nonlinear dynamics of source interactions. A simple circuit analog illustrates this distinction: in figure 3.3 the dependent current source I_S, and other sources in the gray box might be coupled by some complicated nonlinear process that may lead their dynamics to be quite complicated; nevertheless, the net voltage produced by multiple sources will still sum linearly.

CURRENTS AND POTENTIALS IN TISSUE VOLUME CONDUCTORS

OHM'S LAW FOR VOLUME CONDUCTION

Three important new issues arise with the transition from electric circuits to volume conduction. First, while low-frequency current in a copper wire is uniformly distributed over its cross section, current through the head is spread out in complicated spatial patterns determined by both geometric and resistive tissue properties.

The second issue concerns the definition of electric potential. In electric circuits the symbol V normally denotes potential with respect to some arbitrary circuit node where the potential may be set to zero. This practice will not work in a volume

conductor with distributed sources. Thus, for the head volume conductor in EEG applications, we will adopt the symbol Φ rather than V to indicate the (theoretical) *nominal potential with respect to infinity*, where the term *nominal* indicates that this is the potential due only to sources generated by the brain. Note that experimental recordings, whether from inside or outside the skull, measure the experimental potential V, rather than the theoretical potential Φ. V is expected to closely approximate Φ if recordings are mostly free of artifact, other noise sources, and electrode reference distortions. External-noise reduction is greatly facilitated by modern amplifier systems designed to reject potentials that are equal at recording and reference sites (i.e., common mode rejection), and to thereby eliminate (ideally) most environmental (nonbiological) noise sources.

The third issue concerns *spatial scale*. This issue is often ignored in abstract neural network models, but it is critically important in actual physical or biological systems. The spatial scale of electrophysiological measurement spans four or five orders of magnitude, depending on the size and location of the recording electrodes. In practice, all descriptive electrical properties (i.e., potential, current density, resistivity, etc.) must be defined at a specific spatial scale. For example, the resistivity (see below) of a membrane will differ greatly from that of the extracellular fluid, and both will differ from that of a composite large-scale tissue mass.

Ohm's law in volume conductors is a more general statement than it is in its usual form in electric circuits (eq. 3.1). In volume conductors Ohm's law is expressed as a linear relationship between *vector current density* **J** (in microamperes per square millimeter, $\mu A/mm^2$) and electric field **E** (microvolts per millimeter, $\mu V/mm$):

$$\mathbf{J} = \sigma \mathbf{E} \qquad (3.2)$$

Here σ (Siemens/mm, or S/mm, or $ohm^{-1}mm^{-1}$) is the *conductivity* of the physical or biological material. *Conductivity* is typically used in mathematical models. In contrast, experimentalists tend to use its inverse *resistivity,* $\eta \equiv 1/\sigma$ (ohm mm), as the standard parameter. When conductivity is a scalar, equation (3.2) is a vector equation, equivalent to three scalar equations in three directions. Because we are concerned here only with quasistatic (not electromagnetic) fields, the electric field may be expressed conveniently as the gradient of potential

$$\mathbf{E} = -\nabla \Phi = -\left(\frac{\partial \Phi}{\partial x} + \frac{\partial \Phi}{\partial y} + \frac{\partial \Phi}{\partial z} \right) \qquad (3.3)$$

Both electric circuit analysis and electrophysiology are greatly simplified by the introduction of the more simple (scalar) electric potential Φ. The term on the far right side of equation 3.3 involving spatial derivatives applies only in rectangular coordinates. The shorter vector form $(-\nabla \Phi)$ (middle of eq. 3.3) is generally preferred because it is explicitly independent of human choices of coordinate system.

The simple, one-dimensional version of Ohm's law (eq. 3.1) is easily obtained from equations 3.2 and 3.3 for the special case of current passing through a material of constant cross section. This is shown in figure 3.5. Suppose current I is constant across the cross-sectional area A of a cylindrical conductor of resistivity η and length Δx, as in the case of 60-Hz current in a copper wire. In this example, $\mathbf{J}=J_x\mathbf{i}$ and $\mathbf{E}=E_x\mathbf{i}$, where x indicates the direction of current and electric field and $\mathbf{i}$ is a unit vector in the x direction. The x component of current density is $J_x=I/A$. The electric field is approximately $E_x \cong -\Delta\Phi/\Delta x = \left(\Phi_1 - \Phi_2\right)/\Delta x$. Substitution of these relations into equation 3.1 yields

$$\Phi_1 - \Phi_2 = \frac{\eta\Delta xI}{A}$$

(3.4)

In the case of simple wire current, the symbols Φ and V are interchangeable. Comparison of equations 3.1 and 3.4 shows that the resistance of a wire or other cylindrical medium of resistivity η, length Δx, constant cross section A, and constant current density across the cross section is given by

$$R = \frac{\eta\Delta x}{A}$$

(3.5)

Thus, *resistivity* is a basic property of the medium through which current passes. It is determined by interactions between charges in motion and the medium's atomic, molecular, or cellular structure. In contrast, *resistance* depends both on the medium and its geometric properties.

In EEG applications involving head volume conductor models, equation 3.5 reminds us that the resistance of any current path depends on both geometry (tissue boundaries) and tissue resistivity. The former may be obtained by MRI, but it is much more problematic to find the latter. For example, the resistance to current normal to the surface of a skull plug of cross-section A may be expressed as the sum of the resistances of the three skull layers, the middle of which (i.e., cancellous bone) has much lower resistivity than the top and bottom layers (i.e., cortical bone) (Law 1993; Akhtari et al. 2002; Nunez and Srinivasan 2006a).

CURRENT DISTRIBUTION IN THE HEAD

Current flux in the head volume conductor involves several complications not normally present in simple circuits. The most obvious is that current spreads out from sources nonuniformly so that current density $\mathbf{J}(\mathbf{r}, t)$ at each location $\mathbf{r}$ is not generally constant over any cross section A. Also, head resistivity varies with type of tissue so that $\eta = \eta(\mathbf{r})$. That is, the medium is an *inhomogeneous* volume conductor. Here the

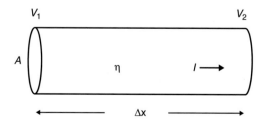

Figure 3.5 *The resistance of a cylindrical conductor of resistivity η also depends on its length Δx and its cross section A. In contrast, resistivity η is simply a property of the medium (e.g., copper wire, salt water, tissue) through which the current passes.*

scalar resistivity is expressed as a function of vector location $\mathbf{r}$; an alternate form is $\eta = \eta(x, y, z)$. Finally, tissue is generally *anisotropic*, meaning that resistivity (or conductivity) is direction dependent. In white matter, for example, resistivity is lower for current flux in directions parallel to axons. In anisotropic tissue (whether homogeneous or inhomogeneous), conductivity is a tensor (or matrix) with matrix elements that may or may not be functions of location $\mathbf{r}$.

In anisotropic conductors, Ohm's law, equation 3.2, involves matrix multiplication. All serious volume-conductor models of the head take into account major inhomogeneities (i.e., among brain, CSF, skull, and scalp tissues). However, because of a paucity of detailed experimental data, nearly all head models assume that these tissues are isotropic. Despite this crude approximation, head volume-conductor models provide semiquantitative predictions of relations between intracranial sources and scalp potentials that are very useful for many applications. For example, even very simple volume-conductor models can provide important "filters" to weed out ill-conceived EEG data reduction methods; that is, if a proposed method does not work even with simple head models, it cannot be expected to work with actual heads.

Despite the complications of conductive inhomogeneity and anisotropy, experiments indicate that living tissue is *linear at macroscopic scales*: Ohm's law (eq. 3.2) is valid, but perhaps only in matrix form. This experimental finding is fully consistent with the nonlinear conductive properties of active membranes: in a tissue volume that is mesoscopic (e.g., 1 mm³) or larger, most externally applied current passes through the extracellular fluid. It is important to note that higher cell density increases mesoscopic resistivity, but the resistivity nevertheless remains linear. *Tissue resistivity can vary widely with measurement scale*: a microelectrode with tip diameter of 10^{-4} to 10^{-3} cm may record potentials based only on extracellular fluid, which has substantially lower resistivity than a mesoscopic or macroscopic tissue mass (i.e., which includes cells). Thus, it makes little sense to speak of tissue "resistivity" without explicit reference to the spatial scale at which this property is defined or measured.

HEAD MODELS OF VOLUME CONDUCTION

Several classes of models have proven valuable in testing our intuitions about volume conduction in heads, and they show that the EEG folklore has often been wrong. The most widely adopted head models are the *three-sphere* and *four-sphere* models. The four-sphere model, portrayed in figure 3.6, consists of an inner sphere (brain) surrounded by three spherical shells representing cerebral spinal fluid (CSF), skull, and scalp layers. The three-sphere model incorporates the CSF as part of the brain; in practice it is about as accurate as the four-sphere model because the largest model errors are caused by inhomogeneity and anisotropy and by uncertainty concerning skull resistivity (Nunez and Srinivasan 2006a).

Cortical mesoscale sources (small arrows in fig. 3.6) send currents into surrounding tissues. These currents form closed loops by returning to their cortical origins. Most of this source current remains inside the skull, but a little reaches the scalp

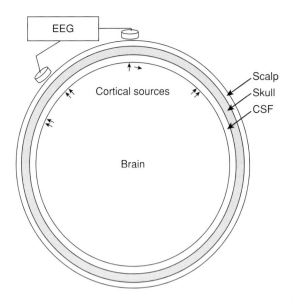

Figure 3.6 The usual four-sphere head model *consists of an inner sphere (brain) surrounded by three spherical shells representing CSF, skull, and scalp layers. The small arrows represent cortical mesoscale sources where closed current loops begin and end. Some of this current reaches the inner dura layer and is recorded as ECoG; much less reaches the scalp to be recorded as EEG.*

and may be recorded as EEG. Cortical morphology, especially the parallel arrangement of pyramidal cells (chapter 2), suggests that source currents tend to flow perpendicular to the local cortical surface. Thus, gyral source currents tend to be perpendicular to the CSF layer, and sulcal source currents tend to be parallel to the CSF layer; however, this geometric picture is very crude given the convoluted nature of cortical folds.

Positive and negative ions travel in opposite directions along current paths such that the numbers of positive and negative charges remain equal in mesoscopic (or even much smaller) volume elements at all locations. This is a standard condition of conductive media called *electroneutrality*. (To imagine this, picture a densely crowded boardwalk on which all men walk north and all women walk south, with much pushing and shoving such that *gender neutrality* is preserved in all large regions of the crowd. If they walk at the same speed, the men and women contribute equally to this "person current.") Although most source current remains inside the skull, a little passes into the scalp before returning to cortex. From a strictly external viewpoint, these are essentially skull current sources, and they produce currents and potentials in the scalp.

Whereas EEG is recorded at the scalp, larger potentials are recorded when electrodes are placed inside the cranium on the cortical surface for ECoG. The ECoG potentials naturally provide better localization of brain dynamics. Even more detail is obtained with smaller electrodes that record LFPs from within cortical tissue. Whereas scalp-recorded EEG measures the activity of synaptic current sources in tissue volumes containing roughly 100 million neurons, intracranial electrodes can record activity in volumes containing perhaps 1–10 million neurons, depending mostly on electrode size and location. It is important to note that intracranial recordings generally obtain *different* information, *not more or better* information, than that obtained from the scalp. To use a standard analogy, scalp

electrodes measure large portions of the forest but no trees, whereas intracranial electrodes measure some individual trees or maybe even a few ants on their leaves.

Although the idealized *n*-sphere models have easily implemented analytic solutions, they provide only crude representation of tissue boundaries. By contrast, *finite-element* and *boundary-element models*, which are substantially more computer intensive, may employ MRI images to locate tissue boundaries more accurately. Are these numerical models more accurate than *n*-sphere models? The answer is not clear, mainly because accurate tissue resistivity is every bit as important as accurate geometry for estimating volume conduction. Tissue resistivity (especially skull resistance) is often poorly known and may vary by 100% or more across subjects or across locations in the same subject. Furthermore, both bulk skull (with three distinct layers) and white matter are substantially anisotropic, meaning that the conductivity of each tissue is an inhomogeneous tensor (or 3×3 matrix), with unknown or poorly known individual components. Some data indicate that, in sharp contrast to equation 3.5, bulk skull plug resistance is uncorrelated to thickness, apparently because thicker skulls may have a disproportionately thick inner layer of cancellous bone, which has relatively high conductivity (Law 1993). This implies that attempts to correct head models by using MRI to find tissue boundaries may achieve only marginal improvements unless much more accurate tissue conductivities are also obtained. Nevertheless, several heroic studies have obtained in vivo measurements of tissue resistivity (e.g., Akhtari et al. 2002; Lai et al. 2005; and others reviewed in Nunez and Srinivasan 2006a). These studies show rather large variation in resistivity estimates, across tissues, across laboratories, and across individual subjects.

POTENTIALS RECORDED INSIDE THE CRANIUM

POTENTIALS AT DIFFERENT SCALES

The incredible fractal-like complexity of cortical tissue, notably the myriad of synapses on branched dendrites, results in complex cortical source distributions and correspondingly complex extracellular potentials. Consider first a thought experiment in which we record and plot a detailed map of potentials at every point within a single cortical macrocolumn of 3 mm height and diameter, with a volume of 85 mm^3. To construct in detail the potentials next to small cell bodies, we might first imagine the microscopic scale and define the ambiguous term "point" as, for example, a cubical voxel (volume element) 0.001 mm on each side. Fully mapping a macrocolumn at this scale would require something like 100 billion microelectrode placements. Figure 3.7 depicts an experiment using a spherical electrode of radius ξ with center located at the tip of the arrow **r**. The volume of the electrode tip is $B = 4\pi\xi^3/3$. The recorded potential is approximately related to our fanciful point potential Φ_p by the following integral over the volume B

$$\Phi(\mathbf{r},t;\xi) \approx \frac{1}{B}\iiint_B \Phi_p(\mathbf{r},\mathbf{r}',t)dB(\mathbf{r}')$$

(3.6)

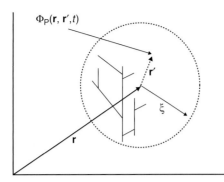

Figure 3.7 $\Phi_P(\mathbf{r},\mathbf{r}',t)$ is the theoretical tissue potential at a point located at $\mathbf{r}+\mathbf{r}'$. Actual measured potentials $\Phi(\mathbf{r},t;\xi)$ that are centered on site $\mathbf{r}$ (tip of $\mathbf{r}$ arrow) depend critically on electrode volume (dashed circle). For a spherical electrode of radius ξ, the volume is $B = 4\pi\xi^3/3$. Given the fractal-like structure of cortical tissue, the dynamic behavior of potentials recorded at different scales may be quite different.

The approximate sign is used in equation 3.6 because, in practice, the electrode will distort the original current distribution and potential. Given the fractal-like nature of cortical anatomy and the fact that intracranial electrophysiology spans three or four orders of magnitude of spatial scale, we expect the dynamic behavior of potentials recorded inside the cranium to be scale sensitive. The magnitude, spatial dependence, and time dependence of intracranial potentials generally depend on the electrode scale (radius = ξ). Potentials recorded at larger scales tend to have smaller magnitudes because larger electrodes tend to pick up more of a mixture of positive and negative source contributions that cancel (as reviewed in Abeles 1982; Nunez 1995). Furthermore, there is no guarantee that the dominant frequencies observed at one scale will closely match frequency spectra recorded at another scale. For example, in brain states with dominant alpha activity, most of the beta and gamma activity recorded with ECoG is typically missing in the simultaneous scalp-recorded EEG, apparently because higher-frequency cortical source regions are much less synchronous and/or smaller than the alpha source regions (Pfurtscheller and Cooper 1975; Nunez 1981, 1995). Potentials that are generated in cortex and recorded from the scalp represent neural activity that has been severely space-averaged due to volume conduction through the intervening tissue. This results in data at scales greater than several centimeters and thus insensitive to electrode size. Equation 3.6 is an example of *experimental coarse-graining* (spatial averaging) of a dynamic variable. Theories of neocortical dynamics often incorporate *theoretical coarse-graining*, to reflect the fact that genuinely useful theory in electrophysiology must be explicitly linked with the appropriate measurement scale. Otherwise, the theory may be little more than mathematical exercise.

MONOPOLE CURRENT SOURCES

Any current source region may be modeled as a sum of distributed point sources (i.e., where current comes from) and sinks (i.e., where current goes to). The potential at distance r from a single point source $I(t)$ in a medium of conductivity σ is given by

$$\Phi(r,t) \cong \frac{I(t)}{4\pi\sigma r} \tag{3.7}$$

Equation 3.7 follows from a simple argument. Surround the point source with an imaginary spherical surface of radius r. Since total current is conserved, the radial current density J_r at this surface equals current divided by surface area, with all current moving in the radial direction. Application of Ohm's law (eq. 3.2) to this current density yields equation 3.7. Let the current source be 4π microamperes (μA), and let cortical resistivity ($\eta = 1/\sigma$) be 3000 ohm mm. The potential in the cortex on a spherical surface of 1.0 mm radius (surrounding the point source) is then approximately 3000 μV, assuming all other sources and sinks are located much farther away (but see caveat 2 in the next paragraph).

Equation 3.7 incorporates several idealizations and thus requires the following caveats: (1) The symbol $\Phi(r,t)$ indicates nominal potential with respect to infinity, approximated with a "distant" (compared to the source region) reference electrode; (2) since all current sources must be balanced by current sinks, equation 3.7 cannot normally be applied in isolation; (3) the distinction in equation 3.6 between a point potential and the potential recorded with an electrode of radius ξ applies; and (4) the medium is assumed to be infinite with constant scalar conductivity σ, that is, no boundary effects due to other tissues are included.

DIPOLE CURRENT SOURCES

The idealized *current dipole* consists of a point source $+I$ and a point sink $-I$, separated by a distance d, as shown on the left side of figure 3.8. However, the word *dipole* has an additional and more general meaning that makes the dipole concept applicable to a wide range of source-sink configurations: nearly any source-sink region where the total source and sink currents are equal (local current conservation) will generate a predominantly dipole potential at distances large compared to the dimensions of the source-sink region. Thus, the collection of equal point sources and sinks shown on the right side of figure 3.8 produces an approximate dipole potential at distances r when r is large compared to d (e.g., $r=3d$ or $4d$ or more, depending on the desired accuracy of the dipole approximation). For this reason, cortical dipoles, and especially dipole layers (sheets), provide the dominant source models for potentials recorded on the scalp. The potential due to either of the source distributions in figure 3.8 may be approximated by

$$\Phi(r,t) \cong \frac{I(t)\overline{d}\cos\theta}{4\pi\sigma r^2} \qquad r \gg d \tag{3.8}$$

Here θ is the angle between the dipole axis and the vector r to the point of measurement. The effective pole separations are $\overline{d}=d$ for the source-sink (fig. 3.8, left) and $\overline{d}<d$ for the distributed sources (fig. 3.8, right). The angular dependence in equation 3.8 is strictly correct only if all sources lie on the vertical axis. However, equation 3.8 provides a reasonable

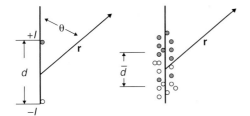

Figure 3.8 *The current dipole (left side of the figure) consists of a point source +I and point sink (negative source, −I) separated by distance d. A mixture of equal numbers of point sources and sinks of equal strength (right side of figure) also produces an approximate dipole potential at moderately large distances (say r > 4d depending on the accuracy of the dipole approximation) but with smaller effective pole separation d̄ < d yielding smaller potentials at the same distance. As sources and sinks become fully mixed, d̄ → 0, which indicates a so-called "closed field" of essentially zero potential external to the source region.*

approximation if the sources approximate a fairly narrow cylindrical region as shown on the right side of figure 3.8. As the average separation between point sources and sinks is reduced, the effective pole separation and external potential also become smaller. The so-called *closed field* of electrophysiology corresponds to the limiting case $\bar{d} \to 0$, which occurs when positive and negative point sources are well mixed, having small average separations. The layered structure of mammalian cortex is critical to the production of scalp potentials: no recordable EEG would be expected if cortical neurons were randomly oriented or if excitatory and inhibitory synaptic action were highly mixed in cortical columns.

The potential due to the two monopoles (the dipole in fig. 3.8, left) or to the source-sink collection (fig. 3.8, right) may be generally expanded in (mathematical) multipole series that include the *dipole* and *quadrupole* terms, in addition to higher-order terms that are nonnegligible close to the source region. Note that use of the term *dipole* in the mathematical expression (expansion) differs from its use when describing the idealized dipole on the left side of figure 3.8. (This is a common source of confusion in electrophysiology.) The monopole term in such expansions is zero, provided that local current is conserved (i.e., when all local point sources are matched by point sinks of equal strength); the dipole potential then becomes dominant.

ACTION POTENTIAL SOURCES

In controlled experiments using isolated axons, classical axon-surface recordings with respect to a distant electrode during the passage of an action potential yield *triphasic* waveforms traveling along the axon. Such *surface potentials* (measured with respect to a distant electrode) are generally in the 100-μV range. By contrast, the corresponding *transmembrane potential* (potential difference between inside and outside the cell) is a traveling monophasic waveform in the 100-mV range; that is, its magnitude is about 1000 times larger. When cell membranes behave as linear conductors (i.e., when Ohm's law is valid), axon current source distribution at membrane surfaces mimics transmembrane potential. However, active membranes or even membranes approaching threshold are inherently nonlinear, meaning Ohm's law is dramatically and selectively violated.

This nonlinearity is immediately evident from the monophasic nature of the transmembrane potential. That is, Ohm's law requires that membrane current source distribution along the axon match the direction (in or out) of transmembrane potential. The latter cannot be strictly monophasic along a linear membrane because membrane source current must have matching sinks somewhere along the axon.

In genuine tissue, the falloff of action potentials with distance from an axon is likely to be very complicated due to axon bending, axon myelination, influence of nearby cells, and other factors. Action potentials in nonmyelinated fibers fall off quite rapidly (perhaps within a few millimeters) with distance from the axon. By contrast, action potentials in large myelinated fibers tend to fall off slowly (over several centimeters) perpendicular to fiber axis (Nunez and Srinivasan 2006a). This raises the question of whether action potentials in *corticocortical fibers* (which form most of the white matter layer just below neocortex) might contribute to the EEG. The answer hinges partly on whether action potentials in enough white matter fibers physically line up and produce synchronous sources distributions that superimpose to produce measurable potentials at the scalp. If this did occur, we might expect very fast (>100 Hz) EEG components (reflecting the passage of the triphasic waveform) as in the example of the brainstem evoked potential. However, the standard view is that cortical synaptic sources are the dominant generators of scalp-recorded EEG. This view is based partly on compelling experimental evidence from animal studies that have used depth probes to map sources (Lopes da Silva and Storm van Leeuwen 1978). Additionally, as discussed in detail in Nunez and Srinivasan (2006a), the assumption that dipole layers of different sizes produced by cortical synapses are responsible for EEG leads to generally correct predictions of the ratios of ECoG to EEG amplitudes observed in different brain states.

LOCAL FIELD POTENTIALS

LFPs are microlevel phenomena recorded within cortex. They are recorded by microelectrodes placed sufficiently far from membrane surfaces to avoid domination by individual neurons, a purposeful reduction in spatial resolution somewhat analogous to the coarse-graining in equation 3.6. The potentials recorded are expected to measure synaptic sources within ~1 mm and action-potential sources within ~0.1 mm of the electrode tips (Leggett et al. 1980; Gray et al. 1995). These potentials are generally low-pass filtered (<350 Hz) (see chapter 7) to remove the fast activity coming from action potential sources. The result is the standard LFP, which can be modeled as a sum over many point sources using equation 3.7. LFPs are expected to be largest in regions where sources are mostly of the same sign, although any current source activity of frequency low enough to survive the low-pass filter can, in theory, contribute to the LFP.

ELECTROCORTICOGRAPHY

ECoG (discussed in more detail in chapter 15) is a mesoscale (intermediate scale) phenomenon that involves placement of electrodes just above the brain's surface on the arachnoid (the middle of the three meningeal membranes that surround the brain and spinal cord), and just below the dura mater (the outermost and thickest of the meninges). Because the electrodes do not penetrate into the brain, ECoG is less invasive than LFP recording and provides spatial resolution intermediate between LFPs and EEG. Before reaching the ECoG electrodes, cortical source currents pass through several layers: the cerebral cortex, the pia mater (the innermost and thinnest of the meninges), the cerebrospinal fluid (CSF), and the arachnoid. Of great importance is that these currents do not pass through the skull. The main differences between ECoG and LFPs include ECoG's larger electrodes, ECoG's larger average source-electrode separation, and the different choices of temporal filtering. ECoG spatial resolution appears to be roughly 2–10 mm, apparently limited partly by source distribution across the 3-mm cortical depth. ECoG is considered the gold standard for identifying cortical tissue prone to epileptic activity and is routinely employed to provide guidance prior to epilepsy surgery (Fisch 1999; Niedermeyer and Lopes da Silva 2005).

INTRASKULL RECORDINGS

Most of the degradation in spatial resolution from ECoG to EEG is due to the intervening skull. Thus, electrodes placed inside the skull but above the dura may provide a good intermediate-resolution option for long-term clinical applications such as BCIs. Such electrodes would be less invasive than ECoG electrodes and might achieve more stable long-term performance.

COMPARISON OF SPATIAL RESOLUTIONS

Table 3.3 lists the estimated (but very approximate) spatial resolution achieved with each of the several recording methods discussed here. The asterisks on high-resolution EEG and high-resolution MEG indicate that their spatial-filtering algorithms are not directly comparable to other methods (see

TABLE 3.3 Estimated spatial resolution of recorded potentials or magnetic fields generated by cortical sources

RECORDING METHOD	TYPICAL SPATIAL RESOLUTION (mm)
Microelectrode of radius ξ	≥ξ
LFP	0.1–1
ECoG	2–5
Intraskull recording	5–10
Untransformed EEG	50
Untransformed MEG	50
High-resolution EEG*	20–30
High-resolution MEG*	Unknown

*Not directly comparable to the other methods listed; see text.

High-Resolution EEG in this chapter). In general, spatial filtering may be applied to data recorded from any system with a sufficiently large number of well-placed sensors in a manner analogous to digital filtering in the time domain. Thus, development of high-resolution versions of MEG is plausible, although the issue of selective sensitivity to different source orientations remains.

BRAIN SOURCES AT MULTIPLE SCALES

EEG GENERATED IN CORTICAL GYRI

Nearly all scalp potentials recorded without averaging originate in cortical *dipole layers* (*sheets*) that occupy at least 10–40 cm² or more of cortical surface (Nunez and Srinivasan 2006a). Furthermore, all other things being equal, the crowns of cortical gyri (see chapter 2) are expected to provide larger contributions than sources in cortical folds. Isolated cortical dipoles, often adopted as models for somatosensory evoked potentials and epileptic spikes, are simply special cases of dipole layers with very small dimensions. Two major reasons for the dominance of synchronous cortical sources are evident. First, potentials generated locally fall off with distance from their source regions, and cortical sources are closest to the scalp. Second, and even more importantly, cortical pyramidal cell morphology allows dipole sources to line up in parallel, potentially creating large dipole layers. Because the dipole vectors in such layers are perpendicular to the cortical surface, gyral crowns are generally more efficient generators of EEG than fissures and sulci in which the dipole layers in opposing cortices tend to cancel each other. When near-parallel sources in contiguous gyral crowns are synchronously active, they add by linear superposition to create relatively large scalp potentials, an effect acknowledged when EEG amplitude reduction is labeled *desynchronization* (chapter 13) (Kellaway 1979; Pfurtscheller and Lopes da Silva 1999).

MULTIPLE SCALES OF CORTICAL SOURCES

The multiple scales of cortical morphology, current sources, and recording electrodes are summarized in tables 3.1 and 3.2, and in figure 3.9. As indicated in figure 3.9, the macrocolumn (mesoscale) in neocortex is defined by the spatial extent of axon branches (seen in the bracketed region E in fig. 3.9) that remain within the cortex (called *recurrent collaterals*). The large pyramidal cell (C) is one of 10^5 to 10^6 neurons in the macrocolumn. Nearly all pyramidal cells send an axon (G) into the white matter, and most of these reenter the cortex at some distant location (*corticocortical fibers*). Each large pyramidal cell has 10^4 to 10^5 synaptic inputs (F and inset) causing microcurrent sources and sinks. A convenient source variable is $s(\mathbf{r},t)$, the total current per unit volume ΔH that crosses a spherical surface centered at location $\mathbf{r}$:

$$s(\mathbf{r},t) = \frac{I(\mathbf{r},t)}{\Delta H}$$

(3.9)

Here the volume ΔH is assumed to be smaller than the measurement volume in equation 3.6. Field measurements can be expected to fluctuate greatly when small electrode contacts (A) are moved over distances of the order of cell body diameters. Small-scale recordings measure space-averaged potential over some volume (B) and depend mostly on the size of the electrode contact. An instantaneous imbalance in sources or sinks in bracketed regions (D) and (E) will cause a diffuse current density **J** and potential difference $\Delta\Phi$ across the cortex.

The conductivity σ (or resistivity η) and other electrical properties of bulk tissue must always refer to space averages over volumes of a certain size. Such parameters have different meanings depending on the measurement scale. A pyramidal cell is a large structure compared to a microelectrode tip. As pictured in figure 3.9, field measurements can be expected to fluctuate greatly when small electrodes (i.e., B, or the individual contacts on A) are moved over distances of the order of cell body diameters. At microelectrode scales, the fundamental electrophysiological parameters are defined separately for intercellular and extracellular fluid and membrane.

Macroelectrode recordings, like those with EEG, present quite a different picture. The scalp electrode measures fields due to neural activity in tissue masses containing perhaps 10^8 neurons. In this case, conductivity must refer to average properties in a large volume of tissue. The conductivity (or resistivity) of tissue can be expected to depend strongly on the packing density of the cells because membranes provide relatively high-resistance current pathways.

At the cell membrane the *microsource function* $s(\mathbf{r}, t)$ includes both active sources at the synapses and passive (return) current from more distant locations on the cell. Thus, microcurrent source-sink separations depend on capacitive-resistive membrane properties of cells within the volume in addition to synaptic action density. As a result a simple model predicts a low-pass filtering effect on scalp (and to a lesser degree ECoG) potentials below perhaps 50–100 Hz due to reduction in average source-sink separations (Nunez and Srinivasan 2006a). Action potentials can contribute to recorded potentials from inside the cranium, but their contribution to (unaveraged) scalp potentials is believed to be small.

MESOSCOPIC SOURCE STRENGTH AS DIPOLE MOMENT PER UNIT VOLUME

Each mesoscale (mm³) volume of human neocortex contains, on average, about 10^5 neurons and 10^9 or so synapses. Each active synapse produces local membrane current, as well as return current from more distant membrane surfaces, as required by current conservation. *Excitatory synapses* produce negative source regions (*sinks*) at local membrane surfaces and distributed positive sources at more distant membrane locations. *Inhibitory synapses* produce current in the opposite direction (i.e., *sources* at local membrane surfaces and *sinks* at more distant locations). Thus, the distribution of passive sources and sinks over each cell depends on both the synapse polarity and the capacitive-resistive properties of the cell and surrounding space.

The *current dipole moment per unit volume* $\mathbf{P}(\mathbf{r}, t)$ of a tissue mass is defined as a weighted space average of all the

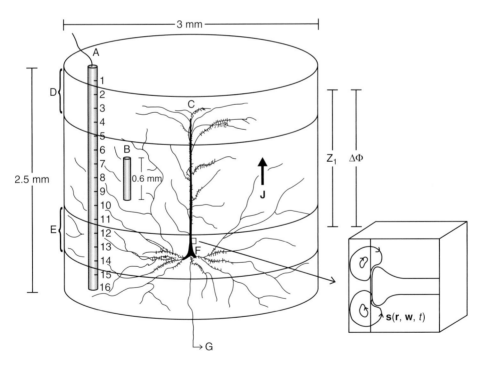

Figure 3.9 The macrocolumn is defined by the spatial extent of axon branches E that remain within the cortex (recurrent collaterals). The large pyramidal cell C is one of 10^5 to 10^6 neurons in the macrocolumn (the figure would be essentially solid black if only as many as 1% were shown). Nearly all pyramidal cells send an axon G into the white matter; most reenter the cortex at some distant location (corticocortical fibers). Each large pyramidal cell has 10^4 to 10^5 synaptic inputs F (and inset) causing microcurrent sources and sinks s(r, w, t), where the vector r locates the tissue volume W (e.g., a macrocolumn, as in fig. 3.10) and the vector w locates microsources within this volume of tissue W. An instantaneous imbalance in sources or sinks in regions D and E (see brackets at left of column) will cause a diffuse current J and potential difference $\Delta\Phi$ across the cortex (z is impedance). Field measurements can be expected to fluctuate greatly when small electrode contacts (at the numbered sites along A) are moved over distances of the order of cell body diameters. Recordings at a somewhat larger scale are represented by region B, which could represent a larger electrode contact. Adapted from Nunez (1995).

micro-sources s(**r**, *t*) within the volume (fig. 3.10). The vector **r** locates the center of the tissue volume or mass (voxel *W*) with respect to an arbitrary coordinate system. The voxel size is also partly arbitrary; that is, dipole moments may be defined at different scales. The vector **w** locates the microsources inside the volume *W*; thus, the notation s(**r**, *t*) is replaced by s(**r**, **w**, *t*) when appropriate. In figure 3.10 the filled circles represent positive sources, and the open circles represent negative sources. With positive sources mostly in the upper part of the tissue mass *W*, **P**(**r**, *t*) is positive. We refer to **P**(**r**, *t*) as a *mesoscopic source function* or *dipole moment per unit volume*. It is defined by the following integral over the tissue volume element *W*:

$$\mathbf{P}(\mathbf{r},t) = \frac{1}{W} \iiint_W \mathbf{w}s(\mathbf{r},\mathbf{w},t)dW(\mathbf{w})$$

(3.10)

Equation 3.10 is useful in EEG when the volume *W* is chosen to roughly match coordinated source activity; *W* may be anything between perhaps the minicolumn to macrocolumn scales (table 3.2). Neocortex may then be treated as a continuum in EEG applications, so that **P**(**r**, *t*) is a continuous *field variable*. There are, however, two limitations to this approach. First, the tissue volume should be large enough to contain many microsources s(**r**, **w**, *t*) due to local synaptic activity as well as their passive return currents; at the same time, its characteristic size should be much smaller than the closest distance to the recording electrode. The former condition suggests that the total strength of microsources will be approximately balanced by an equal strength of microsinks such that the monopole contribution of the tissue volume *W* is approximately zero, that is

$$I_W(\mathbf{r},t) = \iiint_W s(\mathbf{r},\mathbf{w},t)dW(\mathbf{w}) \cong 0$$

(3.11)

This condition is represented symbolically in figure 3.10 with an equal number of open and filled circles. While the volume *W* is partly arbitrary, condition equation 3.11 is more

likely to be satisfied if *W* is a full cortical column of some diameter containing both the soma and dendrites of cortical neurons. The second condition, that the scale of *W* be sufficiently small compared to the recording distance, ensures that the contributions to scalp potential of quadrupole and higher-order terms are negligible. If both conditions on *W* are satisfied, the dipole term is dominant in the general multipole expansion expressing scalp potential.

The volume microsources s(**r**, **w**, *t*) are expressed in microamperes per cubic millimeter ($\mu A/mm^3$), and *mesoscopic source strength* **P**(**r**, *t*) in microamperes per square millimeter ($\mu A/mm^2$), respectively. Thus, **P**(**r**, *t*) has units of current density and has a simple interpretation for the idealized source distribution depicted in figure 3.11 in which inhibitory synaptic activity (which produces current sources) in the lower part of a cortical column is balanced by excitatory synaptic action (which produces current sinks) in the upper part of the column (and with no intermediate sources). In this highly idealized picture, the dipole moment per unit volume **P**(**r**, *t*) is essentially the (negative) diffuse macroscopic current density **J**(**r**, *t*) across the cortex. The two variables **P**(**r**, *t*) and **J**(**r**, *t*) have opposite signs because they essentially represent currents external and internal to the column, respectively. Only a small part of the external current (thin gray arrows outside the column) reaches the scalp to produce EEG.

SCALP-RECORDED POTENTIALS

ALL SCALP RECORDINGS ARE BIPOLAR

Any voltage measurement requires both a *recording electrode* and a *reference electrode*. EEG practitioners have long been perplexed in attempting to find a proper reference electrode for EEG recordings. For ECoG measurements, the reference

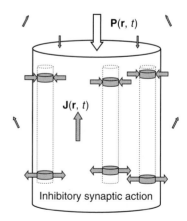

Figure 3.11 *Idealized case providing an intuitive interpretation of dipole moment per unit volume* P(r,t). *In this example, all sources and sinks produced by synaptic action are located in a deep layer (inhibitory-produced sources) and a superficial layer (excitatory-produced sinks) of a cortical column. As a result, the mesosource is* P(r,t)≈−J(r,t), *the diffuse current density (microamperes per square millimeter) between the layers of sources and sinks. The sign change occurs because current from the lower layer exits the column, spreads through distant tissue (including a little to the scalp to yield EEG), and returns through the top of the column to the cortical sinks in the upper layer. The three dashed cylindrical regions represent neural subpopulations within the larger tissue mass.*

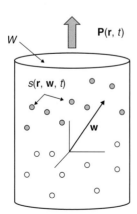

Figure 3.10 *A volume* W *of tissue (e.g., a cortical macrocolumn). The mixture of microsources or sinks s(r,w,t) results in a mesosource (i.e., a dipole moment per unit volume)* P(r,t) *in volume* W. *This mesosource representation is useful for calculating scalp potentials only if* W *is sufficiently large that local current conservation holds, as given by equation 3.11.*

electrode is located outside the skull and may usually be considered effectively "quiet," because the voltages outside the skull are categorically much smaller than inside. In contrast, scalp potentials cannot generally be recorded with respect to some theoretical place called "infinity." This presents a significant challenge for EEG recording.

Suppose $V(\mathbf{r},t)$ is an unknown scalp potential. Each EEG channel records an experimental scalp potential that depends on a *pair* of scalp electrode locations $(\mathbf{r}_n,\mathbf{r}_R)$

$$V(\mathbf{r}_n,\mathbf{r}_R,t) = V(\mathbf{r}_n,t) - V(\mathbf{r}_R,t) \qquad (3.12)$$

Or in shortened notation

$$V_{nR} = V_n - V_R \qquad (3.13)$$

In standard EEG parlance, *reference recordings* involve choosing some fixed location $\mathbf{r}_R$, typically an ear, mastoid, or neck site, and recording all potentials with respect to this fixed site. Unfortunately, $\mathbf{r}_R$ rarely qualifies as a genuinely indifferent reference. Whereas so-called *bipolar recordings* measure the potential difference between two nearby electrodes both of which are presumed to be changing in potential, these recordings are not fundamentally different from referenced recordings, except that bipolar recordings acknowledge the presence and influence of the reference electrode explicitly.

Recording all potentials with respect to some fixed location $\mathbf{r}_R$ is advantageous in that it allows for rereferencing to any other site B. That is, suppose potentials are recorded with respect to site R with a system of N channels and $N + 1$ scalp electrodes. Suppose we wish to find the potentials that would have been recorded had the reference been located at site B. This is accomplished with the following (identity) transformation

$$V_n - V_B \equiv (V_n - V_R) - (V_B - V_R) \qquad (3.14)$$

The first parentheses in equation 3.14 represent the original reference recording; the second parentheses are a single potential difference obtained from the same data set. The left side of equation 3.14 then yields the new reference recording. If the potentials V_B and V_R are free of all artifact (i.e., nonbrain activity such as heart, muscle, or other biological or nonbiological potentials), V_B and V_R are equal to the theoretical nominal potentials with respect to infinity and are given the symbols Φ_B and Φ_R. Equation 3.14 is just one of several EEG data transformations discussed later in this chapter (as well as in chapters 6 and 7).

THE REFERENCE ELECTRODE

The essential feature of a true reference is that it is located far from any sources. Unfortunately, however, the word *far* is often misinterpreted. A true reference (i.e., *at infinity*) must be *electrically far*. This concept and the methods available for realizing it as closely as possible are discussed in detail in chapter 6. As emphasized and illustrated there, the choice of a reference electrode is absolutely crucial to correct interpretation of the EEG signals recorded. Indeed, different reference choices can produce dramatically different, and often misleading, results. Thus, it is essential to choose a reference that is appropriate for the specific recording situation. Chapter 6 describes the different options and discusses the factors important in selecting among them.

THE FORWARD AND INVERSE PROBLEMS IN EEG

THE FORWARD PROBLEM

In EEG theory, the so-called *forward problem* consists of calculating scalp potentials from a known *mesosource function* $\mathbf{P}(\mathbf{r}', t)$, defined in equation 3.10 as the dipole moment per unit volume generated in each mesoscopic tissue voxel located at $\mathbf{r}'$. The nominal macroscopic potential with respect to infinity at any scalp location $\mathbf{r}$ is then given by the following integral over the volume K

$$\Phi(\mathbf{r},t) = \iiint_K \mathbf{G}_K(\mathbf{r},\mathbf{r}') \bullet \mathbf{P}(\mathbf{r}',t) dK(\mathbf{r}')$$
$$(3.15)$$

Here K is the total volume of tissue with active brain sources, generally the entire brain excluding ventricles. All geometric and conductive properties of the head volume conductor are included in the Green's function $\mathbf{G}_K(\mathbf{r},\mathbf{r}')$, which can be viewed as the inverse *electrical distance* (squared) between a source at $\mathbf{r}'$ and a location $\mathbf{r}$ where the potential is obtained. In an infinite, homogeneous, and isotropic volume conductor, the electrical distance equals the actual distance, but this idealization is a poor approximation for genuine heads because of current-path distortions.

Although equation 3.15 may seem complicated, it provides very useful information about the general relationship of potentials to brain sources. Much of this general insight is relatively independent of head-model inaccuracy. Let $\mathbf{P}(\mathbf{r}', t)$ be defined such that the volume W in equation 3.10 is a voxel of 1 mm³. The sources in a 1000-cm³ brain may then be represented by 3 million discrete mesosources $P_k(t)$, taking the three components of the vector $\mathbf{P}(\mathbf{r}', t)$ into account. The potential at any location is simply the weighted linear sum over all sources, so equation 3.15 may then be expressed as a sum of 3 million terms:

$$\Phi_n(t) \cong \sum_{k=1}^{3M} g_{nk} P_k(t)$$
$$(3.16)$$

The fact that EEG may exhibit quite different frequency content at different locations or at different scales is simply the result of the selective weighting g_{nk} of the scalar mesosource components, $P_k(t)$, of each voxel.

For several reasons, scalp (EEG) or cortical-surface (ECoG) potentials are believed to be generated almost exclusively by cortical sources. First, sources close to cortical surfaces are associated with larger Green's functions [i.e., $\mathbf{G}_K(\mathbf{r},\mathbf{r}')$ or g_{nk}]. Second, the large source-sink separations in cortical tissue created by large pyramidal cells yield large mesosources $P_k(t)$, as indicated in equation 3.10. Third, the parallel arrangement of pyramidal cells allows the vectors $\mathbf{P}(\mathbf{r}', t)$ to line up in the smooth parts of cortex (i.e., the gyral crowns). In contrast, in cortical folds (which are also deeper), these vectors may tend to cancel. As a result, for EEG and ECoG, sources in gyral crowns generally generate larger surface potentials than sources in cortical folds.

By contrast, external magnetic fields (detected by MEG) are generated mostly by source vectors *parallel* to the local scalp (and parallel to the plane of the MEG coil). To the extent that cortical folds are perpendicular to local scalp (and perpendicular to the MEG coil), the dipole vectors contributing to MEG tend to come mainly from the sources in the sides of cortical folds if they are not cancelled by sources in the apposing sides. This feature tends to allow MEG data to be fit to localized source models even when the actual sources are widely distributed (an outcome that can be good or bad, depending on the application and on how the data are interpreted).

From these arguments we conclude that cortical anatomy itself is the main determinant of the factors responsible for the relatively large scalp potentials generated by cortical sources. Nevertheless, EEG amplitudes can vary from a few microvolts to more than several hundred microvolts across various brain states. Large scalp potentials require that the mesosources $\mathbf{P}(\mathbf{r}', t)$ be synchronous (i.e., in phase) over large cortical areas. The general rule of the head is that source regions must be synchronous over about 6 cm² or more of cortex in order to be recordable on the scalp without averaging (Cooper et al. 1965; Ebersole 1997; Nunez and Srinivasan 2006a). (The label *synchronously active* in this context is based on cortical surface recordings and should be viewed mainly as a qualitative description.) In the case of dipole layers extending into fissures and sulci, tissue areas larger than 6 cm² are apparently required to produce measurable scalp potentials. The idea that scalp potential magnitudes depend largely on source synchrony is widely recognized in clinical and research EEG environments where amplitude reduction is often characterized as *desynchronization* (Kellaway 1979; Pfurtscheller and Lopes da Silva 1999). EEGs with typical amplitudes in the range 20–100 µV apparently require synchrony over at least several tens of square centimeters of smooth cortical surface. The largest scalp potentials may require synchrony over 50–100 cm² or more (Nunez and Srinivasan 2006a).

Since nearly all EEG signals are apparently generated by cortical sources, it is often convenient to replace equation 3.15 by equation 3.17, which is the integral over the cortical surface, with the mesosource volume elements W in equation 3.10 interpreted as cortical columns, and $\mathbf{P}(\mathbf{r}', t)$ interpreted as a vector everywhere parallel to pyramidal cell axes (i.e., normal to the local cortical surface). Scalp potentials are then expressed in terms of the modified Green's function $\mathbf{G}_S(\mathbf{r},\mathbf{r}')$ and the unit vector $\hat{\mathbf{a}}_s(\mathbf{r}')$, which is everywhere normal to the local cortical surface and may be estimated with MRI images. Scalp potential (eq. 3.15) is then expressed as

$$\Phi(\mathbf{r},t) = \iint_S \mathbf{G}_S(\mathbf{r},\mathbf{r}') \bullet \mathbf{P}(\mathbf{r}',t) dS(\mathbf{r}')$$

$$= \iint_S \mathbf{G}_S(\mathbf{r},\mathbf{r}') \bullet \hat{\mathbf{a}}_s(\mathbf{r}') P(\mathbf{r}',t) dS(\mathbf{r}')$$

(3.17)

(Note that equation 3.17 cannot be applied to ECoG because the electrodes are too close to cortical sources for the dipole approximation to be valid. ECoG depends much more on the details of synaptic source distribution across cortex; such cortical potentials may be estimated from distributed microsources using equation 3.6).

THE INVERSE PROBLEM

The classical *inverse problem* in EEG is concerned with finding the locations and strengths of the current sources on the right side of equations 3.15, 3.16, or 3.17 from discrete samples of the potential V_{nR} (with respect to some reference) on the surface of the volume conductor. That is, the recorded potentials V_{nR} are used to *estimate* the nominal potentials with respect to infinity $\Phi(\mathbf{r},t)$ (i.e., Φ_n in simplified notation). In practice, dipole searches employing sophisticated computer algorithms are based on recordings at perhaps 20–128 or more surface locations, either for fixed time slices (i.e., segments) or over time windows. By contrast to the forward problem, the inverse problem has no unique solution. If one dipole provides a reasonable fit to surface data, two or three or 10 dipoles can provide even better fits. Scalp potentials can always be made to fit a wide range of distributed cortical sources. Within experimental error, any scalp-potential map can be made to fit source distributions that are exclusively cortical, or even made to fit sources that are exclusive to cortical gyri. In the absence of additional information, the constraints (e.g., physiological assumptions) required to obtain these fits cannot generally be expected to be accurate, and the inverse solutions (computed source locations) are generally no better than the physiological assumptions and head-model accuracy. As discussed in Nunez and Srinivasan (2006a), many inverse solutions indicating that EEG generators consist of a few isolated dipoles are inconsistent with known physiology and anatomy. One warning sign of an inadequate solution is failure to show that the estimated source-strength is sufficient to account for scalp-potential magnitudes. Sophisticated computer algorithms are useful only if they are based on sound physiology; sophisticated mathematics can never compensate for unrealistic physical assumptions.

QUANTITATIVE AND HIGH-RESOLUTION EEG

MATHEMATICAL TRANSFORMATIONS OF EEG

Rereferencing of unprocessed EEG data provides the simplest example of the many transformations that may be applied in *quantitative EEG analysis*. Some data transformations have clear physical and physiological motivations; others are purely mathematical. Fourier transforms (see section on *Fourier Transforms* in this chapter) are clearly useful across many applications, mainly because specific EEG frequency bands are closely associated with specific brain states. Other transformations have more limited appeal; in extreme cases they may be no more than mathematics in search of applications. How can we distinguish truly beneficial transformation methods from useless mathematical exercises? One obvious but underused approach is to apply each promising transformation method to several physiologically based dynamic and volume-conduction models. If the method produces transformed variables that reveal important dynamic properties of the *known* sources modeled in these simulations, it may be useful with genuine EEG data; if not, the method is probably not worth using. Note that even simple analytic head models like the *n*-sphere models are quite valuable in such tests even though such head models may not be very accurate. That is, simple head models provide a critical "filter" through which any proposed method should first pass before being tested further. Had this philosophy been applied in EEG over the past 40 years or so (after computers became readily available), the graveyard of erroneous EEG reports would contain far fewer occupants. Examples of appropriate and inappropriate transformations are discussed in (Nunez and Srinivasan 2006a).

The relationships between observed potential differences $V_{nR} = V(\mathbf{r}_i, \mathbf{r}_j, t)$ and brain sources $\mathbf{P}(\mathbf{r}, t)$ depend on the anatomy and physiology of brain tissue and the physics of volume conduction through the human head. *Quantitative EEG analysis* consists of mathematical transformations of recorded potentials to new dependent variables X and independent variables $x_1, x_2, x_3, \ldots$, that is,

$$V(\mathbf{r}_i, \mathbf{r}_j, t) \rightarrow X(x_1, x_2, x_3, \ldots) \qquad (3.18)$$

The transformations in equation 3.18 can provide important estimates of the behavior of source dynamics $\mathbf{P}(\mathbf{r}, t)$ that supplement the estimates provided by the unprocessed data $V(\mathbf{r}_i, \mathbf{r}_j, t)$. In the simple case of transformed electrode references, the new dependent variable X retains identity as an electric potential. With *surface Laplacian* transforms (i.e., in *high-resolution EEG*), X is proportional to the estimated local skull current and brain surface potential. Other transforms include Hilbert transforms, wavelets, principal or independent components analysis, constrained inverse solutions (source localization), correlation dimension estimates, and several measures of phase locking between scalp sites, especially coherence. Coherence estimates are normally based on Fourier transforms (i.e., spectral analysis). These methods are discussed in chapter 7.

FOURIER TRANSFORMS

Historically, and especially before spectral analysis came into more common use in the 1970s, EEG frequency content was often described by simply counting waveform zero crossings. For pure sinusoidal signals, this approach accurately indicates signal frequency; a 10-Hz sine wave has 20 zero crossings per second. However, when the signal contains a mix of frequencies, the number of zero crossings can yield a misleading picture. For example, a mixture of moderate beta (18–30 Hz) and larger alpha (8–12 Hz) oscillations might be classified simply as beta based on visual inspection of zero crossings (Nunez and Srinivasan 2006a).

Fourier (or spectral) analysis expresses any arbitrary time series as a sum of sine waves with different frequencies and phases. The most widely understood and generally practical algorithm is the *fast Fourier transform* (FFT). Each waveform

is expressed in terms of the amplitude or *power* (i.e., amplitude squared) and the *phase* of each frequency component. The phase information is required to estimate coherence between EEG channel pairs for each frequency component. Practical FFT analysis methods are detailed in several texts (Bendat and Piersol 2001; Nunez and Srinivasan 2006a) and are reviewed in chapter 7. The FFT is a starting point for the application of various statistical tools including coherence.

Other approaches to spectral analysis include wavelets (Lachaux et al. 2002), autoregressive models (Ding et al. 2000), and Hilbert transforms (Bendat and Piersol 2001; Le Van Quyen et al. 2001). These methods are sometimes more useful than the FFT with short data epochs. Any of them can be applied to EEG, but interpretation of the transformed variables provided by methods other than FFT may depend on assumptions and parameter choices. These limitations are substantial in some applications and are generally not as widely appreciated as are the minimal limitations of the FFT. Thus, it is often prudent to apply different spectral analysis methods to the same data sets and then compare the results. The validity of each mathematical tool can be assessed by comparing different methods applied to identical data (both genuine and simulated).

EEG PHASE SYNCHRONIZATION AND COHERENCE

In standard EEG terminology, *synchrony* is a qualitative term normally indicating mesosources $\mathbf{P}(\mathbf{r}, t)$ that are approximately *phase-locked* (i.e., synchronized with respect to time), with small or zero phase offsets. In this case, sources tend to add by linear superposition to produce large scalp potentials. Thus, the label *desynchronization* is typically used to indicate the reduction of EEG amplitude, as, for example, in the case of alpha-blocking during eye opening or during execution of certain cognitive tasks.

The term *coherence* refers to the standard mathematical definition, and it is equal to the normalized cross-spectral density function, typically estimated with FFTs. *Coherence* is a measure of phase-locking, specifically the *phase consistency between channel pairs*. Sources that remain synchronous (i.e., have zero or small phase lags) over some period produce large coherence values over the same period. However, depending on their phase offsets, coherent sources may or may not be synchronous: two oscillations that remain approximately 180° out of phase are fully asynchronous but exhibit high coherence. Coherence is a squared correlation coefficient and is expressed as a function of frequency band. For example, when some study subjects perform mental calculations (with eyes closed), many electrode pairs exhibit increased EEG coherence (compared to resting) in the theta and upper alpha (~10 Hz) bands and decreased coherence in the lower alpha band (~8 Hz) (Nunez et al. 2001; Nunez and Srinivasan 2006a).

TRANSIENT AND STEADY-STATE EVOKED POTENTIALS

Averaged *evoked potentials* (EPs) are generated by sensory stimuli such as light flashes, auditory tones, finger pressure, or mild electric shocks. EPs are typically recorded by time-averaging single-stimulus waveforms as an attempt to remove any noise or other sources that are not time-locked to the stimuli. *Event-related potentials* (ERPs) (see chapter 12) are recorded in the same way as EPs, but they normally occur at longer latencies from the stimuli and are more related to *endogenous brain state*. With transient EPs or ERPs, the stimuli consist of repeated short pulses, and the number required to produce an averaged evoked potential may be anywhere from about 10 (for visual EPs) to several thousand (for auditory brainstem EPs). The scalp response to each pulse is averaged over the individual pulses. The EP or ERP in any experiment is a waveform containing a series of characteristic components, or potential peaks (local maxima or minima), typically occurring in the first 0.5 sec after stimulus presentation. A component's amplitude, latency from the stimulus, or covariance (at multiple electrode sites) may be studied, in connection with a cognitive task (e.g., usually for ERPs) or with no task (e.g., usually for EPs) (Gevins et al. 1983 Gevins and Cutillo 1995).

Steady-state visually evoked potentials (SSVEPs) (see chapter 14) use a continuous, sinusoidally modulated stimulus, typically a flickering light produced by special goggles and superimposed on images from a computer monitor that provide a cognitive task. The brain response in a narrow frequency band (often less than 0.1 Hz) around the stimulus frequency is measured. Magnitude, phase, and coherence (in the case of multiple electrode sites) may be related to different parts of the task. SSVEPs have two main advantages over transient ERPs: the large increase in signal-to-noise ratio within the narrow bands studied; and the observation that cognition typically affects select frequency bands. Thus, SSVEP largely avoids the ERP artifact problems that often confound cognitive experiments.

SSVEP coherence reveals that mental tasks consistently involve increased 13-Hz coherence between selected electrodes and decreased coherence between other electrodes (Silberstein et al. 2004). Binocular rivalry experiments using steady-state magnetic-field recordings show that conscious perception of a stimulus flicker is reliably associated with increased cross-hemispheric coherence at 7 Hz (Srinivasan et al. 1999). These data are consistent with the formation of large-scale cell assemblies (e.g., cortical dipole layers) at select frequencies with center-to-center scalp separations of roughly 5–20 cm.

HIGH-RESOLUTION EEG

The process of relating recorded scalp potentials $V(\mathbf{r}_n, \mathbf{r}_R, t)$ to the underlying brain mesosource function $\mathbf{P}(\mathbf{r}, t)$ has long been hampered by reference-electrode distortions and by inhomogeneous current spreading through the head volume conductor. The average reference method (AVE) (chapter 6) provides an approximate solution to the problem of reference-electrode distortions but altogether fails to address the problem of inhomogeneous current spreading. These issues, plus the severe limitations on realistic inverse solutions, provide strong motivation to add *high-resolution EEG* estimates to the standard toolbox. Two distinct approaches are *dura imaging*, in which a head model is employed to find an estimated dural potential map; and the *Laplacian* (Nunez and Srinivasan

2006a), which requires no head model but is approximately proportional to the dural potential when the cortical regions of synchronous sources are not too large (e.g., when they are less than about 40 cm^2 of smooth cortex). The spline Laplacian completely eliminates the reference problem and provides a partial solution to current spreading in the volume conductor. Skull conductivity is lower than that of contiguous tissue by factors of about 10–40; thus, most source current reaching the scalp passes normal to the skull. Based on this factor and Ohm's law, the surface Laplacian L_n at scalp site n is related to the local outer skull potential Φ_{Kn} and the inner skull (i.e., outer CSF) potential Φ_{Cn} by the approximate relation (Nunez and Srinivasan 2006a)

$$L_n \approx A_n \left(\Phi_{Kn} - \Phi_{Cn} \right) \tag{3.19}$$

Here the parameter A_n depends on local skull and scalp thicknesses and resistivities. The interpretation of L_n depends critically on the nature of the cortical sources. With very large dipole layers, the potential falloff through the skull is minimal, so that Φ_{Kn} and Φ_{Cn} have similar magnitudes and the surface Laplacian is very small. Thus, very large dipole layers occupying a substantial portion of the upper cortical surface (as may occur with the global spike and wave of epilepsy, and in the lower-frequency part of the resting alpha-rhythm band) make only small or negligible contributions to the Laplacian. By contrast, when cortical source regions consist of small to moderate-sized dipole layers, the potential falloff through the skull is substantial, such that $\Phi_{Kn} \ll \Phi_{Cn}$. Thus, for small to moderate-sized dipole layers, with diameters less than around 5–10 cm, the negative Laplacian is approximately proportional to the dural surface potential. The Laplacian then acts as a spatial filter that removes low-spatial-frequency scalp signals that are caused by volume conduction or genuine source dynamics. However, it cannot distinguish between these two.

Dura imaging and Laplacian algorithms remove (i.e., filter) genuine large-scale cortical patterns in addition to volume-conduction distortions. Raw scalp potentials and high-resolution EEG are selectively sensitive to source regions of different sizes. Thus, they are complementary measures of neocortical dynamics. High-resolution EEG supplements, but cannot replace, unprocessed potentials.

Over the past 20 years, the author's research groups have tested the Melbourne dura-imaging and the New Orleans spline-Laplacian algorithms in several thousand simulations and with many sets of genuine EEG data (Nunez 1995; Nunez et al. 2001; Nunez and Srinivasan 2006a). When applied to EEG recorded with high-density electrode arrays, these two completely independent algorithms provide nearly identical estimates of dural potential patterns. That is, electrode-by-electrode comparison of the two estimates yields correlation coefficients typically in the 0.85 and 0.95 ranges, with 64 and 131 electrodes, respectively. Note, however, that the actual magnitudes of dura-image and Laplacian variables cannot be directly compared because they have different units, microvolts and microvolts per square centimeter, respectively. In idealized simulations with *n*-sphere models and 131 surface samples, we evaluated algorithm performance by calculating site-by-site correlations between the estimated and actual dural surface potentials produced by a wide range of localized and distributed source patterns in several four-sphere head models. Both algorithms yield typical correlation coefficients ~0.95 in these simulations (Nunez et al. 2001; Nunez and Srinivasan 2006a).

Although dura-imaging and spline-Laplacian algorithms nicely supplement the unfiltered EEG, an additional cautionary note is appropriate. We have cited error estimates in terms of correlation coefficients rather than mean-square errors because correlation coefficients provide the more appropriate test when the high-resolution algorithm precedes normalized operations (e.g., coherence estimates, which are relatively insensitive to local signal magnitudes). Because genuine-tissue properties, such as skull area resistance, are expected to vary over the head surface, the parameter A_n in equation 3.19 must actually vary with location. Thus, the *magnitude* of the Laplacian estimate provides a much less reliable indicator of cortical source patterns than does its sign. Nevertheless, large local Laplacians are normally expected to provide a good indication of local source regions (Nunez and Srinivasan 2006a).

THE BRAIN'S MAGNETIC FIELD

In this chapter, we have emphasized electric (i.e., EEG and ECoG) rather than magnetic (i.e., MEG) recording because the former (particularly in the case of EEG) is inexpensive, far easier to employ than magnetic measures, and widely used for BCIs. A short description of magnetoencephalography (MEG) is included here to provide a somewhat broader perspective on general BCI-related issues.

MEG is an impressive technology for recording the brain's extremely small magnetic fields (Hamalainen et al. 1993). Available since the early 1980s, this technology has been promoted as preferable to EEG for both genuine scientific considerations and poorly justified commercial reasons. MEG is advantageous in that it is selectively sensitive: it is much more sensitive to sources $\mathbf{P}(\mathbf{r},t)$ oriented parallel to its sensor coils (which are placed approximately parallel to the local scalp). This implies that MEG tends to be more sensitive to tangential dipole sources $\mathbf{P}(\mathbf{r},t)$ on sulcal walls and less sensitive to sources along gyral surfaces (although the convoluted geometry of cortex provides exceptions in many regions). By contrast, both the unprocessed EEG and the Laplacian appear to be more sensitive to sources in cortical gyri. Thus, either in the context of source localization or for more general analyses of spatial-temporal patterns, the relative merits of MEG and EEG depend on the nature of the underlying mesosources $\mathbf{P}(\mathbf{r},t)$. However, such source information is almost never available in advance of decisions to choose between EEG and MEG systems.

MEG has certain important advantages and also some disadvantages when compared to EEG. An important advantage of MEG arises from the fact that the skull and other tissues are transparent to magnetic fields, which are therefore minimally distorted between sources and sensors and are apparently close to those produced by sources in a homogeneous sphere. For this reason, there appears to be much less uncertainty in models that relate current sources in the brain (where tissue conductivities and boundaries are known only approximately) to MEG, as compared to EEG. In practice, however, EEG has an important advantage in that scalp electrodes are more than twice as close to the appropriate cortical sources as MEG coils; with today's MEG systems, these coils must be placed 2–3 cm above the scalp. Thus, MEG's advantage of tissue transparency is offset by its disadvantage in sensor location. Its main strength is its selective sensitivity to tangential sources (but mostly those unapposed from the opposite side of a cortical fold) when such sources are of primary interest.

For certain applications, the identification of special source regions may be particularly important. When they are located in fissures or sulci, epileptic foci or primary sensory cortex sources may be difficult or impossible to isolate with EEG because they are masked by larger potentials originating from cortical gyri. One can easily imagine clinical or other applications in which MEG may locate or otherwise characterize such special sources, especially in candidates for epilepsy surgery. It is important to recognize, however, that MEG's advantage in this regard occurs because it is relatively insensitive to gyral sources, not because it is generally more accurate than EEG, which it is not (Malmivuo and Plonsey 1995; Nunez and Srinivasan 2006a).

On the practical side, MEG technology is expensive and cumbersome. It must be used in a magnetically shielded chamber and the coils must be supercooled with liquid helium. These practical disadvantages, in addition to the others discussed in this section, make it a method that can be supportive of, but not likely to be primary to, BCI development.

VOLUME CONDUCTION VERSUS SOURCE DYNAMICS

The physics of EEG is naturally separated into two mostly disparate subtopics: *volume conduction* and *brain dynamics* (or, more specifically, *neocortical dynamics*). *Volume conduction* is concerned with relationships between mesosources $\mathbf{P}(\mathbf{r},t)$ and the resulting scalp potentials; the appropriate expressions are equations 3.15, 3.16, and 3.17, which provide forward solutions. Although the fundamental laws that govern volume conduction (i.e., charge conservation and Ohm's law) are well known, their application to EEG is, in understated physics parlance, *nontrivial*. The time variable in these laws takes on the role of a parameter, and EEG time dependence is just the weighted volume average of all contributing brain sources. This is indicated most clearly in equation 3.16. The resulting simplification of both theory and practice in EEG is substantial: linear superposition of potentials due to multiple sources represents an extremely valuable dry island in the present sea of uncertainty about the details of volume conduction and the dynamic behavior of sources.

Brain dynamics is concerned with the origins of time-dependent behavior of brain current sources. It presents quite a different story. In the simple example of the dependent source in the electric circuit shown in figure 3.3, the functional relationship $I_s = f(V_x)$ originates from hidden interactions between circuit elements. We expect analogous (but far more complicated) phenomena to occur in brains. That is, multiple brain sources interact in cell assemblies (networks) to produce the complex, fractal-like dynamic behavior that is recorded with different methods (and provides neural correlates of consciousness) (Nunez 2010). Although a number of plausible physiologically based mathematical theories have been developed, we are far from any comprehensive theory of brain dynamics (Nunez and Srinivasan 2006b; Nunez 2011). Nevertheless, even very approximate, speculative, or incomplete dynamic theories can have substantial value in supporting general conceptual frameworks and in generating new experiments.

The relationship of the recorded potentials to the full dynamics of the neocortex may be illustrated with an ocean-wave metaphor. Spatial maps of any kind may be expressed as a sum over spatial frequencies in two dimensions in a manner similar to Fourier analysis in the one-dimensional time domain. For example, ocean-wave energy is distributed over more than four orders of magnitude of spatial and temporal frequencies. The longest ocean waves, the tsunamis and tides, have wavelengths of hundreds or thousands of miles. Wind-driven waves have intermediate lengths. Ripples due to surface tension have wavelengths of less than a foot. Similarly, electrophysiology spans about five orders of magnitude of spatial scale (and spatial frequencies) depending on the size and location of electrodes.

Because of poor spatial resolution, EEG is sensitive to only the very longest spatial wavelengths in the full spatial spectrum of cortical dynamics. (The analogous ocean-wave measurement would be surface displacement averaged over ocean patches a thousand or so miles in diameter; only the tides, not the wind-driven waves, would be observed in such experiments.) Intracranial recordings of brain potentials (LFP and ECoG) are sensitive to only a selected part of the cortical spatial spectrum. Electrode size and location determine which part of this spectrum is recorded; and the recording may exclude much of the long-wavelength dynamics. (By analogy, wave-height measurements taken from a ship or low-flying helicopter see mainly wave chop driven by local winds, missing tides and tsunamis entirely. Such small-scale ocean data would fail to match any conceptual framework based on tidal mechanisms.) Thus, dynamic behaviors observed with intracranial recordings may differ substantially from potentials recorded at the scalp.

The author has proposed one possible conceptual framework for the dynamic behavior of cortical mesosources (Nunez 1995, 2010). According to this framework, $\mathbf{P}(\mathbf{r},t)$ is generated by a combination of network (or, more accurately, cell assembly) and global synaptic field sources. The latter are simply the numbers of active excitatory and inhibitory synapses in each tissue volume. The networks may be pictured as *embedded* in global synaptic fields (including standing and traveling waves) analogous to the social networks embedded in a culture. This general idea is demonstrated by human alpha rhythms, which consist of long-wavelength (low spatial frequency) potentials plus more localized (apparent) network activity. The local cortical patches where this activity occurs were recently identified with modern Laplacian methods but were originally found years ago in classical EEG and ECoG studies by the pioneers Grey Walter, Herbert Jasper, and Wilder Penfield (see Nunez and Srinivasan 2006a for overview). Local cortical patches that could reflect the cortical parts of thalamocortical networks produce oscillatory alpha-band activity that may or may not match global alpha frequencies (Nunez 1974, 2000a, 2000b, 2010, 2011). The label *global* suggests dynamics dominated by long spatial wavelengths, implying large contributions to scalp-recorded potentials but much smaller contributions to the Laplacian. Substantial interaction between networks and global synaptic fields is hypothesized, with global fields playing a central role in functional integration of local and regional networks. This general conceptual framework addresses the so-called *binding problem* of brain science: that is, how the unity of conscious perception is brought about by separate and distributed networks perhaps operating in nested hierarchies (Nunez and Srinivasan 2006a, 2006b; Nunez 2010).

SUMMARY

The goal of this chapter has been to provide the reader with the basic information needed to be an effective user of electric- or magnetic-field recording methods in BCI research and development. To this end we have addressed the generation, distribution, and detection of these fields on micro-, meso-, and macroscales, thereby accounting for the multiscale structure of brain tissue. Current sources in the cortex generate potentials that may be recorded at all three scales. The small and intermediate scales represented by LFPs and ECoG activity provide more local details but only sparse spatial coverage. The large-scale EEG covers much of the entire upper-cortical surface, but it yields only very coarse spatial resolution. High-resolution EEG, implemented as either Laplacian and dura image algorithms, can supplement unprocessed EEG, providing somewhat better spatial resolution, but at the cost of eliminating the very large-scale dynamics that may be of interest. Thus, unprocessed and high-resolution EEG provide complementary measures of cortical dynamics. In all cases, the observed dynamic behaviors of recorded potentials or magnetic fields are produced by the weighted linear sums (i.e., linear superposition) of the underlying sources. Different brain regions and measurement scales may exhibit quite different dynamics (e.g., dominant frequencies), but such differences are due only to the different weights in the sums associated with different source locations and recording methods.

Effective use of these methods in BCI research and development also depends on understanding additional practical issues: What are the key features of the electrodes (or magnetic coils) that record these fields? How many are needed, where should they be placed, and how should they be referenced? How should the recorded data be analyzed to maximize the signal-to-noise ratio and to focus on the measures best suited for communication and control? These operational questions are based partly on the fundamentals of brain physics outlined in this chapter and are considered in detail in chapters 6 and 7.

REFERENCES

Abeles M, *Local Cortical Circuits*, New York: Springer-Verlag, 1982.

Akhtari M, Bryant HC, Mamelak AN, Flynn ER, Heller L, Shih JJ, Mandelkern M, Matlachov A, Ranken DM, Best ED, DiMauro MA, Lee RR, and Sutherling WW, Conductivities of three-layer live human skull, *Brain Topography* 14:151–167, 2002.

Bendat JS, and Piersol A, *Random Data: Analysis and Measurement Procedures, 3rd Ed.* New York: Wiley, 2001.

Bertrand O, Perrin F, and Pernier J, A theoretical justification of the average reference in topographic evoked potential studies. *Electroencephalography and Clinical Neurophysiology* 62:462–464, 1985.

Cooper R, Winter AL, Crow HJ, and Walter WG, Comparison of subcortical, cortical, and scalp activity using chronically indwelling electrodes in man, *Electroencephalography and Clinical Neurophysiology* 18:217–228, 1965.

Ding M, Bressler SL, Yang W, and Liang H, Short-window spectral analysis of cortical event-related potentials by adaptive multivariate autoregressive (AMVAR) modeling: data processing, model validation, and variability assessment. *Biological Cybernetics* 83:35–45, 2000.

Ebersole JS, Defining epileptogenic foci: past, present, future, *Journal of Clinical Neurophysiology* 14:470–483, 1997.

Fisch BJ, *Fisch & Spehlmann's EEG Primer*. Amsterdam: Elsevier, 1999.

Gevins AS, Schaffer RE, Doyle JC, Cutillo BA, Tannehill RL, and Bressler SL, Shadows of thought: rapidly changing asymmetric brain-potential patterns of a brief visuo-motor task. *Science* 220:97–99, 1983.

Gevins AS, and Cutillo BA, Neuroelectric measures of mind. In: PL Nunez (Ed), *Neocortical Dynamics and Human EEG Rhythms.* New York: Oxford University Press, pp. 304–338, 1995.

Gray, CM, Maldonado PE, Wilson M, and McNaughton B, Tetrodes markedly improve the reliability and yield of multiple single-unit isolation from multi-unit recordings in cat striate cortex. *Journal of Neuroscience Methods* 63:43–54, 1995.

Hamaleinen M, Hari R, Ilmoniemi RJ, Knuutila J, and Lounasmaa OV, Magnetoencephalography—theory, instrumentation, and applications to noninvasive studies of the working human brain. *Reviews of Modern Physics* 65:413–497, 1993.

Kellaway P, An orderly approach to visual analysis: the parameters of the normal EEG in adults and children. In: DW Klass and DD Daly (Eds) *Current Practice of Clinical Electroencephalography*. New York: Raven Press, pp. 69–147, 1979.

Lachaux JP, Lutz A, Rudrauf D, Cosmelli D, Le Van Quyen M, Martinerie J, and Varela F, Estimating the time-course of coherence between single-trial brain signals: an introduction to wavelet coherence. *Electroencephalography and Clinical Neurophysiology* 32:157–174, 2002.

Lai Y, van Drongelen W, Ding L, Hecox KE, Towle VL, Frim DM, and He B, Estimation of in vivo human brain-to-skull conductivity ratio from simultaneous extra- and intra-cranial electrical potential recordings. *Clinical Neurophysiology* 116:456–465, 2005.

Law S, Thickness and resistivity variations over the upper surface of human skull. *Brain Topography* 3:99–109, 1993.

Legatt AD, Arezzo J, and Vaughan HG, Averaged multiple unit activity as an estimate of phasic changes in local neuronal activity: effects of volume-conducted potentials. *Journal of Neuroscience Methods* 2:203–217, 1980.

Le Van Quyen M, Foucher J, Lachaux J, Rodriguez E, Lutz A, Martinerie J, and Varela FJ, Comparison of Hilbert transform and wavelet methods for the analysis of neuronal synchrony. *Journal of Neuroscience Methods* 111:83–98, 2001.

Lopes da Silva FH, and Storm van Leeuwen W, The cortical alpha rhythm in dog: the depth and surface profile of phase. In: MAB Brazier and H Petsche (Eds) *Architectonics of the Cerebral Cortex*. New York: Raven Press, pp. 319–333, 1978.

Malmivuo J and Plonsey R, *Bioelectromagnitism*. New York: Oxford University Press, 1995.

Niedermeyer E and Lopes da Silva FH (Eds) *Electroencephalography. Basic Principals, Clinical Applications, and Related Fields. 5th Ed.* London: Williams & Wilkins, 2005.

Nunez PL, The brain wave equation: a model for the EEG, *Mathematical Biosciences* 21:279–297, 1974.

Nunez PL, *Electric Fields of the Brain: The Neurophysics of EEG, 1st Ed*, New York: Oxford University Press, 1981.

Nunez PL, Comments on the paper by Miller, Lutzenberger and Elbert, *Journal of. Psycholophysiology* 5:279–280, 1991.

Nunez PL, *Neocortical Dynamics and Human EEG Rhythms,* New York: Oxford University Press, 1995.

Nunez PL, Toward a quantitative description of large scale neocortical dynamic function and EEG (invited target article), *Behavioral and Brain Sciences* 23:371–398, 2000a.

Nunez PL, Neocortical dynamic theory should be as simple as possible, but not simpler (reply to 18 commentaries by neuroscientists), *Behavioral and Brain Sciences* 23:415–437, 2000b.

Nunez, PL, Implications of white matter correlates of EEG standing and traveling waves, *NeuroImage* 57:1293–1299, 2011.

Nunez PL, *Brain, Mind, and the Structure of Reality*, New York: Oxford University Press, 2010.

Nunez PL, and Srinivasan R, *Electric Fields of the Brain: The Neurophysics of EEG, 2nd Ed,* New York: Oxford University Press, 2006a.

Nunez PL, and Srinivasan R, A theoretical basis for standing and traveling brain waves measured with human EEG with implications for an integrated consciousness, *Clinical Neurophysiology* 117:2424–2435, 2006b.

Nunez PL, Wingeier BM, and Silberstein RB, Spatial-temporal structures of human alpha rhythms: theory, micro-current sources, multiscale measurements, and global binding of local networks, *Human Brain Mapping* 13:125–164, 2001.

Pfurtscheller G, and Cooper R, Frequency dependence of the transmission of the EEG from cortex to scalp, *Electroencephalography and Clinical Neurophysiology* 38:93–96, 1975.

Pfurtscheller G, and Lopes da Silva FH, Event related EEG/MEG synchronization and desynchronization: basic principles. *Electroencephalography and Clinical Neurophysiology* 110:1842–1857, 1999.

Silberstein RB, Song J, Nunez PL, and Park W, Dynamic sculpting of brain functional connectivity is correlated with performance, *Brain Topography* 16:240–254, 2004.

Srinivasan R, Nunez PL, and Silberstein RB, Spatial filtering and neocortical dynamics: estimates of EEG coherence. *IEEE Transactions on Biomedical Engineering* 45:814–826, 1998.

Srinivasan R, Russell DP, Edelman GM, and Tononi G, Frequency tagging competing stimuli in binocular rivalry reveals increased synchronization of neuromagnetic responses during conscious perception, *Journal of Neuroscience* 19:5435–5448, 1999.

4 | SIGNALS REFLECTING BRAIN METABOLIC ACTIVITY

NICK F. RAMSEY

Brain activity involves three types of processes: *electrical, chemical,* and *metabolic.* Best known of these is the electromagnetic activity that results in a neuron's action potential, which is itself the result of chemical events occurring in and around the neuron. Action potentials and other neuronal electrical phenomena allow for electrical measurement of brain activity with *electroencaphalography* (EEG), *magnetoencephalography* (MEG), electrocorticography (ECoG), or with microelectrodes implanted in the brain tissue. However, these methods have a variety of disadvantages. EEG and MEG sensors are located far from the neurons, and the signals acquired do not allow precise identification of the active brain areas. In addition, since the orientation of neurons relative to the sensors strongly affects the measurements, some brain regions are less visible to these sensors. Electrodes placed directly on or within the cortex measure electric activity in their immediate vicinity, but they can cover only a very limited part of the brain. Thus, these methods based on electrical signals have significant inherent limitations. Brain activity can also be detected by measuring chemical processes, but the methods for doing so in humans (mainly by *positron emission tomography* [PET]) are still rather crude, involve injection of specially manufactured markers, and have poor temporal resolution. Because of the limitations of electrical and chemical methods, much effort has recently been invested in measuring *metabolic* processes to study brain activity. These *metabolic methods* are the focus of this chapter.

Metabolic processes involve the utilization of energy. When neurons increase their firing rate, they use more energy. This energy is supplied by chemical reactions in and around the neurons. The increased metabolic activity increases the demand for the basic fuels of metabolism: glucose (sugar) and oxygen. This change in demand can be detected because it is accompanied by increased blood flow to the region. Since blood flow in the brain is highly controlled and locally regulated, it acts as a marker for neuronal activity. This chapter explains how signals indicating increased blood flow in the brain (also called the *hemodynamic response*) can, even in humans, be detected and used to construct detailed images of the brain that reveal brain activity.

OVERVIEW OF FUNCTIONAL NEUROIMAGING

RESOLUTION

Ideally, an imaging technique should capture every event in every neuron. Since this is currently not possible, our aims instead are the highest spatial detail and highest temporal detail possible. Spatial and temporal detail are both measured in terms of *resolution,* the distance between two adjacent points in space or time that can be distinguished from each other. For example, in digital photography, a photo taken with a 1-Mpixel camera produces an image consisting of squares and does not show much detail. In contrast, a 10-Mpixel image will have more squares and will display a lot of detail. The size of the squares (much smaller for the higher-resolution image) is called the *resolution.* The term *resolution* is also used in brain imaging. However, since the measurements in brain imaging are in three dimensions, the term *voxel* (volume element) is used instead of *pixel* (picture element). A *spatial resolution* of 1 mm means that each voxel has a size of 1 mm along each side.

Temporal resolution reflects the time it takes to make one measurement. Again using a familiar analogy, this time of digital video recording, we know that more frames per second produce smoother and more detailed moving images and thus give higher *temporal resolution.* Temporal resolution is typically measured in milliseconds (ms) or seconds (s). For both spatial and temporal resolution, a smaller value (in mm or ms) indicates higher resolution; conversely, a larger value indicates poorer resolution.

Although electrical, chemical, and metabolic processes can all be measured with current techniques, they do so with different degrees of resolution and different degrees of overall success depending on the type of process measured and the properties of the measuring technique. Figure 4.1 shows the properties of the most commonly used techniques to measure brain activity. Various chemicals can be imaged with PET, using specially manufactured markers that are injected (Tai and Piccini 2004). However, temporal detail and spatial detail are very poor when compared to images produced by electrical and metabolic methods. It takes tens of minutes to record one PET image of the brain, and the spatial resolution is moderate at best (about 5 mm). In contrast, imaging of electrical processes can give excellent temporal detail. With electrical methods, one can detect and distinguish between two events occurring within a few milliseconds of one another in the same brain region. However, unless one places electrodes within or on the surface of the brain, it is difficult to pinpoint the precise location of this electrical activity, since the flow of current in the brain is affected by less conductive materials like thick membranes and the skull (chapters 3 and 6). Thus, the precise origin of the signals is uncertain, and the images produced by electrical methods have low resolution (1–2 cm).

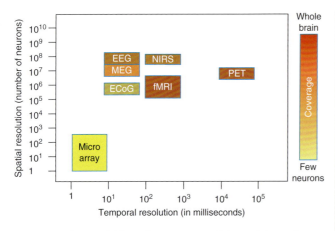

Figure 4.1 *Resolutions of different brain-imaging techniques. Color gradient represents the extent to which the brain can be imaged in one experiment.*

TECHNIQUES FOR IMAGING BLOOD FLOW

The *metabolic processes* that are the focus of this chapter track changes in *blood flow* and are the most recently developed of the relevant imaging techniques. Methods that measure metabolic processes give good spatial resolution (ranging from 5 mm to less than 1 mm), and all brain areas can be imaged. The speed of image capture can be very high, and images can be constructed in less than half a second. However, temporal detail is only moderate because the change in blood flow itself is much slower: it takes about 2 s for a blood vessel to react to the increased oxygen demand, and it takes another 12 s for blood flow to decrease afterward (Donaldson and Buckner 2001). Despite this limitation, the good spatial resolution and broad coverage of the brain make blood-flow imaging an intriguing and useful method for many neuroscientific endeavors. For these reasons, blood-flow imaging has been used increasingly in BCI research.

Currently, there are four major methods used in humans for imaging changes in brain blood flow and its related processes.

- *Functional transcranial Doppler (fTCD):* This method measures changes in blood flow in the major arteries of the brain (Stroobant and Vingerhoets 2000). Of the four metabolic methods listed here, it is the easiest to use because the equipment is mobile and affordable, and because it can be performed with a small probe held against the side of the head (above the cheekbone), allowing for measurements in almost any setting. Although it is quite sensitive, it can only measure differences between the left and right hemispheres. Thus, it is of minimal use for BCI purposes.

- *Positron emission tomography (PET).* In addition to its use in tracking chemical events, this technology can also track blood flow (Fox et al. 1984). However, it is slow, and it requires injection of radioactive compounds. Thus, it has little appeal for BCI applications where speed and ease of use are crucial.

- *Functional near-infrared spectroscopy (fNIRS).* This method measures blood flow by tracking changes in the different forms of hemoglobin (Villringer et al. 1993; Boas et al. 2004). The changes in hemoglobin that accompany brain activity are called the *blood-oxygen-level-dependent (BOLD) response* (Ogawa et al. 1990). fNIRS uses infrared light of specific wavelengths that passes through the skull and back out, where it is detected. It has low spatial resolution (on the order of centimeters) but reasonably good temporal resolution. However, its temporal resolution is limited to several seconds primarily because of the slow rate of the hemodynamic response (Vladislav et al. 2007). Since it is relatively easy and convenient to use, it is an attractive possibility for BCI development.

- *Functional magnetic resonance imaging (fMRI).* fMRI also measures the BOLD response by tracking the changes in blood flow indicated by the relative amounts of the different forms of hemoglobin (Ogawa et al. 1990). fMRI relies on the distinctive responses of different forms of hemoglobin to a high magnetic field. Although this method is expensive and technically demanding, it is the most sensitive of the four hemodynamic methods and has the highest spatial resolution. It is currently the most widely used of the four hemodynamic imaging methods listed here for both basic research and BCI development.

These four methods will be described in greater detail in this chapter, but to do so, we must first discuss the physiological events and the factors that make it possible to obtain images of brain activity based on blood flow. Let us first examine the relationship between blood flow and brain activity.

BLOOD-FLOW RESPONSES TO BRAIN ACTIVITY

Oxygen transport is one of the key functions of blood. Oxygenated blood is pumped from the heart through the arteries to the smallest blood vessels, the capillaries that pass through all the organs and muscles. There, it releases the oxygen that supports metabolic processes, and it absorbs the carbon dioxide produced by metabolic processes. The blood returns to the heart via the veins and then circulates through the lungs where it releases carbon dioxide and picks up molecular oxygen (O_2). The newly oxygenated blood returns to the heart, and the cycle starts again. Each complete cycle takes about one minute. In the blood, the transport of oxygen is carried out by *hemoglobin (Hb),* an iron-containing complex protein that can bind O_2. Hb in the blood exists in two forms: *deoxy-hemoglobin (deoxy-Hb),* which does not contain bound O_2, and *oxyhemoglobin (oxy-Hb),* which does. As blood passes through the lungs, each deoxy-Hb molecule *picks up* four O_2 molecules and thereby becomes oxy-Hb. When the blood passes through organs and muscles, the oxy-Hb *releases* its oxygen and becomes deoxy-Hb.

When a brain region's metabolic activity increases, its oxygen consumption increases. After about a second or so, the neurons begin to absorb more oxygen from the oxy-Hb in the blood of the nearby capillaries (what happens during the delay is not quite clear [see Hyder et al. 2006]). It is estimated that oxygen consumption by neurons accounts for 80% of energy use in brain tissue; in contrast, glial cells account for about 5% and therefore contribute little to metabolic demand (Renaud et al. 2009; Attwell and Iadecola 2002). The capillaries respond to the neurons' increased demand for oxygen by widening to allow more fresh (oxy-Hb-containing) blood to flow into the region. In this process, three important changes occur:

- the amount of blood (blood volume) in the immediate vicinity increases

- the rate of blood flow increases

- *oxy-Hb* delivers oxygen to the cells and becomes *deoxy-Hb*

When brain activity in the region falls back to its baseline level, these three properties also revert back to their original states. The four methods for imaging blood flow discussed in this chapter measure one or more of these three changes.

The two methods most relevant to BCI technology are *functional near-infrared spectroscopy (fNIRS)* and *functional magnetic resonance imaging (fMRI)*. They measure differences in the color (fNIRS) or magnetic properties (fMRI) of Hb in its two states:

- *oxy-Hb is light red, whereas deoxy-Hb is dark red*

- *oxy-Hb is nonmagnetic ("diamagnetic"), whereas deoxy-Hb is slightly magnetic ("paramagnetic")*

Specifically, fNIRS measures the change in near-infrared absorption as oxy-Hb becomes deoxy-Hb, whereas fMRI measures the change in magnetic properties that occurs with change in the relative amounts of oxy-Hb and deoxy-Hb during brain activity.

Brain activity involves communication between neurons. Since a specific communication involves a sender and a receiver (often located in a different part of the brain), it is important to know whether hemodynamic changes are the same for both sender and receiver, or whether they differ. Measuring communication directly is not possible because each neuron is connected to as many as 10,000 other neurons, forming a highly complex system (Buzsaki 2006). Changes in communication can be measured indirectly by measuring single-neuron firing rates or local field potentials (LFPs) (i.e., with microarrays, chapter 5), or by measuring larger-scale field potentials with ECoG (chapter 15) or EEG (chapter 6). Changes in communication can also be measured using fNIRS or fMRI imaging of hemodynamic changes associated with communication. These hemodynamic changes are most pronounced at the receiving end, that is, at the nerve terminals, where presynaptic neurons transfer neurotransmitters to postsynaptic neurons (Logothetis 2008; Attwell and Iadecola 2002). (These terminals

are also largely responsible for the LFPs, and for ECoG and EEG.) Hemodynamic changes are dramatically less pronounced at the sending end, that is, at the neuron cell bodies, which generate the action potentials that travel along the nerve fibers to the terminals (Logothetis 2008). In sum, both the hemodynamic changes and the field potentials measured from the cortex originate mainly from the nerve terminals.

THE FOUR MAJOR METABOLIC NEUROIMAGING METHODS

Let us now examine the four methods of blood-flow measurement in more detail and evaluate their relative merits for BCI use.

FUNCTIONAL TRANSCRANIAL DOPPLER

Blood is supplied to each hemisphere of the brain by three main arteries: the anterior, medial, and posterior cerebral arteries. Each arises from the Circle of Willis below the brain and supplies a specific segment of the hemisphere (fig. 4.2). When a person starts to perform a task, particular areas of the cortex increase their activity level and require more oxygen. This oxygen is delivered by the main arteries, which, in response to the increased demand, increase the supply of oxygen-rich blood by increasing the *rate* of blood flow in those arteries. In *functional transcranial Doppler* (fTCD) imaging, a Doppler probe is placed in contact with the scalp and sends a sound wave of constant frequency (on the order of 2 MHz) to one of the three main cerebral arteries (Stroobant and Vingerhoets 2000). This sound wave enters the head right above the cheekbone through a triangular area of the skull that is sufficiently thin for the sound to pass through. At the same time, the probe detects the reflection of that sound wave. The frequency of the reflected sound indicates the velocity of blood flow in the targeted artery (Stroobant and Vingerhoets. 2000). A change occurs because the traveling blood causes a phase shift in the sound waves, which causes a velocity-specific change in the

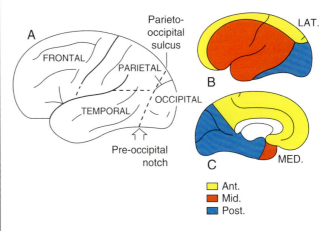

Figure 4.2 *(A) The lobes of the human cerebrum. (B and C) The three main cerebral arteries (see color key) supply different (and partially overlapping) territories. B and C are lateral (LAT) and medial (MED) views, respectively, of the left hemisphere. (Adapted from O'Rahilly et al. 2004.)*

frequency of the sound that the blood reflects back to the probe. fTCD is used clinically to detect abnormal blood flow associated with brain pathology (e.g., stroke). When applied to the measurement of brain function, it relies on the fact that the rate of blood flow to a particular brain area changes when a person starts to perform a task controlled by that brain area (Stroobant et al. 2000).

At any one time, fTCD can target only one artery in each hemisphere. Used in this way, it can, for example, determine a particular person's language lateralization (although language function is located in the left hemisphere in more than 90% of people, in some it is in the right hemisphere, and in others it is bilateral [Deppe et al. 2000]). Despite its usefulness for gaining this type of information, fTCD is unlikely to be useful for BCI purposes because it measures changes that occur only in large areas of brain (i.e., the large areas supplied by each of the three principal arteries). Anything that happens in one of those large areas will increase blood flow, so if fTCD were used for BCI, many different brain functions (including motor imagery and seeing someone else move) would trigger the BCI system and cause frequent false detections.

POSITRON EMISSION TOMOGRAPHY

Positron Emission Tomography (PET) can produce images of chemical processes (Cherry and Phelps 2002) and can also produce images of metabolic processes. It does so by detecting changes in blood flow (Fox et al. 1984). Although PET is very slow in imaging chemical processes (i.e., requiring tens of minutes), it is substantially faster in imaging blood flow (i.e., <1 min).

PET requires the injection of radioactive compounds prepared in an on-site cyclotron that inserts a radioactive atom in a specific marker molecule. (The radioactive isotopes used have short half-lives and are administered at doses small enough to preclude harmful biological effects.) In PET imaging of blood flow, radioactive oxygen (^{15}O) is first inserted into water molecules, making them radioactive. The radioactive water molecules are injected and pass through the body. Since the blood-brain barrier is readily permeable to water, radioactive water in the blood is exchanged with water in the brain. This process occurs in proportion to the level of blood flow. When the brain is active and blood flow to the brain increases, the radioactive water concentrates in the brain.

After injection of the marker, the PET scanner starts to collect images by measuring radiation with a ring of detectors in the scanner. Whenever a radioactive oxygen atom (^{15}O) releases a positron that collides with an electron in the immediate surrounding, the two particles annihilate each other and emit two gamma photons traveling in opposite directions. These gamma photons then hit blocks made of crystals (*scintillators*) that surround the subject's head in the scanner. As the photons impinge on the crystal blocks, a brief flash of light occurs. This flash is detected by high-performance optical cameras arranged directly outside the crystals. Since the two photons travel in opposite directions along a single line, they impinge on two diametrically opposed scintillators. From detections of thousands of such hits, the sources of emission from the brain can then be reconstructed.

The image constructed by the PET scanner displays the density distribution of the radioactive tracers in the brain. When a brain region is active and blood flow in that region increases, more radioactive water enters the brain tissue, and the PET cameras detect the radioactivity to create a brain image. However, since different parts of the brain have different rates of metabolism, the areas with high radioactive-tracer density are not necessarily those that are active. To determine what area(s) are active, it is necessary to collect a reference scan made while the subject is in the scanner but not performing a task. Subtraction of the reference image from the task-activity image generates a difference image, which identifies the areas that are active during the task. Examples of PET images of the brain are shown in figure 4.3.

Temporal resolution for PET is modest, since at least 40 s are needed to collect enough information to construct one

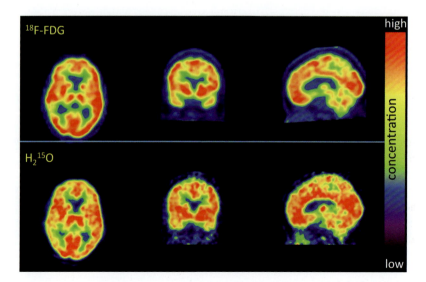

Figure 4.3 *PET images of the brain of one subject. (Top) distribution of ^{18}F-fluorodeoxyglucose (^{18}F-FDG), a radioactive marker of glucose metabolism, showing one slice in each of the transaxial, coronal, and sagittal directions. (Bottom) Distribution of a radioactive marker of cerebral blood flow (^{15}O in water), reflecting brain activity. (Courtesy of B. N. M. van Berckel, Free University Medical Center, Amsterdam, The Netherlands.)*

image. Spatial resolution is about 5 mm. A PET scanner is also expensive because it is necessary to have a cyclotron in the immediate vicinity since ^{15}O decays rapidly, with a half-life of about 2 min. For scanning, this rapid decay is an advantage because it makes multiple scans possible within one session, thus allowing for mapping of different brain functions within an individual. (In contrast, a slow decay would cause radiation from one scan to affect the next.) The expense of the cycloctron and the need for injection of radioactively labeled compounds are significant disadvantages of this method. As a result, interest in ^{15}O-PET imaging diminished when fMRI emerged and developed as a viable imaging method.

FUNCTIONAL NEAR-INFRARED SPECTROSCOPY

FUNCTIONAL NEAR-INFRARED SPECTROSCOPY PRINCIPLES

fNIRS also measures blood flow. It reveals brain activity for only the top few mm of cortex, is noninvasive, and is based on the change in the blood's color when oxygen is delivered to brain tissue (Villringer et al. 1993; Boas et al. 2004). fNIRS is a BOLD-response technology that measures the changes in the relative levels of oxy-Hb and deoxy-Hb during brain activity. Oxygen-rich blood, high in oxy-Hb, is present in the main arteries of the brain, as well as in the smaller arteries and the upstream segments of the capillaries. Oxygen-poor blood, high in deoxy-Hb, is present in the downstream segments of the capillaries as it passes into the venuoles and then into progressively larger veins, the largest of which, the superior venous sinus, runs between the two hemispheres just below the skull.

When an experimental subject performs a particular task, brain activity increases in those brain areas relevant to the task, and the amounts of oxy- and deoxy-Hb change in the immediate vicinity of those areas. In the resting state (before a subject performs a task), there is some baseline neuronal activity, some ongoing metabolic activity, some deoxy-Hb produced, and therefore some presence of baseline deoxy-Hb. When activity in a particular brain region increases during task performance, neuronal and glial metabolism both increase. At first, as the cells take oxygen from the blood to support the increased metabolism associated with neuronal activity, the level of deoxy-Hb increases. The vascular system then responds quickly to prevent oxygen deprivation in downstream brain regions, and in doing so, it supplies much more oxygen-rich blood than is necessary (Fox and Raichle 1986). This surge of fresh blood causes the local concentration of oxy-Hb to increase and the local concentration of deoxy-Hb to effectively drop (almost all deoxy-Hb in the local vicinity is washed away). fNIRS takes advantage of the fact that the relative amounts of oxy-Hb and deoxy-Hb in the area change, and this change is proportional to the level of neuronal activity. The changes in the oxy/deoxy ratio can be detected because the absorbance spectra at near-infrared wavelengths differ for oxy-Hb and deoxy-Hb (Boas et al. 2004). That is,

- deoxy-Hb is dark red; it absorbs light of wavelength around 690 nm (to a greater extent than oxy-Hb does)

- oxy-Hb is light red; it absorbs light of wavelength around 830 nm (to a greater extent than deoxy-Hb does)

In a homogeneous medium, the attenuation of light is expressed by the Beer-Lambert Law (Villringer and Chance 1997), which states that the attenuation, or absorbance, A, is proportional to the concentration of the absorbing molecule:

$$A = c \times \varepsilon \times l \qquad (4.1)$$

where c is the concentration of the absorbing molecule, ε is its absorption coefficient (characteristic for a particular material), and l is the optical path length. A change in the concentration of the absorbing molecule, Δc, will produce a proportional change in absorbance ΔA such that:

$$\Delta A = \Delta c \times \varepsilon \times l \qquad (4.2)$$

A can be detected by the fNIRS sensor at different time points, so ΔA can be determined. Because the head provides a complex heterogeneous medium for the path of light, the Beer-Lambert Law is modified for fNIRS applications (Villringer and Chance 1997) to include additional parameters that account for the effects of light scattering (e.g., signal loss due to rays deflected away from the sensor and increased path length due to rays zigzagging before reaching the sensor). Nevertheless, the Beer-Lambert equation expresses the basic principle underlying fNIRS measurement of changes in brain activity.

In fNIRS, light of wavelengths 690 and 830 nm is shined on the skull with probes positioned on the scalp (fig. 4.4). This light is able to pass through skin and bone to reach the underlying brain tissue. Some of the light is absorbed by the brain tissue. Some of the light is scattered, and part of this scattered light is reflected back out of the head. Less reflection means that more is absorbed. Since deoxy-Hb and oxy-Hb have different patterns of absorbance at 690 and 830 nm, and since

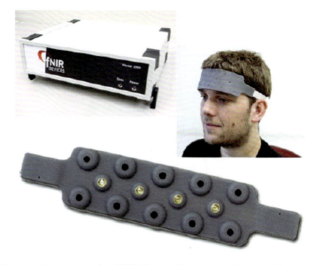

Figure 4.4 An example of an fNIRS device with sources and sensors. The four lights in the middle row are the illuminators, and the two rows at the edges house the 10 detectors. (Reprinted from Biopac Systems; retrieved from fNIRdevices.com.)

the absorbance at a particular wavelength is proportional to the concentration of the absorbing molecules, measurement of the reflected light at wavelengths 690 and 830 nm reveals the concentrations of the absorbing molecules, deoxy-Hb and oxy-Hb, respectively. When brain activity increases, the deoxy-Hb concentration first increases as the blood's Hb releases its oxygen to the cells. This is a small effect and is detected as a small increase in absorbance at 690 nm (indicating more deoxy-Hb). After a few seconds, the flow of fresh oxy-Hb-containing blood to the area increases, and the absorbance at 830 nm (indicating oxy-Hb) therefore increases. This is a much larger effect because it is due primarily to the more than sufficiently increased blood flow to the area (Fox and Raichle 1986).

fNIRS HARDWARE

fNIRS devices consist of light-source/detector pairs (together called sensors) positioned on the head (fig. 4.4). Up to about 52 pairs are currently possible, allowing for measuring a considerable part of the brain surface. As hair obstructs the passage of light (and hair movement disturbs the signal), the best signals are obtained from the forehead. Other positions are possible but require careful repositioning of hair that might obstruct the sources and detectors.

When the light source shines NIR light of a particular wavelength through the skull at an angle, the light passes through to the brain, penetrates a few mm into the cortex, and is reflected back out of the head where it is detected by the detectors located in its path. The deflections of the photons as they cross the interfaces between the different tissues cause them to follow a curvilinear path from the source to the detector. This path is called the *photon banana* (Hongo et al. 1995), and its shape is determined by the optical properties of the tissues. As the distance between the source and the detector increases and absorption increases (due to the longer path length), more of the banana passes through the cortex. This effect is illustrated in figure 4.5. However, although increased source-detector distance increases absorbance (due to longer optical path length), it also results in more light scattering, which degrades fNIRS sensitivity and spatial resolution. Thus, the distance selected is a compromise between these two opposing factors and should be appropriate for the particular application. From data obtained from an array of fNIRS sensors, a map can be constructed of the hemodynamic changes that correlate with task performance. This map looks similar to fMRI maps, although the coverage is limited, and the spatial resolution is much lower (fig. 4.6).

fNIRS is noninvasive, is relatively easy to use, and is portable and inexpensive compared to the other blood-flow measurement technologies. Its temporal resolution is relatively good (on the order of several seconds), but its spatial resolution is relatively low (on the order of cm). Despite its limitations, it has some promise as a method for BCI development. Further details on fNIR techniques as well as fNIRS use for BCIs are discussed in chapter 18.

FUNCTIONAL MAGNETIC RESONANCE IMAGING

The fourth metabolic imaging method that we discuss is *fMRI*, which first emerged as a potentially useful imaging technology in 1990 (Ogawa et al. 1990; Kwong et al. 1992) and has developed very rapidly since then. It provides excellent spatial detail and is now one of the most widely used techniques for imaging brain function. (A significant practical reason for its wide adoption is also the fact that it uses the same MRI scanner that radiologists use for a variety of clinical applications.) fMRI, like fNIRS, is a BOLD-response method since it measures the relative amounts of oxy- and deoxy-Hb in the brain tissue. It is noninvasive.

Before describing fMRI methods and their applicability for BCI technology, we first need to describe the properties of an MRI scanner and the underlying principles of magnetic resonance (see McRobbie et al. 2007 for a detailed explanation of MRI). An MRI scanner consists of six key components:

- a large main magnet
- a radiofrequency transmitter
- a receiver antenna
- gradient coils
- a front-end computer
- a reconstruction computer

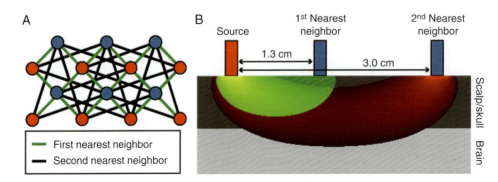

Figure 4.5 Example of an fNIRS sensor scheme. Because a beam of light may scatter before it exits the head, it may be detected by sensors at multiple locations. (A) Possible source-sensor pairings for the 14 sources and sensors shown. (B) Effects of distance between source and sensors (nearby is first neighbor, next is second neighbor). Note the banana shape of the path of the scattered beam from the source to the sensors it reaches. Rays travel farther and deeper for the second neighbor. (Reprinted with permission from Gregg et al. 2010.)

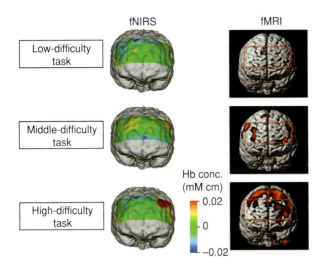

fNIRS   fMRI

Low-difficulty task

Middle-difficulty task

High-difficulty task

Hb conc. (mM cm)

0.02

0

−0.02

Figure 4.6 *Brain-activity maps obtained with fNIRS and fMRI with three levels of difficulty in a mental task. Color indicates strength of the activation (i.e., oxy-Hb concentration). Note difference in spatial detail (resolution) between the two techniques. (Reprinted with permission from Tsunashima and Yanagisawa 2009.)*

THE MAIN MAGNET

The *large main magnet* is an aluminum tube, usually 2 meters long, with a 100-cm wide tunnel running through its center. Wires are wound around the tube to form several rings (fig. 4.7). MRI magnets do not use standard copper wire because the high electric currents required to produce the high magnetic fields needed for imaging would make it difficult to cool the wires and would increase the copper wire's resistance, thereby preventing the creation of the high magnetic field. Instead of copper, MRI magnets use wire made of a *superconducting* material consisting of a combination of niobium-titanium and copper. This superconducting material has zero resistance to electric currents at very low temperatures. In the magnet, the wire is immersed in an aluminum casing that contains liquid helium maintained at −269 degrees Celsius (4 Kelvin). At this temperature, the wire becomes superconducting. That is, it is possible to pass very high electric currents without generating heat, thus creating a very strong magnetic field. The magnetic field that results from passing high electric currents through the cooled superconducting wire is called the B_0 *field*. The strongest magnets currently in use generate a B_0 field of more than 20 Tesla (T). The strongest magnets produce the highest-intensity MRI signals. (Note that the magnetic strength used in human MRI scanners is limited by the need for a tunnel large enough for humans [Robitaille and Berliner 2006]. The strongest magnets currently used in humans have B_0 fields of 11.7 T. Most modern hospitals have a 3-T MRI scanner for clinical diagnosis and research.)

Human tissue itself is not magnetic. However, it is rich in hydrogen. The nucleus of a hydrogen atom (i.e., a proton) has an intrinsic spin that is accompanied by a small magnetic moment (dashed red line pointing up and to the right at the instant depicted in figure 4.8) and an angular momentum. Although these physical properties can be strictly described only by quantum mechanics, it is still possible, under the conditions typically present in an MRI scanner (McRobbie et al. 2007), to describe the properties of a large collection of

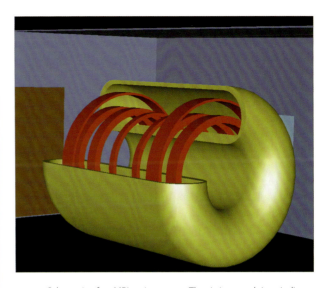

Figure 4.7 *Schematic of an MRI main magnet. The six inner red rings indicate the wire bundles generating the main field (B_0) inside the tunnel. The two outer red rings generate a countering magnetic field to reduce the field outside the scanner, allowing the MRI to be installed in limited space. (Reprinted with permission from Cobham Technical Services; retrieved from http://www.wordsun.com.)*

protons by classic mechanics and electrodynamics. Normally, the tiny magnetic fields created by the many spinning protons (i.e., hydrogen nuclei present in human tissue) cancel one another out because their axes of rotation (and magnetic moments) are randomly oriented due to the Brownian motion of the molecules.

In an external magnetic field, such as the B_0 field of the MRI scanner (dashed vertical blue line in fig. 4.8, conventionally

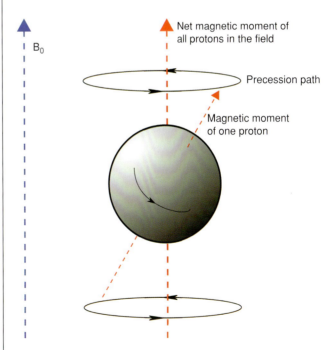

B_0

Net magnetic moment of all protons in the field

Precession path

Magnetic moment of one proton

Figure 4.8 *A hydrogen nuclear proton spins and has a magnetic moment (slanted dashed red arrow) that precesses around the axis of the B_0 field. The behavior of one proton is shown. The net magnetic moment of all the protons in the field (vertical dashed red arrow) aligns with the B_0 field (vertical dashed blue arrow).*

defined as the +z axis), the tiny magnetic moments (e.g., slanted dotted red line in fig. 4.8) that are created by the protons' spin experience a torque that causes them to precess (wobble) around the axis of the B_0 field's magnetic moment (see circular path of this precession in fig. 4.8). The magnetic moments of just over half of these precessing (wobbling) protons (like the proton shown in fig. 4.8) are oriented with the B_0 field; they precess around the +z-axis. The magnetic moments of the remaining protons (not shown in fig. 4.8) precess around the −z-axis. Since these precessions are not in phase with one another, the sum of all the individual proton nuclear moments yields a small *net magnetic moment* that is aligned with the B_0 field (dashed vertical red line in fig. 4.8). It is this small net magnetic moment that allows the tissue to produce an observable signal under the correct conditions. The *frequency of the precession* (wobble) of the protons' magnetic moments is proportional to the strength of the B_0 field: in a higher B_0 field, they precess faster.

Although many atoms other than hydrogen will respond to a magnetic field in this way, hydrogen is by far the dominant contributor to MRI signals for two reasons. First, hydrogen is the most abundant atom in human tissue (about 65% of atoms in biological tissue are hydrogen, predominantly present in water and fat), and second, hydrogen is highly sensitive to energy absorption (which translates to signal strength) in MRI. Nuclei in other atoms such as carbon, phosphorus, and oxygen are protected from magnetic manipulation by the large numbers of electrons surrounding them and acting as a shield. Although these other nuclei are present in the human body and can generate signals for MRI, their detection is quite difficult due to their low abundance and low sensitivity. For these reasons, all current clinical MRI scans are based on signals from hydrogen.

THE RADIOFREQUENCY TRANSMITTER AND RECEIVER ANTENNA

The *radiofrequency (rf) transmitter* is the second essential component of the MRI scanner. It sends brief rf pulses (too small to be noticed by the subject) to the head while it is in the scanner. The rf radiation is generally transmitted with its magnetic component oriented perpendicular to that of the B_0 field. As a result, the net magnetic moment of the sample will now also begin to precess around the axis of the magnetic component of the rf pulse. (This brief rotation of the sample's magnetic moment also serves to bring the axes of precession of the individual nuclear spins into phase coherence.) Typically, the rf pulse is very brief (a few milliseconds) and is terminated when the magnetic moment of the sample has rotated so as to be perpendicular to the static B_0 field. When the pulse is turned off, the protons relax to their original orientation. From an energetic standpoint, this entire cycle represents the excitation of the protons to a higher-energy excited state (net magnetic moment away from the B_0 field toward the rf field) and then a return to the ground state (net magnetic moment aligned with the B_0 field) by relaxation. During the relaxation step, many of the protons emit energy in the form of rf radiation.

The energy, wavelength, and frequency of the rf radiation that is absorbed, and then emitted, by the protons are determined by their gyromagnetic ratio (a constant unique to every atom; e.g., hydrogen's is 2.68×10^8 radian/[T × sec]) and the strength of the static external magnetic field to which they are exposed. In higher magnetic fields the protons absorb rf radiation of higher energy (and therefore higher frequency). Recall that in higher magnetic fields, the protons' magnetic moments also precess (wobble) faster (i.e., at higher frequency). In fact, the frequency of the rf radiation that the protons absorb is exactly equal to the frequency of their precession. This frequency, called the *Larmor frequency*, is described by the *Larmor equation* (see McRobbie et al. 2007). (Note that high magnetic fields have a dramatic effect on the frequency of this precession. In the Earth's magnetic field, the frequency is about 1 Hz, but it is about 64 million Hz in a 1.5-T field.)

The specific Larmor frequency of the rf pulse that is absorbed, and then emitted, by the protons is called the *resonance frequency* (hence the name magnetic *resonance* imaging or *MRI*). Thus, the Larmor frequency can be defined three ways: the frequency of precession (wobble), the frequency of the rf radiation that is absorbed, and the resonance frequency. For each type of nucleus (e.g., hydrogen), this frequency changes in proportion to the exact strength of the surrounding magnetic field. In a higher magnetic field, the protons absorb rf radiation of higher frequency; in a lower magnetic field, the protons absorb rf radiation of lower frequency.

The *receiver antenna* (or *receiver coil*) detects the rf signals emitted by the protons during their relaxation to the ground state.

THE GRADIENT COILS

To identify the areas of the brain responsible for particular signals, the image reconstruction computer needs to be able to distinguish the spatial origins of the detected signals. This information is provided through the contribution of the *gradient coils*. The gradient coils consist of extra magnets lining the inside of the main magnet (fig. 4.9). The gradient-coil

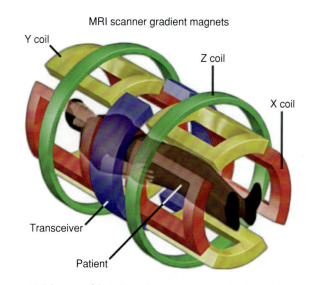

MRI scanner gradient magnets

Y coil

Z coil

X coil

Transceiver

Patient

Figure 4.9 *Schematic of the MRI gradient coils. Each set of coils (coded by color here) creates an additional magnetic field: x for right-to-left, y for front-to-back, and z for foot-to-head. (Reprinted from http://www.magnet.fsu.edu.)*

magnets are weak compared to the main magnet, but by adding to the B_0 field, they can create a *gradient* of magnetic fields across the imaged tissue.

In an MRI scanner, when the gradient magnets are switched on, different portions of the brain experience different magnetic-field strengths due to the *combined* effect of the B_0 field and the gradient coils. Since different magnetic-field strengths give different Larmor frequencies, the protons in different locations in the brain will absorb (and then emit) rf radiation of different frequency. Thus, in each voxel, the protons will absorb, and then emit, the rf radiation that has exactly the resonance (Larmor) frequency corresponding to its local magnetic field, which is the combined result of the B_0 field and the gradient coils.

THE FRONT-END COMPUTER AND THE RECONSTRUCTION COMPUTER

The *front-end computer* controls the *pulse sequence* (also called the *scanning protocol*), which is a complex sequence of, and combination of, rf pulses and gradient-coil settings used during a scan. There are many different pulse sequences, each of which results in a different type of image (i.e, anatomical, blood flow, tumor detection, edema, etc.). For fMRI, only a few pulse sequences can be used, and the one most widely used is called *echo-planar imaging* (see Bandettini 2001).

The pulse sequence produces not only a gradient of field strengths (and thus a gradient of Larmor frequencies), but it also affects the relaxation times of the protons differently in different locations. The *reconstruction computer* (or *reconstructor*) uses this information about the exact distribution of the magnetic fields (created at each location by the gradient coils) and the relaxation characteristics of the protons (manipulated by the pulse sequence) to relate specific signals to particular locations of origin.

fMRI MEASUREMENT OF THE BOLD RESPONSE

fMRI methodology produces maps of the *hemodynamic response* to brain activity, based on the effect that local deoxy-Hb has on the magnetic field. As noted earlier in this chapter, the hemodynamic effect generates the BOLD signal that was first described by Ogawa et al. (1990). The key principle is that deoxy-Hb (which is paramagnetic) provides a disturbance *additional* to the magnetic field created by the main magnet and the gradient coils. Deoxy-Hb changes the strength of the magnetic field in its immediate vicinity, so that the actual local field strength is slightly lower than that predicted by the pulse sequence. This decrease, due to the presence of deoxy-Hb, is revealed as a tiny dark spot in the reconstructed image. The intensity of the dark spot is correlated with the amount of deoxy-Hb present.

Since fMRI scanning is very fast (it takes only seconds to make an image of the whole brain, and on some scanners it takes even less than a second), it is possible to create a series of images (i.e., a *movie*) of the brain, based on the amount of deoxy-Hb at specific locations in the brain over time. As described in this chapter's section *Brain Activity and Blood Flow*, brain activity causes changes in the amounts of oxy- and deoxy-Hb. At first, as oxygen is released to the cells, deoxy-Hb increases, causing a darkening of the active part of the brain image. Then, as the blood vessels respond to the cells' need for oxygen, a surge of fresh blood causes the concentration of deoxy-Hb to decline, thereby causing the image to brighten at the location of brain activity. Hence, during initiation of brain activity, the image first darkens (due to higher concentration of deoxy-Hb) and then brightens (due to lower concentration of deoxy-Hb). The increase in brightness is proportional to the amount of brain activity. Thus, maps of brain activity can be created based on the changes in brightness of the fMRI image. A set of such maps is shown in figure 4.10. In this way, fMRI images can reveal the brain areas that are active during performance of specific tasks.

Effective functional neuroimaging with fMRI requires many scans because the BOLD effect is small and because head movements, respiration, and blood-vessel pulsations introduce considerable noise in the images (Jones et al. 2008). A variety of software packages are available for fMRI data analysis;

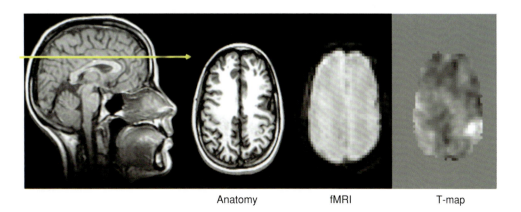

Anatomy   fMRI   T-map

Figure 4.10 *fMRI scans of a study subject during right-hand finger tapping. The yellow arrow in the left image indicates the location and plane of the brain "slice" imaged for fMRI. The image labeled anatomy shows the anatomical scan used for the display of activation. The image labeled fMRI shows an fMRI scan. The image labeled T-map shows the T-map for the task. The level of gray intensity indicates the strength of activation (white indicates an increase in activity; black, a decrease in activity). In the images labeled anatomy, fMRI, and T-map, the left side of the images is the right side of the brain (radiological orientation).*

these incorporate algorithms that reduce the impact of noise. The most widely used programs are SPM (http://www.fil.ion.ucl.ac.uk/spm/), AFNI (http://afni.nimh.nih.gov/afni), FSL (http://www.fmrib.ox.ac.uk/fsl/), and the commercial program Brainvoyager (http://www.brainvoyager.com/). These programs all generate brain-activity maps based on statistical measures such as t- or F-statistics. The activity maps for each subject are typically called t-maps (Ramsey et al. 2002). In a *t-map*, every voxel has a value that reflects the amount of signal change attributable to the task performed during the scan, divided by the unexplained variability of the signal. A *higher t-value* means that the activity change stands out more prominently from the noise.

TASK DESIGN FOR METABOLIC NEURAL IMAGING

These techniques all produce functional images of the brain. What the resulting maps represent depends on the task the subject is performing during image acquisition. Thus, experimental tasks are designed to reveal the specific parts of the brain that perform particular functions (Ramsey et al. 2002). This *task design*, or *paradigm design,* is a field in its own right and merits some discussion here (Donaldson and Buckner 2001).

One main goal of functional neuroimaging is to reveal which parts of the brain perform a particular function. For example, in reading a book, it is not only the language network that is active, but also visual systems, memory systems, and even motor systems, all of which must participate in order to read, comprehend, and interpret text, to move one's eyes back and forth, and to flip pages. Suppose that we want to learn which parts of the brain are involved in language. We may perform fMRI scans while a person reads in the scanner. However, scans of this activity alone would not provide informative activity maps because the brain is always active, even during sleep or during anesthesia. When a person performs a task, many brain regions may be involved. What is needed is to find the *changes* in the image that coincide with reading.

This is typically accomplished by designing a task that is presented to the subject, usually with the use of specific software such as "Presentation" (http://www.neurobs.com/) or "Eprime" (http://www.pstnet.com/). For example, while in the scanner, the subject might first see a blank screen for 30 s, then see text to read for 30 s, and then a blank screen. This cycle would repeat several times. Subsequent analysis would calculate, for each voxel in the scans, the correlation between the task (reading versus watching a blank screen) and the intensity of the signal. The stronger the correlation, the more likely it is that the voxel in the image is involved in the reading task. The voxels are then superimposed on an anatomical scan to produce a map of brain activity related to reading (fig. 4.11).

Although this map reveals the anatomical location of the brain regions that are active in reading, it also includes areas that are merely correlated with the task but not necessarily specific to language (e.g., the visual systems). To separate

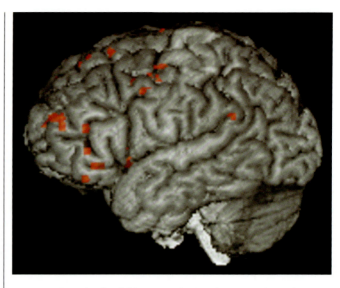

Figure 4.11 *Example of an fMRI-generated image during a reading task in a healthy volunteer. The view is from the left. Anterior is to the left. Significant activity is shown in red.*

out those systems, one can replace the blank screen in the task with random drawings. With this task design, the visual system would be activated during the entire task and can be subtracted out to produce an activity map showing language areas only.

BCI APPLICATIONS OF fNIRS AND fMRI

Metabolic functional imaging methods such as fNIRS or fMRI can, in principle, be used as the basis for BCI technology. Examples of this are discussed in greater detail in chapters 18 and 22. As with all BCI methods, it is essential that signals be processed in real time so that feedback to the user can be provided in real time. From the studies discussed in chapters 18 and 22, it has become evident that people can learn to regulate specific aspects of their brain activity as detected by fNIRS or fMRI, if they are given real-time feedback.

In a typical BCI experiment, the subject first performs a *localizer* task, in which brain activity is recorded during performance of a specific task (e.g., imagining hand movement), alternated with a control task or rest period. The data are processed, and a t-map is created to identify the brain areas involved in the task. Next, a brain region is selected either based on the location where the subject's brain is activated by the localizer task or based on an anatomical atlas of predefined brain regions, or a combination of the two. In subsequent imaging sessions the subject performs the same or a similar task and receives immediate fNIRS- or fMRI-based feedback regarding the level of the signal in the region of interest. This feedback might, for example, be in the form of visual presentation of a vertical bar representing the level of activity in the region. The subject tries to regulate the height of that bar, perhaps based on mental imagery. The task can be a BCI-related task such as moving a computer cursor to a target (e.g., Wolpaw et al. 2002), or moving a cursor to play a game of Pong™. With continued training, the subject's control of the brain activity tends to improve. Control developed in this way might be applied to an fMRI- or fNIRS-based BCI.

fNIRS-BASED BCIs

BCIs using fNIRS certainly have the potential to provide very basic communication capability to people with severe disabilities (Coyle et al. 2007). Major advantages of fNIRS are that it is noninvasive, portable, and relatively inexpensive. However, its temporal resolution is limited since it measures the BOLD response. Moreover, fNIRS imaging of blood flow is inferior to that of fMRI both in spatial resolution and in that it reveals activity for only the top few mm of cortex. Nevertheless, in the future, with increases in the number of sensors and with standardization of placement methods, fNIRS-based BCIs might constitute a practical option for people who need a basic communication system. These issues and possibilities are discussed further in chapter 18.

fMRI-BASED BCIs

Realistically, fMRI-based BCIs are at present not very practical due to the high expense and bulk of the equipment, the need for liquid helium to cool the superconducting coils, and the need for an rf-shielded chamber. (Nevertheless, in the case of patients in a vegetative state, fMRI signal modulation can be useful [Monti et al. 2010]).) Although fMRI imaging itself is fast, the BOLD response that it measures is slow (with a delay of several seconds), so fMRI feedback is relatively slow compared to feedback in BCIs that use electrical signals.

Nevertheless, since fMRI activity correlates closely with electrical activity in the cortex (Ramsey et al. 2006, Hermes et al. 2011), fMRI imaging can help to identify the most promising brain regions for BCIs that use other imaging methods. This could be particularly valuable for supporting development and use of invasive BCIs. Microelectrode arrays (chapters 5 and 16) cannot be implanted throughout the entire cortex, so it will be essential to develop methods for selecting the best areas prior to implantation. For a prospective BCI user, fMRI could identify the best areas for implanting arrays. In addition, fMRI-based training prior to implantation might lead to the identification of brain areas that were not considered promising prior to the training.

Such fMRI-aided preimplantation localization could be especially valuable in BCI approaches that target higher cortical functions such as language (Brumberg et al. 2010), particularly because cortical localization for these functions varies widely across individuals. Thus, preimplantation guidance that can be provided by fMRI is likely to be important. Moreover, because it is noninvasive, fMRI can also be used in large control studies aimed at identifying brain areas and functions and in developing training protocols that may then be used for BCIs for people with disabilities.

Recent studies suggest that with the use of advanced multivariate pattern analysis (e.g., Kamitani and Tong 2006), such fMRI localization might become far more precise in the future. Miyawaki et al. (2008) recently showed that with pattern analysis they could determine which of a set of complex shapes (e.g., letters) a subject was looking at. One can imagine that with extensive further development, it may be possible for fMRI analysis to identify specific words a person wants to communicate or specific actions to implement.

PROMISING FUTURE DEVELOPMENTS

Several areas of inquiry are likely to be particularly important as BCI technology and metabolic methods develop further. fMRI allows investigators and study subjects to discover the tactics that work best for them in gaining control of signals from specific cortical regions; the regions can then be targeted as implantation sites for microelectrodes (or sensor placement for a noninvasive portable fNIRS system). fMRI can also track the changes in brain activity that occur following practice and can be used to identify the factors that contribute to those changes. Thus, because it allows some of the key issues for implanted systems to be investigated noninvasively in healthy subjects and in individual patients, and over many brain areas, fMRI is likely to play an important role in the development of invasive BCIs.

Improved spatial resolution will play a critical role in the importance of fMRI's contribution to BCI technology. The strength of the MRI magnet determines the spatial detail of fMRI brain maps. With the advent of 7-T systems for human use, it is already clear that functional maps can be obtained with high spatial detail (at 1 mm resolution), a level of detail not possible with standard 3-T fMRI scanners. These higher-resolution maps provide even greater detail by distinguishing the different gray-matter layers (Siero et al. 2011) and indicate that brain functions may be more highly localized than previously thought (Formisano et al. 2003). Further research on functional resolution with high-field fMRI will provide information on the optimal spatial detail for intracranial BCIs, so that it may be possible for an intracranial BCI to obtain output commands with multiple degrees of freedom from a single small multielectrode intracortical microarray (Hatsopoulos and Donoghue 2009) or from one of the newly developed high-density cortical surface (ECoG) arrays (e.g., as in Leuthardt et al. 2009).

High-field MRI systems are currently being used to develop *new signal modalities* including new methods for imaging brain function. These include molecular imaging to measure neurochemical processes directly, as is done in MRI measurement of neurotransmitters and intracellular metabolic processes (Jasanoff 2010; Zhu et al. 2011). The neurochemical MRI modality is likely to be much more complex than the electrophysiological modality, as each neuron may use more than one neurotransmitter, and each transmitter may relate differently to brain activity. fMRI may also be used to measure electrophysiological events directly (so-called *neuronal-current fMRI*). Thus far, this possibility been demonstrated only in in vitro experiments (Petridou et al. 2006). If the neuronal-current fMRI approach works in humans, it would eliminate the issues introduced by the delayed response of blood vessels that is inherent in BOLD fMRI, and it would improve the accuracy of localization. At this time, neither neurochemical nor neuronal current MRI is yet available for use in humans.

SUMMARY

Although most BCIs use electrical signals as measures of brain activity, metabolic signals can also be used. At present, two metabolic methods used for BCIs are *functional near-infrared spectroscopy (fNIRS) imaging* and *functional magnetic resonance imaging (fMRI)*. Both methods measure the hemodynamic response: they track changes in the relative amounts of deoxy- and oxy-hemoglobin to measure changes in cerebral blood flow and thereby infer changes in brain activity. The temporal resolution of both methods is limited by the fact that the hemodynamic response itself is slow; it is much slower than the signals measured by electrical BCI methods. Spatial resolution for fMRI is high (on the order of 1 mm), but it is low for fNIRS (on the order of cms). Whereas fMRI can image the entire brain, fNIRS is limited to the top few mm of the cortex, just below the skull. On the other hand, fMRI is very expensive, cumbersome, and technically complex, whereas fNIRS is inexpensive and portable. At present, fMRI is likely to be most useful as a noninvasive method for localizing (and possibly training) brain function prior to implantation of microarrays or other invasive BCI devices, whereas fNIRS may serve in simple BCI systems that provide basic communication and that are practical for long-term home use by people with severe disabilities.

REFERENCES

Attwell D, Iadecola C (2002) The neural basis of functional brain imaging signals. Trends Neurosci 25:621–625.

Bandettini PA (2001) Selection of the optimal pulse sequence for functional MRI. In Functional MRI: An Introduction to Methods, Jezzard P, Matthews PM, Smith SM (Eds). Oxford: Oxford University Press.

Boas DA, Dale AM, Franceschini MA (2004) Diffuse optical imaging of brain activation: approaches to optimizing image sensitivity, resolution, and accuracy. NeuroImage 23(1):S275–288.

Brumberg JS, Nieto-Castanon A, Kennedy PR, Guenther FH (2010) Brain-computer interfaces for speech communication. Speech Commun 52(4):367–379.

Buzsaki G (2006) Rhythms of the Brain. Oxford: Oxford University Press.

Cherry S, Phelps M (2002) Imaging brain function with positron emission tomography, In Brain Mapping: The Methods, Toga AW, Mazziotta JC (Eds), San Diego, Academic Press.

Coyle SM, Ward TE, Markham CM (2007) Brain-computer interface using a simplified functional near-infrared spectroscopy system. J Neural Eng 4(3):219–226.

Deppe M, Knecht S, Papke K, Lohmann H, Fleischer H, Heindel W, Ringelstein EB, Henningsen H (2000) Assessment of hemispheric language lateralization: a comparison between fMRI and fTCD. J Cereb Blood Flow Metab 20:263–268.

Donaldson DI, Buckner RL (2001) Effective paradigm design. In Functional MRI: An Introduction to Methods, Jezzard P, Matthews PM, Smith SM (Eds). Oxford: Oxford University Press.

Formisano E, Kim DS, Di Salle F, van de Moortele PF, Ugurbil K, Goebel R (2003) Mirror-symmetric tonotopic maps in human primary auditory cortex. Neuron 13;40(4):859–869.

Fox PT, Mintun MA, Raichle ME, Herscovitch P (1984) A noninvasive approach to quantitative functional brain mapping with H$_2$(15)O and positron emission tomography. J Cereb Blood Flow Metab 4(3):329–333.

Fox PT, Raichle ME (1986) Focal physiological uncoupling of cerebral blood flow and oxidative metabolism during somatosensory stimulation in human subjects. Proc Natl Acad Sci USA 83(4):1140–1144.

Gregg NM, White BR, Zeff BW, Berger AJ, Culver JP (2010) Brain specificity of diffuse optical imaging: improvements from superficial signal regression and tomography. Front Neuroenerget 2:14.

Hatsopoulos NG, Donoghue JP (2009) The science of neural interface systems. Annu Rev Neurosci 32:249–266.

Hermes D, Miller KJ, Vansteensel MJ, Aarnoutse EJ, Leijten FSS, Ramsey NF (2011) Neurophysiologic correlates of fMRI in human motor cortex. Human Brain Mapping (Epub ahead of print june 20, 2011)

Hongo K, Kobayashi S, Okudera H, Hokama M, Nakagawa F (1995) Noninvasive cerebral optical spectroscopy: depth-resolved measurements of cerebral haemodynamics using indocyanine green. Neurol Res 17(2): 89–93.

Hyder F, Patel AB, Gjedde A, Rothman DL, Behar KL, Shulman RG (2006) Neuronal–glial glucose oxidation and glutamatergic–GABAergic function. J Cereb Blood Flow Metab (2006) 26:865–877.

Jasanoff A (2010) MRI contrast agents for functional molecular imaging of brain activity. Curr Opin Neurobiol 17(5):593–600.

Jolivet R, Magistretti PJ, Weber B (2009) Deciphering neuron-glia compartmentalization in cortical energy metabolism. Front Neuroenerg 1:4.

Jones TB, Bandettini PA, Birn RM (2008) Integration of motion correction and physiological noise regression in fMRI. NeuroImage 42(2):582–590.

Kamitani Y, Tong F (2006) Decoding seen and attended motion directions from activity in the human visual cortex. Curr Biol 16:1096–1102.

Kwong HK, Belliveau JW, Chesler DA, Goldberg IE, Weiskoff RM, Poncelet BP, Kennedy DN, Hoppel BE, Cohen MS, Turner R, Cheng H, Brady TJ, Rosen BP (1992) Dynamic magnetic resonance imaging of human brain activity during primary sensory stimulation. Proc Natl Acad Sci USA 89:5675–5679.

Leuthardt EC, Freudenberg Z, Bundy D, Roland J (2009) Microscale recording from human motor cortex: implications for minimally invasive electrocorticographic brain-computer interfaces. Neurosurg Focus 27(1):E10.

Logothetis NK (2008) What we can do and what we cannot do with fMRI. Nature 453(7197):869–878.

McRobbie DW, Moore EA, Graves MJ, Prince MR (2007) MRI, from picture to proton. Cambridge: Cambridge University Press.

Miyawaki Y, Uchida H, Yamashita O, Sato MA, Morito Y, Tanabe HC, Sadato N, Kamitani Y (2008) Visual image reconstruction from human brain activity using a combination of multiscale local image decoders. Neuron 60(5):915–929.

Monti MM, Vanhaudenhuyse A, Coleman MR, Boly M, Pickard JD, Tshibanda L, Owen AM, Laureys S (2010) Willful modulation of brain activity in disorders of consciousness. N Engl J Med 362(7):579–589.

Ogawa S, Lee TM, Kay AR, Tank DW (1990) Brain magnetic resonance imaging with contrast dependent on blood oxygenation. Proc Natl Acad Sci USA. 87(24):9868–9872.

O'Rahilly RR, Müller F, Carpenter SJ, Swenson RS (2004) Basic human anatomy. http://www.dartmouth.edu/~humananatomy.

Petridou N, Plenz D, Silva AC, Loew M, Bodurka J, Bandettini PA (2006) Direct magnetic resonance detection of neuronal electrical activity. Proc Natl Acad Sci USA. 103(43):16015–16020.

Ramsey NF, Hoogduin H, Jansma JM (2002) Functional MRI experiments: acquisition, analysis and interpretation of data. Eur Neuropsychopharmacol. 12(6):517–526.

Ramsey NF, van de Heuvel MP, Kho KH, Leijten FS (2006) Towards human BCI applications based on cognitive brain systems: an investigation of neural signals recorded from the dorsolateral prefrontal cortex. IEEE Trans Neural Syst Rehabil Eng 14(2):214–217.

Robitaille PM, Berliner LJ (2006) Ultra high field magnetic resonance imaging. Berlin: Spinger.

Siero JCW, Petridou N, Hoogduin H, Luijten PR, Ramsey NF (2011) Cortical depth-dependent temporal dynamics of the BOLD response in the human brain. J Cereb Bloodflow Metab (Epub ahead of print april 20, 2011)

Stroobant N, Vingerhoets G (2000). Transcranial Doppler ultrasonography monitoring of cerebral hemodynamics during performance of cognitive tasks. A review. Neuropsychol Rev 10, 213–231.

Tai YF, Piccini P (2004) Applications of positron emission tomography (PET) in neurology. J Neurol Neurosurg Psychiatry 75:669–676.

Toronov VY, Zhang X, Webb AG (2007) A spatial and temporal comparison of hemodynamic signals measured using optical and functional magnetic resonance imaging during activation in the human primary visual cortex. NeuroImage 34:1136–1148.

Tsunashima H, Yanagisawa K (2009) Measurement of brain function of car driver using functional near-infrared spectroscopy (fNIRS). Comp Intell Neurosci, Article 164958.

Villringer A, Chance B (1997) Non-invasive optical spectroscopy and imaging of human brain function. Trends Neurosci 20(10):435–442.

Villringer A, Planck J, Hock C, Schleinkofer L, Dirnagl U (1993) Near infrared spectroscopy (NIRS): a new tool to study hemodynamic changes during activation of brain function in human adults. Neurosci Lett 14;154 (1–2):101–104.

Wolpaw JR, Birbaumer N, McFarland DJ, Pfurtscheller G, Vaughan TM (2002) Brain–computer interfaces for communication and control. Clin Neurophysiol 113:767–791.

Zhu H, Edden RAE, Ouwerkerk R, Barker PB (2011) High resolution spectroscopic imaging of GABA at 3 Tesla. Magn Reson Med 65:603–609.

PART III. | BCI DESIGN, IMPLEMENTATION, AND OPERATION

5 | ACQUIRING BRAIN SIGNALS FROM WITHIN THE BRAIN

KEVIN J. OTTO, KIP A. LUDWIG, AND DARYL R. KIPKE

The *neural interface* component of a brain-computer interface (BCI) is the hardware device that detects brain signals so they can be sent to other components of the BCI for analysis and translation into useful commands. Since different BCI systems record different brain signals from different areas at different resolutions either noninvasively or invasively and use them to control different types of effectors (e.g., computer cursor, switch, robotic arm), it is inevitable that BCI designs and functional requirements vary over a broad range. The design and functional requirements of a particular BCI are driven by the BCI's intended use and its intended target population, people with severe disabilities. A BCI system that provides cursor control for people with amyotrophic lateral sclerosis will have a much different design and different functional requirements from one that is to control an anthropomorphic arm and hand for an otherwise able-bodied amputee.

One of the major challenges in designing BCI systems is to develop effective and versatile neural interfaces to detect the neural signals that then undergo signal transduction to support the BCI system's functional requirements. To accomplish this, several primary requirements must be met:

- the interface must be safe
- the neural signals must have sufficient information to support BCI use
- the interface must be reliable
- the degree of invasiveness must not exceed what is absolutely necessary

In light of these requirements, research and development of neural interface technologies have been guided by the broad strategic goal of improving information content and reliability, while minimizing risk and complexity. Since the characteristics of the neural interface often become the rate-limiting factor in a BCI's performance, careful and appropriate design of the neural interface is critical.

BCI neural interfaces currently fall into three major classes:

- electroencephalographic (EEG) scalp electrode arrays that attach noninvasively to the skin to record field potentials with relatively low information content from very large and widely distributed sets of neurons and synapses
- electrocorticographic (ECoG) electrode arrays that are surgically positioned on the brain surface to record field potentials with moderate information content from smaller more localized sets of neurons and synapses
- miniaturized *microelectrode arrays* that are surgically inserted into the cerebral cortex to record neuronal action potentials (spikes) from individual neurons and/or local field potentials (LFPs) from small highly localized sets of neurons and synapses and that yield high information content.

The typical strategy in engineering a neural interface is to strive for the least invasive type that can provide brain signals with information content sufficient for controlling the effector with the required reliability, safety, longevity, and cost-effectiveness (Wolpaw et al. 2002; Wolpaw 2004).

This chapter focuses on *intracortical* BCI neural interfaces that use microelectrode arrays permanently implanted in movement-related areas of cerebral cortex to record from (and possibly also to stimulate) individual neurons or local populations of neurons. A *microelectrode array* is designed to penetrate into the cerebral cortex and be positioned in close proximity to the targeted neuronal population. The term *microelectrode array*, or sometimes just *microelectrode*, is used as the general term to refer to any of several types of implantable, multisite recording microelectrodes, including microwire arrays, Utah electrode arrays, and Michigan arrays.

A microelectrode array detects the neural signals that are then sent to other components of the BCI system for processing. Thus, the microelectrode array is the intracortical BCI's *signal transduction component*. To create a complete intracortical BCI neural interface system, the microelectrode arrays must be integrated with highly specialized low-power electronics for signal conditioning and communication, flexible multichannel cables to connect the microelectrode and electronics, and associated hermetic packaging to protect the electronics and interconnects. The underlying premise driving development of microscale neural interfaces for BCI systems is that these interfaces can ultimately record neural signals with the high information content needed for control of high-dimensionality prosthetic limbs and associated effectors.

Design of useful microscale interfaces for implantation in the brain is particularly challenging because the microenvironment surrounding the interface is exquisitely sensitive to the properties of the microelectrode. Adverse tissue responses can occur, and the physiological states of nearby neurons and local neuronal networks can be affected. To be of practical use, an implanted microelectrode must be reliable and long lasting, and must function with high fidelity and with little adverse tissue reaction.

Although engineering BCI intracortical neural interfaces presents many challenges, a viable path for achieving this goal exists. This path is based on current understanding of microscale neural interfaces and implantable microelectrodes, biological information about the brain tissue surrounding microscale implants, and ongoing progress in the sophisticated neurotechnology underlying implantable devices.

The outlook has brightened over the last 5-10 years through steady advances in the collective understanding of microscale neural interfaces and high-quality microelectrode technologies. Advanced next-generation microelectrode technologies and materials are enabling new strategies and paradigms that have the potential to avoid both biological failure (i.e., tissue damage or poor functionality) and device failure. These approaches make it more probable that performance can achieve the ideal of 100% of the electrode sites working 100% of the time for multiple decades in an individual using a high-dimensional BCI.

This chapter describes and discusses the current state of intracortical neural interface technologies for BCI applications. The first section provides an overview of the various intracortical microelectrode technologies now in use and under continuing development. The second section discusses the basic principles of extracellular neural recording and microelectrode-array design and analysis. The third section discusses the performance of current types of implantable microelectrode arrays. The fourth section discusses the local brain tissue responses associated with these devices. The final section discusses strategies for improving implantable microelectrode performance through advanced designs and technologies.

OVERVIEW OF IMPLANTABLE MICROELECTRODES FOR BCIs

The fundamental technical requirement for an intracortical BCI neural interface is the ability to record neuronal spike activity and/or LFPs from the target neural population with sufficient quality, information content, stability, reliability, and longevity to meet the needs of the BCI system. Intracortical interfaces are of particular interest because they may be the best method for acquiring the high-information content signals needed for applications such as controlling a robotic arm with multiple degrees of freedom.

The various types of actual and proposed intracortical BCI interfaces have developed largely from the rich history of implantable microelectrodes used in neuroscience research dating back over 60 years. In the 1950s, Strumwasser (1958) implanted several 80-μm stainless-steel wires into the reticular formation of squirrels and recorded multiunit spike activity for 4 days. This approach was later improved by etching smaller-diameter (30-μm) platinum wires to a sharpened tip, enabling single-unit recordings for over 3 days, and functional implant durations of 3 months (Burns et al. 1973). Although it was

hypothesized that the small diameter of these platinum microelectrodes would provide better single-neuron recording, their fragility prevented pia mater penetration; and a harpoon-like wire was needed to mechanically stiffen the microelectrode during insertion. The first successful chronic microelectrode arrays consisted of five insulated tungsten microwires etched to sharpened tips bundled in plastic tubing (Marg and Adams 1967). Although these devices provided more control of electrode spacing and implantation, their fabrication was fairly labor intensive, and there was high manufacturing variability. The seminal studies in direct brain control with intracortical signals used microwire arrays of this kind (Fetz 1969; Schmidt et al. 1977).

GENERAL CHARACTERISTICS OF MICROELECTRODE ARRAYS

There is now a reasonably well-developed design space for chronic microelectrode arrays in terms of materials, fabrication technologies, packages, and component integration. In the categorization scheme depicted in figure 5.1, a given microelectrode array is first categorized by whether it is designed and fabricated using bundles of microwires or through micro-electro-mechanical systems (MEMS) microfabrication processes, a broad class of technologies involving microfabrication of silicon and polymer structures for miniaturized sensors, actuators, and integrated microsystems. MEMS microelectrode arrays are micro-machined at wafer level from silicon and/or polymer substrates, whereas microwire arrays are assembled from individual microwires. A microelectrode array is further categorized by the details of its fabrication process (e.g., planar, thin-film, or a bulk micro-machined MEMS process), its materials (e.g., platinum or iridium electrode sites, polymer or inorganic dielectric), and its assembly/packaging. Various microelectrode array designs have been validated to varying degrees through research use in animals and/or early clinical testing of intracortical BCIs in humans. Several of these designs are described in this chapter in more detail.

To understand the functional requirements of microelectrode arrays and how these requirements are met by different types of devices, it is useful to consider a canonical microelectrode array that has the following five primary functional components.

- An array of *electrode sites* (or *contacts*) that are the location of biopotential signal transduction for recording. The sites are in direct contact with brain tissue and support charge transfer and capacitive current at their surface. The most important factors in determining their electrical characteristics are the site material and the area, roughness, and shape of the contact surface.

- The *lead* (or *trace*) that electrically connects the electrode site to the separate electronics interface. The lead is buried in the dielectrics

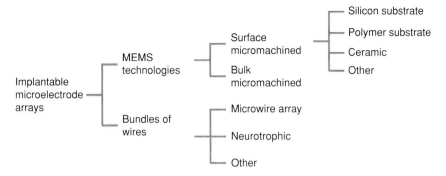

Figure 5.1 Taxonomy of common implantable microelectrode arrays for BCI neural interfaces, based on their primary fabrication method and primary material. The first level differentiates between bundles of microwires and MEMS technologies. The second and third levels involve progressively more specialized processes and materials.

(see next item) and does not come into direct contact with tissue. Its primary requirements are: a sufficiently low resistance to minimize signal loss between the electrode contact and the electronics; sufficient flexibility and robustness to avoid both breakage and mechanical stress on the electrode contact; a compatible and consistent fabrication process; and negligible corrosion or cytotoxicity if the surrounding dielectric covering is partially or fully breached.

- The *dielectric,* which is the material, or composite material, that electrically insulates each individual lead from the surrounding tissue. The primary requirements are to maintain sufficiently high electrical insulation between the lead and the surrounding tissue and to have sufficient flexibility, strength, and robustness to remain intact for long implant times. The dielectric is generally characterized by its dielectric constant, leakage resistance, and shunt capacitance, as well as the degree to which it degrades over time in tissue. Although it may be acceptable for dielectric characteristics to change over time, the changes must be predictable and not cause significant loss of function (e.g., a conductance path to tissue).

- The *substrate*, which is the component that provides the structural integrity of each tine or shank of the electrode array. Not all types of microelectrode arrays have a distinct substrate component; in some cases the dielectric material and/or the leads provide both electrical insulation and structural support. The substrate can also provide an additional moisture barrier between the dielectric layer and tissue.

- Optional surface *coatings*, which may be used to modify particular electrical, mechanical, or biological characteristics of a microelectrode array. Typically, a microelectrode's substrate/ dielectric and its electrode sites are in contact

with the brain, and the substrate/dielectric surface area is usually significantly larger than the total surface area of all the electrode sites. A functionalized dielectric coating may be used to provide an additional moisture barrier between the tissue and the lead, to fine-tune device-tissue interface properties (e.g., roughness or lubricity), or to attenuate or control tissue reactions. Additionally, an electrode site coating can be used to fine-tune the electrical characteristics of the site (e.g., to lower its impedance, to sense neurochemicals, or to deliver small doses of drugs).

These five primary components are interrelated through materials, fabrication process compatibility, and application requirements. For example, high-temperature silicon-oxide and silicon-nitride thin films are often suitable long-term dielectrics, but the high temperature at which these films must be deposited precludes the use of metal leads (or traces). The alternative is to use conductive polysilicon traces, but the tradeoff is that polysilicon has higher resistivity than thin-film metals.

MICROWIRE ARRAYS

Microwire arrays (fig. 5.2) continue to be a very important technology for intracortical BCI neural interfaces. There are many approaches to making microwire arrays, all of which take the approach of assembling small-diameter (usually 10–100 μm) insulated wires into structured bundles. The precision and consistency of the bundle vary with the intricacy of the assembly process. In these arrays, the recording sites are the exposed tips of the individual microwires. The wires are typically made of tungsten, platinum, or platinum/iridium with a thin insulating coating of parylene, epoxylite, or Teflon™. Although the microwire itself is a mature technology, notable innovations have been made in the methods for fabricating more precise arrays with more microwires (Nicolelis and Ribeiro 2002; Nicolelis et al. 2003; Williams et al. 1999), for machining the wire tips (Bullara et al. 1983), and for producing "floating" arrays (i.e., arrays that are not rigidly anchored to

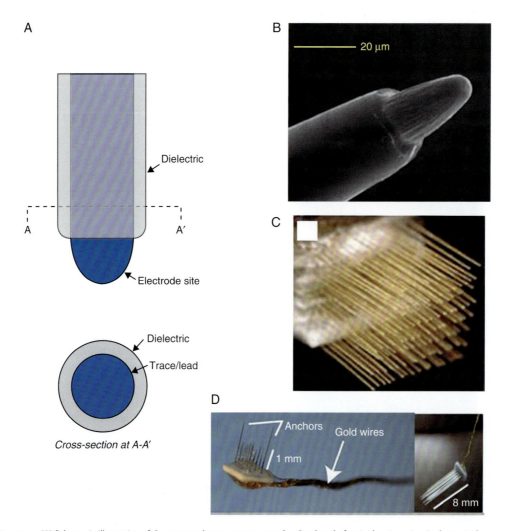

Figure 5.2 Microwire arrays. (A) Schematic illustration of the structural components near the distal end of a single microwire. In the typical case, the uninsulated tip of the microwire is the electrode site; the insulated aspect of the microwire serves as the interconnect component; and the insulative coating is the dielectric layer. Microwires do not have a separate substrate component. (B) Scanning electron micrograph of the tip of a typical platinum-iridium (PtIr) microwire formed through laser ablation of the insulation at the tip and electrochemical shaping of the tip (Cogan 2008). (C) Bundle of precisely arranged microwires forming a Microwire arrays (Nicolelis et al. 2003). (D) Microwire arrays with a ceramic platform and multiwire gold interconnect to create a "floating" implantable array for recording and stimulating (Musallam et al. 2007).

bone or dura) (Musallam et al. 2007; Rennaker et al. 2005). Twisted microwires (i.e., two microwires to form a stereotrode, or four wires to form a tetrode) (Gray et al. 1995; McNaughton et al. 1983) are used extensively in neuroscience research to create a cluster of multiple, closely spaced sites at the end of a single multistrand wire. Tetrodes have not been emphasized in BCI research because clustered sites are not thought to significantly improve the recording of unit activity from the target pyramidal cells in the cerebral cortex (due to the size of these cells and their moderate packing compared to other parts of the brain). Nevertheless, the tetrode configuration does improve single-unit discrimination in some areas of the brain, such as the hippocampus.

NEUROTROPIC (CONE) ELECTRODE

The *neurotrophic electrode* (also called the *cone* electrode) is a particular class of microwire-based electrode with a unique bioactive design strategy that induces neuronal processes to grow close to the microwires (Brumberg et al. 2010; Kennedy 1989). The neurotrophic electrode consists of several microwires inserted into a small glass cone that is open on both ends and filled with a neurotrophic material. When this electrode assembly is implanted in cerebral cortex, neuronal processes grow, over several weeks, into and through the cone so that a few neuronal processes are close to the microwires within the cone (Kennedy et al. 1992). The neurotrophic design concept is unique among microelectrode technologies in that the cone creates a relatively closed environment for the neural interface and that the neurotrophic material induces targeted neuronal plasticity to establish a long-term, bioactive neural interface. Although neurotropic electrodes record reliably and with high signal quality, their disadvantage compared to higher channel-count microelectrode arrays is that each electrode assembly records from relatively few neurons.

MEMS-BASED MICROELECTRODES

MEMS-based microelectrodes include the Utah electrode array, the Michigan-style probe, and others. MEMS technology represents a broad class of technologies involving microfabrication of silicon and polymer structures for miniaturized sensors, actuators, and integrated microsystems. MEMS-based methods use significantly different microfabrication technologies from microwire arrays to create various types of implantable microelectrode arrays that are functionally equivalent to microwire arrays in terms of neural recording and stimulation. MEMS technologies use a broad range of conductive and dielectric materials to make microelectrode arrays in many sizes and architectures. These can be fabricated with high precision and consistency. The microfabrication and assembly of MEMS arrays is generally more complex than that of microwire arrays. These processes involve detailed sequences of selective deposition or removal of patterned thin films of conductive or dielectric materials on a substrate, and/or bulk micromachining of materials through etching, grinding, or sawing.

UTAH ELECTRODE ARRAY

The *Utah electrode array* (fig. 5.3) is a well-known MEMS microelectrode array that has been systematically developed and refined over nearly 20 years (Bhandari et al. 2010; Campbell et al. 1991; S. Kim et al. 2009). At present, it is probably the most widely used type of implantable microelectrode array for intracortical BCI neural interfaces. This device is fabricated by micro-machining monocrystalline silicon blocks to form an archetypal bed-of-nails architecture (fig. 5.3). Each rigid conical shank (or *tine*) of the Utah array has approximately one conical recording site at its tip, making it functionally similar to a single microwire. In earlier versions of Utah arrays the site material was platinum and the dielectric was polyimide (Campbell et al. 1991), but recent fabrication developments have now transitioned to sputtered iridium oxide and parylene (Bhandari et al. 2010). The typical arrangement is a 10×10 array of tines, with tine lengths of 1.5–2.0 mm, regularly spaced at 400 μm, resulting in a 4 mm × 4 mm footprint on the cortical surface. The Utah array is typically attached to skull-mounted interface electronics (Nurmikko et al. 2010), to a connector through a thin wire cable (Rousche and Normann 1998), or to an electronics chip attached directly to the bond pads (S. Kim et al. 2009). The array is surgically implanted into cortex using a well-described surgical procedure and a specialized, high-velocity inserter (Rousche and Normann 1992). The Utah array has extended the design space of comparable microwire arrays

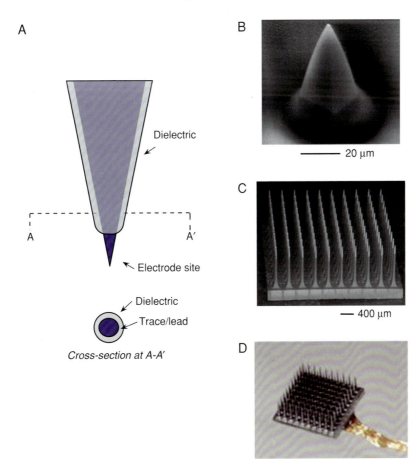

Figure 5.3 The Utah electrode array (UEA). (A) Schematic illustration of the structural components near the distal end of a single tine of the UEA. The uninsulated tip of the doped silicon tine is the electrode site; the insulated aspect of the tine serves as the interconnect component; the thin-film parylene coating and silicon nitride are the dielectric component; the silicon tine itself is the substrate. (B) Scanning electron micrograph of the tip of a UEA tine (Bhandari et al. 2010). (C) Scanning electron micrograph of the bottom (brain) side of the typical 10 × 10 UEA (100 tines, with 400-μm separation) illustrating the "bed of nails" structure (Bhandari et al. 2010). (D) UEA bonded to multiwire gold interconnect cable to create a "floating" implantable array for intracortical recording and stimulation (Donoghue et al. 2007).

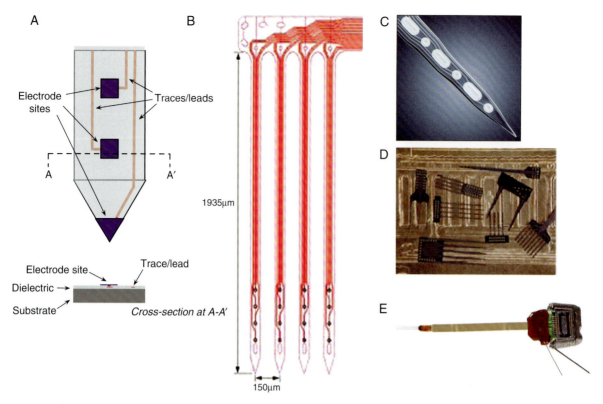

Figure 5.4 *The planar Michigan-style electrode array. (A) Schematic illustration of the structural components near the distal end of a single shank of a typical planar Michigan-style electrode. The electrodes are a thin layer of metal sites at prescribed positions along the shank. Thin-film polysilicon or metal traces connect each electrode site to a separate bond pad at the back end of the probe. The traces are buried in thin-film inorganic (typically silicon nitride and/or silicon dioxide) and/or organic layers that comprise the dielectric component. The silicon back side of the electrode is the substrate. (B) Design layout of a typical Michigan electrode having four shanks, each with four sites. (C) Scanning electron micrograph of the tip of a shank on a Michigan electrode showing six precisely arranged electrode sites. (D) Examples of eight different site and shank designs for intracortical recording. (E) Michigan-style electrode array connected to a flexible thin-film polymer ribbon cable to create a "floating" implantable array for intracortical recording and stimulation. (Courtesy of NeuroNexus, Ann Arbor, MI.)*

through its very precise and reproducible geometry and packaging. Thus, for example, tine lengths, intertine spacing, and total tine number may be readily varied. A clinical-grade version of the Utah array was used in a seminal study of intracortical BCIs in humans (Hochberg et al. 2006), and a number of animal studies describe the use and performance of the Utah array in chronic cortical recording (Suner et al. 2005) and stimulation applications (Rousche and Normann 1999).

MICHIGAN-STYLE PROBE

The *Michigan-style probe* (fig. 5.4) is another well-known type of MEMS microelectrode array. The seminal *Michigan* probe is a planar device having a boron-diffused silicon substrate, a silicon dioxide and silicon nitride dielectric stack, polysilicon traces, and iridium electrode sites (Anderson et al. 1989; BeMent et al. 1986; Hetke et al. 1990; Najafi et al. 1990; Wise et al. 1970; Wise and Angell 1975; Wise et al. 2004). Through a sustained development program, this base MEMS technology has since been expanded to broader types of electrode designs, materials, and microfabrication techniques to result today in a broad-based Michigan-style microelectrode platform technology that is used in a wide range of neural structures for diverse neural interface applications.

In the canonical form, the Michigan-style probe technology creates an array of planar electrode sites on thin (i.e., nominally

5–50 μm thick) planar penetrating shanks (fig. 5.4A,B). The probes are fabricated through lithographic patterning of thin films of dielectrics and conductors on a silicon substrate to form very precise arrays of recording (and/or stimulation) sites. An integrated or separate thin-film ribbon cable, or interconnect, is bonded to the penetrating probe to connect to another connector or to an electronics interface. This technology has a broad design space that allows designs that have almost any reasonable one-, two-, or three-dimensional layout of electrode sites across one or more planar shanks. Michigan-style probes offer unique advantages over alternative types of electrode technologies. These include greater site-packing density, reduced tissue displacement per site, reproducibility, and precise two- and three-dimensional geometries. Michigan-style probe technologies have been successfully commercialized and validated in neuroscience research. The in-vivo performance of various types of Michigan probes is well described (e.g., Csicsvari et al. 2003; Drake et al. 1988b; Kipke et al. 1991; Ludwig et al. 2006; Vetter et al. 2004a), and ongoing development is directed at translating this technology for clinical applications, including BCI systems.

OTHER MEMS-BASED PROBES

Since the seminal Michigan probe first established the feasibility of planar, thin-film microelectrode arrays (Drake et al.

1988), the broad class of photolithographically defined, planar MEMS technology has been advanced by a number of research groups (Han and McCreery 2008; Kewley et al. 1997; Kovacs et al. 1994; McCarthy et al. 2011a; McCarthy et al. 2011b; McCreery et al. 2007; Moxon et al. 2004; Muthuswamy et al. 2005; Neves 2007). There are now various microfabrication processes, assembly technologies, and integrated microsystems that significantly expand the design space of this class of micro-electrode array technology.

Interest in developing implantable microelectrode arrays that are more flexible and robust than thin silicon probes has motivated the development of thin-film polymer and hybrid polymer-silicon microelectrode arrays (Fernandez et al. 2009; Guo et al. 2010; Lee et al. 2004a; Rousche et al. 2001; Schuettler et al. 2005; Seymour and Kipke 2007; Seymour et al. 2009; Seymour et al. 2011; Stieglitz et al. 2000; Yu et al. 2009). It has been suggested that the lower elastic modulus improves the flexibility of these materials to reduce the elastic mismatch with brain tissue and provide enhanced compliance that may minimize the motion of the device relative to the surrounding cortex (Lee et al. 2005; Subbaroyan et al. 2005). As discussed in this chapter, this approach may help to reduce the reactive tissue response (Fernandez et al. 2009; Mercanzini et al. 2008).

In sum, over the past two decades it has become clear that chronic intracortical neural recording is both technologically feasible and useful for basic neuroscience studies and in neuro-prosthetic applications and that microelectrode technologies make this possible. The current challenges are to increase reliability, longevity, and signal fidelity, as well as overall safety.

BASIC CONCEPTS OF NEURAL RECORDING WITH CHRONICALLY IMPLANTED MICROELECTRODES

No matter what the source of the brain signals or the recording techniques on which a BCI is based, a BCI's efficacy is a function of the *quality* of the recorded neural signals used as an input to the system. In this context it is useful to consider the *fidelity* of the neural recording, that is, the extent to which the characteristics of the recorded signal match the underlying neuronal signal source(s). In the simplest formulation, maximizing the information content of the cortical-control signal for input to a BCI is an exercise in attaining sufficient neural recording fidelity.

The overall strategy to attain sufficient fidelity of chronic extracellular neural recording is to maximize and maintain sensing of the neuronal signals of interest by the electrodes and to reduce the obscuring sources of noise. This involves using microelectrode arrays that have sufficient selectivity, sensitivity, and stability to record large-amplitude signals from the targeted neuronal populations, while also minimizing the interfering and additive noise sources. To address this issue effectively, it is important to understand how a recording microelectrode registers signals, the factors that influence neuronal signal characteristics in chronic neural recordings, and the factors that influence the contributions of noise sources in these recordings.

HOW A RECORDING MICROELECTRODE REGISTERS SIGNALS

The biopotential at the electrode surface is the combined result of neural signal sources in the vicinity of the electrode site that are conducted through the encompassing brain tissue from their points of origin to the electrode surface (Bretschneider and De Weille 2006). The neural signal sources are membrane currents that underlie action potentials and synaptic potentials among the neurons of interest. Brain tissue is a volume conductor that, to a first approximation, is assumed to be linear, resistive, and homogeneous, but not necessarily isotropic (see chapter 3, this volume). The numerous sources and sinks from active neurons (and glia cells) within a brain region are assumed to combine linearly to create a fluctuating electric field that is sampled by the small area of the electrode site. For implanted electrodes the biopotential characteristics (e.g., spike amplitudes and waveforms and local field potential spectra) may be affected by reactive tissue responses that develop over time and that change the local tissue conductivity. They can also be affected by neuronal damage, degeneration, or morphology changes that may develop from the presence of the microelectrode array.

The biopotential at the microelectrode site is transduced to an electronic current in the electrode trace by complex, but well-described electrochemical processes at the electrode-tissue interface (Cogan 2008; Merrill et al. 2005; Robinson 1968). This signal transduction occurs through two types of reversible electrode-electrolyte interface currents. The first is a capacitive displacement current resulting from the intrinsic capacitance of the electrode-tissue interface. The second is a chemical current resulting from intrinsic oxidation-reduction reactions at the electrode surface. Extracellular spike recording occurs mainly through capacitive currents because of the small amount of charge displacement in the small and fast extracellular spikes. Extracellular action potentials have amplitudes of about 50–500 µV and bandwidth of about 500–5000 Hz. Local field potentials relevant to BCIs have amplitudes of about 10–800 µV and bandwidth of about 0.1–200 Hz. Recording local field potentials may, in general, involve both capacitive displacement currents and oxidation-reduction currents depending on the bandwidth and amplitude of the signals.

The lumped-element functional model shown in figure 5.5 provides useful representations of the primary functional elements of chronic extracellular neural recording. This model represents extracellular recording from K neurons using an electrode array containing L electrode sites and a separate electrode site to provide the voltage reference signal. Each recording channel has three functional submodels arranged in series (see fig. 5.5A): *biopotential sensing* to represent the summation of biopotentials within the recording volume of an electrode site; *neural interface tissue impedance* to represent the conductivity of the local tissue surrounding an electrode site; and an *electrode-tissue interface* to represent electrochemical and electrical characteristics of the electrode.

In its simplest formulation (fig. 5.5A), the *biopotential-sensing submodel* can be considered as a summation node to linearly combine neural sources scaled by source amplitude and inverse distance from the electrode. A higher level of detail would also include integration of biopotentials across the electrode site, which becomes important when considering recording selectivity and sensitivity. Note that in this treatment, the electrode site is *not* considered to be a simple point but rather a surface having a particular geometric surface area. (This is important, because, for example, a 750 μm^2 circular site has a diameter of 30 μm, which is a significant dimension relative to the size, location, and packing density of neurons, and the distribution of charge on the electrode surface.) Intrinsic neural noise that results from neural activity that is either too small or too distant to be identified or that is unrelated to BCI control is represented by the $V_{neu\text{-}ns}$ input to the summation node. Extrinsic biological noise associated with voltage perturbations caused by muscle activation (e.g., electromyographic activity [EMG] from cranial or extraocular muscles), by eye movements (electrooculographic activity [EOG]), by heartbeats (electrocardiographic activity [ECG]), and motion artifacts are represented by the lumped input, $V_{bio\text{-}ns}$.

The *neural interface tissue impedance submodel* (fig. 5.5B) represents the tissue impedance surrounding an electrode site due to the localized reactive tissue response. Although the extent of the localized tissue impedance variations and the corresponding effects on chronic neural recordings are not fully understood, the model in figure 5.5B captures two of the observed characteristics of tissue impedance: a resistive component associated with conductance pathways in the extracellular space and a complex impedance component associated with cellular encapsulation around the electrode site.

The biopotential signal transduction at the *electrode-tissue interface* and transmission of the resulting electronic signal through the electrode traces to the electronics interface are represented with the lumped-element equivalent circuit submodel shown in figure 5.5C (Merrill et al. 2005; Robinson 1968). The voltage source, E_{hc}, represents the half-cell potential of the electrode-tissue interface. The capacitor, C_{dl}, represents the double layer capacitance. The resistor, R_{ct}, represents the resistance to the transfer of charge that occurs through Faradaic currents. The constant phase element (CPE) impedance represents charge-transfer variations resulting from the surface morphology of the electrode site and the ion-diffusion nonlinearities in the diffusion region. The resistor, R_s, represents the resistance to ion movement in the diffusion region. The capacitor, C_{sh}, and resistor, R_{sh}, represent the *shunt or leakage pathways* from the insulated electrode traces to the bulk tissue. The resistor, R_t, represents the resistance in the electrode trace from the electrode site to electronics interface. The voltage source, $v_{elec\text{-}ns}$, represents the lumped electrode intrinsic noise sources that arise from several biophysical and electrical phenomena. The primary source is associated with the electrode-tissue interface and caused by Brownian motion of electrons, drift and diffusion of charged ions due to concentration gradients, and oxidation/reduction reactions occurring at the electrode/electrolyte interface (Hassibi et al. 2004; Kovacs 1994; Robinson 1968; Schmidt and Humphrey 1990; Shoham and Nagarajan 2003). The magnitude of the noise depends on the site material, size, and surface morphology, and contamination.

Additional noise sources include random fluctuations and instability in the half-cell potential caused by disturbances of the double-layer capacitance and contamination of the electrode surface, thermal noise (also referred to as Johnson or Nyquist noise) due to the random motion of electrons in the electrode trace, and frequency-dependent 1/f noise (also referred to as flicker or pink noise). To a reasonable first approximation, these noise sources can be modeled as thermal (Johnson, 2005) noise and represented by the voltage source, $v_{elec\text{-}ns} = (4kTZ\Delta f)^{0.5}$, where k is Boltzmann's constant, T is Kelvin temperature, Z is electrode magnitude impedance, and Δf is the frequency range of interest.

This functional systems-level model of extracellular neural recording is useful for associating electrode performance characteristics, such as recording selectivity, sensitivity, and signal-to-noise ratios, with electrode design and usage parameters, such as electrode site size, electrode materials, and placement of electrode sites within the targeted brain region. However, the model's structure and assumptions do not map directly to underlying detailed biophysical mechanisms (e.g., biopotential sampling, resistive paths through the neural interface, and electrode site morphology are interrelated with complex spatial and electrical characteristics). More sophisticated models require finite-element analysis of the neural sources, neural interface tissue impedance, and electrode-electrolyte interface.

FACTORS THAT INFLUENCE NEURAL SIGNAL FIDELITY IN CHRONIC NEURAL RECORDINGS

In the context of electrode design and analysis, neural signal fidelity can be considered in terms of general sensor attributes of *sensitivity*, *selectivity*, and *stability*.

Recording sensitivity can be defined as the ratio of the differential change in the recorded signal (i.e., V_{e2} in fig. 5.5A) to a differential change in the underlying signal source (i.e., V_{neu}). Under this definition, the maximum sensitivity is 1 (i.e., all differential charge of an input spike is transduced to the differential charge of an output spike in the electrode trace). Sensitivity varies inversely with electrode site size because the relative contribution of any one targeted neural signal source in the transduced signal generally decreases as biopotentials are integrated across a larger site area. Sensitivity is also affected by the shunt pathway (C_{sh} and R_{sh}), resistive losses in the tissue (R_{int} and R_s), and resistive losses in the electrode trace (R_t).

Recording selectivity can be defined as the degree to which an electrode preferentially records a targeted group of neuron signal sources and excludes unwanted neural signal sources. As such, selectivity varies inversely with electrode site size because a larger sensing area will tend to integrate biopotentials from more neural signal sources.

Recording stability can be defined as the degree to which the functional characteristics of the electrode array—including biopotential sensing, neural interface tissue impedance, and electrode-tissue interface components—do not change over time. Well-designed electrodes have relatively stable electrode-tissue interface characteristics (which suggests that recording

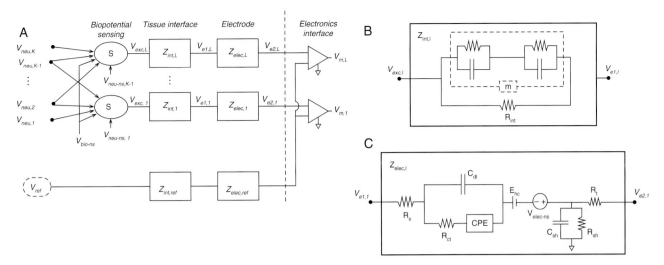

Figure 5.5 *Lumped-element functional models of neural recording with a microelectrode array. (A) System model of extracellular neural recording from K neurons with an electrode array with L channels. The three components for each channel are biopotential sensing (S), tissue interface impedance ($Z_{int,j}$), and electrode equivalent impedance ($Z_{elec,j}$) (note that j can range from 1 to L). (B) Lumped-element equivalent circuit for impedance changes in the neural interface associated with reactive tissue responses. This model incorporates adjacent cellular layers of glia and macrophages as a membrane capacitance, a membrane conductance resistance, and a membrane area-scaling term (m) related to encapsulation thickness and cell-to-cell adhesion within the cellular layer. The extracellular pathway between cells is defined as a resistance. (C) Lumped-element equivalent circuit for the microelectrode site. R_s, access resistance of the site; C_{dl}, the double-layer capacitance; R_{ct}, the charge-transfer resistance; CPE (constant phase element), the generalized phase shift (time delay) associated with site morphology, diffusion limitations, and associated interface complexities; voltage source E_{hc}, half-cell potential of the electrode-electrolyte interface; $v_{elec-ns}$, additive noise sources in the interface; C_{sh}, shunt capacitance; R_{sh}, leakage resistance; R_t, electrode trace resistance.*

stability depends mainly on the Biopotential Sensing and Tissue Interface blocks shown in fig. 5.5). Stability can be affected by variability in the neural signal source, which can occur if a neuron is damaged or degenerates, or undergoes morphological or electrophysiological changes. It can also be affected by time-varying changes in reactive tissue responses around the electrode.

Thus, the basic strategy for optimizing neural signal fidelity is to design electrodes to have sufficient sensitivity, selectivity, and stability to maximize the contributions of neural signals of interest and minimize the contributions of the various noise sources (see next section). That is, the strategy is the familiar one of maximizing the signal-to-noise ratio. The primary factors in neural signal amplitude are the distance of the neuron from the electrode site, the magnitude and spatial distribution of its current sources and sinks, and the size of the electrode site. The largest deflections in extracellular potentials occur close to the largest membrane current, which, under typical circumstances, is assumed to be the point of origin of the action potential, the cell body/axon hillock. The extracellular potential falls off with distance from a current source as $1/r$ (i.e., with r the distance from source to electrode site). For neurons with morphology and channel distributions that approximate a localized and paired current source and sink (i.e., a current dipole, as is typically assumed for spiking cortical pyramidal cells), the extracellular interactions between source and sink lead to a fall-off in extracellular potential as roughly $1/r^2$. In addition, neurons with larger cell bodies and dendritic processes tend to have larger membrane currents compared to smaller neurons. These factors contribute to causing spike

recordings to be biased toward larger neurons over smaller neurons, and toward neurons that are closer to electrode sites over neurons that are farther from electrode sites. In order to maximize recording selectivity and sensitivity, the electrode site size should be matched to the cell sizes, cell-packing density, and current source amplitudes.

FACTORS THAT INTRODUCE NOISE IN CHRONIC RECORDINGS

Intrinsic *electrode* noise is minimized first through appropriate selection of materials and electrode design to lower the electrode impedance (i.e., noise power varies with impedance). The trace resistance can be reduced through proper selection of trace material and size, and the shunt pathways can be minimized through selection of high-quality dielectric materials (which can generally be accomplished without performance trade-offs). The double-layer capacitance and charge-transfer resistance are a function of material and site size. The spreading resistance is a function of site size. The net trade-off is that increasing site size to lower electrode impedance has the general effect of decreasing recording selectivity and sensitivity. Advanced microelectrode site materials, such as iridium oxide thin-films (Cogan et al. 2009) and conductive polymers (Abidian et al. 2010; Abidian et al. 2009; Ludwig et al. 2011; Ludwig et al. 2006; Venkatraman et al. 2011), can significantly lower electrode impedance without changing the electrode site size.

Intrinsic neural noise sources can be minimized by increasing recording selectivity and by positioning the electrode site close to the neurons of interest. However, this generally involves minimizing the electrode site area, which usually causes higher electrode impedance (and thus, intrinsic electrode noise) and lower recording stability.

The contributions of *extrinsic biological noise* can be minimized through appropriate signal referencing and signal conditioning (Horsch and Dhillon 2004; Kovacs 1994; Linderman et al. 2006; Ludwig et al. 2009; Schmidt and Humphrey 1990; Shoham and Nagarajan 2003; Webster 1998). The importance of proper referencing is discussed extensively in chapters 3, 6, and 15 in this volume (also see Donoghue 2007). Typically, referencing is accomplished either by recording from an additional microelectrode site or by recording from a relatively large electrode positioned in a location with minimal neural activity; the recording from the additional reference is subtracted to remove correlated noise across channels (Blanche et al. 2005; Henze et al. 2000; Ludwig et al. 2009; Nelson et al. 2008; Vetter et al. 2004b; Webster 1998; Williams et al. 1999). Each type of configuration involves associated trade-offs.

An alternative solution is to use a common average reference (AVE or CAR), commonly employed in EEG to help detect small signals in very noisy recordings (Cooper et al. 2003; Offner 1950; Osselton 1965) (see chapters 6 and 7, this volume). Unlike more complex posthoc methods of removing noise from recorded signals (Aminghafari et al. 2006; Bierer and Andersen 1999; Oweiss and Anderson 2001), CAR is a computationally simple technique and therefore amenable to incorporation into the recording hardware (i.e., on-chip) and to real-time BCI applications. As its name implies, the recordings from all the microelectrodes are *averaged*, and the average is used as the reference to be subtracted from each individual site (Ludwig et al. 2009). Through the averaging process, signal or noise that is common to all sites (i.e., correlated) (e.g., 60-Hz noise or motion artifact) remains on the CAR and can thus be eliminated from each site's recording.

CHRONIC RECORDING PERFORMANCE OF INTRACORTICAL MICROELECTRODE ARRAYS

A steadily growing body of evidence indicates that reliable chronic recording of information-rich neural activity is feasible with intracortical microelectrode arrays. However, the present technologies do not yet achieve the chronic performance levels that are possible. In addition to various material- and device-related failures, biological processes also contribute substantially to the degradation of recording performance.

A concise general description of the chronic-recording performance of intracortical microelectrode arrays is challenging because of the inherent complexity and variability of chronic microscale neural interfaces and because of the difficulty of quantitatively assessing recording performance. Looking across many studies using several types of microelectrode technologies, and considering the highest-quality microelectrodes and implant techniques, four general observations emerge (Hochberg et al. 2006; Jackson and Fetz 2007; Kim

et al. 2008; Kipke et al. 2003; Liu et al. 1999; Maynard et al. 1997; McCreery et al. 2004; Nicolelis et al. 2003; Rousche and Normann 1998; Santhanam et al. 2006; Suner et al. 2005; Vetter et al. 2004b; Ward et al. 2009; Williams et al. 1999).

The first observation is that recording performance (i.e., signal longevity, reliability, and quality) generally degrades over weeks to months, such that the information-rich neural signals required for high-dimensional BCI control diminish and are eventually lost. The second is that chronic recordings over time typically do not fail completely; there are usually some remaining neural signals available across an array, typically lower-quality multineuron activity or LFPs. The third observation is that over time, neural signals from a particular microelectrode, or from a microelectrode array as a whole, are generally variable and not reliable; good and bad recording days often alternate, with little ability to predict, observe, or control the transition. The fourth observation, coming usually from anecdotal reports and representing the exception rather than the rule, is that there are particular cases in which single-neuron recording is stable, at a particular site or at least somewhere on the array, for long periods of time (i.e., one to several years).

Meaningful assessment of chronic-recording performance over time involves evaluation of several interrelated recording characteristics, including *signal quality, array yield, signal stability, recording longevity,* and *overall reliability*. Although there are not yet definitive, universally accepted quantitative measures of these characteristics, a growing literature is beginning to quantify electrode performance in these terms (Kipke et al. 2003; Liu et al. 1999; Liu et al. 2006; Nicolelis et al. 2003; Suner et al. 2005; Vetter et al. 2004a). Qualitative inferential comparisons among different types of microelectrode arrays are common, but meaningful quantitative comparisons are limited because of different experimental preparations, techniques, and analysis algorithms (Polikov et al. 2005; Suner et al. 2005; Ward et al. 2009; Williams et al. 1999). Moreover, development of relevant performance measures for recording LFPs is particularly problematic because the amplitude and bandwidth characteristics of these signals make it difficult to distinguish them from nonneural background noise. Thus, LFP recording performance is typically assessed indirectly by measuring the performance of BCIs that use these signals.

SIGNAL QUALITY

For action potential (spike) recordings, *signal quality* is typically expressed as a signal-to-noise ratio, in which the signal is defined as the amplitude of identified spikes, and the noise level is defined in terms of either the root-mean-square (RMS) level of the recording after the identified spikes are removed, or as 2–6 standard deviations from the average signal level. Signal quality is important for intracortical BCI applications because it directly affects the reliability of the spike trains (i.e., the timing of identifiable single-neuron or multineuron spike activity) that provide inputs to BCI decoding algorithms (see chapters 7, 8, 16, 17, in this volume). In typical cases, signal-to-noise ratios of about 2.5 to 4 (i.e., spike amplitudes 2.5–4.0 times higher than the RMS noise level) are interpreted as multineuron activity and accepted as the lowest useful level of spike activity. Signal-to-noise ratios greater than about 4.0 are interpreted as single-neuron activity. Most microelectrode sites with useful signals have multineuron activity or one or two discriminable single neurons plus multineuron activity.

ARRAY YIELD

The *array yield* is operationally defined as the fraction of electrodes on an array that record discriminable spike activity (or appropriate LFPs) of sufficient quality over a given time interval. Array yield is important because it measures the number of spike trains providing input to the BCI decoding algorithm. In studies in rats the daily array yield over postimplant periods of weeks to several months was typically 50–90% (Vetter et al. 2004a; Ward et al. 2009). Comparable array yields have been reported in nonhuman primate studies (Nicolelis et al. 2003; Suner et al. 2005). Initial studies of intracortical BCIs in humans showed similar daily array yields over a period of several months (Hochberg et al. 2006). Both within and across studies, the large variability in array yield reflects the current limited ability to make precise a priori assumptions about a particular level of chronic recording performance.

SIGNAL STABILITY

Signal stability can be defined as the likelihood of recording the same set of putative neurons on a given microelectrode site over specified time periods. Signal stability is important because it directly relates to the day-to-day consistency of spike discrimination settings and BCI decoding algorithms. If neural signals are highly stable, spike discrimination settings will require minimal adjustment, and decoding algorithms will receive consistent sets of inputs from day to day. Although fraught with caveats, signal stability is typically measured by tracking the consistency of brief (about 1-ms) extracellular spike waveforms, sometimes augmented with spike train statistics such as the interspike intervals (Chestek et al. 2007; Dickey et al. 2009). It is particularly difficult to confirm that day-to-day recordings of an action potential with a stable voltage-time wave shape are from the same neuron over time.

In a landmark study, Harris et al. (2000) used simultaneous intracellular recordings and extracellular tetrode recordings to investigate the reliability of manual spike sorting by experienced operators. Despite the experience of the operators and the availability of multidimensional tetrode recordings, significant rates (as high as 30%) of both Type I (false-positive) and Type II (false-negative) errors were found. Additionally, the measured waveform features of the extracellular spike waveforms were found to change up to 30% over a 24-hr period (Santhanam et al. 2007). Thus, it appears that not only are there inherent technical difficulties in recording from the putative same neuron (judged by its spike waveform), but it is also difficult to discern the discrimination errors. Nevertheless, and regardless of confidence in, or ability to, record from individual neurons over short and long time frames, significant levels of BCI control have been achieved with chronic recordings and have been found to be quite robust (Chestek et al. 2007; Ganguly and Carmena 2009; Heliot et al. 2010; Hochberg et al. 2006; Santhanam et al. 2006; Velliste et al. 2008).

LONGEVITY OF RECORDING

Recording longevity can be operationally defined as the length of time over which the neural recordings maintain consistent recording quality, array yield, and stability characteristics. A number of investigators have recently reported viable neuronal recordings extending over months or longer using microwire arrays (Nicolelis et al. 2003), ceramic-substrate arrays (Moxon et al. 2004), Utah arrays (Suner et al. 2005), and Michigan arrays (Vetter et al. 2004a). A recent, systematic study was conducted to compare objectively the performances of these various microelectrode arrays (Ward et al. 2009). This report confirmed the various longevities previously reported and indicated largely comparable performance of the different microelectrode technologies. However, this comparative-performance study was conducted using rat brain exclusively, and therefore did not take into account some of the potential failure modes for implants in larger brains (e.g., high acceleration movements of the head in nonhuman primates [Santhanam et al. 2007]).

OVERALL PERFORMANCE

In addition to considering the chronic performance of microelectrode arrays, it is important to consider the performance of the intracortical implant procedure itself. What risks are associated with receiving an intracortical BCI neural interface; and what is the likelihood of the implant attaining and maintaining a useful level of function? Most of the animal studies in this area have not been designed to address these questions in a comprehensive manner, and the relevant clinical experiences have been limited. An ad hoc, qualitative assessment across animal studies, combined with one of the few studies to report both implant successes and failures (Williams et al. 1999), suggests that in experienced labs with validated protocols and trained personnel, roughly 60–90% of implants result in at least a nominal level of useful performance. The most important salient aspect of this assessment is that while the likelihood is high, it is well below 100%. That is, any given implant procedure is likely to be successful to some degree, but success is not guaranteed. Although clinical studies to date have been very limited, they support this general observation (Hochberg et al. 2006).

Taken as whole, the animal and human studies to date suggest that long-term, information-rich neural recordings from intracortical electrodes are ultimately feasible. Nevertheless, the transition of BCI intracortical neural interfaces from research grade to clinical grade has yet to be accomplished. This transition involves two classes of tasks: first, to increase the number of sites on an array that record viable signals, to improve the recording fidelity signal on each of these sites, and to increase day-to-day recording stability; second, to increase the longevity and reliability of the recordings from weeks to months and (eventually) to decades.

BRAIN-TISSUE RESPONSES TO INTRACORTICAL MICROELECTRODE ARRAYS

In addition to assessing chronic recording performance, intracortical microelectrode arrays must be evaluated with regard to any localized tissue responses that occur around the implant. Although the detailed relationships between brain-tissue responses (i.e., histology) and chronic neural recording performance (i.e., function) are not well understood, it is reasonable to expect that they are closely related because functional characteristics result directly from the state of the neurons within the field of interest and from the electrical characteristics of the electrode-tissue interface (Liu et al. 2006; Nicolelis et al. 2003; Polikov et al. 2005; Rousche and Normann 1998; Schwartz et al. 2006; Williams et al. 1999; Biran et al. 2005; Purcell et al. 2009a; Purcell et al. 2009b; Silver and Miller 2004). Although elucidation of these reactive processes is just beginning, it is generally expected that better understanding of the dynamic biological processes surrounding a microscale neural interface will guide development of advanced microelectrode designs that are better able to record chronically from information-rich sources. This will be necessary if intracortical recording is to be used for controlling BCIs, particularly those capable of complex applications (i.e., multidimensional movement control).

The common working hypothesis is that degradation of recording performance over time is caused by deleterious brain-tissue responses, and improvement of long-term recording performance involves attenuating, mitigating, or appropriately guiding these brain-tissue responses (Kennedy et al. 1992; Lee et al. 2004b; Maynard et al. 1997; Rousche et al. 2001; Shain et al. 2003; Stensaas and Stensaas 1978; Suzuki et al. 2003; Takeuchi et al. 2004; Zhong and Bellamkonda 2007). In this section of the chapter we review current understanding of the complex and nuanced relationship between the electrode-brain microenvironment and a microelectrode's functional performance.

THE MICROENVIRONMENT SURROUNDING AN IMPLANTED MICROELECTRODE ARRAY

The brain and spinal cord are enclosed within the meningeal membranes and cushioned by cerebrospinal fluid. In a typical region of brain, cells (i.e., neurons and glia) fill about 78% of the volume, microvasculature about 2%, and extracellular space about 20% (Nicholson and Syková 1998; Tsai et al. 2009). In humans, the average cell density across cortex is about 100,000 cells/mm³, with significant variations among cortical regions and among layers within a region (reviewed in Tsai et al. 2009). The average neuronal density is about 30,000 neurons/mm³ (Tsai et al. 2009), resulting in a glial to neuronal cell ratio of about 2:1. The vasculature length in human cortex is about 0.4 m/mm³. In mouse, average microvessel diameter is about 4 μm, and the average distance from any spot in cortex to the closest vessel is 13 μm (Tsai et al. 2009). The overall composition of brain tissue in the cerebral cortex is illustrated in figure 5.6, which shows a detailed image of the microenvironment of the rat cerebral cortex at the scale of a typical implantable microelectrode shank.

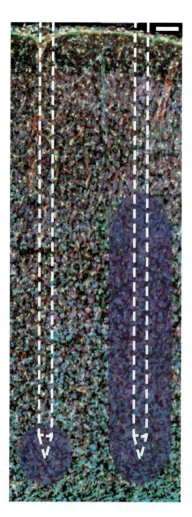

Figure 5.6 Brain tissue microenvironment around a microelectrode implanted in rat cerebral cortex, with cortical surface at the top. The image is a montage of 64 three-dimensional images collected on a Zeiss LSM META system with spectral unmixing. Cyan, CyQuant-labeled cell nuclei; purple, NeuroTrace-labeled Nissl substance; yellow, Iba1-labeled microglia; red, GFAP-labeled astrocytes; green, EBA-labeled blood vessels. (Image courtesy of C. Bjornsson, Rensselaer Polytechnic Institute, modified for this chapter [Tsai et al. 2011].) To illustrate the scale of implanted microelectrodes relative to the density of the primary brain-tissue elements, the outline shapes (dotted lines) of two typical microelectrode shanks/tines (50-μm diameter and 400-μm separation) are superimposed on the montage. The left microelectrode depicts a single site at the tip (e.g., a microwire or Utah electrode array). The right microelectrode depicts a tip site and an array of sites along the shank (e.g., a Michigan-style electrode array). Their respective approximate recording volumes (i.e., about 100-μm radius from electrode site) are shown in blue.

It is important to note that, through the course of normal activity, the brain and spinal cord move relative to the skull and vertebrae (e.g., with respiration, heartbeat, bodily movements). This movement is particularly prominent in primates.

LOCALIZED TISSUE DAMAGE ASSOCIATED WITH MICROELECTRODE INSERTION

Implanting a microelectrode array into the cerebral cortex requires incising, or at least penetrating, the meninges, including the dura mater, the arachnoid, and the pia mater. Arachnoidal penetration releases cerebrospinal fluid, and arachnoidal and pial penetration disrupts vasculature. Cortical insertion displaces or damages neurons, glia, and intracortical microvasculature.

The localized injury response due to microelectrode array insertion starts immediately. This localized response involves the four primary constituent elements in the microenvironment: neurons, reactive cells (i.e., microglia, macrophages, and astrocytes), blood vessels, and extracellular matrix. Given the packing density of blood vessels and the size and shape of microelectrodes, the initial electrode insertion penetrates the blood-brain barrier (BBB) at some point, resulting in edema as well as a release of erythrocytes and macrophages into brain tissue (Schmidt et al. 1993). The simple presence of a typical microelectrode shank (nominally 15×50 μm, inserted 2.5 mm into cerebral cortex) would be expected to displace or destroy about 120 glia, about 60 neurons, and about 80 tiny blood vessels.

In addition to this volumetric estimation of the cellular, vascular, and extracellular damage, compressive damage occurs due to the viscoelastic nature of the neural tissue. Bjornsson et al. (2006) used a novel ex-vivo preparation to compare the tissue distortion in thick slices from rat brains as a function of insertion speed and device sharpness. By fluorescently labeling the vasculature and observing the tissue deformation via microscopy, they reported that damage due to severing, rupturing, and dragging of vasculature was common as far as 300 μm away from the insertion site. The acute tissue disruption and damage from microelectrode-array insertion has also been studied by measuring changes in local pH levels in the extracellular space surrounding the electrode shank as a function of insertion speed (fig. 5.7) (Johnson et al. 2007).

Despite these observations of the local tissue injury typically incurred by microelectrode array insertion, it is particularly noteworthy that adjacent electrode tracks from the same array can show very different tissue reactions (Rousche and Normann 1998; Williams et al. 2007), and that different ranges of tissue damage can be observed at different locations on a single electrode track (Stensaas and Stensaas 1976). These findings suggest that the heterogeneity of the tissue at the microscale level results in variable localized injuries. Kozai et al. (2010) used a two-photon imaging technique to produce a 3-D reconstruction of the subsurface neurovasculature prior to inserting an electrode and showed that proper selection of the insertion location based on this imaging could produce a >80% reduction in vascular damage. This suggests that imaging or other preimplant information may lessen localized tissue damage due to insertion.

In sum, it appears that, regardless of the mitigation strategies that might be used to minimize insertion damage, some initial vascular damage and subsequent BBB disruption are unavoidable given the size, stiffness, and sharpness of current types of implantable microelectrode arrays. In addition to rupturing the BBB barrier, array insertion injures or destroys neurons, oligodendrocytes, astrocytes, and microglia and thus initiates some degree of initial reactive tissue response. In the presence of a chronically implanted array, the initial response perpetuates inflammation and subsequent tissue responses, leading to a chronic brain tissue response. Interestingly, the tissue damage decreases if the array is removed (Biran et al. 2005).

CHRONIC BRAIN-TISSUE RESPONSES

The chronic tissue response is a time-varying, complex sequence of events that involves many signalling molecules and cell types. The chronic inflammation that follows device insertion is not unique to microscale devices such as

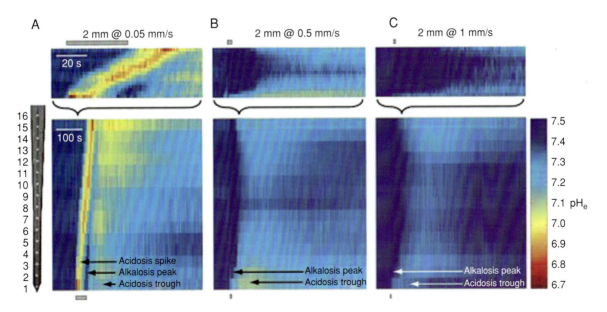

Figure 5.7 *Insertion damage measured by spatiotemporal variations in extracellular pH (pHe) levels along an electrode shank inserted 2 mm deep at three different speeds (A, 0.05 mm/sec; B, 0.50 mm/sec; C, 1.00 mm/sec). Spatiotemporal pHe plots reveal more robust longer-term acidosis with slow insertion speed (e.g., A), as well as variability in the response along the probe shank. The upper plots give a detailed picture of the pHe response during the act of insertion (duration of insertion indicated by gray bars at bottom). The lower plots show a 10-min response window. A triphasic acidic–alkaline–acidic waveform, which includes substantial longer-term acidosis, is evident following the slowest insertion (A). Insertion speeds of 0.50 and 1.00 mm/sec (B and C) typically elicited a biphasic alkaline–acidic waveform with a muted acidosis trough. (From Johnson et al. 2007, with permission.)*

microelectrode arrays. It also occurs with implantation of electrodes for deep brain stimulation (Haberler et al. 2000; Moss et al. 2004; Nielsen et al. 2007). However, due to the small size of the microscale devices, and especially because of their use in recording rather than stimulation, the chronic brain tissue responses due to this persistent neuroinflammation are likely to affect their performance and reliability over the long term.

CELLULAR RESPONSES

Microglia are the first class of cells that respond in the localized injury after device insertion. Within the first day activated microglia are observed around the implanted devices (Szarowski et al. 2003). Cytokines and chemokines, the inflammatory molecules that activate the *microglia*, are present near to and adsorbed onto the implanted device. The microglia change from a ramified (i.e., resting) morphology into an amoeboid morphology similar to that of macrophages (Fawcett and Asher 1999). In this activated state microglia behave similarly to macrophages, propagating the inflammatory cascade through the release of additional cytokines and through attempting to phagocytize the implanted device. Using the immunostain ED-1, which is specific for both microglia and macrophages, Winslow and Tresco (2010) determined that these cell types were still active 12 weeks after insertion of a typically sized microwire but that they were largely confined to an area <100 μm from the electrode (see fig. 5.8A,B). This finding suggests persistent neuroinflammation. In the same study, the presence of IgG immunoreactivity surrounding the

electrode tracks confirmed this conclusion and indicated leakiness in the BBB as well.

Astrocytes are a second class of cells that participate in the localized injury response. Astrocytes typically perform supportive roles for the neuronal environment, regulating nutrients and neurotransmitters, as well as helping to form the BBB. During a chronic tissue response, and apparently due to the same cytokine signaling to which the microglia respond, astrocytes assume a reactive phenotype characterized by hypertrophy, proliferation, and secretion of various neuronal growth inhibitory molecules (e.g., NG2 chondroitin-sulfate proteoglycans [Levine 1994] or Nogo protein [GrandPre et al. 2000]). During this activation, the astrocytes can form a *glial sheath* around the microelectrode (Edell et al. 1992; Turner et al. 1999) (see fig. 5.8C,D), which is probably part of the process of reformation of the BBB during which reactive astrocytes up-regulate gap junction proteins (connexins) to enable the formation of tight junctions (Haupt et al. 2007).

Neurons themselves can also be affected by the chronic tissue response. Although a related signal cascade has not been defined, the tissue response is typically accompanied by long-term neuronal death or damage in the area adjacent to the microelectrode, creating what may be referred to as neuronal kill-zone, or perhaps more accurately, a neuronal depletion zone (Biran et al. 2005; Edell et al. 1992; Polikov et al. 2005) (see fig. 5.8E). This finding was subsequently correlated with chronic local inflammation around the electrodes (McConnell et al. 2009a). In addition to the anatomical depletion zone,

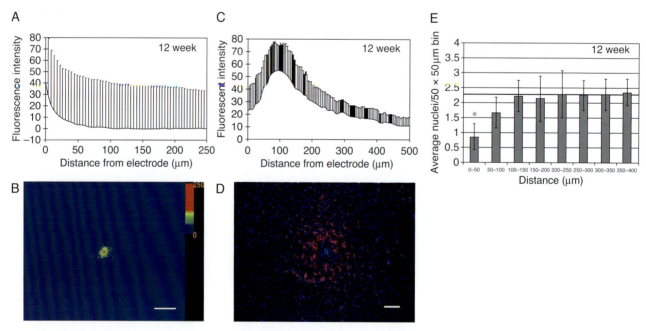

Figure 5.8 Chronic tissue responses from microwire implants in rat motor cortex 12 weeks after implantation. (A) Microglia as a function of distance from the implant, as indicated by average ED-1 immunoreactivity (+ standard deviation). (B) Average surface plot for ED-1 immunoreactivity showing symmetrical distribution around the microwire. Scale bar = 100 μm. (C) Astrocytes as a function of distance from the implant as indicated by average glial fibrillary acidic protein (GFAP) immunoreactivity (+ standard deviation). (D) Representative horizontal section illustrating the hypertrophic astrocyte response, as indicated by GFAP immunoreactivity (pink). DAPI (4′,6-diamidino-2-phenylindole) staining (blue) indicates the presence of additional cell types near the electrode-tissue interface. Scale bar = 100 μm. (E) Average number (± standard deviation) of NeuN-labeled neuronal cell bodies as a function of distance from the implant. There is a significant decrease (*p ≤ 0.05) in the number of neuronal nuclei within 50 mm of the microwire, as compared to the average number in unimplanted tissue (indicated by the light gray horizontal line). (From Winslow and Tresco 2010, with permission.)

physiological (i.e., functional) effects may also develop, either through network restructuring due to synaptic damage or through creation of *silent neurons* (Henze et al. 2000).

Oligodendrocytes have also recently been shown to contribute to the reactive tissue response. Loss of myelin occurs around devices implanted for 2, 4, and 12 weeks (e.g., Winslow and Tresco 2010). These effects also extend along a cortical column, suggesting widespread physiological influence (Woolley et al. 2009). Demyelination, a hallmark of many neurodegenerative diseases, causes slowing of action potential conduction and thereby disrupts normal function. One possible (although unproven) mechanism of neuronal silencing is based on Hebbian dynamics (Hebb 1949). The hypothesis is that the synaptic inputs from these slowed axons, because they no longer synchronize with inputs from other axons, gradually weaken to the point that the neurons giving rise to these slowed axons are essentially disconnected from the network.

EXTRACELLULAR MATRIX CHANGES

Extracellular matrix changes may also occur in response to injury from penetrating electrodes. In spinal cord injury, glial scar formation is associated with production of extracellular matrix proteins (e.g., $\gamma1$ laminin, type IV collagen, $\alpha1$ laminin) by reactive astrocytes (Liesi and Kauppila 2002). Several reports suggest that these extracellular matrix changes also occur with penetrating injury in the cortex (Liu et al. 1999; Stensaas and Stensaas 1976) and that they probably contribute to the observed increases in the impedance spectra. However, due partly to a lack of adequate methods, there are little data that directly address the role of extracellular matrix changes associated with chronic microelectrode arrays.

ASSESSING TISSUE RESPONSE OVER TIME

Several recently developed histological methods are helping to elucidate changes at the cellular level and in the extracellular matrix. For example, a new device-extraction histological method avoids the potential for artifactual overlabelling of the tissue near the microelectrode array by immunohistochemical antibodies and biomarkers. Although in situ histology (e.g., fig. 5.9) (Woolley et al. 2011) can provide detail at the level of the interface that cannot be gathered with traditional methods, such in-situ methods provide only end-point data. In contrast, in-vivo imaging (e.g., Kleinfeld and Griesbeck 2005) can repeatedly assess the chronic tissue response as it develops over time. As this technique develops further, it may provide enhanced information regarding the timing and composition of the chronic reactive tissue response over the lifetime of the array.

Figure 5.10 gives a qualitative summary of the reactive tissue responses resulting from chronic implantation of a microelectrode into cerebral cortex from the time of electrode insertion through 6 weeks after implantation.

ASSESSING THE EFFECT OF TISSUE RESPONSE ON MICROELECTRODE PERFORMANCE

The acute and chronic tissue responses discussed above may affect electrode performance. Measuring the impedance of the

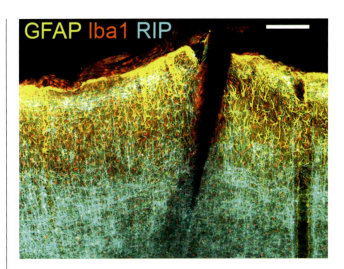

Figure 5.9 *In situ histological image of neural interface microenvironment with electrode placed in motor cortex. Single optical section (approximately 50 µm into a 300-µm-thick sagittal section through the motor cortex) at the site of a silicon Michigan microelectrode array implanted 1 week prior to imaging. Yellow, GFAP; red, ionized calcium-binding adaptor molecule 1 (Iba1); cyan, receptor-interacting protein (RIP). Scale bar=200 µm. (From Woolley et al. 2011.)*

device-tissue interface in vivo is a way to assess the effect of chronic tissue response on performance (Grill and Mortimer 1994). Williams et al. (2007) observed a gradual and significant increase in tissue impedance over the first seven days after implantation of a microwire array in somatosensory cortex of the rat. This increase did not occur for all arrays; rather, it occurred for those that exhibited an extensive GFAP reaction in post-mortem histology, indicating a high degree of encapsulation.

A lumped-parameter circuit model was developed to delineate the real and imaginary contributions to the impedance from the electrode, the cells, and the extracellular space (Williams et al. 2007). Subsequently, McConnell et al. (2009a) described a more detailed model to quantitatively correlate impedance parameters with histological measures of GFAP and 4,6-diamidino-2-phenylindole (DAPI). The results of these impedance studies have been corroborated by the observation in glial cell cultures of three-dimensional, high-density glial growth around neural probes (Frampton et al. 2010). Increased glial sheathing was correlated with increased impedance (Frampton et al. 2010). These studies provide longitudinal data that corroborate earlier histological observations regarding the progression of the stereotypical chronic brain tissue response to an implanted microelectrode array.

IMPORTANT REMAINING QUESTIONS

Several important questions remain to be answered concerning the chronic brain-tissue response to an implanted microelectrode array and its effect on electrode performance.

Does the astrocyte sheath progressively condense in the area surrounding a microelectrode array, and does it thereby increase the tissue impedance between neuronal signal sources and electrode sites? Some of the earlier studies involving earlier types of microelectrode arrays and insertion techniques support this hypothesis (Turner et al. 1999; Williams et al. 2007). However, several recent studies that use current types of microelectrodes

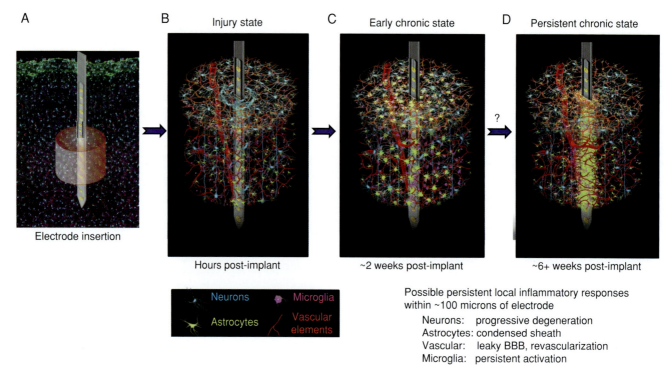

A   B   Injury state   C   Early chronic state   D   Persistent chronic state

Electrode insertion

Hours post-implant   ~2 weeks post-implant   ~6+ weeks post-implant

Neurons   Microglia

Astrocytes   Vascular elements

Possible persistent local inflammatory responses within ~100 microns of electrode

Neurons: progressive degeneration
Astrocytes: condensed sheath
Vascular: leaky BBB, revascularization
Microglia: persistent activation

Figure 5.10 *Summary of typical chronic brain-tissue responses to an implanted microelectrode in cortex. The chronic phase involves varying degrees of dynamic neuroinflammatory processes triggered by reaction to the implanted electrode as a foreign body. (A) Acute injury response characterized by cellular damage, local bleeding, localized ischemia, and edema develops immediately after electrode insertion. (B) The early phase of the chronic response involves activated microglia (purple) and reactive astrocytes (yellow), accompanied by some degree of damage or loss of neurons (blue). (C and D) The chronic response persists throughout the lifetime of the implant and involves a spectrum of responses, which may include progressive neuronal degradation, condensation of reactive astrocytes into a sheath around the electrode, ongoing low-level microglia activation, and a leaky blood-brain barrier. The factors leading to progressive encapsulation of the electrode by reactive cells, including condensation of reactive astrocytes (illustrated by transition from panel C to panel D), are not completely understood. Encapsulation seems to be a function of electrode design, surgical techniques, and localized characteristics of the electrode-tissue microenvironment. (From the authors, in collaboration with W. G. Shain, University of Washington, Seattle.)*

and techniques (McConnell et al. 2009b; Winslow et al. 2010; Winslow and Tresco 2010) suggest that progressive encapsulation through a condensing astrocyte sheath is not inevitable.

What is the actual cause of the gradual loss of signal over time? Is it neuronal degeneration, silent neurons, or disconnected neurons? Recent demyelination data suggest that the latter two may have a prominent role in the loss of signal (Winslow and Tresco 2010).

Is the persistence of the inflammatory and microglial components of the chronic tissue response the cause of recording unreliability and failure? Several studies indicate persistent inflammation with chronic neural microimplants (Winslow and Tresco 2010; Woolley et al. 2009; Biran et al. 2005; Polikov et al. 2005; Szarowski et al. 2003; Turner et al. 1999). Careful experimental studies of effectors known to trigger various tissue response processes are likely to guide development of electrode designs and techniques that minimize deleterious tissue responses.

METHODS TO ADDRESS DEGRADATION OF SIGNAL QUALITY CAUSED BY TISSUE RESPONSE

Although there is growing understanding of the response of brain tissue to a chronically implanted microelectrode array, direct and detailed information providing mechanistic links between the chronic tissue state (i.e., histology) and the concurrent recording characteristics of the microelectrode (i.e., function) is relatively sparse, and the causative links now drawn are mainly inferential. The progressive degradation of neural recording characteristics probably results from a complex interplay of multiple mechanisms. Several putative mechanisms are discussed here.

Since the brain reacts to the typical implanted microelectrode array as a foreign object, the constitutive properties of the device (e.g., its materials, mechanical characteristics, shape, and size) are all expected to determine the brain's reactive response to some degree. In accord with *biocompatibility* considerations of material-host responses, high-quality microelectrode materials can be selected so that the microelectrode remains intact within the brain and does not elicit significant deleterious biological responses to the materials themselves (Kipke et al. 2003; Stensaas and Stensaas 1978). Appropriate materials include thin-film dielectrics made of parylene C or silicon-oxide, and electrode sites made of platinum, platinum/iridium, iridium, or poly(3,4-ethylenedioxythiophene) (PEDOT) (Abidian et al. 2009; Cogan et al. 2009; Ludwig et al. 2011; Ludwig et al. 2006; Wilks et al. 2009). Although these materials do not at this time seem to cause functional loss, it is possible that they do induce deleterious responses that might become apparent as microelectrode technologies continue to be refined.

Biofouling (i.e., the adsorption of molecules to the electrode sites) has been hypothesized to be a cause of the chronic tissue response and degradation of recording. One approach to determining the effect of biofouling on device performance is to remove the biofouling at some point after implantation. This has been achieved by passing small amounts (hundreds of nA) of direct current from the electrode sites to a distant ground (Johnson et al. 2005; Otto et al. 2006). Although this produces significant reductions in impedance, and occasionally, the reappearance of large-amplitude neural signals from individual microelectrode sites, this approach is not a viable long-term solution to biofouling because its repeated use would be likely to progressively degrade the electrochemical state of the electrode site.

An alternative approach is to minimize biofouling by coating the device with anti-biofouling materials prior to insertion. These coatings may block the initial protein adsorption of the cytokines and chemokines and thereby create a *stealth environment* for the microelectrode array (i.e., in which the microelectrode array and/or site is not sensed by nearby neurons and glia). The most successful anti-biofouling agent used thus far is polyethylene glycol (PEG) (Alcantar et al. 2000). Recent in-vitro results indicate that coating with PEG reduces protein adsorption on the microelectrode surface (Sommakia et al. 2009). This suggests that PEG may prevent the initial precursor proteins that cause biofouling from adsorbing onto the microelectrode array. Whereas these initial results are encouraging, the longevity of these coatings in vivo is still unknown.

Another promising point of inquiry is the *mechanical mismatch* between the relatively soft brain and the relatively stiff electrode. Typical microelectrodes are 3–6 orders of magnitude stiffer than brain tissue, creating a mechanical mismatch. For example, the elastic moduli of silicon and polyimide are 166 gigapascals (GPa) and 2.5 GPa, respectively, while the estimated elastic modulus of brain tissue is only about 5 kPa (comparable to room temperature gelatin). It has been difficult to test directly and in isolation the hypothesis that this mismatch causes tissue damage and tissue response. Several modeling studies have reported simulations showing higher strain fields near the tip of stiff electrodes compared to less stiff electrodes (Lee et al. 2005; Subbaroyan et al. 2005). The effect of the softness of the electrode surface has also been studied, but, as with electrode stiffness, the effects of electrode softness have been difficult to isolate and measure. The addition of a relatively soft hydrogel coating does not appear to significantly affect the tissue response (Kim et al. 2010). Although stiffness and hardness are likely to be factors in performance degradation, recent results showing minimal tissue responses to conventional stiff and hard electrode types (Winslow et al. 2010), suggest that they are not major factors.

Micromotions, operationally defined as small (i.e., submicron to micron) movements of the electrode relative to the surrounding tissue, may also have a role in signal degradation. These movements may be caused by normal brain pulsations (e.g., respiratory and cardiac) and by movements of the brain associated with bodily movements, and they may be exacerbated by tethering of the array to the dura or the skull and by the mechanical mismatch of the electrodes relative to the brain.

The movements of the electrodes relative to the brain tissue have been hypothesized to induce a chronic inflammatory response due to repeated cellular disruption or strain. Whereas this is a reasonable hypothesis, the micromotions that actually occur in vivo have not been precisely measured or linked to particular brain-tissue response processes (Liu et al. 2006; Schmidt and Humphrey 1990; Subbaroyan et al. 2005).

STRATEGIES FOR DEVELOPING NEXT-GENERATION INTRACORTICAL BCI INTERFACES

The engineering science behind implantable microelectrode technologies and applications has advanced to the point of enabling data-driven, rational development of next-generation intracortical BCI interfaces. This heralds a remarkable new era in the arc of microelectrode technologies that began over 50 years ago when readily available laboratory materials and techniques were used to make the early microwire arrays. The scientific results from these early studies sparked the introduction of newly developed MEMS technologies to enable the development of more sophisticated and specialized types of microelectrodes, thereby significantly expanding the microelectrode design space. Now, the primary challenges have moved beyond simply making high-quality microelectrode arrays and getting them into the brain. Rather, the challenge now is to develop advanced designs, materials, and techniques that more effectively integrate with the brain at cellular and subcellular scales and that function reliably for many years. As this advanced functionality brings emerging clinical applications into focus, the additional challenge of clinical translation of the microelectrode technology comes to the forefront.

Advanced strategies for microelectrode design that maximize the quality, stability, and reliability of neural recordings can produce high-fidelity neural recordings. In addition, innovative approaches to signal processing will also further improve the quality of signals going into the neural decoding algorithms. These include topics addressed in other chapters such as referencing strategies, multichannel denoising and filtering techniques, and blended approaches that combine spike recordings with local field potentials (e.g., Gaumond et al. 2004; Ludwig et al. 2009).

A general strategy is starting to emerge for developing next-generation intracortical microelectrode arrays. This strategy has four coupled elements.

MINIMALLY DAMAGING SURGICAL INSERTIONS AND IMPLANTS

Although injury associated with microelectrode insertion and implantation is not a definitive predictor of long-term chronic performance, the components of the initial injury (i.e., bleeding on the brain surface, meningeal reaction, intracortical microhemorrhages, cellular damage) drive inflammatory responses and tissue-repair processes in the early postimplantation period. There is limited, if any, capacity to restore lost or damaged neurons in the electrode's microenvironment.

Insertion approaches that minimize damage include precise control of the insertion trajectory, position, speed, and depth, as well as well-designed electrode leading edges. After implantation the microelectrode array should be able to move with small, normal brain movements. Finally, dural sealing and/or repair are essential in order to prevent fluid seepage from the microelectrode insertion point and to minimize dural adhesions to the electrode interconnects outside the brain (Nunamaker and Kipke 2010; Nunamaker et al. 2011).

MICROELECTRODE ARRAYS WITH ADVANCED CONSTITUTIVE PROPERTIES

There is a compelling data-driven and intuitive rationale for developing microelectrodes that are smaller, more flexible, and perhaps have open mesh-like architectures. At the same time, the microelectrodes must have suitable electrical characteristics for high-quality bioelectrical signal transduction and connection to electronics. They must also have sufficient strength and robustness for surgical handling and insertion into the cortex. Finally, the microelectrode arrays and their coatings must have sufficient integrity to remain intact and functional for long periods of time.

In one in-vivo study, researchers investigated in rat subcutaneous tissue the effect of single polymer fibers with diameters of 2–27 μm (Sanders et al. 2000). The results showed a marked decrease in capsular thickness around fiber diameters in the 2.1 to 5.9-μm group. Other studies showed that the geometric dimensions of adhesive substrate patterns determined whether apoptosis (programmed cell death) occurred, and affected growth by controlling cellular spreading (Chen et al. 1997; Chen et al. 2004; Turner et al. 2000). These results led to the hypothesis that microelectrodes with dimensions of less than 7 μm would significantly reduce the brain-tissue response by preventing cellular adhesion to and growth on the electrode surface.

This hypothesis was confirmed in a cross-disciplinary study that added a thin (5-μm) polymer lateral extension to a conventional microelectrode shank. Called the *subcellular edge electrode*, or SEE probe (see fig. 5.11A), this device was produced in several different forms, and the chronic tissue responses they induced in rat cerebral cortex were evaluated (Seymour and Kipke 2007; Seymour et al. 2011). As shown in figures 5.11C and D, the SEE probe induced significantly less encapsulation than a conventional shank electrode, and preserved healthy neurons in the surrounding tissue. One particularly striking result was a significant decrease in encapsulation density around the lateral edge of the thin platform: encapsulation density at the lateral platform edge was reduced to about 50% of the level around the conventional microelectrode shank. Moreover, neuronal loss was significantly reduced: within the first 25 μm it was 30–48% less than for the conventional shank. These findings led to further technology development to make functional versions with an open architecture and with small electrode sites positioned on the lateral edge (see fig. 5.11B). Initial short-term in-vivo testing of this subcellular edge electrode found that the edge sites recorded, on average, higher amplitude spikes than nearby planar control sites. This electrode technology continues to be developed for chronic recording applications.

MICROELECTRODE ARRAYS WITH BIOACTIVE SURFACES

In addition to meeting stringent size, mechanical, and electrical requirements, the surfaces of a microelectrode array should be designed to interface with the surrounding cells and extracellular substances in a manner that localizes and minimizes foreign-body responses and that promotes tissue integration. This might be achieved with thin, conformal coatings (Pierce et al. 2009) and/or precisely controlled surface morphologies for the dielectric and substrate components and for the electrode sites. The basic strategy is to attenuate proinflammatory signalling, reduce biofouling, maintain the BBB, and promote neuronal growth and maintenance (Azemi et al. 2011; He et al. 2006; He et al. 2007).

ACTIVE CONTROL OF LOCALIZED BRAIN-TISSUE RESPONSES

Beyond designs and technologies for the microelectrode array itself, an additional innovative direction would be active management of localized, dynamic brain-tissue responses. Such interventions would most probably employ localized or systemic delivery of therapeutics targeting localized inflammatory processes (Abidian et al. 2010; Abidian et al. 2009; Anderson 2008; Purcell et al. 2009b). This concept may extend to feedback control based on electrode functional performance, local tissue conditions, or the state of the subject. The strategy would be to facilitate self-repair of the intracortical interface. This strategy might become a component of intracortical implant systems that are capable of reliable, stable functional performance over years to decades.

LOOKING TO THE FUTURE

What is the developmental path from the current state of microelectrode technology to realization of a clinical-grade intracortical BCI neural interface that is used to control a lifelike prosthetic arm and hand with normal movement? Ongoing research and development should be increasingly driven by the results of highly focused engineering and scientific studies of critical biological processes and device technologies. As such, improved methods for quantitative analysis of the tissue responses around a chronic microelectrode array are needed to evaluate their relationship to recording performance. Investigation of detailed mechanisms of electrode performance (and failure) must extend beyond correlational analysis of tissue responses and electrode-array performance. Furthermore, as we seek to develop microelectrode arrays that will function for decades in humans, it will be critical to have improved methods to evaluate safety and effectiveness, including perhaps accelerated lifetime testing.

Finally, although the focus of this chapter has been on neural recording, recent advances in neural interface technology

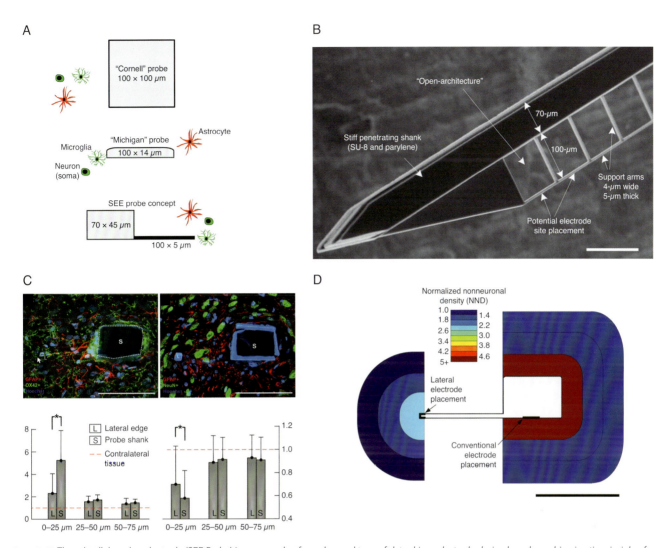

Figure 5.11 *The subcellular edge electrode (SEE Probe) is an example of an advanced type of data-driven electrode design based on a biomimetic principle of subcellular size to modulate the foreign body response. (A) Schematic cross sections of a relatively thick silicon probe (Cornell probe) (top); a Michigan silicon probe (middle); and the SEE probe concept (bottom), shown with the relative sizes of cells. The upper two structures were found to have a similar tissue response after 4 weeks (Szarowski et al. 2003). The SEE probe lateral platform has subcellular dimensions; note the large size of the microglia relative to the 5-μm edge. (B) Scanning electron micrograph of a prototype SEE probe having a conventional-sized stabilizing shank with a thin, lattice-like lateral platform. The scale bar equals 100 μm. (C) Qualitative and quantitative results around two nonfunctional SEE probes. Top left: GFAP (red) and OX42 (green) antibodies label astrocytes and microglia, respectively (scale bar = 100 μm). Top right: GFAP (red) and NeuN (green) label astrocytes and neuronal cell bodies, respectively (scale bar = 100 μm). Bottom left: normalized mean nonneuronal density as a function of distance from probe interface (p < 0.05). Bottom right: Mean neuronal density as a function of probe interface (p < 0.05). The advanced architecture featuring dimensions less than 7 μm and large perforations in the substrate improved the chronic neural interface through reduced encapsulation and reduced neuronal loss. (D) Schematic illustration of electrode placement, comparing SEE and conventional probes, and showing the corresponding average nonneuronal density regions. Histological results indicated that the best electrode placement would be at the lateral edge. (Scale bar = 100 μm.) (Seymour and Kipke 2007; Seymour et al. 2011.)*

and pilot studies in nonhuman primates and humans (Bak et al. 1990; Bartlett et al. 2005; Bradley et al. 2005; Schmidt et al. 1996) suggest that intracortical electrical microstimulation may be a valuable method for providing sensory feedback in a BCI (see chapter 16, in this volume). Microstimulation requires only an energy source, uses the same physical encoding parameters to interface with every sensory system (i.e., stimulus frequency, duration, shape, and amplitude in volts or amperes), and provides stimuli that can be highly controlled in location, temporal characteristics, and other parameters (Koivuniemi et al. 2011; Koivuniemi and Otto 2011; Romo et al. 1998; Rousche and Normann 1999; Rousche et al. 2003; Salzman et al. 1990; Scheich and Breindl 2002; Talwar et al.

2002). Several recent studies integrating cortical microstimulation into a BCI task (Fitzsimmons et al. 2007; Marzullo et al. 2010; O'Doherty et al. 2009) showed that, in some cases, response latencies are shorter than with natural sensory stimulation. These reports indicate the potential value of intracortical microstimulation for providing sensory feedback in a variety of tasks. On the other hand, cortical microstimulation is highly artificial in that it bypasses earlier precortical stations of sensory processing and simply translates peripheral differences in sensation location and strength into differences in the location and strength of cortical stimulation. Thus, its usefulness for BCI applications remains to be determined. Whereas numerous physiological and technical issues remain to be resolved, intracortical microstimulation, perhaps delivered by the same microelectrode arrays used to record, could provide an important additional feature for the development of BCI systems capable of complex control applications.

SUMMARY

A wide variety of different microelectrode designs have proved capable of recording intracortical signals safely and effectively for prolonged periods. The results suggest that chronic recording of neural spike trains from many (e.g., 200+) microelectrodes simultaneously for periods of months to years should be technologically feasible. Thus, practical BCI systems that use these signals appear to be attainable. At the same time, if clinically practical intracortical BCIs are to be realized, the reliability, stability, and signal quality of the implanted devices have to be substantially improved. The current science and technology base is sufficiently mature and robust to support progressive advances to implantable microelectrode arrays that meet the necessary clinical requirements. Success will depend on careful science and engineering approaches that incorporate knowledge of the relevant and most critical biological, physical, and chemical factors, and their interrelationships.

REFERENCES

Abidian, M. R., Corey, J. M., Kipke, D. R., and Martin, D. C. (2010), Conducting-polymer nanotubes improve electrical properties, mechanical adhesion, neural attachment, and neurite outgrowth of neural electrodes, *Small,* 6 (3), 421–429.

Abidian, M. R., Ludwig, K. A., Marzullo, T. C., Martin, D. C., and Kipke, D. R. (2009), Interfacing conducting polymer nanotubes with the central nervous system: Chronic neural recording using poly (3,4-ethylenedioxythiophene) nanotubes, *Adv Mater,* 21 (37), 3764–3770.

Alcantar, N. A., Aydil, E. S., and Israelachvili, J. N. (2000), Polyethylene glycol-coated biocompatible surfaces, *J Biomed Mater Res,* 51 (3), 343–351.

Aminghafari, M., Cheze, N., and Poggi, J. M. (2006), Multivariate de-noising using wavelets and principal component analysis, *Comp Stat Data Anal,* 50, 2381–2398.

Anderson, D. J. (2008), Penetrating multichannel stimulation and recording electrodes in auditory prosthesis research, *Hear Res,* 242 (1–2), 31–41.

Anderson, D. J., Najafi, K., Tanghe, S. J., Evans, D. A., Levy, K. L., Hetke, J. F., Xue, X. L., Zappia, J. J., and Wise, K. D. (1989), Batch-fabricated thin-film electrodes for stimulation of the central auditory system. *IEEE Trans Biomed Eng,* 36 (7), 693–704.

Azemi, E., Lagenaur, C. F., and Cui, X. T. (2011), The surface immobilization of the neural adhesion molecule L1 on neural probes and its effect on neuronal density and gliosis at the probe/tissue interface, *Biomaterials,* 32 (3), 681–692.

Bak, M.J., Girvin, J. P., Hambrecht, F. T., Kufta, C. V., Loeb, G. E., and Schmidt, E. M. (1990), Visual sensations produced by intracortical microstimulation of the human occipital cortex., *Med Biol Eng Comput,* 28 (3), 257–259.

Bartlett, J. R., DeYoe, E. A., Doty, R. W., Lee, B. B., Lewine, J. D., Negrao, N., and Overman, W. H., Jr. (2005), Psychophysics of electrical stimulation of striate cortex in macaques, *J Neurophysiol,* 94 (5), 3430–3442.

BeMent, S. L., Wise, K. D., Anderson, D. J., Najafi, K., and Drake, K. L. (1986), Solid-state electrodes for multichannel multiplexed intracortical neuronal recording, *IEEE Transact Biomed Eng,* 33 (2), 230–241.

Bhandari, R., Negi, S., and Solzbacher, F. (2010), Wafer-scale fabrication of penetrating neural microelectrode arrays, *Biomed Microdevices,* 12 (5), 797–807.

Bierer, S. B., and Andersen, D. J. (1999), Multi-channel spike detection and sorting using an array processing technique, *Neurocomputing,* 26–27, 947–956.

Biran, R., Martin, D. C., and Tresco, P. A. (2005), Neuronal cell loss accompanies the brain tissue response to chronically implanted silicon microelectrode arrays, *Exp Neurol,* 195 (1), 115–126.

Bjornsson, C. S., Oh, S. J., Al-Kofahi, Y.A., Lim, Y. J., Smith, K. L., Turner, J. N., De, S., Roysam, B., Shain, W., and Kim S. J. (2006), Effects of insertion conditions on tissue strain and vascular damage during neuroprosthetic device insertion, *J Neural Eng,* 3, 196–20

Blanche, T. J., Spacek, M. A., Hetke, J. F., and Swindale. (2005), Polytrodes: High-density silicon electrode arrays for large-scale multiunit recording, *J Neurophysiol,* 93 (5), 2987–3000.

Bradley, D. C., Troyk, P. R., Berg, J. A., Bak, M., Cogan, S., Erickson, R., Kufta, C., Mascaro, M., McCreery, D., Schmidt, E. M., Towle, V. L., and Xu, H. (2005), Visuotopic mapping through a multichannel stimulating implant in primate V1, *J Neurophysiol,* 93 (3), 1659–1670.

Bretschneider, F., and De Weille, J.R. (2006), "Electrochemistry," in *Introduction to electrophysiological methods and instrumentation,* Amsterdam: Elsevier, 103–130.

Brumberg, J. S., Nieto-Castanon, A., Kennedy, P. A., and Guenther, F. H. (2010), Brain-computer interfaces for speech communication, *Speech Commun,* 52 (4), 367–379.

Bullara, L. A., McCreery, D. B., Yuen, T.G., and Agnew, W. F. (1983), A microelectrode for delivery of defined charge densities, *J Neurosci Methods,* 9 (1), 15–21.

Burns, B. D., Stean, J. P., and Webb, A. C. (1973), Recording for several days from single cortical neurones in the unrestrained cat, *J Physiol,* 231 (1), 8P–10P.

Campbell, P. K., Jones, K. E., Huber, R. J., Horch, K. W., and Normann, R. A. (1991), A silicon-based, three-dimensional neural interface: Manufacturing processes for an intracortical electrode array, *IEEE Trans Biomed Eng,* 38 (8), 758–768.

Chen, C. S., Tan, J., and Tien, J. (2004), Mechanotransduction at cell-matrix and cell-cell contacts, *Annu Rev Biomed Eng,* 6, 275–302.

Chen, C. S., Mrksich, M., Huang, S., Whitesides, G. M., and Ingber, D. E. (1997), Geometric control of cell life and death, *Science,* 276 (5317), 1425–1428.

Chestek, C. A., Batista, A. P., Santhanam, G., Yu, B. M., Afshar, A., Cunningham, J. P., Gilja, V., Ryu, S. I., Churchland, M. M., and Shenoy, K. V. (2007), "Single-neuron stability during repeated reaching in macaque premotor cortex," *J Neurosci,* 27 (40), 10742–10750.

Chestek, C. A., Cunningham, J. P., Gilja, V., Nuyujukian, P., Ryu, S. I., and Shenoy, K. V. (2009), Neural prosthetic systems: current problems and future directions, *Conf Proc IEEE Eng Med Biol Soc,* 2009, 3369–3375.

Cogan, S. F. (2008), Neural stimulation and recording electrodes, *Annu Rev Biomed Eng,* 10, 275–309.

Cogan, S. F., Ehrlich, J., Plante, T. D., Smirnov, A., Shire, D. B., Gingerich, M., and Rizzo, J. F. (2009), Sputtered iridium oxide films for neural stimulation electrodes, *J Biomed Mater Res B Appl Biomater,* 89B (2), 353–361.

Cooper, R., Binnie, C. D., Osselton, J. W., Prior, P. F., and Wisman, T. (2003), EEG, pediatric neurophysiology, special techniques and applications, in Binnie, C. D., Cooper, R., Mauguiere, F., Osselton, J. W., Prior, P. F., and Tedman, B. M. (Eds.), *Clinical Neurophysiology, Vol 2.* Amsterdam: Elsevier BV, 8–103.

Csicsvari, J., Henze, D. A., Jamieson, B., Harris, K. D., Sirota, A., Bartho, P., Wise, K. D., and Buzsaki, G. (2003), Massively parallel recording of unit and local field potentials with silicon-based electrodes, *J Neurophysiol,* 90 (2), 1314–1323.

Dickey, A. S., Suminski, A., Amit, Y., Hatsopoulos, N. G. (2009), Single-unit stability using chronically implanted multielectrode arrays, *J Neurophysiol,* 102 (2), 1331–1339.

Donoghue, J. P., Nurmikko, A., Black, M., and Hochberg, L. R. (2007), Assistive technology and robotic control using motor cortex ensemble-based neural interface systems in humans with tetraplegia, *J Physiol,* 579 (Pt 3), 603–611.

Drake, K. L., Wise, K. D., and Farraye, J. (1988), Performance of planar multi-site microprobes in recording extracellular single-unit intracortical activity, *IEEE Trans Biomed Eng,* 35 (9), 719–732.

Edell, D. J., Toi, V. V., McNeil, V. M., and Clark, L. D. (1992), Factors influencing the biocompatibility of insertable silicon microshafts in cerebral cortex, *IEEE Trans Biomed Eng,* 39 (6), 635–643.

Fawcett, J. W., and Asher, R. A. (1999), The glial scar and central nervous system repair, *Brain Res Bull,* 49 (6), 377–391.

Fernandez, L. J., Altuna, A., Tijero, M., Gabriel, G., Villa, R., Rodriguez, M. J., Batlle, M., Vilares, R., Berganzo, J., and Blanco, F. J. (2009), Study of functional viability of SU-8-based microneedles for neural applications, *J Micromechan Microeng,* 19 (2), 025007.

Fetz, E. E. (1969), Operant conditioning of cortical unit activity, *Science,* 163 (870), 955–958.

Fitzsimmons, N. A., Drake, W., Hanson, T. L., Lebedev, M. A., and Nicolelis, M. A. (2007), Primate reaching cued by multichannel spatiotemporal cortical microstimulation, *J Neurosci,* 27 (21), 5593–5602.

Frampton, J.P., Hynd, M. R., Shuler, M. L., and Shain, W. (2010), "Effects of glial cells on electrode impedance recorded from neural prosthetic devices in vitro," *Ann Biomed Eng*, 38 (3), 1031–1047.

Ganguly, K., and Carmena, J. M. (2009), Emergence of a stable cortical map for neuroprosthetic control, *PLoS Biol*, 7 (7), e1000153.

Gaumond, R. P., Clement, R., Silva, R., and Sander, D. (2004), Estimation of neural energy in microelectrode signals, *J Neural Eng*, 1 (3), 127–134.

GrandPre, T., Nakamura, F., Vartanian, T., and Strittmatter, S. M. (2000), Identification of the Nogo inhibitor of axon regeneration as a Reticulon protein, *Nature*, 403 (6768), 439–444.

Gray, C. M., Maldonado, P. E., Wilson, M., and McNaughton, B. (1995), Tetrodes markedly improve the reliability and yield of multiple single-unit isolation from multi-unit recordings in cat striate cortex, *J Neurosci Methods*, 63 (1–2), 43–54.

Grill, W. M., and Mortimer, J. T. (1994), Electrical properties of implant encapsulation tissue, *Ann Biomed Eng*, 22 (1), 23–33.

Guo, L., Meacham, K. W., Hochman, S., and DeWeerth, S. P. (2010), A PDMS-based conical-well microelectrode array for surface stimulation and recording of neural tissues, *IEEE Trans Biomed Eng*, 57 (10), 2485–2494.

Haberler, C., Alesch, F., Mazal, P. R., Pilz, P., Jellinger, K., Pinter, M. M., Hainfellner, J. A., and Budka, H. (2000), No tissue damage by chronic deep brain stimulation in Parkinson's disease, *Ann Neurol*, 48 (3), 372–376.

Han, M. and McCreery, D. B. (2008), A new chronic neural probe with electroplated iridium oxide microelectrodes, *Conf Proc IEEE Eng Med Biol Soc*, 2008, 4220–4221.

Harris, K. D., Henze, D. A., Csicsvari, J., Hirase, H., and Buzsaki, G. (2000), Accuracy of tetrode spike separation as determined by simultaneous intracellular and extracellular measurements, *J Neurophysiol*, 84 (1), 401–414.

Hassibi, A., Navid, R., Dutton, R. W., and Lee, T. H. (2004), Comprehensive study of noise processes in electrode electrolyte interfaces, *J Appl Physics*, 96 (2), 9.

Haupt, C., Witte, O. W., and Frahm, C. (2007), Up-regulation of Connexin43 in the glial scar following photothrombotic ischemic injury, *Mol Cell Neurosci*, 35 (1), 89–99.

He, W., McConnell, G. C., and Bellamkonda, R. V. (2006), Nanoscale laminin coating modulates cortical scarring response around implanted silicon microelectrode arrays, *J Neural Eng*, 3, 316.

He, W., McConnell, G. C., Schneider, T. M., and Bellamkonda, R.V. (2007), A novel anti-inflammatory surface for neural electrodes, *Adv Mater*, 19 (21), 3529–3533.

Hebb, D.O. (1949), *The organization of behavior: A neuropsychological theory*, New York: Wiley.

Heliot, R., Ganguly, K., Jimenez, J., and Carmena, J. M. (2010), Learning in closed-loop brain-machine interfaces: Modeling and experimental validation, *IEEE Trans Syst Man Cybern B Cybern*, 40 (5), 1387–1397.

Henze, D. A., Borhegvi, Z., Csicvari, J., Mamiya, A., Harris, K. D., and Buzsaki, G. (2000), Intracellular features predicted by extracellular recordings in the hippocampus in vivo, *J Neurophysiol*, 84 (1), 390–400.

Hetke, J. F., Najafi, K., and Wise, K. D. (1990), Flexible miniature ribbon cables for long-term connection to implantable sensors, *Sens Actuat A–Physical*, 23 (1–3), 999–1002.

Hochberg, L. R., Serruya, M. D., Friehs, G. M., Mukand, J. A., Saleh, M., Caplan, A. H., Branner, A., Chen, D., Penn, R. D., and Donogue, J. P. (2006), Neuronal ensemble control of prosthetic devices by a human with tetraplegia, *Nature*, 442 (7099), 164–171.

Horsch, K. W., and Dhillon, G. S. (2004), *Neuroprosthetics theory and practice*, *Series on bioengineering and biomedical engineering*, River Edge, NJ: World Scientific.

Jackson, A., and Fetz, E. E. (2007), Compact movable microwire array for long-term chronic unit recording in cerebral cortex of primates, *J Neurophysiol*, 98 (5), 3109–3118.

Johnson, M. D., Kao, O. E., and Kipke, D. R. (2007), "Spatiotemporal pH dynamics following insertion of neural microelectrode arrays," *J Neurosci Methods*, 160 (2), 276–287.

Johnson, M. D., Otto, K. J., and Kipke, D. R. (2005), Repeated voltage biasing improves unit recordings by reducing resistive tissue impedances, *IEEE Trans Neural Syst Rehabil Eng*, 13 (2), 160–165.

Kennedy, P. R. (1989), The cone electrode: A long-term electrode that records from neurites grown onto its recording surface, *J Neurosci Methods*, 29 (3), 181–193.

Kennedy, P. R., Mirra, S. S., and Bakay, R.A. (1992), The cone electrode: Ultrastructural studies following long-term recording in rat and monkey cortex., *Neurosci Lett*, 142 (1), 89–94.

Kewley, D. T., Hills, M. D., Borkholder, D. A., Opris, I. E., Maluf, N. I., Storment, C. W., Bower, J. M., and Kovacs, G. T. A. (1997), Plasma-etched neural probes, *Sens Actu A: Physical*, 58 (1), 27–35.

Kim, D. H., Wiler, J. A., Anderson, D. J., Kipke, D. R., and Martin, D. C. (2010), Conducting polymers on hydrogel-coated neural electrode provide sensitive neural recordings in auditory cortex, *Acta Biomater*, 6 (1), 57–62.

Kim, S, Bhandari, R., Klein, M., Negi, S., Rieth, L., Tathireddy, P., Toepper, M., Oppermann, H., and Solzbacher, F. (2009), Integrated wireless neural interface based on the Utah electrode array, *Biomed Microdev*, 11 (2), 453–466.

Kim, S. P., Simeral, J. D., Hochberg, L. R., Donoghue, J. P., and Black, M. J. (2008), Neural control of computer cursor velocity by decoding motor cortical spiking activity in humans with tetraplegia, *J Neural Eng*, 5 (4), 455–476.

Kipke, D. R., Vetter, R. J., Williams, J. C., Hetke, J. F. (2003), Silicon-substrate intracortical microelectrode arrays for long-term recording of neuronal spike activity in cerebral cortex, *IEEE Trans Neural Syst Rehabil Eng*, 11 (2), 151–155.

Kipke, D.R., Clopton, B.M., and Anderson, D.J. (1991), Shared-stimulus driving and connectivity in groups of neurons in the dorsal cochlear nucleus, *Hearing Res*, 55 (1), 24–38.

Kleinfeld, D. and Griesbeck, O. (2005), From art to engineering? The rise of in vivo mammalian electrophysiology via genetically targeted labeling and nonlinear imaging, *PLoS Biol*, 3 (10), e355.

Koivuniemi, A.S. and Otto, K.J. (2011), "Optimized waveforms for electrical microstimulation of auditory cortex," *IEEE Transactions in Neural Systems and Rehabilitation* (In press).

Koivuniemi, A.S., Wilks, S.J. Woolley, A.J., and Otto, K.J. (2011), "Neural microstimulation and interfacial quality effects," *Progress in Brain Research* (In press).

Kovacs, G. T., Storment, C. W., Halks-Miller, M., Belcynski, C. R., Jr., Della Santina, C. C., Lewis, E. R., and Maluf, N. I. (1994), Silicon-substrate microelectrode arrays for parallel recording of neural activity in peripheral and cranial nerves, *IEEE Trans Biomed Eng*, 41 (6), 567–577.

Kovacs, G. T. A. (1994), Introduction to the theory, design, and modeling of thin-film microelectrodes for neural interfaces, in Stenger, D. A., and McKenna, T. (Eds.), *Enabling technologies for cultured neural networks*, New York: Academic Press, 121–165.

Kozai, T. D., Marzullo, T. C., Hooi, F., Lanhals, N. B., Majewska, A. K., Brown, E. B., and Kipke, D. R. (2010), Reduction of neurovascular damage resulting from microelectrode insertion into the cerebral cortex using in vivo two-photon mapping, *J Neural Eng*, 7 (4), 046011.

Lee, H., Bellamkonda, R. V., Sun, W., and Levenston, M. E. (2005), Biomechanical analysis of silicon microelectrode-induced strain in the brain, *J Neural Eng*, 2 (4), 81–89.

Lee, K., He, J., Clement, R., Massia, S., and Kim B. (2004a), Biocompatible benzocyclobutene (BCB)-based neural implants with micro-fluidic channel, *Biosens Bioelectron*, 20 (2), 404–407.

Lee, K. K., He, J. P., Singh, A., Massia, S., Ehteshami, G., Kim, B., and Raupp, G. (2004b), Polyimide-based intracortical neural implant with improved structural stiffness, *J Micromechan Microeng*, 14 (1), 32–37.

Levine, J. M. (1994), Increased expression of the NG2 chondroitin-sulfate proteoglycan after brain injury, *J Neurosci*, 14 (8), 4716–4730.

Liesi, P., and Kauppila, T. (2002), Induction of type IV collagen and other basement-membrane-associated proteins after spinal cord injury of the adult rat may participate in formation of the glial scar, *Exp Neurol*, 173 (1), 31–45.

Linderman, M. D., Gilja, V., Santhanam, G., Afshar, A., Ryu, S., Meng, T. H., and Shenoy, K. V. (2006), Neural recording stability of chronic electrode arrays in freely behaving primates, *Conf Proc IEEE Eng Med Biol Soc*, 1, 4387–4391.

Liu, X., McCreery, D. B., Bullara, L. A., and Agnew, W. F. (2006), Evaluation of the stability of intracortical microelectrode arrays, *IEEE Trans Neural Syst Rehabil Eng*, 14 (1), 91–100.

Liu, X., McCreery, D. B., Carter, R. R., Bullara, L. A., Yuen, T. G., and Agnew, W. F. (1999), Stability of the interface between neural tissue and chronically implanted intracortical microelectrodes," *IEEE Trans Rehabil Eng*, 7 (3), 315–326.

Ludwig, K. A., Langhals, N. B., Joseph, M. D., Richardson-Burns, S. M., Hendricks, J. L., and Kipke, D. R. (2011), Poly(3,4-ethylenedioxythiophene) (PEDOT) polymer coatings facilitate smaller neural recording electrodes, *J Neural Eng*, 8 (1), 014001.

Ludwig, K. A, Mirriani, R. M., Langhals, N. B., Joseph, M. D., Anderson, D. J., and Kipke, D. R. (2009), Using a common average reference to improve cortical neuron recordings from microelectrode arrays, *J Neurophysiol*, 101 (3), 1679–1689.

Ludwig, K. A., Uram, J. D., Yang, J., Martin, D. C., and Kipke, D. R. (2006), Chronic neural recordings using silicon microelectrode arrays electrochemically deposited with a poly(3,4-ethylenedioxythiophene) (PEDOT) film, *J Neural Eng*, 3 (1), 59–70.

Marg, E., and Adams, J. E. (1967), Indwelling multiple micro-electrodes in the brain, *Electroencephalogr Clin Neurophysiol,* 23 (3), 277–280.

Marzullo, T. C., Lehmkuhle, M. J., Gage, G. J., and Kipke, D. R. (2010), Development of closed-loop neural interface technology in a rat model: Combining motor cortex operant conditioning with visual cortex microstimulation, *IEEE Trans Neural Syst Rehabil Eng,* 18 (2), 117–126.

Maynard, E. M., Nordhausen, C. T., and Normann, R. A. (1997), The Utah intracortical electrode array: A recording structure for potential brain-computer interfaces, *Electroencephalogr Clin Neurophysiol,* 102 (3), 228–239.

McCarthy, P.T., Otto, K.J., and Rao, M.P. (2011a), "Robust penetrating micro-electrodes for neural interfaces realized by titanium micromachining," *Biomedical Microdevices,* 13:503–515.

McCarthy, P.T., Rao, M.P., and Otto, K.J. (2011b), "Simultaneous recording of rat auditory cortex and thalamus via a titanium-based multi-channel, microelectrode device," *Journal of Neural Engineering,* 8 046007.

McConnell, G. C., Butera, R. J., and Bellamkonda, R. V. (2009a), Bioimpedance modeling to monitor astrocytic response to chronically implanted electrodes, *J Neural Eng,* 6 (5), 055005.

McConnell, G. C., Rees, H. D., Levey, A. I., Gutekunst, C. A., Gross, R. E., and Bellamkonda, R. V. (2009b), Implanted neural electrodes cause chronic, local inflammation that is correlated with local neurodegeneration, *J Neural Eng,* 6 (5), 056003.

McCreery, D., Lossinsky, A., and Pikov, V. (2007), Performance of multisite silicon microprobes implanted chronically in the ventral cochlear nucleus of the cat, *IEEE Trans Biomed Eng,* 54 (6 Pt 1), 1042–1052.

McCreery, D. B., Pikov, V., Lossinsky, A., Bullara, L., and Agnew, W. (2004), Arrays for functional microstimulation of the lumbrosacral spinal cord, *IEEE Trans Neural Syst Rehabil Eng,* 12 (2), 195–207.

McNaughton, B. L., O'Keefe, J., and Barnes, C. A. (1983), The stereotrode: A new technique for simultaneous isolation of several single units in the central nervous system from multiple unit records, *J Neurosci Methods,* 8 (4), 391–397.

Mercanzini, A., Cheung, K., Buhl, D. L., Boers, M., Maillard, A., Colin, P., Bensadoun, J., Bertsch, A., and Renaud, P. (2008), Demonstration of cortical recording using novel flexible polymer neural probes, *Sens Actuat A: Physical,* 143 (1), 90–96.

Merrill, D. R., Bikson, M., and Jeffreys, J. G. R. (2005), Electrical stimulation of excitable tissue: design of efficacious and safe protocols, *J Neurosci Methods,* 141 (2), 171–198.

Moss, J., Ryder, T., Aziz, T. Z., Graeber, M. B., and Bain, P. G. (2004), Electron microscopy of tissue adherent to explanted electrodes in dystonia and Parkinson's disease, *Brain,* 127 (Pt 12), 2755–2763.

Moxon, K. A., Leiser, S. C., Gerhardt, G. A., Barbee, K. A., and Chapin, J. K. (2004), Ceramic-based multisite electrode arrays for chronic single-neuron recording, *IEEE Trans Biomed Eng,* 51 (4), 647–656.

Musallam, S., Bak, M. J., Troyk, P. R., and Andersen, R. A. (2007), A floating metal microelectrode array for chronic implantation, *J Neurosci Methods,* 160 (1), 122–127.

Muthuswamy, J., Okandan, M., Gilletti, A., Baker, M. S., and Jain, T. (2005), An array of microactuated microelectrodes for monitoring single-neuronal activity in rodents, *IEEE Trans Biomed Eng,* 52 (8), 1470–1477.

Najafi, K., Ji, J., and Wise, K. D. (1990), Scaling limitations of silicon multi-channel recording probes, *IEEE Trans Biomed Eng,* 37 (1), 1–11.

Nelson, M. J., Pouget, P., Nilsen, E. A., Patten, C. D., and Schall, J. D. (2008), Review of signal distortion through metal microelectrode recording circuits and filters, *J Neurosci Methods,* 169 (1), 141–157.

Neves, H. (2007), Advances in cerebral probing using modular multifunctional probe arrays, *Med Device Technol,* 18 (5), 38–39.

Nicholson, C., and Syková, E. (1998), Extracellular space structure revealed by diffusion analysis, *Trends Neurosci,* 21 (5), 207–215.

Nicolelis, M. A., Dimitrov, D., Carmena, J. M., Crist, R., Lehew, G., Kralik, J. D., and Wise, S. P. (2003), Chronic, multisite, multielectrode recordings in macaque monkeys, *Proc Natl Acad Sci USA,* 100 (19), 11041–11046.

Nicolelis, M. A., and Ribeiro, S. (2002), "Multielectrode recordings: The next steps," *Curr Opin Neurobiol,* 12 (5), 602–606.

Nielsen, M. S., Bjarkam, C. R., Sorensen, J. C., Bojsen-Moller, M., Sunde, N. A., and Ostergaard, K. (2007), Chronic subthalamic high-frequency deep brain stimulation in Parkinson's disease—a histopathological study, *Eur J Neurol,* 14 (2), 132–138.

Nunamaker, E. A. and Kipke, D. R. (2010), An alginate hydrogel dura mater replacement for use with intracortical electrodes, *J Biomed Mater Res B Appl Biomater,* 95 (2), 421–429.

Nunamaker, E. A., Otto, K. J., and Kipke, D. R. (2011), Investigation of the material properties of alginate for the development of hydrogel repair of dura mater, *J Mech Behav Biomed Mater,* 4 (1), 16–33.

Nurmikko, A. V, Donoghue, J. P., Hochberg, L. R., Patterson, W. R., Song, Y., Bull, C. W., Borton, D. A., Laiwalla, F., Park, S., Ming.,Y., and Aceros, J. (2010), Listening to brain microcircuits for interfacing with external world—Progress in wireless implantable microelectronic neuroengineering devices, *Proc IEEE,* 98 (3), 375–388.

O'Doherty, J. E., Lebedev, M. A., Hanson, T. L., Fitzsimmons, N. A., and Nicolelis, M. A. (2009), A brain-machine interface instructed by direct intracortical microstimulation, *Front Integ Neurosci,* 3, 20.

Offner, F. F. (1950), The EEG as potential mapping: The value of the average monopolar reference, *Electroencephalogr Clin Neurophysiol,* 2 (1–4), 213–214.

Osselton, J. W. (1965), Acquisition of EEG data by bipolar unipolar and average reference methods: a theoretical comparison, *Electroencephalogr Clin Neurophysiol,* 19 (5), 527–528.

Otto, K. J., Johnson, M. D., and Kipke, D. R. (2006), Voltage pulses change neural interface properties and improve unit recordings with chronically implanted microelectrodes, *IEEE Trans Biomed Eng,* 53 (2), 333–340.

Oweiss, K. G., and Anderson, D. J. (2001), Noise reduction in multichannel neural recordings using a new array wavelet denoising algorithm, *Neurocomputing,* 38–40, 1687–1693.

Pierce AP, SS Sommakia, JL Rickus, and KJ Otto. (2009), "Thin-film silica sol-gel coatings for neural microelectrodes," *Journal of Neuroscience Methods,* 180:106–110.

Polikov, V. S., Tresco, P. A., and Reichert, W. M. (2005), Response of brain tissue to chronically implanted neural electrodes, *J Neurosci Methods,* 148 (1), 1–18.

Purcell, E. K., Seymour, J. P., Yandamuri, S., and Kipke, D. R. (2009a), "In vivo evaluation of a neural stem cell-seeded prosthesis," *J Neural Eng,* 6 (2), 026005.

Purcell, E. K., Thompson, D. E., Ludwig, K. A., and Kipke, D. R. (2009b), Flavopiridol reduces the impedance of neural prostheses in vivo without affecting recording quality, *J Neurosci Methods,* 183 (2), 149–157.

Rennaker, R. L., Ruyle, A. M., Street, S. E., and Sloan, A. M. (2005), An economical multi-channel cortical electrode array for extended periods of recording during behavior, *J Neurosci Methods,* 142 (1), 97–105.

Robinson, D. A. (1968), The electrical properties of metal microelectrodes, *Proc IEEE,* 56 (6), 1065.

Romo, R., Hernandez, A., Zainos, A., and Salinas, E. (1998), Somatosensory discrimination based on cortical microstimulation, *Nature,* 392 (6674), 387–390.

Rousche, P. J., and Normann, R. A. (1992), A method for pneumatically inserting an array of penetrating electrodes into cortical tissue, *Ann Biomed Eng,* 20 (4), 413–422.

Rousche, P. J., and Normann, R. A. (1998), Chronic recording capability of the Utah intracortical electrode array in cat sensory cortex, *J Neurosci Methods,* 82 (1), 1–15.

Rousche, P. J., and Normann, R. A. (1999), Chronic intracortical microstimulation (ICMS) of cat sensory cortex using the Utah intracortical electrode array, *IEEE Trans Rehabil Eng,* 7 (1), 56–68.

Rousche, P. J., Otto, K. J., and Kipke, D. R. (2003), "Single electrode micro-stimulation of rat auditory cortex: An evaluation of behavioral performance," *Hearing Res,* 179 (1–2), 62–71.

Rousche, P. J., Pellinen, D. S., Pivin, D. P., Jr., Williams, J. C., Vetter, R. J., and Kipke, D. R. (2001), Flexible polyimide-based intracortical electrode arrays with bioactive capability, *IEEE Trans Biomed Eng,* 48 (3), 361–371.

Salzman, C. D., Britten, K. H., and Newsome, W. T. (1990), Cortical micro-stimulation influences perceptual judgements of motion direction, *Nature,* 346 (6280), 174–177.

Sanders, J. E., Stiles, C. E., and Hayes, C. L. (2000), Tissue response to single-polymer fibers of varying diameters: Evaluation of fibrous encapsulation and macrophage density, *J Biomed Mater Res,* 52 (1), 231–237.

Santhanam, G., Ryu, S. I., Yu, B. M., Afshar, A., and Shenoy, K. V. (2006), A high-performance brain-computer interface, *Nature,* 442 (7099), 195–198.

Santhanam, G., Linderman, M. D., Gilja, V., Afshar, A., Ryu, S. I., Meng, T. H., and Shenoy, K. V. (2007), HermesB: A continuous neural recording system for freely behaving primates, *IEEE Trans Biomed Eng* 54 (11), 2037–2050.

Scheich, H., and Breindl, A. (2002), An animal model of auditory cortex prostheses, *Audiol Neuro-Otol,* 7 (3), 191–194.

Schmidt, E. M., Bak, M. J., Hambrecht, F. T., Kufta, C. V., O'Rourke, D. K., and Vallabhanath, P. (1996), Feasibility of a visual prosthesis for the blind based on intracortical microstimulation of the visual cortex, *Brain,* 119 (Pt 2), 507–522.

Schmidt, E. M., Bak, M. J., McIntosh, J. S., and Thomas, J. S. (1977), "Operant conditioning of firing patterns in monkey cortical neurons," *Exp Neurol,* 54 (3), 467–477.

Schmidt, E., and Humphrey, D. R. (1990), Extracellular single-unit recording methods, in *Neurophysiological techniques,* edited by Boulton B, Baker B, and Vanderwolf H. Clifton, NJ: Humana Press, 1990, 1–64.

Schmidt, S., Horch, K. W., and Normann, R. A. (1993), Biocompatibility of silicon-based electrode arrays implanted in feline cortical tissue, *J Biomed Mater Res,* 27 (11), 1393–1399.

Schuettler, M., Stiess, S., King, B. V., and Suaning, G. J. (2005), Fabrication of implantable microelectrode arrays by laser cutting of silicone rubber and platinum foil, *J Neural Eng,* 2 (1), S121–128.

Schwartz, A. B., Cui, X. T., Weber, D. J., and Moran, D. W. (2006), Brain-controlled interfaces: Movement restoration with neural prosthetics, *Neuron,* 52 (1), 205–220.

Seymour, J. P., Elkasabi, Y. M., Chen, H. Y., Lahann, J., and Kipke, D. R. (2009), "The insulation performance of reactive parylene films in implantable electronic devices," *Biomaterials,* 30 (31), 6158–6167.

Seymour, J. P., and Kipke, D. R. (2007), Neural probe design for reduced tissue encapsulation in CNS, *Biomaterials,* 28 (25), 3594–3607.

Seymour, J. P., Langhals, N. B., Anderson, D. J., and Kipke, D. R. (2011), Novel multi-sided, microelectrode arrays for implantable neural applications, *Biomed Microdevices.* Epub 2011, February 08.

Shain, W., Spataro, L., Dilgen, J., Haverstick, K., Retterer, S., Isaacson, M., Saltzman, M., and Turner, J. N. (2003), Controlling cellular reactive responses around neural prosthetic devices using peripheral and local intervention strategies, *IEEE Trans Neural Syst Rehabil Eng,* 11 (2), 186–188.

Shoham, S., and Nagarajan, S. (2003), The theory of central nervous system recording, in Horch, K. W., and Dhillon, G. S. (Eds.), *Neuroprosthetics: Theory and Practice,* Singapore: World Scientific Publishing, 448–465.

Silver, J., and Miller, J. H. (2004), Regeneration beyond the glial scar, *Nat Rev Neurosci,* 5 (2), 146–156.

Sommakia, S., Rickus, J. L., and Otto, K. J. (2009), Effects of adsorbed proteins, an antifouling agent and long-duration DC voltage pulses on the impedance of silicon-based neural microelectrodes, *Conf Proc IEEE Eng Med Biol Soc,* 2009, 7139–7142.

Stensaas, S. S., and Stensaas, L. J. (1976), The reaction of the cerebral cortex to chronically implanted plastic needles, *Acta Neuropathol,* 35 (3), 187–203.

Stensaas, S. S., and Stensaas, L. J. (1978), Histopathological evaluation of materials implanted in cerebral-cortex. *Acta Neuropathologica,* 41 (?), 145–155.

Stieglitz, T., Beutel, H., Schuettler, M., and Meyer, J. (2000), Micromachined, polyimide-based devices for flexible neural interfaces, *Biomedical Microdevices,* 2 (4), 283–294.

Strumwasser, F. (1958), "Long-term recording" from single neurons in brain of unrestrained mammals, *Science,* 127 (3296), 469–470.

Subbaroyan, J., Martin, D. C., and Kipke, D. R. (2005), A finite-element model of the mechanical effects of implantable microelectrodes in the cerebral cortex, *J Neural Eng,* 2 (4), 103–113.

Suner, S., Fellows, M. R., Vargas-Irwin, C., Nakata, G. K., and Donoghue, J. P. (2005), Reliability of signals from a chronically implanted, silicon-based electrode array in non-human primate primary motor cortex, *IEEE Trans Neural Syst Rehabil Eng,* 13 (4), 524–541.

Suzuki, T., Mabuchi, K., and Takeuchi, S. (2003), A 3D flexible parylene probe array for multichannel neural recording, *Conference Proceedings. First International IEEE EMBS Conference on, Neural Engineering* 154–156.

Szarowski, D. H., Andersen, M., Retterer, S., Spence, A. J., Isaacson, M., Craighead, H. G., Turner, J. N., and Shain, W. (2003), Brain responses to micro-machined silicon devices, *Brain Res,* 983 (1–2), 23–35.

Takeuchi, S., Susuki, T., Mabuchi, K., and Fujita, H. (2004), 3D flexible multi-channel neural probe array, *J Micromechan Microeng,* 14 (1), 104.

Talwar, S. K., Xu, S., Hawley, E. S., Weiss, S. A., Moxon, K. A., and Chapin, J. K. (2002), Rat navigation guided by remote control, *Nature,* 417, 37–38.

Tsai, P. S., Kaufhold, J. P., Blinder, P., Friedman, B., Drew, P. J., Karten, H. J., Lyden, P. D., and Kleinfeld, D. (2009), Correlations of neuronal and microvascular densities in murine cortex revealed by direct counting and colocalization of nuclei and vessels, *J Neurosci,* 29 (46), 14553–14570.

Tsai, C.-L., Lister, J. P., Bjornsson, C. S., Smith, K., Shain, W., Barnes, C. A., and Roysam, B. (2011), Robust, globally consistent, and fully-automatic multi-image registration and montage synthesis for 3-D multi-channel images, *J Microsc,* Epub 2011 Mar 1.

Turner, A. M., Dowell, N., Turner, S. W., Kam, L., Isaacson, M., Turner, J. N., Craighead, H. G., and Shain, W. (2000), Attachment of astroglial cells to microfabricated pillar arrays of different geometries, *J Biomed Mater Res,* 51 (3), 430–441.

Turner, J. N., Shain, W., Szarowski, D. H., Andersen, M., Martins, S., Isaacson, M., and Craighead, H. (1999), Cerebral astrocyte response to micromachined silicon implants, *Exp Neurol,* 156, 33–49.

Velliste, M., Perle, S., Spalding, M. C., Whitford, A. S., and Schwartz, A. B. (2008), Cortical control of a prosthetic arm for self-feeding, *Nature,* 453 (7198), 1098–1101

Venkatraman, S., Hendricks, J., King, Z., Sereno, A., Richardson-Burns, S. Martin, D., and Carmena, J. (2011), In vitro and in vivo evaluation of PEDOT microelectrodes for neural stimulation and recording, *IEEE Trans Neural Syst Rehabil Eng.* Epub 2011, Jan 31

Vetter, R.J., Williams, J. C., Hetke, J. F., Nunamaker, E. A., and Kipke, D. R. (2004a), Chronic neural recording using silicon-substrate microelectrode arrays implanted in cerebral cortex, *IEEE Trans Biomed Eng,* 51 (6), 896–904.

Vetter, R.J., Williams, J. C., Hetke, J. F., Nunamaker, E. A., and Kipke, D. R. (2004b), Spike recording performance of implanted chronic silicon-substrate microelectrode arrays in cerebral cortex, *IEEE Trans Neural Syst Rehabil Eng,* 52 (1), 896–904.

Ward, M. P., Rajdev, P., Ellison, C., and Irazoqui, P. P. (2009), Toward a comparison of microelectrodes for acute and chronic recordings, *Brain Res,* 1282, 183–200.

Webster, J. G. (1998), *Medical instrumentation—Application and design,* 3rd ed. New York: John Wiley & Sons.

Wilks, S.J., Richardson-Burns, S.M., Hendricks, J.L., Martin, D.C., and Otto, K.J. (2009), "Poly(3,4-ethylene dioxythiophene) (PEDOT) as a microneural interface material for electrostimulation," *Frontiers in Neuroengineering,* 3:3.

Williams, J. C., Hippensteel, J. A., Dilgen, J., Shain, W., and Kipke, D. R. (2007), "Complex impedance spectroscopy for monitoring tissue responses to inserted neural implants," *J Neural Eng,* 4 (4), 410–423.

Williams, J. C., Rennaker, R. L., and Kipke, D. R. (1999), Long-term neural recording characteristics of wire microelectrode arrays implanted in cerebral cortex, *Brain Res Proto,* 4 (3), 303–313.

Winslow, B D, Christensen, M. B., Yang, W. K., Solzbacher, F., Tresco, P. A. (2010), A comparison of the tissue response to chronically implanted Parylene-C-coated and uncoated planar silicon microelectrode arrays in rat cortex, *Biomaterials,* 31 (35), 9163–9172.

Winslow, B. D., and Tresco, P. A. (2010), Quantitative analysis of the tissue response to chronically implanted microwire electrodes in rat cortex, *Biomaterials,* 31 (7), 1558–1567.

Wise, K. D., Anderson, D. J., Hetke, J. F., Kipke, D. R., and Najafi, K. (2004), Wireless implantable microsystems: High-density electronic interfaces to the nervous system, *Proc IEEE,* 92 (1), 76–97.

Wise, K. D., and Angell, J. B. (1975), A low-capacitance multielectrode probe for use in extracellular neurophysiology, *IEEE Trans Biomed Eng,* 22 (3), 212–219.

Wise, K. D., Angell, J. B., and Starr, A. (1970), An integrated-circuit approach to extracellular microelectrodes, *IEEE Trans Biomed Eng,* 17 (3), 238–247.

Wolpaw, J. R. (2004), Brain-computer interfaces (BCIs) for communication and control: A mini-review, *Suppl Clin Neurophysiol,* 57, 607–613.

Wolpaw, J. R., Birbaumer, N., McFarland, D. J., Pfurtscheller, G., and Vaughan, T. M. (2002), Brain-computer interfaces for communication and control, *Clin Neurophysiol: J Int Fed Clin Neurophysiol,* 113 (6), 767–791.

Woolley, A. J., Desai, H., Steckbeck, M. A., Patel, N., and Otto, K. J. (2010), Characterizing tissue around intracortical microelectrode interfaces using imaging strategies which minimize morphological disruption, *40th Annual Meeting of the Society for Neuroscience,* San Diego, CA.

Woolley, A. J., Desai, H., Steckbeck, M. A. Patel, N., and Otto, K. J. (2011), In situ characterization of the brain-microdevice interface using Device Capture Histology, *Journal of Neuroscience Methods,* 201, 67–77.

Yu, Z., Graudejus, O., Lacour, S. P., Wagner, S., and Morrison, B III. (2009), Neural sensing of electrical activity with stretchable microelectrode arrays, *Conf Proc IEEE Eng Med Biol Soc,* 2009, 4210–4213.

Zhong, Y., and Bellamkonda, R. V. (2007), Dexamethasone-coated neural probes elicit attenuated inflammatory response and neuronal loss compared to uncoated neural probes, *Brain Res,* 1148, 15–27.

6 | ACQUIRING BRAIN SIGNALS FROM OUTSIDE THE BRAIN

RAMESH SRINIVASAN

Most brain-computer interfaces (BCIs) determine their user's wishes by recording electromagnetic signals noninvasively from sensors on or above the scalp. As described in chapter 3 of this volume, the two principal noninvasive extracranial methods that are used for BCIs are electroencephalography (EEG) and magnetoencephalography (MEG). Chapter 3 describes the generation of EEG and MEG signals by the dipole current sources produced by neural activity and the principles that determine their distribution through the head. This chapter addresses the methods for recording these signals. EEG is the main focus because it is by far the most commonly used noninvasive BCI methodology. EEG is inexpensive, convenient, and amenable to diverse environments and has been developed commercially into portable and even wireless designs for a wide variety of purposes. EEG in general and EEG-based BCI technology in particular have generated a substantial body of theoretical and practical research literature. In contrast, only a few research groups are actively working on MEG-based BCIs, because MEG instrumentation is expensive, cumbersome, and not practical for everyday use. As a result, at least to date, MEG is used mainly as a research tool for BCI technology.

In the first part of this chapter we consider practical aspects of EEG and MEG recordings. In the remainder we consider the critical physical issues associated with use of these methods. These issues will be addressed by using both real EEG data and simulations in idealized physical models of the head to clarify the key features of EEG and MEG signals. Physical models of EEG and MEG recordings underlie *source analysis* methods and are constructed based on the fundamental properties of the electric and magnetic fields generated by current sources in the brain. We focus on the two main practical issues in the acquisition of EEG signals: reference location and number of electrodes. The models will help us understand the impact that these two experimental parameters have on spatial properties of recordings. We conclude by considering alternative choices regarding data-acquisition strategy in the specific context of BCI applications.

EEG RECORDING

EEG ELECTRODES

Every EEG recording involves at least three electrodes: a ground electrode and two recording electrodes. Figure 6.1 depicts EEG recording from a human subject who is conductively isolated from the ground of the power supply. The ground electrode is connected to the amplifier ground, which is isolated from the ground of the power supply. As described in detail in chapter 3, potential differences $V_2(t) - V_1(t)$ measured on the scalp are generated by brain *current sources* $P(\mathbf{r}, t)$ (current dipole moments per unit volume) and by biological artifacts. Environmental electric and magnetic fields can also generate scalp potentials, mostly due to capacitive coupling of body and electrode leads to ambient electromagnetic fields (e.g., from power lines and other electric equipment.)

In figure 6.1, the potentials at scalp locations 1 and 2 with respect to an external ground ("infinity") are given by $V_1(t) + V_{CM}(t)$ and $V_2(t) + V_{CM}(t)$, respectively, where $V_{CM}(t)$ is the *common mode potential* (the potential common to both locations that is caused mostly by power-line fields). Electrocardiographic (ECG) signals and other factors can also make contributions. EEG systems as exemplified by figure 6.1 use *differential amplifiers*, which are designed to reject the (spatially constant) common-mode potential $V_{CM}(t)$ and amplify the potential difference between pairs of scalp locations such that the output voltage $E(t)$ is proportional to scalp potential differences generated within the body (Kamp et al., 2005), that is,

$$E(t) = A[V_2(t) - V_1(t)] \tag{6.1}$$

where A is the total system *gain* typically due to several amplifier stages. The ground electrode that is placed on the scalp, nose, or neck provides a reference voltage to the amplifier to prevent amplifier drift and to facilitate better common-mode rejection. As shown in figure 6.1, the ground serves as a reference for the differential amplifier. The remaining unwanted contribution from the common-mode signal is due mainly to unequal contact impedances of the two recording electrodes (Ferree et al., 2001).

Traditional EEG practice provides guidelines for contact impedances, typically requiring impedances of less than 10 kΩ (Picton et al., 2000). This can be achieved by abrading the scalp at the electrode site and using a conductive gel or paste between the electrode and the scalp. When using modern amplifiers that have large input impedances (e.g., 200 MΩ), electrode-contact impedances of ~30–50 kΩ (relatively large compared to traditional guidelines) can easily be tolerated without degrading EEG quality (Ferree et al., 2001); the only noticeable effect is to increase power-line artifacts at 50 Hz (Europe, Asia, Africa, Oceania) or 60 Hz (North and South America), which

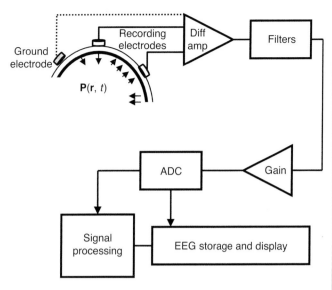

Figure 6.1 *The major components of a typical EEG recording system are shown. Electrodes record scalp signals due to brain current sources (arrows); the signals are passed through differential amplifiers sensitive to potential differences between electrode pairs and insensitive to common-mode potentials (the generally much larger, spatially constant potentials over the scalp). Modern EEG systems record simultaneously from about 32–131 scalp locations. Analog filters low-pass filter (see chapter 7) the input signal, typically removing substantial EEG power above about 50 or 100 Hz. High-pass analog EEG filters typically remove substantial power below about 0.5 Hz (depending on the application). A notch filter (chapter 7) may or may not be used to remove the power-line frequency (e.g., 60 Hz in the United States, 50 Hz in Europe and Asia). The scalp signal is substantially boosted by amplifier gains (e.g., amplified 20,000 times). In modern EEG systems the amplified analog signals are sampled and digitized, and numbers are assigned to successive segments of the waveforms. This step is called analog-to-digital conversion (ADC). It requires calibration by measuring the ADC output produced by a known calibration signal. EEG waveforms may then be displayed on a computer screen and stored for additional processing. In BCI systems, online processing of the EEG signals often starts with frequency analysis (using the fast Fourier transform [FFT] or another method) of each data channel. See chapter 7 for more information about low-pass, high-pass, and notch filtering as well as the FFT and other frequency analysis methods. (Adapted from Cadwell and Villarreal, 1999, and Fisch, 1999.)*

can easily be removed from the data by online analog filters or by postprocessing with digital filters (see chapter 7, in this volume). This tolerance for higher-impedance electrode contacts that is provided by high-input-impedance amplifiers allows the use of electrodes embedded in small sponges containing conductive saline solution. These sponge-saline electrode systems have higher contact impedance than the conductive-gel electrode systems traditionally used for EEG. On the other hand, application of the electrodes is significantly faster: a large number (e.g., 128) of sponge-saline electrodes can be placed in 15 minutes, as compared to 20 minutes or more with conventional gel electrodes. The major disadvantage of sponge-saline electrodes is their limited recording time (about an hour) because impedances rise as the sponges dry.

Both conductive-gel and sponge-saline electrode systems use metallic electrodes usually made from tin (Sn), silver/silver-chloride (Ag/AgCl), gold (Au), or platinum (Pt). Sn electrodes are the least costly but introduce low-frequency noise

below 1 Hz. In applications where low-frequency recordings are essential (e.g., most event-related potential [ERP] recordings; see chapters 12 and 14, in this volume), Ag/AgCl electrodes are typically used. Most commercial EEG electrode systems use Ag/AgCl electrodes. Au electrodes also minimize drift and show less high-frequency noise than Ag/AgCl electrodes.

Conductive-gel and sponge-saline electrodes are often referred to as *wet electrodes*. Because of the inconvenience and messiness of the typical electrode gels and the short useful lifespan of the electrode saline solutions, there has been much interest in recent years in developing *dry electrodes*, electrodes that do not require the low-impedance contact with the scalp that gel and mild skin abrasion provide to wet electrodes. The sensor material of a dry electrode can be an inert metal (e.g., platinum, gold, or stainless steel) or even an insulator. Whichever material is used, there is generally a capacitive coupling between the skin and the electrode. A number of different dry electrodes have been described (Taheri et al., 1994; Searle et al., 2000; Popescu et al., 2007; Matthews et al., 2007; Sullivan et al., 2008; Sellers et al., 2009; Gargiulo et al., 2010; Grozea et al., 2011), and several are available from commercial vendors (e.g., Nouzz [http://nouzz.com], Quasar [http://www.quasarusa.com]). However, problems related to movement, environmental noise, and degradation of the sensor materials in contact with sweat on the skin have been identified but are not yet adequately resolved. Thus, although anxiously awaited by many in the EEG community, dry-electrode technology is still evolving. For the practicality of noninvasive BCIs, the successful development of dry electrodes could represent an extremely significant advance.

It is also worth noting that several options that reduce (but do not eliminate) the need for conductive gel (or saline) and skin abrasion are currently available (Brunner et al., 2011). *Active electrodes*, electrodes that amplify the EEG signal at the electrode, are offered by many commercial vendors (although they are typically quite expensive). Another option is active shielding of the connection between the electrode and the amplifier in order to prevent capacitive coupling with the environment (Twente Medical Systems International, http://www.tmsi.com).

BIPOLARITY OF EEG RECORDING

As emphasized in chapter 3, it is important to recognize that *there are no monopolar recordings in EEG. All EEG recordings are bipolar*: it is always necessary to use electrode pairs to measure scalp potentials because such recording depends on current passing through a measuring circuit (Nunez and Srinivasan, 2006), and each electrode in the pair is active (i.e., its voltage fluctuates over time). Thus, no EEG recording measures the voltage difference between an active electrode and an inactive, or unchanging, electrode. Typically, one of the two electrodes is designated as the *recording electrode* and the other electrode is designated the *reference electrode*. In reality, the EEG signal depends equally on the potentials at both the recording electrode and the reference electrode positions.

In most EEG practice, the potentials at all the other (typically 32–256) electrodes are recorded with respect to one electrode selected as the reference electrode. Any particular choice of reference placement has advantages and disadvantages that depend on the locations of the sources generating the EEG signals. Because we usually do not know with precision the locations of the sources before recording EEG, it is often not obvious in advance which will be the best reference location. References are frequently chosen without clear understanding of the biases they impose on the recording. For example, many researchers have used and may still use the linked-ears or linked-mastoids reference, but there is minimal theoretical justification for this choice. Another popular choice is the common-average reference. The properties of these two popular reference choices are discussed in detail later in this chapter. Fortunately, it is possible to reference all the electrodes to a single electrode, and then, by simple subtraction in postprocessing, change the effective reference to another recording site. Other simple linear transformations are also possible and often useful, including the nearest-neighbor (Hjorth) Laplacian and common-average reference (discussed later in this chapter and in chapter 7, this volume). Thus, when all electrodes are referenced to a single electrode during recording, the choice of that reference electrode can be arbitrary since the data can easily be rereferenced in postrecording data processing.

EEG ELECTRODE MONTAGE

The positions of the electrodes are referred to collectively as the *electrode montage.* In practice, these vary considerably across laboratories. Standard electrode-placement strategies use the International 10–20, 10–10, and 10–5 placement systems shown in figure 6.2 (Oostenveld and Praamstra, 2001). These montages are based on systematic extensions of the standard clinical-EEG 10–20 electrode montage (Kiem et al., 1999), and they are widely (but not universally) used. The basis of these standard electrode placements is to define contours between skull landmarks (e.g., nasion and inion) and to subdivide the resulting contours in proportional distances. The standard 10–20 system uses proportional distances of 20% of the total length along contours between skull landmarks, whereas the 10–10 and 10–5 systems use 10% and 5% distances, respectively. Figure 6.2 shows the standard 10–20 system consisting of 21 electrodes indicated by black circles. The standard nomenclature used to identify electrodes by the major skull bones is indicated on each of these electrodes (AES, 1994). Note that electrodes on the left side are odd-numbered, whereas electrodes on the right side are even-numbered, and that midline electrodes are indicated by z. The 10–10 system consists of 74 electrodes: it includes the 10–20 electrodes (black circles) as well as 53 additional electrodes (gray circles). Possible intermediate electrodes defined by the 10–5 system are indicated by dots or open circles. The 68 open-circle electrodes (named by extending the standard nomenclature), combined with the 10–10 system, comprise a subset of 142 electrodes that provides a more complete and homogeneous coverage of the head (Oostenveld and

Praamstra, 2001). EEG caps with 128 of these electrodes are widely available commercially. It should be noted that for large numbers of channels (>64), other placement systems have been developed, with the goal of obtaining more regularly spaced sampling of scalp potentials, an approach that is potentially advantageous for source localization and high-resolution EEG methods (Tucker, 1993).

SAMPLING RATE

EEG signals are detected by the electrodes, amplified and filtered by analog circuits, and then digitized. The analog circuits remove both low- and high-frequency noise and all signal components that have frequencies greater than the Nyquist limit (see chapter 7, in this volume), which is defined by the sampling rate of the analog-to-digital converter (ADC). The discrete sampling of continuous signals is a well-characterized problem in time-series acquisition and analysis (Bendat and Piersol, 2001). As discussed in chapter 7, the central concept is the *Nyquist criterion:* $f_{dig} > 2f_{max}$ where f_{dig} is the digitization (i.e., sampling) rate and f_{max} is the highest frequency present in the signal. For example, if the highest frequency in a signal is 20 Hz (20 cycles per second), a minimum sampling rate of 40 Hz (one sample every 25 msec) is required. This frequency ensures that each peak and each trough in the 20-Hz oscillation is sampled once so that we can detect that oscillation. Sampling at a lower rate will cause *aliasing*, defined as the misrepresentation of a high-frequency signal as a low-frequency signal because the sampling rate of the ADC is lower than the Nyquist limit. If a time series has been aliased by undersampling, no digital signal processing method can undo the aliasing because the information necessary for accurate representation of the time series is not present in the digitized data.

In conventional digital EEG practice, a sampling rate is selected and the aliasing error is avoided by applying a low-pass filter (see chapter 7, in this volume) to the analog signal. (As the name implies, a low-pass filter allows only signals of frequency below a given value to pass.) This filter eliminates power (i.e., amplitude squared) at frequencies greater than the maximum frequency determined by the Nyquist limit. In practice, it is most common to use what is termed the *Engineer's Nyquist criterion* (or *the Engineer's Nyquist limit*) by which the low-pass filter is typically applied with a cutoff frequency that is 2.5 times smaller than the sampling rate (e.g., if the frequencies of interest are less than 30 Hz, the cut-off frequency is 30 Hz, and the sampling rate is at least 75 Hz). This more restrictive limit, the *Engineer's Nyquist limit*, is used to account for the possibility of *phase-locking* between the sampling and high-frequency components of the signal (Bendat and Piersol, 2001). (Phase locking occurs if the ADC and a high-frequency component of the signal are synchronized.) That is, if phase-locking occurs and the ADC rate is only twice that of the component, the component will always be sampled at the same points in its cycle, and this will produce a distorted measure of its amplitude. For example, if it is always sampled at its negative and positive peaks, its measured power will be falsely high, whereas if it is always sampled at its zero-crossings, its power will be

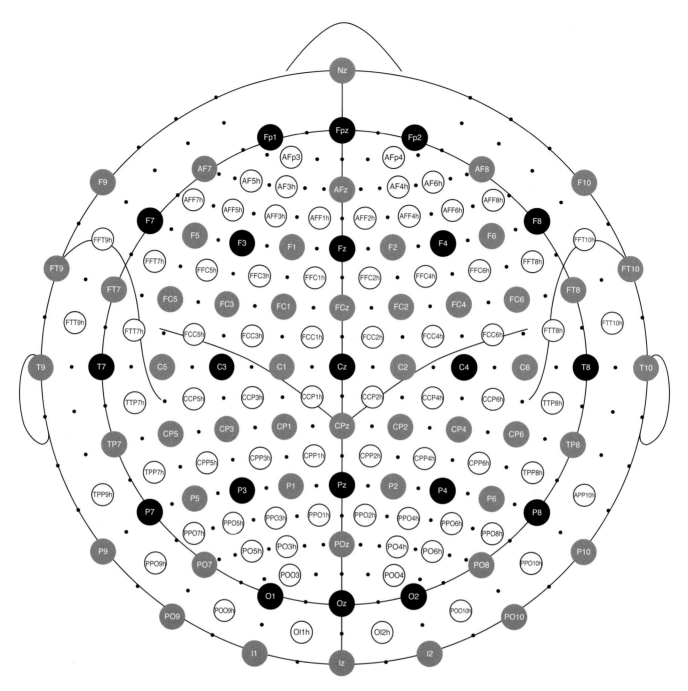

Figure 6.2 *The standard 10–20, 10–10, and 10–5 electrode montages. The 10–20 montage is indicated by the 21 electrodes shown as black circles. The 10–10 montage (totalling 74 electrodes) consists of the 21 electrodes of the 10–20 montage (black circles) plus 53 additional electrodes indicated in gray. The additional electrodes of the 10–5 montage are indicated by the black dots and the open circles. The 68 open circles and the 74 10–10 electrodes together comprise a 142-channel montage that provides a more complete and homogeneous coverage of the head. The nomenclature for the standard 10–20 and 10–10 and 10–5 extensions is indicated. Note that electrodes on the right side have even numbers and electrodes on the left side have odd numbers, while electrodes along the midline are indicated by z. (Reproduced with permission from Ooostenveld and Praamstra, 2001.)*

measured as zero. Using the Engineer's Nyquist criterion prevents such distortion.

Typically, the analog signal from each EEG channel is *sampled* 200–1000 times/sec, *digitized* (assigned numbers proportional to instantaneous amplitude), and *converted* from ADC units to volts. In conventional clinical EEG practice, these samples are then stored on a disk. In BCI applications and in certain clinical applications, they are also processed online (see chapters 7 and 8, in this volume) to produce a real-time output.

AVOIDING, RECOGNIZING, AND ELIMINATING NONBRAIN SIGNALS (ARTIFACTS)

Nonbrain physiological sources make substantial (and undesirable) contributions to EEG recordings. These include primarily signals from cranial muscle activity (measured by electromyography [EMG]), eye movements (measured by electrooculography [EOG]), and heart muscle activity (measured by electrocardiography [ECG]). EMG artifacts are broadband high-frequency artifacts observed above ~10 Hz. EOG artifacts generated by eye blinks or eye movements and ECG artifacts generated by the heart have stereotypical waveforms that can be easily identified in an EEG record (Fisch, 1999). Mechanical effects from electrode or cable movement typically induce low-frequency (<2 Hz) oscillations, abrupt baseline shifts, or high-frequency transients (*electrode pops*). As noted earlier, higher electrode impedance will increase power-line (50–60 Hz) artifacts. Other kinds of environmental sources can also contaminate EEG recordings. One obvious consequence of all of these artifacts is potentially to reduce the signal-to-noise ratio for the EEG features used to produce BCI outputs. Moreover, artifacts (especially EMG) masquerading as EEG can give the false impression of EEG-based BCI control and/or interfere with the user's acquisition of actual EEG-based BCI control (e.g., McFarland et al., 2005). Although nonbrain activity may be useful for some purposes (e.g., EMG switches for assistive communication), in the context of BCI research and development, nonbrain activity constitutes artifact that needs to be avoided, detected, and eliminated.

Many of the potential artifacts in EEG signals occur at higher frequencies (e.g., power-line noise (50/60 Hz) and EMG activity). This suggests the possibility of using the amplifier's low-pass filter to remove the high-frequency artifacts. However, the choice of filter settings requires careful consideration. Clearly, a low-pass filter must be set to ensure removal of power at frequencies above the Nyquist criterion. However, severe low-pass filtering increases the risk of allowing muscle artifact (i.e., EMG) to masquerade as EEG. This can occur because EMG is normally recognized by its power at high frequencies (well above the EEG frequency range); removal of high-frequency EMG by a low-pass filter will actually prevent recognition of EMG artifacts present in the low-frequency range. As a result, the remaining low-frequency EMG can be mistaken for EEG (Fisch, 1999). For example, suppose that an analog filter is used to remove most power at frequencies greater than 30 Hz, thereby obtaining a much cleaner-looking EEG signal. The remaining signal might well contain significant muscle artifact in the 8–30 Hz range (the mu and beta bands), and it will be much more difficult to recognize this artifact without the higher-frequency information to provide guidance. In particular, such subtle muscle artifacts could substantially reduce the signal-to-noise ratio in the beta band or even the mu band. It is important to recognize that EMG artifact can contaminate EEG signals even when they are recorded over central head areas (e.g., Goncharova et al., 2003).

Many commercial EEG systems have *notch filters* (see chapter 7, in this volume) to remove power-line interference (60 Hz in North and South America; 50 Hz in Europe, Asia, Africa, and Oceania). On the other hand, the appearance of such noise serves as a warning that electrode impedance has risen (or that the electrode may even have lost contact entirely). Thus, automatic removal of power-line noise takes away a useful check on system function. Furthermore, if EEG processing and analysis are based on FFT or other spectral-analysis methods, the presence of moderate 60-Hz noise has

no practical effect on the lower frequencies that contain most of the EEG information. This suggests that the best strategy (particularly for BCI research studies) for minimizing contamination with artifact is to identify useful EEG features in frequency bands that are less likely to have artifacts and to carry out the comprehensive topographic and spectral analyses needed to distinguish EEG from non-EEG (particularly EMG) signals.

MEG RECORDING

In addition to the generation of *electrical* signals, brain-current sources can also generate an external *magnetic* field that can be detected with specialized sensors. Detection of these magnetic signals is performed by MEG (see chapter 3, this volume) (see Hamaleinen et al., 1993, for a detailed review). MEG methods record the small magnetic field generated by the brain using a superconducting quantum interference device (SQUID) magnetometer. SQUID devices were first used to detect the magnetic field of the brain in the 1970s (Cohen, 1972) and are sensitive detectors of magnetic flux. As discussed in chapter 3, it is important to recognize that the magnetic fields associated with brain activity are not coupled to the brain's electrical fields; that is, they are not the more familiar electromagnetic fields

When compared to EEG recording, MEG has advantages and disadvantages. For BCI applications, a major disadvantage of MEG is that the magnetic fields associated with brain current sources are very small relative to the ambient magnetic-field variations that are outside experimental control (e.g., fluctuations in the Earth's magnetic field). Moreover, MEG (like EEG) has the usual problems of noise from power-line fields. Thus, as typically used, an MEG SQUID coil is able to detect the small magnetic field generated by the brain only when the subject is placed in a specially shielded chamber, usually made of high-permeability mu-metal (Hamaleinen et al., 1993), in order to minimize contamination of the recording by the external magnetic field. Superconductivity is essential to the function of the SQUID coils, so the coils are maintained at very low temperatures in a helium-containing insulated (Dewar) chamber. The main practical effect of this elaborate system is that the measurement point is about 1–2 cm above the scalp surface. This substantial distance from the sources of brain activity reduces spatial resolution significantly.

Individual SQUID coils, called *magnetometers*, can be arranged in different configurations to accommodate different purposes. The simplest configuration is a single magnetometer. An array of 100–200 magnetometers can provide coverage of the entire head. Each one detects only the radial component of the magnetic field generated by brain sources. Another common coil configuration is an *axial gradiometer*, which consists of a *pick-up coil* and a *compensation coil* located above the pick-up coil; the two coils are wound in opposite directions to cancel noise produced by nonbrain magnetic fields. Although both the simple magnetometer and the axial-gradiometer coil configurations have spatial resolution comparable to (but sometimes poorer than) EEG (Malmivuo and Plonsey, 1995; Srinivasan 2006; Srinivasan et al., 2007), they are both more sensitive than EEG to a particular subset of sources. Whereas EEG detects activity from both tangential and radial sources, MEG is sensitive to sources oriented tangentially to the detectors and is blind to sources pointed radially (Nunez and Srinivasan, 2006). This property of MEG is identically valid in spherical models of the head (see chapter 3 in this volume) and is approximately valid in realistic models that include the fields produced by return currents. MEG's preferential sensitivity for tangential sources has particular value in studies of primary sensory areas of the brain that are located in sulcal folds oriented tangential to the MEG coils (Hamaleinen et al., 1993). This preferential sensitivity to tangential sources, discussed in more detail later in this chapter, accounts for the main practical distinction between EEG and MEG.

A recently developed MEG system implements a *planar gradiometer*; it consists of two adjacent coils (with parallel axes) wound in opposite directions. This configuration measures the gradient of the radial component of the magnetic field in one direction. The *planar gradiometer* strategy is similar to the bipolar EEG recording strategy (see *EEG Reference Electrode Selection*, in this chapter) and imparts to MEG a potentially much higher spatial resolution than is possible with conventional MEG.

A major advantage of MEG over EEG is that MEG provides a true field measure at a specific point, whereas EEG measures the potential difference between two points on the head. Thus, MEG does not require the choice of a reference sensor. As explicated in the *EEG Reference Electrode Selection* section of this chapter, reference selection is a critical factor in EEG recording, since an improper choice can result in data that are misleading or even entirely useless. Furthermore, MEG is less distorted by the head openings and other tissue inhomogeneities that can distort EEG. (Because current follows the paths of lowest resistance, such irregularities may cause EEG electrodes to record substantial scalp currents produced by sources located far from the recording sites.) These and other considerations such as signal-to-noise ratio and electrode density must be taken into account when assessing the relative advantages and disadvantages of EEG and MEG for a particular application. Other practical issues, such as temporal filtering and analog-to-digital conversion (ADC) are identical for EEG and MEG.

COMPARISON OF EEG AND MEG IN SENSITIVITY AND SPATIAL RESOLUTION

To some degree, EEG and MEG complement each other in their sensitivities to cortical activity. This is illustrated in figure 6.3 in which each arrow indicates a cortical dipole. In cortex, EEG is most sensitive to correlated dipoles located in cortical *gyri* (e.g., regions a–b, d–e, and g–h in fig. 6.3). EEG is less sensitive to correlated dipoles located in cortical *sulci* (e.g., region h–i). It is insensitive to *apposing* sets of correlated dipoles (i.e., sets that cancel each other due to their opposite orientations) located in sulci (regions b–c–d and e–f–g) and randomly oriented dipoles (region i–j–k–l–m). In contrast, MEG is most sensitive to correlated and minimally opposed

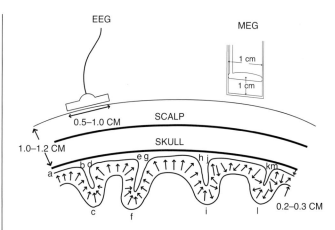

Figure 6.3 *Sources of EEG and MEG signals. Neocortical sources can be pictured generally as dipole layers (or dipole sheets) that fold in and out of cortical fissures and sulci, with mesoscale source strength (see chapter 3, in this volume) varying as a function of cortical location. EEG is most sensitive to correlated dipole layers in gyri (such as regions a–b, d–e, and g–h), less sensitive to correlated dipole layers in sulci (such as region h–i) and insensitive to opposing dipole layers in sulci (such as regions b–c–d and e–f–g) and randomly oriented dipoles (such as region i–j–k–l–m). MEG is most sensitive to correlated and minimally opposed dipole layers in sulci (such as region h–i) and much less sensitive to all the other sources shown, which are radial, opposing, or randomly oriented dipole layers.*

dipoles located in sulci (e.g., region h–i) and much less sensitive to all the other dipoles shown (i.e., radial, random, or apposed dipoles). Subcortical structures such as the thalamus make negligible contributions to EEG and MEG signals because of their smaller surface areas and greater distances from the sensors (Nunez, 1981).

It is not generally true that MEG has better spatial resolution than EEG, despite the fact that this idea has entered into the common folklore of the neuroscience community. This reality can be appreciated by direct examination of the properties of volume conduction in EEG and field spread in MEG (Malmivuo and Plonsey, 1995; Srinivasan et al., 2007). Figure 6.4 shows the sensitivity distributions for a single EEG electrode (yellow circle in figure inset) and a single MEG coil (small green line seen exterior to the head in inset). For this figure Srinivasan et al. (2007) defined a sensitivity function that describes the contribution of sources at each location to the signal recorded by the sensor. Figure 6.4A shows that the EEG electrode is most sensitive to sources in the gyral crown closest to the electrode. Although sensitivity falls off with distance from the electrode, gyral crowns distributed elsewhere over the hemisphere contribute roughly half the potential of the crown directly beneath the electrode. Sources along sulcal walls, even when close to the electrode, contribute much less to the EEG than sources in the gyral crowns. Figure 6.4B shows the sensitivity of the same electrode after applying a Laplacian transformation (see *Surface Laplacian* section later in this chapter; see chapters 3 and 7, in this volume). As expected, the sensitivity of the EEG Laplacian is highest for the gyral crown directly beneath the electrode. At the same time, the Laplacian is far less sensitive to distant gyral crowns and thereby provides a far more localized measure of source activity. Figure 6.4C shows the sensitivity distribution of an MEG coil located 2 cm above the EEG electrode. The sensitivity function has local

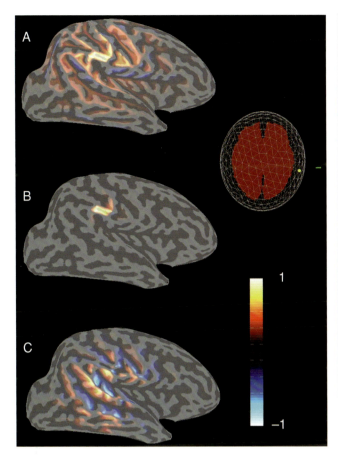

Figure 6.4 Brain sensitivity distributions associated with (A) the raw scalp EEG, (B) a surface Laplacian of scalp EEG, and (C) MEG, for a single EEG electrode location (yellow circle at right inset) and a single magnetic coil position (green line at right inset). The cortical surface was constructed from the MRI of one subject. Simulated dipole sources P(r, t) (dipole moment per unit volume, 100,000 in one hemisphere) were assumed to be normal to the local cortical surface. Scalp surface potentials, scalp Laplacians, and surface normal magnetic fields due to each dipole were calculated at the electrode and coil locations shown in the inset based on a concentric three-ellipsoid head model. (See Srinivasan et al., 2007, for details of these simulations.) The potentials, Laplacians, and magnetic fields were normalized with respect to their maximum values (i.e., +1 and −1 on the scale bar) so that the relative sensitivity of the three measurements could be compared. (A) The EEG electrode is most sensitive to the gyral sources under the electrode, but this electrode is also sensitive to large source regions in relatively remote gyral crowns; it is much less sensitive to sources in cortical folds. (B) The Laplacian is most sensitive to gyral sources under the electrode; sensitivity falls off very rapidly at moderate and large distances. (C) The MEG is most sensitive to sources in cortical folds that tend to be tangential to MEG coils. Maximum MEG sensitivity occurs in folds that are roughly 4 cm from the coil in directions tangent to the surface. Regions in blue provide contributions to MEG of opposite sign to those of yellow/orange, reflecting dipoles on opposite sides of folds; these tend to produce canceling magnetic fields at the coil.

maxima on sulcal walls. Since apposing dipoles in sulcal walls (e.g., regions b–c–d and e–f–g in fig. 6.3) have opposite effects on the coil because of the reversal in source orientation, opposing sulcal walls with correlated activity are expected to make only small or negligible contributions to MEG.

It is clear from figure 6.4 that the MEG coil, like the EEG electrode, is sensitive to a wide area of the cortex. Indeed, estimates of the area of sensitivity (Srinivasan et al., 2007; Malmivuo and Plonsey, 1995) indicate that MEG is sensitive to

a somewhat wider region of cortex than EEG. This effect is a direct consequence of the greater distance between sources and sensors in MEG than EEG. The recent developments in MEG hardware (i.e., planar gradiometer coils) potentially provide much better spatial resolution (analogous to the role played by close bipolar EEG recordings). Nevertheless, even with advances in MEG recording technology, the main differences between EEG and MEG are not related to spatial resolution. *The main difference between EEG and MEG is that they are preferentially sensitive to different sources.* The choice of method depends on the location, orientation, and size of the source region, which is rarely known in advance. The main advantage of MEG for source localization is that the model of the spread of the magnetic field is much simpler and better understood than models of volume conduction of electric current. The main disadvantage of MEG is the cost and complexity of the instrumentation as compared to EEG.

EEG REFERENCE ELECTRODE SELECTION

CHOICE OF A REFERENCE ELECTRODE SITE

One of the most important issues in any EEG recording strategy is the choice of reference-electrode location. Figure 6.5 shows examples of a visual evoked potential (VEP) recorded at a right occipital electrode (O_2 in the 10–20 electrode system; location X in figure 6.5A and 6.5C), with the reference mathematically (see *Bipolarity of EEG Recording* section above and chapter 3, in this volume) shifted to different electrode positions. Because the occipital cortex contains striate and extrastriate visual areas, the VEP is reasonably expected to include signals generated by sources in occipital cortex. Figure 6.5A shows the VEP with the reference mathematically shifted to each of three different electrodes within 2.7 cm of the vertex electrode (C_Z), which was the reference-electrode position used for the recording. The VEP is often characterized in terms of the magnitude of the positive and negative voltage peaks. The amplitude of the first positive deflection, peaking at approximately 120 msec poststimulus, is reduced by about one-third as the reference site is changed from the midline position (1) to either of the other two positions (2, 3). Amplitude differences are also evident at other peaks in the evoked-potential waveform. Figure 6.5B shows the same VEP with the reference site shifted to three midline frontal locations (4, 5, 6) separated from one another by less than 2.7 cm. The first positive peak is reduced in comparison to reference positions near the vertex shown in figure 6.5A, and the shape of the evoked potential is considerably altered between 100 and 350 msec poststimulus. When the reference is located at frontal sites, the VEP is dominated by a faster oscillation than that seen in the waveform obtained when the reference is close to the vertex (compare figs. 6.5A and 6.5B). Figure 6.5C shows the VEP with the reference site mathematically shifted to the left mastoid (7) or temporal electrodes (8, 9). The positive peak occurring 120 msec poststimulus is no longer distinguishable from noise, and the first distinct peak occurs 200 msec poststimulus. Thus, both the amplitude and temporal structure of the VEP recorded at a location over the occipital lobe can be altered

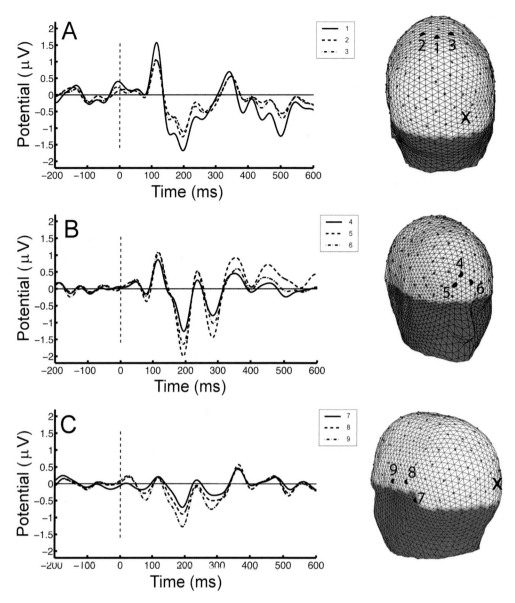

Figure 6.5 *Influence of the reference-electrode site on the visual evoked potential (VEP). The original VEP (A) was recorded at the occipital location O_2 (site X on the head in A) with respect to a Cz reference (site 1). All other sites in the three images were also recorded with respect to the Cz reference. This allowed the VEP to be referenced not only to site 1 but also to be rereferenced to sites 2 and 3 in A, to sites 4, 5, and 6 in B, and to sites 7, 8, and 9 in C. This produced nine examples of the VEP, shown in the traces on the left. As discussed in detail in the text, it is clear that the choice of the reference location has a substantial influence on VEP waveforms, even when the references are located seemingly far from the primary visual cortex under O_2. (Adapted with permission from Nunez and Srinivasan, 2006.)*

considerably by the choice of reference site. Which is the true VEP? The answer is *all of them*. VEPs depend on the location of *both* the so-called recording electrode *and* the so-called reference electrode. The different waveforms and peak amplitudes seen in figure 6.5 suggest that the sources and/or the volume currents caused by visual stimuli are not tightly confined to primary visual cortex, and thus that both electrodes (i.e., the so-called recording electrode *and* the so-called reference electrode) may be affected by them. VEP sources may be widely distributed, and/or the head volume conductor may provide low-resistance pathways over large distances. In fact, both of these possibilities probably occur and affect the VEPs.

Is there an ideal, or correct, reference position? Although the EEG folklore suggests that an *inactive* electrode is the ideal reference electrode, this notion stems from the unfounded idea that if a recording electrode is near a *generator* (i.e., a dipole source) and the reference electrode is far from it, the reference electrode can be considered to be at an infinite distance and therefore to be inactive. If this idealized picture were accurate, one could truly record potentials with respect to a standard zero-potential reference. However, the so-called *inactive* electrode may or may not be a good reference. Whether or not it is depends partly on the size of the generator region, which itself depends on several factors. Dipole layers of synchronous and partly aligned cortical neurons that extend over large areas of the cortical surface appear to be the primary generators of scalp EEG; thus, generator dimensions can easily be as large as tens of centimeters. With head diameters on the order of

20 cm, it is generally not possible to find a point on the head at a sufficiently large distance from the generator regions to be considered to be at an infinite distance away. Because of volume conduction, locating a reference electrode at a place where there is no underlying generator is not sufficient for it to be considered at infinity. Furthermore, low-resistance current paths in an inhomogeneous or anisotropic head can make electrical distances shorter than actual distances. Even if there is no generator activity directly beneath the electrode, for a reference to be considered at infinity, the *electrical distance* between the reference and recording electrodes must be very large in comparison to the generator region.

Because all sources and sinks of interest in EEG are located in the head, which is partly isolated (electrically) from the body except for the relatively narrow path through the neck, the current produced by brain sources is expected to be mostly confined to the head (Nunez and Srinivasan, 2006). We expect minimal current flow through the relatively narrow neck region. (Indeed, if neck geometry did not severely restrict neck currents, scalp potentials would often be greatly contaminated by ECG sources, which are about 100 times stronger than EEG sources.) Thus, for EEG, a reference on the neck is essentially the same as a reference anywhere on the body (if we disregard the minimal additional series resistance of the rest of the body) (Nunez and Srinivasan, 2006).

A REFERENCE ELECTRODE TEST

A simple test can reveal whether any candidate reference location can be considered a true reference (i.e., at infinity). Suppose, for example, that we suspect that there is beta activity localized in right motor cortex. If this assumption of a localized generator region is correct, any location on the left side of the head might qualify as a suitable reference. We might, for example, choose a putative reference over left prefrontal cortex. The critical reference test is to see whether the appearance of the beta activity remains constant as we change the reference location from left frontal to, for example, left temporal or left mastoid or left neck. If the amplitude and frequency are unchanged with such changes of reference location, then the *true reference test* is passed. If, on the other hand, the recorded beta activity changes as the reference location changes, the candidate reference location fails the true reference test, probably because the postulate of a localized source region is incorrect.

The examples of a VEP recorded at the occipital channel shown in figure 6.5 indicate that none of the reference sites examined passes the true reference test. The peak amplitudes and temporal waveforms change with the reference location. For each set of reference locations (fig. 6.5A, B, or C), shifting the reference locally even among the three closely spaced electrodes has substantial effects on the peak amplitudes and frequency content of the VEP. The implication is that, with each of these reference locations, the potential difference between the recording electrode and the reference electrode reflects a somewhat different set of sources. The distribution of sources underlying this VEP example may be sufficiently large and widely spread to prevent any location on the head from qualifying as at infinity.

The unavoidable conclusion is that no sufficiently distant reference point is generally available in EEG recording. We rarely know in advance where EEG sources are located (or if they are indeed localized at all), and thus we rarely know whether a true reference location exists or, if it does, where it is. Even in cases where the sources are truly localized, their locations must be known in advance in order to choose the appropriate reference. Thus, the (perhaps painful) truth about EEG references is that there is no essential difference between recording and reference electrodes: in EEG, we measure potential *differences* between two locations on the head, and these differences depend on the locations of both electrodes, as well as on the brain source configurations and locations. That is, every EEG recording is a *bipolar recording*: it reflects the voltage *difference* between two active electrodes.

CLOSELY SPACED ELECTRODES

In spite of the fact that all EEG recordings are in fact bipolar, EEG terminology usually uses the term *bipolar recording* to refer to the special case of measuring the potential difference between *two electrodes that are relatively close to one another*. Today, the term bipolar recording is used most commonly in clinical environments. As two electrodes are moved closer and closer together, they provide a progressively better (or more fine-grained) estimate of the local gradient of the potential (i.e., voltage) along the scalp surface on the line between the two electrodes. As discussed in chapter 3, the electric field is proportional to current density along the scalp surface. When the two electrodes are placed close together, the recorded potential difference is roughly proportional to the current density tangential to the scalp. The current flows from higher to lower potential.

Bipolar recordings with closely-spaced electrodes (i.e., <2–3 cm apart) are better for localizing sources (at least idealized superficial sources) than are recordings that use a single fixed reference at some relatively distant location. The use of bipolar electrode pairs for measuring local tangential electric fields is an improvement over distant-reference recordings in the sense that both electrodes are explicitly acknowledged to be active (and the reference issue becomes moot). If the bipolar pair crosses isopotential lines, it senses current flow from regions of higher to lower potential. In contrast, if the bipolar pair is placed along an isopotential line, zero potential difference is recorded. Clinical electroencephalographers often use different bipolar pairs to emphasize different sources, and to make qualitative judgments of their orientation and localization based on long experience with such methods (Pilgreen, 1995; Fisch, 1999). In addition, raw EEG may be recorded with respect to a distant fixed reference and later converted to bipolar recordings by subtraction (see *Bipolarity of EEG Recording* section above and chapter 3, this volume), provided that the recording electrodes were placed sufficiently close together.

Figure 6.6 provides an example of three additional sets of VEP recordings, this time using bipolar electrode pairs. Each set consists of VEPs from 6 different bipolar pairs. Each pair consists of a fixed (central) recording electrode (X in the figure) and an electrode at one of six surrounding positions, all at a distance of ~2.7 cm from X. In each plot, the six black curves indicate the bipolar potentials, while the thick gray line is the mean of all six bipolar potentials. These bipolar VEPs are considerably different from the VEPs shown in figure 6.5, which used distant references. Peaks are still evident at 100 and 200 msec poststimulus, but the slower oscillation evident in figure 6.5A and the potentials at 300 msec or later are reduced in each set of bipolar VEPs shown in figure 6.6. The positive peak at 120 msec poststimulus is clearest in figure 6.6B, where five of the six bipolar pairs exhibit a positive peak. The bipolar VEPs in figure 6.6B are generally larger than the bipolar VEPs in figures 6.6A and C. This implies that some of the source

activity is localized in brain tissue immediately beneath the central electrode (X) of figure 6.6B. In figures 6.6A and C, the different bipolar pairs show 120-msec peaks of opposite polarity, and these average to near zero (i.e., the gray traces). This implies the presence, at the central (X) electrodes of figures 6.6A and C, of tangential currents passing from regions of higher potential to lower potential. Thus, although the bipolar VEPs reveal a source below the central electrode of figure 6.6B, they provide little evidence for sources below the central electrode of figure 6.6A or 6.6C.

The analysis of close bipolar pairs illustrated in figure 6.6 can be an effective strategy to identify local generators. By

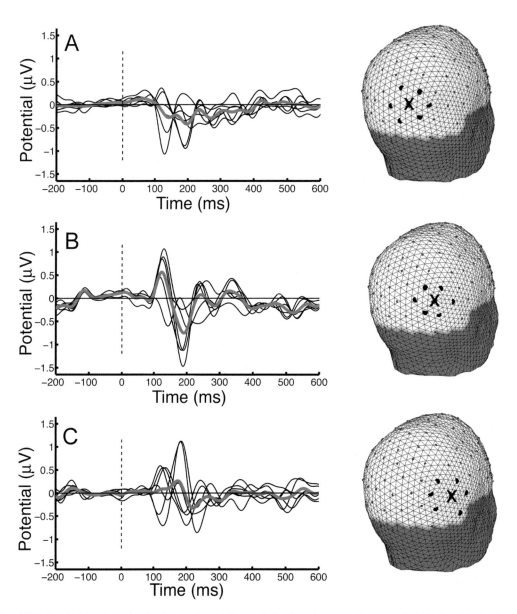

Figure 6.6 Examples of VEPs from bipolar electrode pairs. Starting from VEPs recorded with a reference at the vertex, the VEPs from bipolar electrode pairs were calculated by taking the difference between the VEP recorded at the central electrode in each set (referenced to the vertex) and the VEP at each of the six surrounding electrodes (also referenced to the vertex). In this way the effect of the original (i.e., the vertex) reference electrode cancels exactly. The separation distance between bipolar electrode pairs is 2.7 cm. Each plot (A, B, C) corresponds to a different right-posterior-area location of the center electrode in each set. The six different black VEPs in each plot come from the six bipolar pairs for the set of placements shown at the right. The thick gray line in each plot is the average of its six bipolar VEPs. See text for discussion.

placing the reference electrode nearby rather than at a distant location on the head, we limit the sensitivity of each pair of electrodes mainly to local sources. In fact, when 32 or fewer electrodes are available, closely spaced bipolar recordings are perhaps the best option available to improve the spatial resolution of the EEG (Srinivasan et al., 1996). Closely related to this strategy is the Hjorth or nearest-neighbor Laplacian (Hjorth, 1975) discussed in this chapter.

LINKED-EARS AND LINKED-MASTOIDS REFERENCE

The *linked-ears* or *linked-mastoids reference* is a popular reference strategy. However, the main reason for their widespread use appears to be tradition rather than a compelling theoretical justification. That is, there is no compelling reason to believe that this reference approximates an ideal reference (i.e., a reference at infinity).

Published EEG studies typically implement the linked-ears or linked-mastoids reference in two major ways. One, which we call the *physically linked-ears* (or the *physically linked-mastoids*) *reference*, is to physically link the ears (or mastoids) by a wire and use this wire as the reference. Alternatively, with the *mathematically linked-ears (or mastoid) reference,* each scalp potential (V_x) is recorded with respect to a reference placed at one ear ($V_x - V_{Ear1}$), with the potential at the second ear measured with respect to the first ear ($V_{Ear2} - V_{Ear1}$). The mathematically linked-ears reference is calculated by subtracting half this potential difference from each scalp potential, creating an artificial reference at the average potential of the two ears or mastoids.

It is now widely appreciated that the physically linked reference is actually a *random reference*, meaning that the effective reference site generally varies across subjects and/or over time in the same subject because of unequal electrode contact impedances (Nunez, 1991; Nunez and Srinivasan, 2006). Furthermore, the relatively low (~10–20 kΩ) impedance of the electrode contrasts sharply with the high-input impedance of modern amplifiers. (The goal of high-input impedance is to limit drastically the current flowing across the scalp-electrode boundary; in this way, the act of measuring the scalp voltage has a negligible effect on that voltage.) Physically linking the ears or mastoids permits more current to flow across these scalp-electrode boundaries, tending to make the scalp potential artificially similar on the two sides of the head.

As a result of these complications of the physically linked reference, use of the mathematically linked reference has gained in popularity. The mathematically linked reference is calculated to create an artificial reference at the average potential of the reference sites 1 and 2 (which are on the left and right ear, or left and right mastoids):

$$(V_n - V_1) - \left(\frac{V_2 - V_1}{2}\right) \equiv V_n - \left(\frac{V_2 + V_1}{2}\right) \tag{6.2}$$

Although the mathematically linked reference has been proposed as a solution to the reference problem, it actually falls quite short of this goal. Potential differences between electrode pairs depend on head-current patterns due to sources that are not necessarily close to the electrodes. With linked references, potentials depend on head currents at three different locations (i.e., the two ears and the recording-electrode position). This may further complicate, rather than simplify source-distribution estimates. The apparent symmetry of equation 6.2 is misleading: a linked reference may artificially correlate potentials recorded near the mastoid regions and thereby yield erroneous estimates of hemispheric source asymmetries (Srinivasan et al., 1998a).

COMMON AVERAGE REFERENCE

The average reference (AVE) (also called the *common-average reference* [CAR] or *global-average reference*) is now widely used in EEG studies. This *AVE reference* does have some theoretical justification (Bertrand et al., 1985). When one records data from N electrodes, the measured potentials V_n ($n = 1, 2, . . . N$) are related to the scalp potential $\Phi(r)$ (with respect to infinity) by

$$V_n = \Phi(r_n) - \Phi(r_R) \tag{6.3}$$

where r_n is the position of the nth electrode and r_R is the reference-electrode site. If we designate the average of these measured potentials as V_{AVG}, the potential at the reference site can be written in terms of the scalp potentials as

$$\Phi(r_R) = \frac{1}{N} \sum_{n=1}^{\infty} \Phi(r_n) - V_{AVG} \tag{6.4}$$

The first term on the right side of equation 6.4 is the average of the scalp surface potentials at all recording sites. Theoretically, this term vanishes if the electrodes are positioned such that the mean of the potentials approximates a surface integral over a closed surface containing all current within the volume. Because only minimal current flows from the head through the neck even with the reference electrode placed on the body, it is a reasonable approximation to consider the head to be a closed volume that confines all current. As a consequence of current conservation, the surface integral of the potential over a volume conductor containing dipole sources must be zero (Bertrand et al., 1985). In this case, then, the reference potential can be estimated by the second term on the right side of equation 6.4 (i.e., by averaging the measured potentials and changing the sign of this average). This reference potential can be added to each measurement V_n using equation 6.3, thereby estimating the reference-free potential $\Phi(r_n)$ (i.e., the potential with respect to infinity, at each location).

Because we cannot measure the potentials on a closed surface surrounding the brain, the first term on the right side of equation 6.4 will generally not vanish. For example, the distribution of potential on the underside of the head (within the neck region) cannot be measured. Furthermore, the average potential for any group of electrode positions (given by the second term on the right side of equation 6.4), can only approximate the surface integral over the volume conductor. Thus, this is expected to be a very poor approximation if applied with the standard 10–20-electrode system. As the number of electrodes increases to 64 or more, the error in the approximation is expected to decrease. Thus, like any other choice of reference, the average reference provides biased estimates of reference-independent potentials. Nevertheless, when used in studies with large numbers of electrodes (e.g., 128 or more) that are spread widely over the head, the average reference seems to perform reasonably in providing reference-independent potentials (i.e., in approximating an ideal reference) (Srinivasan et al., 1998a).

Figure 6.7 illustrates a simulation of scalp potentials generated by two dipole sources, one radial (i.e., perpendicular) to the scalp and one tangential (i.e., parallel) to the scalp. The radial source (i.e., the lateral blue minus sign in fig. 6.7A) is located at a depth comparable to that of the surface of a cortical gyrus located just beneath the skull. The tangential dipole (i.e., the medial red plus and blue minus signs in fig. 6.7A) is located somewhat deeper, at a depth comparable to that of a gyrus located in the superficial part of the medial wall of one of the cerebral hemispheres. Figure 6.7A shows the location of the two sources (blue and red symbols) and the reference-independent potentials (with respect to infinity) obtained from 111 electrode locations on the surface of the outer sphere in a four concentric-spheres head model (see chapter 3, in this volume). The average nearest-neighbor (center-to-center) separation

between these electrodes is 2.7 cm. The topographic maps are interpolated from the potentials calculated at the electrode positions. The positive lobe (solid lines) and negative lobe (dashed lines) of the potential distribution associated with this tangential dipole are readily apparent, and reverse over the midline. The radial dipole (negative at the surface) generates a more restricted potential distribution close to the right mastoid electrode.

Figure 6.7B shows the potential distribution if the reference electrode is placed at the vertex, indicated by an X. Directly above the center of the tangential dipole, the potential generated by the tangential dipole is zero and a small positive potential is contributed by the radial dipole. This small positive contribution by the radial dipole results in an apparent asymmetry in the potential distribution due to the tangential dipole, with a reduced magnitude of the positive peak on the right side of the array and an increase in the magnitude of the negative peak. Figure 6.7(C and D) shows the potential distribution when the reference is placed at the left and right mastoid, respectively. The left mastoid reference produces little change from the potential distribution seen in 6.7A, since the potential at the left mastoid is close to zero. By contrast, placing the reference electrode at the right mastoid (fig. 6.7D) significantly distorts the potentials by adding a positive potential to all locations. This effect is also present, but with smaller

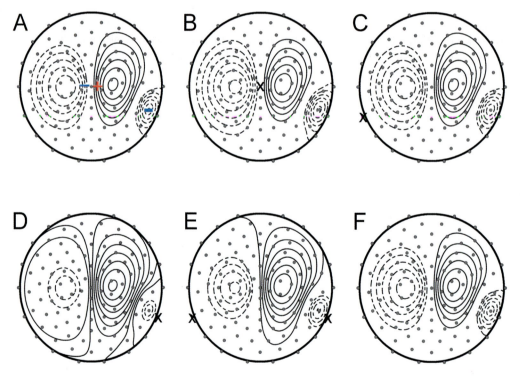

Figure 6.7 *Simulated potential maps on the surface of a four-sphere head model (see chapter 3). It shows two dipole sources: one tangential (located 3.2 cm below the scalp) (indicated by the blue minus sign and red plus sign close to the vertex) and one radial (located 1.4 cm below the scalp and indicated by the blue minus sign near the right lateral edge of the head). The tangential source has twice the strength of the radial source. Potentials were calculated at 111 surface sites derived from a 128-channel array centered at the vertex and covering the area subtended by an angle of 109° from the vertex. The simulated electrode positions are indicated in the figure by the small gray circles. Topographic maps of the potential distribution were obtained from a spline interpolation (Srinivasan et al., 1996). (A) Potential map with respect to infinity with the dipoles indicated. (B) Potential map with reference (indicated by X) located at the vertex. (C) Potential map with reference (X) located at the left mastoid electrode. (D) Potential map with reference (X) located at the right mastoid electrode. (E) Potential map with respect to the mathematically linked (averaged) mastoids (X and X). (F) Average (AVE) reference potential map obtained by first calculating the potentials at 110 electrode sites with respect to the vertex, then calculating the average reference, and finally rereferencing every site to this average reference. See text for discussion.*

magnitude, when a mathematically linked-mastoids reference is used, as shown in figure 6.7E (with the linked-mastoids reference computed from 110 electrodes using the vertex-referenced potentials). In contrast, the AVE reference shown in figure 6.7F provides potentials that closely approximate those provided by the ideal reference shown in figure 6.7A. Thus, as the close similarity of figures 6.7A and F indicates, the AVE reference works well, at least in this example.

One concern often expressed about the AVE reference is that the presence of strong sources deep in the brain may result in major misinterpretations of recorded data. In most EEG recordings there are few if any electrodes on the lower surface of the head. Thus, a dipole near the center of the head and oriented toward the vertex contributes more positive potential to the array of electrodes than negative potential. By using the AVE reference, we force the potential distribution to have a mean of zero over the portion of the head covered by the electrodes (typically 50–70% of the head surface). However, although the average reference can distort potentials generated by deep sources (Junghofer et al., 1999), the impact of this distortion is usually small since EEG potentials generated by deep sources are usually much smaller than those generated by superficial sources. In one study spherical splines were fit to the voltage at superior electrodes to approximate the potential at inferior sites due to deep sources, thereby improving the estimate of the average reference (Ferree, 2006).

It is important to emphasize that the effectiveness of the AVE reference depends on the number and distribution of the electrodes that compose it, as well as on the nature and number of the sources. Although the AVE reference offers theoretical as well as practical advantages, it is effective only if it uses a sufficient number of electrodes (e.g., 64 to 128 or more) distributed over the entire scalp, including (if practical) locations on the lower surface of the head. Practical considerations that limit electrode placements on the lower surface of the head include artifacts such as muscle activity.

THE MODEL-BASED REFERENCE

A more recent approach to the reference problem is to base the reference on a head model. This method is called the *reference electrode standardization technique* (REST) (Yao, 2001; Yao et al., 2005). The basic idea is to first define *equivalent sources*, sources that can account for the recorded scalp potential distribution. Next, these fictitious sources are used to find the corresponding reference potential with respect to infinity. The philosophical approach of this method differs from the inverse problem (discussed in chapter 3, in this volume) in that no close relationship between the equivalent sources and genuine brain sources is ever claimed (Nunez, 2010).

COMPARISON OF AVE AND REST

Aside from artifact and external noise, AVE errors are due to limited electrode density and incomplete electrode coverage (i.e., sampling only the upper part of head). If these errors were fully eliminated (which is only possible in detached heads), AVE would provide the desired gold standard, that is, a reference

method essentially equivalent to a reference at infinity. REST can also suffer errors due to electrode density and electrode coverage and can suffer additional errors due to head-model uncertainty. This latter additional source of error may discourage implementation of REST and is perhaps the reason it was not used earlier.

However, this aversion to REST is generally not warranted because the three error sources are correlated; in particular, the coverage error is expected to become progressively smaller as the head model improves. Thus, if the head model is sufficiently accurate, it is possible for REST (even with its three sources of error) to be more accurate than AVE (with only its two error sources). From this argument we see that the choice between AVE and REST largely depends on the accuracy of a *genuine* (as opposed to an idealized) head model. Because the accuracy of REST in genuine heads is currently unknown, one plausible strategy is to apply both AVE and REST to the same data sets (Nunez, 2010). Any result that changes substantially when AVE is replaced by REST (or vice versa) may be suspect.

SUMMARY OF REFERENCE ELECTRODE STRATEGIES

In summary, no matter which reference strategy is used, we record the potential at one head location with respect to some other head location. By definition this potential difference is the result of integration of the electric field over any path connecting the reference point and the point in question. The potential is not a unique characteristic of a single point but rather a characteristic of the path between two points.

The changes in the recorded potentials that result from changing the reference location make intuitive sense since any change involves subtracting the potential at one location on the head from all the other potentials. This has an impact not only on the estimated spatial properties of the EEG but also on its temporal properties, since the potential at the reference location can be expected to vary over time. This impact is evident in figure 6.5, where the time course of the VEP depends on the position of the reference electrode. The main point is that any specific reference, including the mathematically linked-ears or linked-mastoids reference, contributes potentials from distant sites to the potential obtained from each so-called recording electrode. The specific effects of any choice of reference will depend on the configuration of the EEG sources. An average reference based on many electrodes spread widely over the head provides a good estimate of reference-independent potentials because it integrates many possible paths to the point.

SPATIAL SAMPLING OF EEG

In addition to reference selection, the other important practical issue for any EEG recording is the number of electrodes needed to obtain an accurate spatial representation of the relevant EEG and the locations for their placement. We consider this problem in terms of the Nyquist theorem: *to represent a continuous signal by discrete sampling, the sampling rate must exceed twice the highest frequency in the signal* (see chapter 7, in this volume). In other words, to avoid aliasing, at least two samples per cycle are required. This requirement is quite familiar to researchers who digitally sample time series. Moreover, the Nyquist criterion for discrete sampling of any analog signal applies not only to *temporal* sampling but also to *spatial* sampling.

In EEG recording, the scalp-surface potential at any point in time is a continuous field that varies over the surface of the head. The electrode array provides a discrete sampling of this field and is therefore subject to the Nyquist criterion. However, unlike the time series of a single amplifier channel, which is continuous, the spatial signal is discrete (i.e., it is acquired only at a limited number of points on the head). Whereas the temporal signal can be easily low-pass filtered by analog filters to meet the Nyquist criterion as dictated by the sampling rate, the raw spatial signal cannot be treated in the same manner because no continuous representation of the spatial signal is ever available. As a consequence of this limitation, any aliasing caused by under-sampling (i.e., by too widely spaced electrodes) cannot be undone. Thus, it is essential that adequate spatial sampling of the potentials be accomplished from the outset.

The highest spatial frequency that can be observed without aliasing is determined by the electrode density (assuming a relatively uniformly distributed electrode placement) and electrode size. If the EEG contains signals with spatial frequencies that are too high for the electrode density, the signals will be *spatially aliased*. They will appear in topographical maps or spatial spectra as signals of lower spatial frequency and will thereby distort spatial maps of potential, coherence, and other measures. In this context, it is important to note that when the EEG is spatially under-sampled (e.g., with only one recording electrode and one reference electrode), the measured *time series* is a valid measurement of the potential difference between the two sites, but the *spatial distribution* of the potential is unknown.

To illustrate spatial-sampling issues further, let us consider the problem of discrete sampling of the potential distribution on a spherical surface containing dipole current sources. Any distribution on a spherical surface can be expressed as a sum of *spherical harmonics* Y_{nm}. Y_{nm} are the natural basis set for functions defined on a sphere, analogous to the Fourier series for functions defined on a time interval that is used in spectral analysis of EEG time series (see chapters 3 and 7, in this volume). The n and m indices of the Y_{nm} functions denote spatial frequencies in the two surface directions (e.g., north/south and east/west). Index n defines the angle θ which is essentially latitude (but measured from the north pole [(e.g., the vertex {electrode Cz}], rather than from the equator). Index m defines the angle φ, which is essentially longitude. Any potential distribution due to dipole sources in a spherical-head model may be represented by a double sum of spherical harmonic functions over the two indices (Arfken, 1985). Thus, a potential distribution for which n is 4 and m is 3 rises and falls exactly four times as one moves around the sphere from the north pole to the south pole and back to the north pole, and it rises and falls exactly three times as one moves once around the equator.

Examples of spherical harmonics with $n = 4, 5, 7,$ or 9, and with m fixed at 3 are shown in figure 6.8. The left column (fig. 6.8A) shows each spherical harmonic under assumptions of perfect sampling, while the middle and right columns show the same spherical harmonic discretely sampled with 111 simulated electrodes (fig. 6.8B) or with only 36 simulated electrodes (fig. 6.8C). The samples are assumed to cover the upper part of the sphere (with the north pole at the vertex) to a maximum latitude somewhat below the equator ($0 \leq θ \leq 109$ deg). With the 111 electrode positions, the average (center-to-center) nearest-neighbor separation between electrodes is 2.7 cm (somewhat less than that of the 10–10 system); with the 36 electrode positions, the average separation is 5.8 cm (similar to the spacing of the 10–20 system). The topographic maps shown in Figure 6.8 were produced by interpolation (Srinivasan et al., 1996). The figure shows that discrete sampling distorts the spherical harmonics as n increases. In the figure, both the 36- and 111-electrode arrays accurately represent the $n = 4$ spherical harmonic (i.e., compare the maps at the tops of the three columns). However, for the $n = 5$ spherical harmonic, the 111-electrode array (column B of the $n = 5$ row of topographies) gives an accurate representation, but the 36-electrode array produces serious aliasing (see column C of the $n = 5$ row of topographies). For the $n = 7$ spherical harmonic, the 111-electrode array again gives an accurate representation, but it loses spatial detail (i.e., begins to produce aliasing) with the $n = 9$ spherical harmonic. Thus, as n increases, aliasing can create the erroneous appearance of spatial frequencies lower than the actual spatial frequencies. That is, aliasing distorts EEG components that have relatively focused spatial distributions so that they appear to have broader less focused distributions.

From these examples it is evident that the highest spatial frequency present in the EEG determines the sampling density needed to accurately reflect its spatial distribution. Although time series can be filtered by anti-aliasing filters applied according to the Nyquist criterion (e.g., low-pass analog filtering of signals below 40 Hz to permit sampling at 100 Hz), an equivalent process of spatial filtering is not possible for the sampling by individual scalp electrodes because such sampling is inherently discrete. If the number of electrodes is insufficient, spatial maps of the potentials are unavoidably aliased (e.g., the lower three maps for 36 electrodes in fig. 6.8C).

For scalp-recorded EEG, power at higher spatial frequencies is severely limited by the blurring of brain potentials due to the intervening tissues of the head. This limitation actually makes the problem of discrete sampling of scalp potentials more manageable. The effect of volume conduction through the cerebrospinal fluid (CSF), skull, and scalp is that it spatially low-pass filters the cortical potentials (Srinivasan et al., 1996; Nunez and Srinivasan, 2006). That is, nature has conveniently provided us with an analog low-pass spatial filter in the form of the poorly conducting skull! However, note that whereas this low-pass filter is present in EEG recordings, it is absent in electrocorticographic (ECoG) recordings (see chapter 15, in this volume). This can add substantially to the problem of spatial aliasing of ECoG mapping in animals and humans. (On the other hand the absence of this natural low-pass spatial filter in

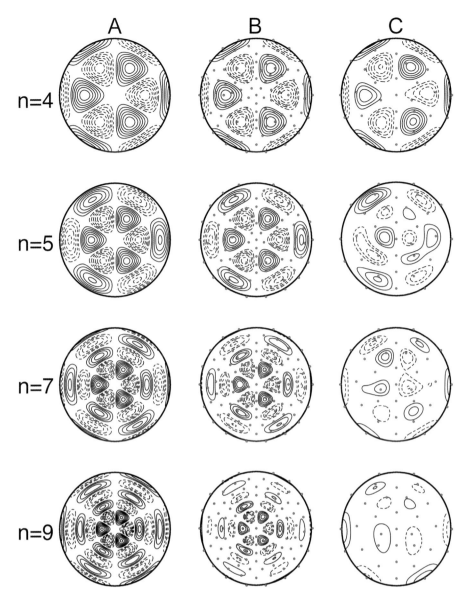

Figure 6.8 *Illustration of the impact of electrode density on the spatial distributions calculated for potentials of different spatial frequencies. The vertex (i.e., the north pole) is the center. The circle extends to 19° below the equator. The spherical harmonic index m (i.e., longitude) of the potentials is fixed at 3. Each row corresponds to a potential with a different value (i.e., 4, 5, 7, or 9) of the spherical harmonic index n (i.e., latitude). Column A is the gold standard, that is, the potential distributions plotted with infinite (i.e., perfect) sampling. Columns B and C are the maps obtained by sampling the potential distributions with 111 electrodes (B; 2.7-cm spacing) or 36 electrodes (C; 5.8-cm spacing), respectively, and spline interpolation. Gray circles indicate the electrode positions. See text for discussion.*

ECoG recording allows it to measure accurately signals with higher spatial frequencies, which is one of its major advantages over EEG recording [see chapter 15, in this volume].)

In conclusion, we note that appropriate application of the Nyquist criterion in choosing the density and location of EEG electrode arrays requires a priori knowledge of the spatial spectrum of the EEG and of the source distributions. Such information is not generally available, in part because knowledge of the adequate number of electrodes for a specific EEG signal would first require over-sampling of the potential distribution to determine the highest spatial frequencies present in the data. One study using very closely spaced needle electrodes suggested that a spacing of 1.9–2.7 cm (Spitzer et al., 1989) is adequate to avoid aliasing somatosensory evoked potentials. This corresponds to 128–256 electrodes covering the upper surface of the head. Srinivasan et al. (1998b) and Nunez and Srinivasan (2006) have used volume-conduction models to obtain estimates of the highest spatial frequencies that can be expected to contribute significantly to EEG signals. Using these values, they have calculated that 128–256 electrodes are needed to produce adequate spatial sampling of scalp potentials.

HIGH-RESOLUTION EEG METHODS

The poor spatial resolution of EEG could limit EEG-based BCI development, particularly when the BCI protocol seeks to use signals from particular localized cortical areas (e.g., the hand region of primary motor cortex). In addressing this limitation, *high-resolution EEG methods* may have greater value than source-localization methods. In fact, high-resolution methods have already been applied successfully in BCI research (McFarland et al., 2006). High-resolution EEG methods are based on a conceptual framework that differs substantially from that of EEG source-localization methods (Nunez and Srinivasan, 2006). Because scalp-recorded EEG is not by itself sufficient information to estimate the distribution of sources within the head, source-localization methods must rely on assumptions about the numbers and nature of sources. In contrast, high-resolution EEG methods do not need to make assumptions about the sources. Instead, they focus on increasing the sensitivity of each electrode.

The EEG signal recorded at each electrode is a spatial average of active current sources distributed over a volume of brain space. The size and shape of this volume depend on a number of factors including the volume conduction properties of the head and the choice of reference electrode. The contribution of each source to this spatial average depends on the *electrical* distance between source and electrode, the source orientation, and the source strength. When two electrodes are very closely spaced, they record similar signals because they reflect the average activity in largely overlapping tissue volumes. High-resolution EEG methods improve spatial resolution by reducing the effective volume that each electrode averages.

SURFACE LAPLACIAN

The *surface Laplacian* (see also chapter 7, in this volume) improves spatial resolution by making the electrode more sensitive to activity from sources that are superficial, radial, and localized underneath the electrode and less sensitive to activity from sources that are deep or broadly distributed (i.e., of low spatial frequency). The *surface Laplacian* is the second spatial derivative of the scalp potential in both surface directions (latitude and longitude on a sphere). It is an estimate of current density entering (or exiting) the scalp through the skull (Srinivasan et al., 2006; Nunez and Srinivasan, 2006). The Laplacian method requires only that the outer surface shape of the volume conductor (i.e., the head) be specified; typically a best-fit spherical surface is adopted. One of the complicating factors in interpreting scalp EEG involves reference-electrode effects: at each instant, the potential recorded at the reference electrode is subtracted from potentials recorded at all the other electrodes. Since the surface Laplacian is a (second) spatial derivative, the potential common to all electrodes is automatically removed in the Laplacian estimate. Thus, the reference electrode can be moved to any position on the head without influencing the surface Laplacian. At the same time, because the surface Laplacian estimates derivatives of the potential along the scalp surface, high-density electrode arrays are generally recommended to obtain good spatial resolution with modern Laplacian algorithms (i.e., 64–131 electrodes or more) (Srinivasan et al., 1996). Nevertheless, the Laplacian at a given

electrode can be estimated with as few as five electrodes using a nearest-neighbor Laplacian, that is, a finite difference approximation of the second derivative (Hjorth, 1975). While this is a crude estimate of the Laplacian as compared to more accurate but computationally intensive methods, the nearest-neighbor Laplacian is potentially a very useful solution for BCI applications because it requires only five electrodes localized to a limited scalp area and can be computed easily and efficiently in real time (e.g., as a part of actual BCI operation).

In effect, the surface Laplacian algorithm acts as a band-pass spatial filter that tends to emphasize sources focused in the underlying superficial cortex. Extensive simulation studies of the surface Laplacian have been conducted using dipole sources in spherical and realistically shaped head models (Srinivasan et al., 1996; Srinivasan et al., 1998; Nunez and Srinivasan, 2006; Srinivasan et al., 2007). The surface Laplacian appears to effectively limit the sensitivity of the electrode to compact sources located within a distance of 2–3 cm. Figure 6.4B demonstrates the enhanced spatial resolution afforded by the surface Laplacian in a simulation with a realistic head model. Here the Laplacian focuses the sensitivity of the electrode to the gyral surface directly beneath the electrode. The part of the EEG signal removed by the Laplacian filter is not as well localized; it may be generated by very deep sources (less likely) or by coherent sources distributed over large cortical areas (e.g., entire cortical lobes) (more likely). In the latter case, the question of EEG source localization is essentially irrelevant, since the sources themselves are not well localized but are, instead, regional or even global (Nunez, 2000). In sum, the surface Laplacian filter is a useful tool that achieves high-resolution EEG by reducing the volume of the tissue that produces the activity detected at each electrode location.

SUMMARY

Electroencephalography is the principal noninvasive BCI method. Magnetoencephalography may also be used. Both EEG and MEG have comparable spatial resolution. They differ principally in that they are preferentially sensitive to different brain sources. EEG emphasizes synchronized dipole sources in superficial gyral surfaces and larger dipole layers that generate larger scalp potentials. In contrast, MEG emphasizes sources in the sulcal walls, which are tangential to the scalp and thus tangential also to the coils.

It is not clear what role MEG can have in practical BCI applications because of the expense and inconvenience of the need to cool the superconducting coils and to isolate the subject in a magnetically shielded room in order to detect the brain's magnetic fields, which are very small relative to environmental magnetic fields. Nevertheless, MEG may be valuable in laboratory-based studies aimed at developing new BCI protocols and/or in locating brain areas relevant for other BCI methodologies, particularly those that require implantation of recording arrays.

EEG recording requires careful attention to electrode application, number, and location, to sampling rate, to reference choice, and to contamination by nonbrain artifacts. Mild skin abrasion and conductive gel are generally needed to obtain adequately low electrode impedance. Dry electrode technology is under development.

To avoid temporal aliasing of the EEG, the sampling rate should exceed the Engineer's Nyquist Criterion, that is, it should be at least 2.5 times the highest frequency to which the recording amplifier is sensitive. Similarly, electrode density on the scalp should be high enough to prevent spatial aliasing of the relevant EEG features. The recognition of nonbrain artifacts (e.g., EMG) requires adequately comprehensive spatial and frequency analyses.

Reference selection is critical. An ideal, completely inactive reference site is not obtainable. Nevertheless, with many electrodes (128 or more) distributed widely over the scalp and the average reference (AVE) method (also called the common-average reference [CAR]), it is possible to closely approximate reference-independent EEG recording. However, although this approach may be ideal for research or clinical purposes, it is impractical for BCIs intended for long-term use in daily life. In such situations a very small number of electrodes (e.g., five), portability, ease of use, and capacity for rapid online processing are highly desirable or even essential. Thus, because the EEG recording in practical BCI systems is necessarily bipolar, it is probably best to incorporate a *variety* of promising bipolar strategies into BCI research. In this regard, high-resolution EEG methods such as the surface Laplacian have potential advantages, especially when a specific cortical area (e.g., motor cortex) produces the signals used by the BCI (e.g., McFarland et al., 2008).

REFERENCES

American Electroencephalographic Society. Guideline thirteen: Guidelines for standard electrode position nomenclature. *J Clin Neurophysiol* 11:111–113, 1994.

Arfken G. *Mathematical Methods for Physicists*, 3rd ed. Orlando, FL: Academic Press, 1985.

Bendat JS, and Piersol A. *Random Data: Analysis and Measurement Procedures*, 3rd ed. New York: Wiley, 2001.

Bertrand O, Perrin F, and Pernier J. A theoretical justification of the average reference in topographic evoked potential studies. *Electroencephalogr Clin Neurophysiol.* 62:462–464, 1985.

Brunner P, Bianchi L, Guger C, Cincotti F, and Schalk G. Current trends in hardware and software for brain–computer interfaces (BCIs). *J Neural Eng.* 8, 025001, 2011.

Cadwell JA, and Villarreal RA, Electrophysiological equipment and electrical safety. In: Aminoff MJ (Ed), *Electrodiagnosis in Clinical Neurology* 4th ed. New York: Churchill Livingstone, 15–33, 1999.

Cohen D Magnetoencephalography: Detection of brain's electrical activity with a superconducting magnetometer. *Science* 175:664–666, 1972.

Cohen D, Cuffin BN, Yunokuchi K, Maniewski R, Purcell C, Cosgrove GR, Ives J, Fein G, Raz J, Brown FF, and Merrin EL, Common reference coherence data are confounded by power and phase effects. *Electroencephalogr Clin Neurophysiol* 69:581–584, 1988.

Ferree TC. Spherical splines and average referencing in scalp EEG. *Brain Topogr.* 19(1/2):43–52, 2006.

Ferree TC, Luu P, Russell GS, and Tucker DM, Scalp electrode impedance, infection risk, and EEG data quality. *Clin Neurophysiol.* 112:536–544, 2001.

Fisch BJ, *Fisch & Spehlmann's EEG Primer*, Amsterdam: Elsevier, 1999.

Gargiulo G, Calvo RA, Bifulco P, Cesarelli M, Jin C, Mohamed A, and van Schaik A. A new EEG recording system for passive dry electrodes *Clin Neurophysiol.* 121:686–693, 2010.

Goncharova II, McFarland DJ, Vaughan TM, and Wolpaw JR. EMG contamination of EEG: Spectral and topographical characteristics. *Clin Neurophysiol.* 114:1580–1593, 2003.

Grozea C, Voinescu CD, and Fazli S. Bristle-sensors - low-cost flexible passive dry EEG electrodes for neurofeedback and BCI applications. *J Neur Engin.* 8(2):025008, 2011.

Hamaleinen M, Hari R, Ilmoniemi RJ, Knutila J, and Lounasmaa OV. Magnetoencephalography: Theory, instrumentation, and applications to noninvasive studies of the working human brain. *Rev Modern Physics.* 65:413–497, 1993

Hjorth B. An on-line transformation of EEG scalp potentials into orthogonal source derivations. *Electroencephalogr Clin Neurophysiol.* 39:526–530, 1975.

Junghofer M, Elbert T, Tucker DM, and Braun C. The polar average reference effect: A bias in estimating the head surface integral in EEG recording. *Clin Neurophysiol.* 119(6):1149–1155, 1999.

Kamp A, Pfurtscheller G, Edlinger G, and Lopes da Silva FH, Technological basis of EEG recording. In Niedermeyer E, and Lopes da Silva FH. (Eds), *Electroencephalography. Basic Principals, Clinical Applications, and Related Fields.* 5th ed. London: Williams & Wilkins, 127–138, 2005.

Klem GH, Lüders HO, Jasper, H.H. and Elger, C., The ten-twenty electrode system of the International Federation. *Electroencephalogr Clin Neurophysiol Suppl.* 52:3–6, 1999.

Malmivuo J, and Plonsey R. *Bioelectromagnetism*. New York: Oxford University Press, 1995.

Matthews R, McDonald NJ, Hervieux P, Turner PJ, and Steindorf MA. A wearable physiological sensor suite for unobtrusive monitoring of physiological and cognitive state. Engineering in Medicine and Biology Society. EMBS. *29th Annual Int Conf IEEE*, 5276–5281, 2007.

McFarland DJ, Krusienski DJ, Wolpaw JR. Brain-computer interface signal processing at the Wadsworth Center: Mu and sensorimotor beta rhythms. *Prog Brain Res.* 159:411–419. 2006.

McFarland DJ, Sarnacki WA, Vaughan TM, and Wolpaw JR. Brain-computer interface (BCI) operation: Signal and noise during early training sessions. *Clin Neurophysiol.* 116:56–62, 2005.

Murias M, *Oscillatory brain electric potentials in developmental psychopathology and form perception*, PhD Dissertation, University of California, Irvine, 2004.

Nunez, PL. *Electric fields of the brain: The neurophysics of EEG*, New York: Oxford University Press, 1981.

Nunez PL, A method to estimate local skull resistance in living subjects. *IEEE Trans Biomed Eng.* 34:902–904, 1987.

Nunez PL, REST: A good idea but not the gold standard. Clinical Neurophysiology, 121:2177–2180, 2010.

Nunez PL. Toward a quantitative description of large-scale neocortical dynamic function and EEG. *Behav Brain Sci.* 23(3):371–398, 2000.

Nunez PL, and Srinivasan R. *Electric Fields of the Brain: The Neurophysics of EEG*, 2nd ed. New York: Oxford University Press, 2006.

Nunez PL, Srinivasan R, Westdorp AF, Wijesinghe RS, Tucker DM, Silberstein RB, and Cadusch PJ, EEG coherency I: Statistics, reference electrode, volume conduction, Laplacians, cortical imaging, and interpretation at multiple scales. *Electroencephalogr Clinical Neurophysiology* 103: 516–527, 1997.

Oostenveld R, and Praamstra P, The 5% electrode system for high-resolution EEG and ERP measurements, *Clin Neurophysiol.* 112:713–719, 2001.

Picton TW, Bentin S, Berg P, Donchin E, Hillyard SA, Johnson R Jr, Miller GA, Ritter W, Ruchkin DS, Rugg MD, and Taylor MJ, Guidelines for using human event-related potentials to study cognition: Recording standards and publication criteria *Psychophysiology* 37:127–152, 2000.

Pilgreen KL, Physiologic, medical and cognitive correlates of electroencephalography. In: Nunez PL (Au), *Neocortical Dynamics and Human EEG Rhythms*. New York: Oxford University Press, 195–248, 1995.

Popescu F, Fazli S, Badower Y, Blankertz B, and Muller KR. Single trial classification of motor imagination using 6 dry EEG electrodes. *PLoS One* 2(7): e637, 2007.

Searle A, Kirkup L. A direct comparison of wet, dry and insulating bioelectric recording electrodes. *Physiol Meas.* 22:71–83, 2000.

Sellers EW, Turner P, Sarnacki WA, Mcmanus T, Vaughan TM, and Matthews R. A novel dry electrode for brain–computer interface. In *Proceedings of the 13th International Conference on Human–Computer Interaction: Part II. Novel Interaction Methods and Techniques.* Berlin: Springer, 623–631, 2009.

Spitzer AR, Cohen LG, Fabrikant J, and Hallett M, A method for determining the optimal interelectrode spacing for cerebral topographic mapping. *Electroencephalogr Clin Neurophysiol* 72:355–361, 1989.

Srinivasan R. Anatomical constraints of source models for high-resolution EEG and MEG derived from MRI. *Technol Cancer Res Treat.* 5:389–399, 2006.

Srinivasan R, Nunez PL, and Silberstein RB, Spatial filtering and neocortical dynamics: Estimates of EEG coherence. *IEEE Trans Biomed Eng.* 45:814–826, 1998a.

Srinivasan R, Nunez PL, Tucker DM, Silberstein RB, and Cadusch PJ, Spatial sampling and filtering of EEG with spline Laplacians to estimate cortical potentials. *Brain Topogr.* 8:355–366, 1996.

Srinivasan R, Tucker DM, and Murias M. Estimating the spatial nyquist of the human EEG. *Behav Res Methods Instrum Comput.* 30:8–19, 1998b.

Srinivasan R, Winter WR, Ding J, Nunez PL. EEG and MEG coherence: Estimates of functional connectivity at distinct spatial scales of neocortical dynamics. *J Neurosci Methods.* 166:41–52, 2007.

Sullivan TJ, Deiss SR, Jung TP, and Cauwenberghs G. A brain–machine interface using dry-contact, low-noise EEG sensors. In *2008 IEEE International Symposium on Circuits and Systems,* 1986–1989, 2008.

Taheri A, Knight R, and Smith R, A dry electrode for EEG recording. *Electroencephalogr Clin Neurophysiol.* 90:376–383, 1994.

Tucker DM. Spatial sampling of head electrical fields: The geodesic sensor net. *Electroencephalogr Clin Neurophysiol.* 87:154–163, 1993.

7 | BCI SIGNAL PROCESSING: FEATURE EXTRACTION

DEAN J. KRUSIENSKI, DENNIS J. McFARLAND, AND JOSÉ C. PRINCIPE

The purpose of a BCI is to detect and quantify characteristics of brain signals that indicate what the user wants the BCI to do, to translate these measurements in real time into the desired device commands, and to provide concurrent feedback to the user. The brain-signal characteristics used for this purpose are called *signal features*, or simply *features*. *Feature extraction* is the process of distinguishing the pertinent signal characteristics from extraneous content and representing them in a compact and/or meaningful form, amenable to interpretation by a human or computer. Feature extraction is the focus of this chapter. Figure 7.1 shows the overall structure of a BCI and the place that feature extraction (shaded in red in the figure) occupies in this structure. It occurs after signals have been acquired, and it prepares the signals for translation into BCI output commands. The process of feature extraction does this by isolating the important features of the signals from superfluous corrupting information or interference, typically referred to as *noise*.

The *signal-to-noise ratio* (SNR) of a measurement is simply the ratio of the *signal power to the noise power*. Power, which is proportional to the squared amplitude, is a measure of energy per unit time. Power is universally used to quantify and relate arbitrary electrical signals such as audio, communications, and electroencephalogram (EEG). A high SNR indicates minimal corruption of the signal of interest by background noise.

In discussing feature extraction, it is important to understand the difference between *noise* and *artifacts*. Both noise and artifacts can contaminate the signal. Noise is due to background *neurological* activity. In contrast, artifacts are due to sources unrelated to the neurological activity and are not intrinsic to the expected measurement of this activity. Artifacts can be due to biological or external sources, such as eye blinks or artificial respirator activity. Artifacts typically combine additively in the measurement of the desired signal, often completely masking the signal. Thus, it is important to note that the SNR may not directly apply to artifacts.

A *fundamental signal feature* is simply a direct measurement of the signal (e.g., the voltage difference between a pair of electrodes at a particular time after a sensory stimulus). By themselves, fundamental signal features usually provide limited relevant information about typically complex brain signals. Thus, it is more common for BCIs to use features that are linear or nonlinear combinations, ratios, statistical measures, or other transformations of multiple fundamental features detected at multiple electrodes and/or multiple time points. Such complex features, if selected appropriately, can reflect the user's desires more accurately than the fundamental features themselves. Most features used in BCI applications are based on spatial, temporal, and/or spectral analyses of brain signals or the relationships among them. Furthermore, in order to determine the user's wishes as accurately as possible, most BCIs extract a number of features simultaneously. This set of features is referred to as a *feature vector*.

To be effective for BCI applications, a feature should have the following attributes:

- its spatial, temporal, spectral characteristics, and dynamics can be precisely characterized for an individual user or population of users

- it can be modulated by the user and used in combination with other features to reliably convey the user's intent

- its correlation with the user's intent is stable over time and/or can be tracked in a consistent and reliable manner

Figure 7.1 shows a block diagram of a BCI system with emphasis on its signal-processing aspects. First, the analog brain signals measured from the sensors are amplified to levels suitable for electronic processing (and they may also be subjected to an analog filter); these signals are then digitized and transmitted to a computer. The digitized signals then pass to an optional signal-conditioning stage, which acts to enhance the signals and/or remove extraneous information. Otherwise, the digitized signals are grouped into *sample blocks* comprised of the current (and possibly previous) consecutive digitized values. The feature extraction and conditioning algorithm analyzes each incoming sample block from one or more signal channels to produce the features that constitute the feature vector. This analysis can involve any of a wide variety of possible spatial, temporal, and/or spectral transformations. This feature vector is then passed to the feature translation stage, in which it is converted into device commands and feedback to the user.

This chapter reviews signal amplification/digitization and then focuses in some detail on *feature extraction*. *Feature*

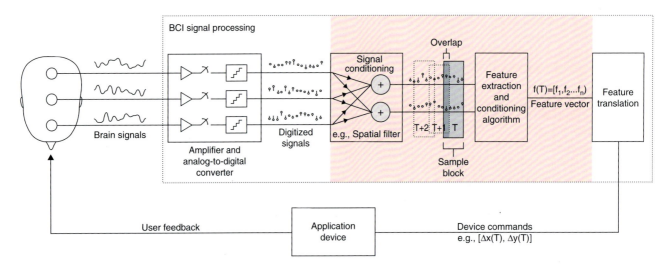

Figure 7.1 *A block diagram of a BCI system, with the portion representing feature extraction shaded in red. Brain signals are recorded by one of a variety of methods. They are amplified and digitized, then conditioned (e.g., spatial filtering) and, in blocks of consecutive samples (with the sample block currently being processed numbered as T in the diagram, the subsequent sample block numbered T+1, etc.), sent to the feature extraction (e.g., frequency analysis) and conditioning (e.g., normalization) algorithm. This results in a single feature vector for each consecutive sample block processed (i.e., a function T) that is translated into a device command (e.g., amount of vertical displacement from the previous cursor position, also a function of T). An application device executes the command and sends feedback to the user, completing the closed loop.*

translation will be covered in chapter 8. Nevertheless, it is important to recognize that feature extraction constitutes the transformation of fundamental signal characteristics to produce a feature vector, whereas feature translation is merely the transformation of this feature vector into a form that is appropriate for device control. Thus, in certain designs (e.g., artificial neural networks; see chapter 8, this volume), a single transformation is used to convert the digital signals directly into device commands, and there is no clear distinction between the extraction and translation stages.

As the first stage in the signal processing that converts brain signals into actions that accomplish the user's intent, feature extraction is critically important. Accurate and robust feature extraction simplifies the subsequent translation stage and produces more accurate and reliable actions and more natural feedback to the user. On the other hand, it is possible to compensate for somewhat poor or nonspecific feature extraction by using a more complex translation algorithm to produce equally effective results. It is important to recognize that feature extraction and translation go hand-in-hand and that practical BCI systems balance the emphasis between these two stages and ensure that they work together effectively.

The presentation in this chapter focuses on well-established feature-extraction methods that are applied to EEG, electrocorticogram (ECoG), or single-neuron recordings. It is meant to serve as an introduction to and reference for common BCI feature-extraction methods. Most methods of feature extraction that appear in the BCI literature are based on, or are closely related to, the methods presented in this chapter.

The chapter is written and organized assuming that readers have an understanding of college-level linear algebra and calculus, basic probability and statistics, negligible signal processing or machine-learning background, and basic knowledge gained from previous chapters. It begins with an overview of some basic principles of digital signal processing and a discussion of common techniques used to enhance signals prior to feature extraction. It then covers method selection, typical processing protocols, and major established methods for BCI feature extraction.

PRINCIPLES OF SIGNAL PROCESSING

ANALOG-TO-DIGITAL CONVERSION

Electrical signals recorded from the brain are on the order of microvolts (µV) to millivolts (mV) and are typically *amplified*, using a standard biosignal amplifier, to higher voltages suitable for processing and storage. Most modern biosignal amplifiers also *digitize* the signal using an *analog-to-digital converter* (ADC); if the amplifier itself does not perform this digitization, a separate ADC is necessary to process and store the signal using a computer. Analog-to-digital conversion consists of two consecutive steps: *sampling* and then *quantization*.

SAMPLING

Sampling is the process of capturing the value (typically voltage, but possibly a value originating from other signal measures such as blood flow) of a continuous analog signal at specific instants in time. The signal values at these instances in time are known as *samples*. In conventional ADCs, samples are uniformly spaced in time. This spacing or *sampling rate* is measured in Hertz (Hz) (samples/second). For example, an analog signal sampled at 100 Hz will produce a digital signal comprised of 100 consecutive samples uniformly spaced over a 1-sec interval, with values corresponding to the analog signals at the consecutive sampled time points. The higher the sampling rate, the better the time resolution and the more accurately the sampled signal represents the original analog signal. However, in many cases perfect reconstruction of the analog signal can be achieved with a certain minimum sampling rate. The *Nyquist-Shannon sampling theorem* is used to find that minimum acceptable sampling rate. It states that perfect reconstruction can be achieved only by sampling the analog signal at a rate that is at least double the highest frequency of the analog signal. This threshold is known as the *Nyquist sampling rate* (or *Nyquist criterion* or *Nyquist limit*). If the sampling rate for a particular signal is less than the Nyquist sampling rate, the information contained in the sequence of samples is distorted and not representative of the true spectral characteristics of the original signal.

The distortion that can occur due to a sampling rate that is less than the Nyquist criterion is known as *aliasing*. The concept of aliasing can be visualized using the classic example of a rotating fan and a strobe light in a dark room. The fan rotates at a constant rate (analogous to an analog signal that oscillates at a constant frequency). The strobe flashes (potentially independent of the fan rate) at a constant rate (analogous to the digital sampling rate). If the strobe light is set to flash at the same rate as the fan, the fan will appear motionless. This is obviously not representative of the true motion of the fan, and it is thus a form of aliasing.

To prevent aliasing, analog signals are often low-pass filtered (see section *Digital Filtering* in this chapter) prior to sampling to ensure that there are no frequency components above the imposed Nyquist limit. This filter is known as an *anti-aliasing filter*. To understand this, let us consider an example using EEG. In scalp-recorded EEG, little observable activity occurs above 80 Hz. Therefore, an anti-aliasing filter at 80 Hz could be applied (but is not necessary if there is no signal power above 80 Hz in the raw EEG), and a sampling rate of 160 Hz would be sufficient to digitize and perfectly reconstruct this signal. A sampling rate above this 160 Hz is also acceptable but is unnecessary and will require more data-storage space.

QUANTIZATION

Quantization is the conversion of each sample (e.g., its analog voltage) into a binary number for processing and storage in a computer. The number, k, of binary *bits* used for quantization determines the number of possible discrete amplitude values used to represent the digital signal. These discrete amplitude values are called *quantization levels*. The number of quantization levels equals 2^k. For example, an 8-bit ADC produces 2^8 (i.e., 256) quantization levels, and a 16-bit converter produces 2^{16} (i.e., 65,536) levels. These quantization levels are usually uniformly spaced over the analog voltage range of the ADC. Each sample of the analog voltage is normally rounded to the nearest quantization level. The more quantization levels used, the more accurate is the digital-amplitude representation of the original analog signal. For example, if the voltage range of the ADC is ±5 V (giving a range of 10 V), the quantization

levels of an 8-bit ADC (which has 256 quantization levels) are 39 mV apart (because 10 V divided by 256 equals 39 mV); the levels of a 16-bit ADC (which has 65,536 quantization levels) are only 0.153 mV (or 153 μV) apart. It should be noted that the analog signal amplification and the voltage range of the ADC should be coordinated in order to distribute the quantization levels over the full expected amplitude range (called the *dynamic range*) of the analog signal. Otherwise, if the dynamic range of the amplified analog signal is smaller than the voltage range of the ADC, only the lowest quantization levels will be used, resulting in suboptimal amplitude resolution. This can be mitigated somewhat by overcompensating when one is selecting the bits of resolution for the ADC, that is, by selecting an ADC resolution that will be sufficient in cases where the dynamic range of the signal may drop below the expected voltage range of the ADC. On the other hand, if the dynamic range of the amplified analog signal is larger than the voltage range of the ADC, all voltages above the largest positive and negative quantization levels will be mapped to those levels, respectively. This results in a digitized signal with *clipping distortion*, leaving square-like clipping artifacts in which the peaks of the signal exceed the largest quantization levels.

The number of bits in the ADC also affects the SNR, which is commonly measured in decibels (dB):

$$SNR(dB) = 10 \log_{10}\left(\frac{P_{signal}}{P_{noise}}\right) = 20 \log_{10}\left(\frac{A_{signal}}{A_{noise}}\right)$$

(7.1)

where P is the power and A is the amplitude of the signal or noise. The noise in this case represents the quantization error caused by rounding. For instance, an 8-bit ADC uses one bit for the sign (polarity) and 7 bits for the amplitude. The well-accepted rule of thumb is that 6 dB of SNR are obtained for each bit in an ADC. Thus, for the 7 bits for amplitude, the SNR is approximately 6 dB/bit × 7 bits ≈ 40 dB. Using this value SNR = 40 dB to equal the right-hand term in equation 7.1, and solving equation 7.1 for the ratio A_{signal}/A_{noise}, we get 100. This means that, for an 8-bit ADC, the captured digital-signal amplitude will be approximately 100 times the quantization noise amplitude.

At the same time, it should also be noted that higher sampling rates and finer quantization require more digital storage space. Thus, an effective BCI system requires a sampling rate and quantization level that adequately capture the analog signal but that are also practical in terms of the necessary hardware and software. The binary value assigned to each digital sample can be mapped back to the corresponding voltage value for signal visualization and processing. Figure 7.2 illustrates the sampling and quantization process. Additional details regarding sampling and quantization theory can be found in (Proakis 2007).

FOURIER ANALYSIS

Much of signal-processing theory is rooted in *Fourier analysis*, which transforms a *time-domain* (i.e., time on the *x*-axis) signal into its equivalent *frequency-domain* (i.e., frequency on the

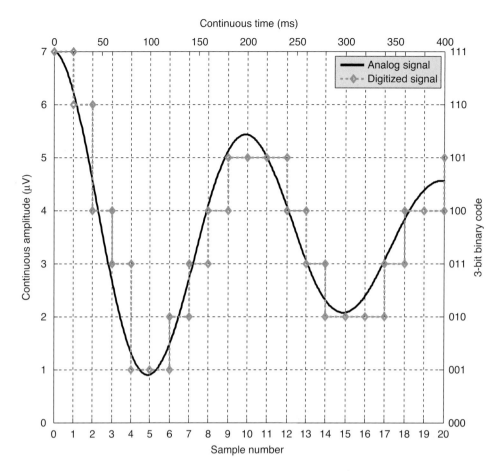

Figure 7.2 *A basic 3-bit binary encoding of an analog signal. Note that the digital samples exist only at the sample instants corresponding to the sample number; the dashed line is provided for illustration purposes.*

x-axis) representation. The primary utility of Fourier analysis is to decompose a signal into individual sinusoidal components that can be isolated and evaluated independently. Using Fourier analysis, practically any signal can be accurately represented as the sum of a number (possibly an infinite number) of amplitude-scaled and time-shifted sinusoids at specific frequencies. This is illustrated in figure 7.3, which shows the successive approximations of a neuronal action potential (left column) and a bipolar pulse (right column) by sums of sinusoids. Note that the continuous signals (top row) are better approximated as more sinusoids (e.g., the third and particularly the fourth row) are used for modeling.

In order to model these continuous signals, it is necessary to properly adjust the phase and the magnitude of each sinusoid. For an arbitrary signal $x(t)$, the *magnitude* (scale) and *phase* (shift) of the sinusoid at each frequency [ω (*radians*) = $2\pi f (Hz)$] required to represent an arbitrary signal can be determined from the *Fourier transform*:

$$X(\omega) = \int_{-\infty}^{\infty} x(t)e^{-j\omega t}dt = \int_{-\infty}^{\infty} x(t)[\cos \omega t + j \sin \omega t]dt$$

$$= \underbrace{\int_{-\infty}^{\infty} x(t)\cos \omega t dt}_{a(\omega)} + j \underbrace{\int_{-\infty}^{\infty} x(t)\sin \omega t dt}_{b(\omega)}$$

$$= a(\omega) + jb(\omega)$$

(7.2)

The magnitude and phase for each sinusoidal component are given as:

$$Magnitude: \quad |X(\omega)| = \sqrt{a^2(\omega) + b^2(\omega)}$$

(7.3a)

$$Phase: \quad \theta = \arg(X(\omega)) = \tan^{-1}\left(\frac{b(\omega)}{a(\omega)}\right)$$

(7.3b)

The Fourier transform represents a conversion from the time domain to the frequency domain. Note that the magnitude and phase representations produce real numbers. These values can be plotted with respect to frequency in order to visualize the frequency content of a signal. The inverse Fourier transform can be computed from the magnitude and phase to perfectly reconstruct the signal in the time domain. The original time-domain signal is reconstructed from the scaled and shifted sinusoids at each frequency as follows:

$$x(t) = \int_{-\infty}^{\infty} |X(\omega)|\cos(\omega t + \theta(\omega))d\omega$$

(7.4)

The Fourier transform for digital signals (with finite frequency resolution given by the inverse of the number of samples times the sampling period) can be efficiently implemented using a computer via the fast Fourier transform algorithm (FFT). More detail regarding Fourier methods is provided in

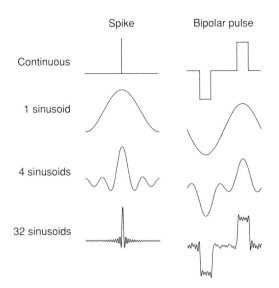

Spike Bipolar pulse

Continuous

1 sinusoid

4 sinusoids

32 sinusoids

Figure 7.3 Modeling of continuous signals using Fourier analysis. A spike and a bipolar pulse are shown in the top row of the figure. The second row shows an approximation with a single sinusoid, with a single cycle in the interval shown. The next row shows the sum of sinusoids with 1, 2, 3, and 4 complete cycles (i.e., four sinusoids having uniformly spaced frequencies) in the interval. Note that these four sinusoids are orthogonal (i.e., uncorrelated) in the interval shown. The last row shows the sum of 32 orthogonal sinusoids. Note that the continuous signals are better approximated as more sinusoids are used for modeling.

the section on *Fast Fourier Transform* in this chapter and in Proakis and Manolakis (2007).

DIGITAL FILTERING

Digital filters are central to digital signal processing. They modify the frequency content of a digital signal by attenuating some frequencies (or frequency ranges) and amplifying others. Each successive sample of a digitized signal is passed through a digital filter to produce a new value as the output.

Given a digital signal $x[n]$, each input sample of $x[n]$ enters the filter sequentially (note that n is now used to denote the sample number of the digital signal, which is analogous to t for continuous time signals). The digital filter's output $y[n]$ at any given time point is simply a weighted sum of the current and past input (and possibly past output) samples:

$$y[n] = \sum_{l=0}^{M} b_l x[n-l] - \sum_{l=1}^{N} a_l y[n-l]$$

(7.5)

where $x[n-l]$ is the lth past input sample, $y[n-l]$ is the lth past output sample, b_l and a_l are scalar weights for each input and output sample, respectively, and M and N are the number of input and output sample weights employed by the filter, respectively. The resulting filter output $y[n]$ is a digital signal having the same number of samples as $x[n]$, where the first sample of $y[n]$ corresponds to the first sample of $x[n]$. Past input and output values of the filter are commonly initialized to zero. Filters that depend only on current and past input and past output samples are referred to as *causal filters*. For

most practical (i.e., real-time) applications, causal filters are necessary because future input and output samples are not yet available.

The simplest example of a digital filter is the computation of a uniform moving average. In computing a uniform moving average, the digital signal passes through the filter, and the filter output at a particular instant is equal to the sum of the past N consecutive samples each weighted by $1/N$ (this is the equivalent of calculating the current output sample as the average of the N past samples). In this case the amplitudes of signal frequencies that have a period less than N (i.e., "high" frequencies) tend to average to zero or to be attenuated at the filter output. This occurs because, for these high frequencies, N samples include samples from both the positive and negative halves of each cycle, which tend to cancel each other and thereby reduce the average value yielded by the filter. The amplitudes of signal frequencies having periods greater than N (i.e., "low" frequencies) tend to be preserved because N is not long enough to contain samples from both halves of the cycle, and thus the majority of the samples are of the same polarity, and the magnitude of the filter output tends to be larger relative to the output for higher frequencies. Since higher frequencies are attenuated and lower frequencies are preserved, the computation of a uniform moving average is known as a *low-pass filter*. In a similar fashion, a simple *high-pass filter* can be constructed by alternating the polarity of the sample weights for successive input samples. In this case constant and slowly varying signals will average toward zero at the filter output, and more rapid signal fluctuations will be preserved. In sum, by properly adjusting the length of the filter (i.e., N, the number of successive samples included) and the weights assigned to successive samples, very specific ranges of signal frequencies can be amplified, attenuated, preserved, and/or eliminated. Thus, digital filters can enhance, isolate, or eliminate signal phenomena that have power at particular frequencies. In addition to low-pass and high-pass, the other two most common types of filters are *bandpass* and *notch (band reject)*. A bandpass filter preserves signal power within a specified continuous frequency range, while attenuating signal power outside of this range. A notch filter is the converse of a bandpass filter; it attenuates signal power within a specified continuous frequency range, while preserving signal power outside of this range.

Figure 7.4 illustrates the *magnitude response* for each of the four common filter types. The *magnitude response* indicates the amplitude scale factor, or gain, that the filter applies to an input signal of a particular frequency. Actual filters produce a rapidly changing response rather than an abrupt cutoff in the frequency domain. Although it is not possible to create an ideal filter having magnitude response with a perfect threshold at a particular frequency (i.e., a step discontinuity), it is possible to achieve sufficient approximations for most practical purposes.

Any of the four common filter types, as well as others, can be realized using equation 7.5. However, there are some tradeoffs, depending on whether or not the filter employs *feedback* of past outputs. If the filter does not employ feedback of past outputs (i.e., $a_l = 0$), the filter is known as a *finite impulse*

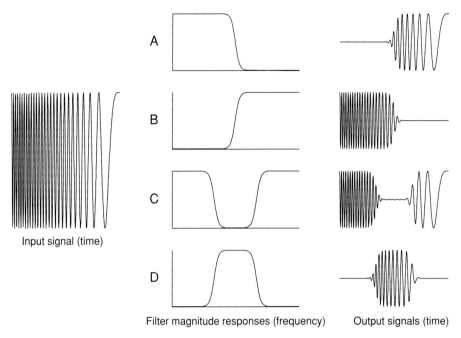

Figure 7.4 *The signal on the left has a frequency that decreases linearly with time (known as a chirp signal) (x-axis is time). The middle column (x-axis is frequency) shows the magnitude response (i.e., the amplitude scale factor, or gain, applied) for each of the four filters: (A) low-pass; (B) high-pass; (C) bandstop/notch; and (D) bandpass. The signals in the right column (x-axis is time) are the outputs when the filters of the middle column are applied to the signal in the left column.*

response filter. If the filter does employ feedback of past outputs (i.e., $a_i \neq 0$), the filter is known as an *infinite impulse response filter*. These two fundamental linear digital filter structures are described here, and additional details regarding digital-filter design can be found in Proakis and Manolakis (2007).

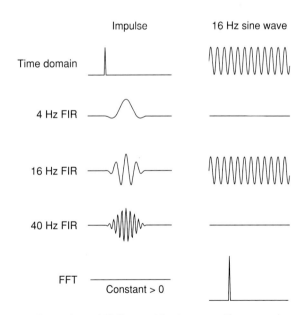

Figure 7.5 *Comparisons of FIR filters and Fourier spectra. The top row shows two time-domain waveforms (impulse and sine wave). The next three rows illustrate the outputs after passing these time-domain signals through a 4-, 16-, and 40-Hz FIR bandpass filter, respectively. The bottom row shows the corresponding Fourier-based spectra. Note that the impulse (left column) produces output at all frequencies, whereas the sine wave (right column) produces output at frequency corresponding to the frequency of the input. Thus, considering the output of only a single FIR filter or spectral bin can be misleading. It is always advisable to examine the entire spectrum.*

FINITE IMPULSE RESPONSE FILTERS

A finite impulse response (FIR) filter is a weighted moving-average filter without feedback of past outputs. The term *finite* is used to describe this filter because a single sample entering the filter is guaranteed to affect the resulting output signal for a time no longer than the order of the filter (i.e., the duration of the time period from which the filter obtains the samples used to determine each output sample). Since there is no output feedback in an FIR filter (i.e., the output is not used in the calculation of subsequent outputs), it is stable; that is, the output signal amplitude cannot grow without bound if the input is amplitude-limited. Moreover, FIR filters can be designed with a *linear phase response*. This means that any time delay introduced by the filter will be the same for all frequencies; thus, the filter does not distort the morphology of the output signal with frequency-dependent delay. This property is particularly advantageous when the signal of interest is characterized or distinguished by its shape (i.e., by the relative amplitudes of consecutive samples). The primary disadvantage of FIR filters is that filter length increases with increasing sharpness of the desired magnitude response transition. Very long filter lengths are needed to achieve very sharp transitions in the magnitude response that approach those provided by ideal filters. This is a key consideration for real-time BCI implementations because longer causal FIR filters will result in longer time delays of the output. For a causal FIR filter with symmetric weights, the time delay of the output in samples will correspond to roughly half the filter length.

Figure 7.5 shows the outputs of three different FIR filters (bandpass of 4-, 16-, and 40-Hz) and a Fourier spectrum, given two different time-domain input signals (impulse and 16-Hz sine wave). The impulse produces an output in each of the FIR filters, as well as a uniform value across the Fourier spectra.

In contrast, the sine wave produces an output only in the FIR filter with the same frequency characteristics and a narrow peak in the Fourier spectra. Thus, considering the output of only a single FIR filter or spectral bin can be misleading. It is always advisable to examine the entire spectrum.

INFINITE IMPULSE RESPONSE FILTERS

An *infinite impulse response* (IIR) filter can be thought of as combination of two FIR filters, one that combines the current and past inputs and one that combines the past outputs. The IIR filter output is the sum of the two FIR filter outputs. The term *infinite* is applied to this filter because a single input sample will affect an infinite sequence of output samples through its role in determining the outputs that constitute the feedback. The primary advantage of IIR filters is that they are capable of producing sharp transitions in the magnitude response using relatively few properly weighted input and output samples. However, in contrast to FIR filters, IIR filters can be unstable because of their use of feedback. Thus, they must be designed so as to promote stability. In addition, IIR filters tend to have a nonlinear phase response; that is, different frequencies will experience different time delays unless specifically designed otherwise. Depending on the application, this phase distortion may not be of particular concern for feature extraction since compensations for the nonlinear phase characteristics can be achieved during feature translation.

THE THREE STEPS OF FEATURE EXTRACTION

The process of feature extraction is discussed here as a three-step procedure:

- signal conditioning to reduce noise and to enhance relevant aspects of the signals
- extraction of the features from the conditioned signals
- feature conditioning to properly prepare the feature vector for the feature-translation stage

FIRST STEP: SIGNAL CONDITIONING

The first step of feature extraction is called *signal conditioning* or *preprocessing*. This step enhances the signal by preemptively eliminating known interference (i.e., artifacts) or irrelevant information, and/or by enhancing spatial, spectral, or temporal characteristics of the signal that are particularly relevant to the application. It is common to have some prior knowledge about the general signal characteristics relevant for a particular application, and this knowledge is used in conditioning. Signal conditioning can include a number of different procedures that can primarily be categorized as:

- frequency-range prefiltering
- data decimation and normalization

- spatial filtering
- removal of environmental interference and biological artifacts

FREQUENCY-RANGE PREFILTERING

Signals are often prefiltered to eliminate frequencies that lie outside the frequency range of the brain activity most relevant to the application. Depending on the application and the available hardware, this prefiltering can be performed before or after the signal is digitized. For example, because the observed signal power in EEG decreases as 1/frequency and the skull and scalp tissue provide additional signal attenuation, scalp-recorded EEG frequencies above 40 Hz have a very low signal-to-noise ratio and thus may not be very useful for BCI applications. Additionally, EEG low-frequency drift produced by the amplifier is sometimes present in EEG and can distort signal visualization. When combined with an ADC of limited amplitude range, a reduction in amplification may be necessary, thus reducing the amplitude resolution of the digitized signal. As a result, it is common at the beginning of EEG feature extraction to apply a 0.5–40 Hz (or narrower if possible) bandpass filter to isolate the relevant brain activity. For instance, 8–12 Hz bandpass can be applied to isolate mu-band activity, or 8–30 Hz can be applied to include both mu- and beta-band activity. In contrast, for evoked potentials such as the P300 (see chapter 12, in this volume), it is prudent to use a high-pass cutoff of 0.1–0.5 Hz to preserve the characteristic low-frequency information of the response (typically with a low-pass cutoff between 5–40 Hz, depending on the nature of the evoked response). In general, the width of the filter should be set conservatively to prevent unnecessary loss of information, which can also be beneficial for offline analysis of the signals.

DATA DECIMATION AND NORMALIZATION

If the signal is digitized at a rate that is higher than the Nyquist rate required to capture the relevant activity, it may be advantageous to *decimate* the sampled signal to the minimum effective sampling rate for more efficient processing and storage. *Decimation* is the elimination of samples in a periodic fashion. For example, the decimation of a signal by a factor of two will eliminate every other sample, effectively halving the sampling rate and the length of (i.e., the number of samples in) the signal. However, just as with sampling in analog-to-digital conversion, it is important to avoid aliasing (see section on *Sampling* earlier in this chapter). To avoid aliasing, the signal should be low-pass filtered before decimation, with a cutoff frequency equal to one-half of the decimated sampling frequency.

The most common way to *normalize* a set of signals is to subtract from each signal its mean value and then scale the resulting signals by dividing by its variance. Signal normalization can be useful when one is comparing different signals that have differences in mean values or dynamic (i.e., amplitude) ranges that are not relevant to the particular application. For example, EEG signals recorded over two brain areas often differ markedly in amplitude range, but the signal dynamics within these ranges may be of primary interest for a given BCI application, not the actual difference in the respective signal amplitude values. Normalization can also be used to adjust signals that are affected by unintended electrode impedance differences (which are obviously not relevant to the application). By converting the signals to the same scale, normalization can potentially simplify the analysis and interpretation of the signals and the subsequent processing steps. At the same time, however, normalization must be used with caution since it does eliminate the potentially useful amplitude differences within a set of signals.

SPATIAL FILTERING

In methods that measure electrical signals from the scalp or within the head, the quantity measured is the electrical potential difference (in volts) between two electrodes, and the voltage signal obtained is commonly called a *channel*. Each channel reflects the voltage fields produced by multiple proximal brain sources and sometimes by nonbrain sources as well (e.g., muscle activity, 60-Hz artifacts, etc.). The sensitivity of a channel to different brain sources depends on the sizes and orientations of the sources in relation to the locations of the channel's two electrodes. Thus, by properly selecting the pairs of electrodes that comprise each channel, it is possible to make the channel more sensitive to some sources and less sensitive to others. If all the channels recorded have one electrode in common, it is possible to reconstruct any desired alternative set of channels by weighting and combining the channels after digitization. This procedure is known as *spatial filtering*. The common electrode, called the *reference electrode*, or *reference*, is usually placed at a location that is relatively inactive, or insensitive, with regard to brain activity, and in this case the recording is termed *monopolar* (even though, as explained in detail in chapters 3 and 6, *all* voltage recordings, strictly speaking, are bipolar.) When both electrodes in a channel are affected by brain activity, the recording is typically termed *bipolar*.

Spatial filters are generally designed to enhance sensitivity to particular brain sources, to improve source localization, and/or to suppress certain artifacts. Most commonly, spatial filters are selected as linear combinations (i.e., weighted sums) of channels and can be represented in matrix form:

$$\begin{bmatrix} y_{11} & y_{12} & \cdots & y_{1P} \\ y_{21} & y_{22} & & \\ \vdots & & \ddots & \\ y_{M1} & & & y_{MP} \end{bmatrix} = \begin{bmatrix} w_{11} & w_{12} & \cdots & w_{1N} \\ w_{21} & w_{22} & & \\ \vdots & & \ddots & \\ w_{M1} & & & w_{MN} \end{bmatrix} \begin{bmatrix} x_{11} & x_{12} & \cdots & x_{1P} \\ x_{21} & x_{22} & & \\ \vdots & & \ddots & \\ x_{N1} & & & x_{NP} \end{bmatrix}$$

(7.6)

or equivalently in matrix notation:

$$Y = WX \qquad (7.7)$$

where each row of X consists of P consecutive digital signal samples from one of N channels, each row of W is a set of N channel weights that constitute a particular spatial filter, and each row of Y is a resulting spatially filtered channel (M spatially filtered channels × P samples). Essentially, each spatially filtered channel of Y is a weighted sum of the all of the channels in X, where the channel weights are defined by the corresponding row in W. There are several common approaches for

determining the set of spatial-filter weights W. These approaches fall into two major classes: data-independent and data-dependent spatial filters.

Data-Independent Spatial Filters

Data-independent spatial filters typically use fixed geometrical relationships to determine the spatial-filter weights and thus are not dependent on the data being filtered. These filters have certain local or global characteristics that, although somewhat generic, can be extremely effective in many applications. McFarland et al. (1997) describe the value of appropriate data-independent spatial filtering for BCIs. Figure 7.6 illustrates the characteristics of several of these filters: the *common-average reference* and two *surface Laplacian spatial filters* (small and large).

A *common-average reference* (CAR or AVE) spatial filter is realized by recording all channels with a common reference, computing at each time point the global mean of all the digitized channels, and then subtracting that mean from each individual channel. This tends to reduce the impact of artifacts that are similar across all channels (e.g., 60-Hz power-line interference).

A *surface Laplacian spatial filter* is based on a computation of the second spatial derivative. If the channels have been recorded with a common reference, this computation is effectively equivalent to taking a central channel of interest and subtracting the mean of all the channels at some fixed radial distance from this central channel. Although this simplified Laplacian filter is effective and commonly used, more elaborate Laplacian filters can be constructed based on the precise spatial-derivative derivation. Spatially adjacent channels tend to be highly correlated since they have similar positions relative to many brain sources. By eliminating this correlated activity, a Laplacian filter emphasizes highly localized activity (i.e., activity that is not the same at both locations). Thus, the fixed radial distance of the filter should be set based on the spatial characteristics of the activity of interest.

Data-Dependent Spatial Filters

In contrast to the generalized data-independent filters, *data-dependent* spatial filters are derived directly from each BCI user's data. Although these filters tend to be more complex in terms of derivation and spatial geometries, they can produce more precise results for a particular user or application. This is particularly useful in cases where little is known about the exact characteristics of the relevant brain activity. Data-dependent filters are derived by placing an objective constraint on the weight matrix W from equation 7.7. Because Y consists of linear combinations of the original channels, the constraints on W are typically designed to linearly combine the original channels X to produce fewer, more meaningful and/or localized channels in Y, effectively reducing the dimensionality of the problem. Three common methods for deriving data-dependent spatial filters are discussed here:

- principal components analysis (PCA)

- independent component analysis (ICA)

- common spatial patterns (CSP)

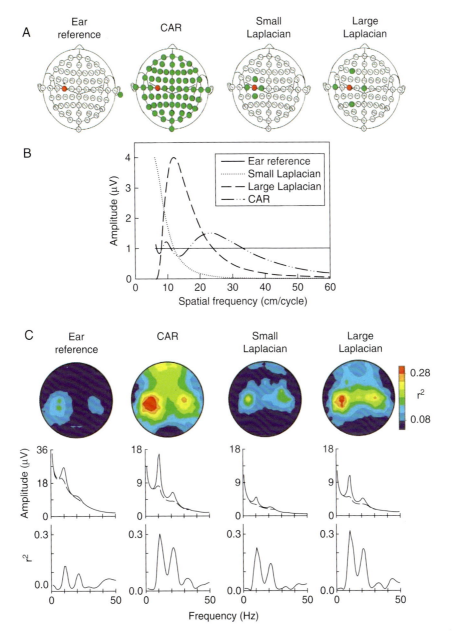

Figure 7.6 *Comparison of four spatial filters. Sixty-four channel EEG data, collected while well-trained subjects were moving a cursor to targets on the top or bottom edge of a video monitor using sensorimotor rhythms, were analyzed offline using four spatial filters. (A) Electrode locations used by four different spatial filters for EEG recorded from C3 (red). For the common average reference (CAR) and Laplacian methods, EEG at the green electrodes is averaged and subtracted from EEG at C3. (B) Spatial bandpass. For each method, the trace shows the square root of the root-mean-square values (amplitude, mV) of a signal that varies sinusoidally in amplitude across the scalp as its spatial frequency varies from 6 cm, twice the interelectrode distance (i.e., the highest spatial frequency that would not cause spatial aliasing), to 60 cm (i.e., approximate head circumference). (C) Average r^2 topography, and amplitude and r^2 spectra for each spatial filter method for trained BCI users at the frequency and electrode location, respectively, used online (r^2 is the proportion of the variance of the signal feature that is accounted for by the user's intended cursor direction toward the target). Each method is applied to the same body of data. With each method, EEG control (measured as r^2) is focused over sensorimotor cortices and in the mu- and beta-rhythm frequency bands. In this example using sensorimotor rhythms, the value of r^2 is highest for the CAR and large Laplacian spatial filters and lowest for the ear reference. (Adapted from McFarland et al. 1997. Reprinted with permission from Clinical Neurophysiology.)*

Principal Component Analysis. Given a set of spatial signals, a specific linear combination of these signals (i.e., a spatial filter) can be determined such that the resulting signals account for the highest proportion of the amplitude variance of the set of original signals. Because EEG channels tend to be highly correlated, PCA can be useful for localizing and enhancing certain brain activity, particularly when amplitude variance is correlated with the BCI task conditions.

PCA determines a set of weights W that transform the set of channels X into a set of new channels Y having the same dimensionality (i.e., W is a square matrix), such that the filtered signal in Y associated with the first principal component (row of weights in W) is the linear combination of the signals in X that produces maximum amplitude variance. When applying PCA, the resulting principal components are orthogonal to each other; that is, the resulting output channels are uncorrelated with each other. Each successive principal component accounts for a smaller portion of the amplitude variance of the original channels. Because the first few principal components usually capture most of the variance of the channels in *X*, the remaining components are typically discarded. By keeping only the signals in *Y* that represent the dimensions accounting for the most variance in *X*, the dimensionality of the problem can be greatly reduced. That is, a typically large number of original (input) channels is reduced to a smaller number of output channels (e.g., a large portion of the variance of 64 input channels may be captured in five or fewer output channels after PCA). Ideally, this process discards very little relevant information, but this is not guaranteed.

One disadvantage of PCA for discriminating different types of brain activity in a BCI application is that, since no information about BCI task conditions is used to derive the weight matrix *W*, the resulting PCA signals accounting for the largest amplitude variance may not be correlated with the task conditions. For instance, if all of the original channels are corrupted with significant 60-Hz line noise compared to the EEG signal power, it is likely that this 60-Hz signal will appear as a top PCA component although it would be independent of any BCI task conditions. Thus, the drawback in PCA is that a comparatively low-power channel that is highly correlated with the task conditions may not be included in the top set of PCA components. Dien et al. (2003) discuss the application of both spatial and temporal PCA for detecting event-related potentials in EEG.

Independent Component Analysis. Although the channels resulting from PCA are uncorrelated, they are not necessarily statistically independent. To be statistically independent, the joint probability distribution function $F_{XY}(x, y) = \Pr\{X \leq x, Y \leq y\}$ of channels x and y must satisfy the following:

$$F_{XY}(x, y) = F_X(x)F_Y(y)$$

(7.8)

In contrast, to be uncorrelated, the expected value of the channels must satisfy the following:

$$E\{XY\} = E\{X\}E\{Y\}$$

(7.9)

Thus, independence is a stricter constraint on the statistical relationship between channels than uncorrelatedness. Assuming that particular sources of brain activity are localized and function independently, identifying a spatial filter that produces independent channels is important because it is theoretically more likely to identify the channels sensitive to different signal-generating sources within the brain. ICA seeks to determine the weight matrix *W* that produces independent channels in *Y*. Because the resulting spatial weights tend to correspond to localized activity, this process can also be understood as a form of source separation or source localization. As with PCA, an application might use only the most relevant ICA components (i.e., the channels that correlate well with the BCI task conditions) in order to reduce the dimensionality.

In general, ICA presents a significant challenge in BCI applications. Not only are the algorithms relatively complex, but the number of independent sources must be accurately approximated to effectively isolate the intended source information. In addition, the maximum number of independent sources that can be identified is limited to the number of channels in *X*. When the number of original channels is much greater than the number of expected independent sources and/or the channels are highly correlated, it is common to use PCA prior to ICA to remove the irrelevant channels and streamline the ICA processing. Hyvärinen (1999) provides a useful survey of ICA algorithms, and Makeig et. al. (2000) discuss the application of ICA for a BCI.

Common Spatial Patterns. CSP is an approach closely related to PCA, except that the task-condition labels (e.g., movement vs. rest, move cursor right vs. move cursor left, etc.) are incorporated when determining *W* such that the corresponding components produce minimum variance for one condition and maximum variance for the other, and vice versa. In this way the CSP spatial filters are optimal for discriminating between two task conditions. For CSP, the channels in *X* are first bandpass-filtered, which makes the variance equivalent to band power (see the discussion of band power in this chapter's section on *Frequency [Spectral] Features*). As with PCA and ICA, only the relevant CSP components are retained. Since the reduced CSP signal matrix is already optimized for discriminating the task conditions, the resulting CSP projections can be fed directly to the translation algorithm without further feature extraction. Also, by inverting the filtering matrix *W* and spatially plotting its components, it is possible to visualize the actual spatial patterns corresponding to the different task conditions. Müller-Gerking et al. (1999) discuss basic use of CSP for BCI applications, whereas Lemm et al. (2005) and Dornhenge et al. (2006) discuss extensions of basic CSP methodology.

DETECTION AND REMOVAL OF ENVIRONMENTAL INTERFERENCE AND BIOLOGICAL ARTIFACTS

Environmental interference is an artifact in brain-signal recordings not attributable to biological sources. It includes interference from environmental factors such as power-lines or other electrical sources in the environment. *Biological artifacts* arise from biological sources such as muscle (electromyographic) (EMG) activity, eye movement (electrooculographic) (EOG) activity, heart-beat (electrocardiographic) (ECG) activity, respiratory activity, etc. We will discuss the most commonly encountered interference and biological artifacts. Other kinds of nonbrain noise can usually be addressed with methods similar to those described here.

50/60-Hz Power-Line Interference

Power-line interference is generated by the electrical systems in buildings. The electrical and/or magnetic fields created by these systems may create electrical fields in the body that are detected by electrodes used to record brain signals, particularly EEG electrodes. This interference manifests itself as a continuous sinusoidal signal at 50 Hz (in Europe and Asia) or 60 Hz (in North and South America). Significant power-line interference often results from high electrode impedance or impedance mismatch involving the electrodes of individual channels or the ground electrode. Some degree of power-line interference is often unavoidable, particularly in home or other nonlaboratory environments in which BCIs are often used. However, even when this interference is obvious in the recorded channels, it may not impair feature extraction if it is stable over time and consistent across channels, or if it is not within the frequency range most relevant for the BCI application. If power-line interference is a significant problem, a *bandstop* (or *notch*) filter can be applied to eliminate a narrow frequency band (e.g., 55–65 Hz) that encompasses the power-line interference. With multichannel recordings, Laplacian and CAR spatial filters can remove power-line interference that is common to all the channels without the need for frequency filtering.

Interference from EMG and EOG Activity and Eye Blinks

EMG activity is electrical activity generated by muscle contractions. It is typically manifested as spectrally broadband activity that often varies substantially from moment to moment. EOG activity is the electrical activity generated by eye movements. For obvious reasons, this interference tends to be prominent in frontal EEG activity. Similarly, eye blinks create a large transient frontal pulse that can also affect more posterior channels. EMG, EOG, and eye-blink artifacts are problems mainly for EEG. They are absent or minimal in ECoG or intracortical signals, which are typically of much higher amplitude than EEG and are largely shielded from contamination by the skull.

In EEG recording, EMG is typically the most significant artifact because it is often difficult to remove or even to fully recognize. In scalp EEG recording, cranial EMG activity is most prominent around the periphery (i.e., frontal, temporal, occipital) and can easily exceed brain activity in amplitude. EMG can also contaminate EEG recorded from more central head regions (Goncharova et. al. 2003). Since EMG is broadband (from the mu/beta range up to several hundred Hz), it is often difficult to detect and difficult to remove using a frequency filter and can easily masquerade as EEG. It therefore presents a considerable challenge in BCI recording. Often, it can be recognized only with sufficiently comprehensive topographical analysis (Goncharova et. al. 2003).

Spatial filtering may be useful for reducing EMG, EOG, or eyeblink artifacts. For example, the spatial filter weights might be derived from a regression with respect to frontal temporal electrodes (if temporal EMG is present), or based on electrodes placed next to the eyes (if EOG is present). Since most of the power for EOG and eye-blink artifacts is usually in low frequencies (~1 Hz), a high-pass or bandpass filter can be used to remove these artifacts, as long as the BCI-relevant EEG signals are not also of low frequency.

SECOND STEP: EXTRACTING THE FEATURES

After the initial signal conditioning step has optimized the signal by enhancing its most relevant features and/or reducing artifacts, the next step of feature extraction measures or *extracts* the chosen features. This section introduces the process of feature extraction with emphasis on methods widely used and/or particularly appropriate for BCI applications. The methods are described in terms of processing a single channel, but they can be generalized to multiple channels.

METHOD SELECTION

Most BCI applications to date have used components of brain signals that are clearly characterized spatially, spectrally, and temporally (e.g., sensory evoked potentials or sensorimotor rhythms). In these situations, the known characteristics of the components and the specific BCI application usually dictate a logical starting point for feature extraction. For example, because sensorimotor rhythms are amplitude modulations at specific frequencies over sensorimotor cortex, it is logical to extract frequency-domain features using processing parameters appropriate to the characteristic dynamics of these rhythms. In contrast, in more exploratory situations, when less is known about the optimal feature choice, it is preferable to first assess potential features in both time and frequency domains, and it may be worthwhile initially to construct a feature vector that includes features extracted in both time and frequency domains. In the long run, however, it is best to eliminate features that are redundant or less relevant to the application. Since feature extraction and translation need to work together, the choice of translation algorithm may affect the choice of feature-extraction method, and vice versa. McFarland et al. (2006) and Bashashati et al. (2007) provide comprehensive surveys of BCI feature-extraction methods and translation algorithms.

BLOCK PROCESSING

For most BCI applications, it is highly desirable for the processing to occur in real time (i.e., rapidly enough to sustain an ongoing interaction between the user and the system that accomplishes the user's intent). Prior to feature extraction, the incoming signal samples are commonly segmented into consecutive, possibly overlapping, sample blocks (see fig. 7.1). A feature vector (i.e., the values of one or more features) is created from the signal samples within each individual sample block. The feature vectors from the successive sample blocks are then fed to the translation algorithm, which produces a device command or user feedback corresponding to each sample block or corresponding to sets of consecutive sample blocks. For efficient online implementation, the length and overlap of these sample blocks should fit the relevant temporal dynamics of the signal, the feature-extraction method, the nature of the application, and the concurrent user feedback, as well as the available processing power. For example, for BCI cursor control, it is not normally necessary to compute a new feature vector (and thus a cursor movement) for each new input sample, since the sampling rate is usually much higher (e.g., 128 Hz) than an acceptable cursor movement rate (e.g., 20 movements/sec). Computing feature vectors more frequently than needed for the application is generally a needless expenditure of computational time and power.

For some applications, it is not necessary to compute feature vectors for every sample block. For instance, in the case of transient stimulus-locked responses such as stimulus-evoked potentials like the P300 response (see chapter 12, this volume), it is important to compute the feature vectors only for a defined period after (and perhaps also before) each stimulus. Additionally, for some applications, feature vectors for a number of successive sample blocks are averaged to improve the signal-to-noise ratio before being processed by the translation algorithm to produce output.

TIME (TEMPORAL) FEATURES
Peak-Picking and Integration
Peak-picking and *integration* are two of the most straightforward and basic feature-extraction methods. Peak-picking simply determines the minimum or maximum value of the signal samples in a specific time block (usually defined relative to a specific preceding stimulus) and uses that value (and possibly its time of occurrence) as the feature(s) for that time block. Alternatively, the signal can be averaged or integrated over all or part of the time block to yield the feature(s) for the block. Some form of averaging or integration is typically preferable to simple peak-picking, especially when the responses to the stimulus are known to vary in latency and/or when unrelated higher-frequency activity is superimposed on the relevant feature. Moreover, these same methods can be applied for tracking transient amplitude peaks in the frequency domain. Farwell and Donchin (1988) used these straightforward methods with considerable success in the first P300-based BCI.

Correlation and Template-Matching
The similarity of a response to a predefined template might also be used as a feature. Computing the similarity, or correlation, of a response to a template is essentially equivalent to FIR filtering using the template as the filter weights. For a given response, the output of the template filter will be high for the segments that closely resemble the template and low for segments that differ from the template. Wavelet analysis (see section on *Time-Frequency Features* in this chapter) can be considered a variation of this method; it uses templates with specific analytical properties to produce a frequency decomposition related to Fourier analysis. Krusienski et al. (2007) and Serby et al. (2005) apply a template scheme to a sensorimotor rhythm-based BCI and a P300-based BCI, respectively.

FREQUENCY (SPECTRAL) FEATURES
Much brain activity manifests itself as continuous amplitude- and frequency-modulated oscillations. Therefore, it is often advantageous to accurately track these changes in the frequency domain. Although the Fourier transform is the most common method for converting from the time domain to the frequency domain, there are several alternatives that have characteristics that are particularly desirable given specific constraints or specific objectives. These include:

- band power
- fast Fourier transform (FFT)
- autoregressive (AR) modeling

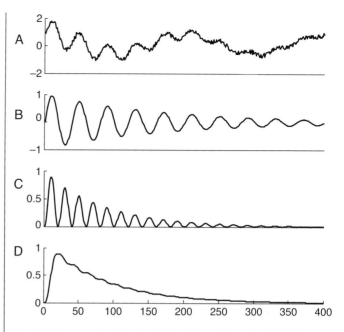

Figure 7.7 *The procedure for extracting bandpower from a signal. (A) The original signal. (B) The result after applying a bandpass filter to the data in A. (C) The result after squaring the amplitude of B. (D) The final bandpower result after smoothing C with a low-pass filter. The x-axis is time.*

Band Power
One of the most straightforward and intuitive methods for tracking amplitude modulations at a particular frequency is to first isolate the frequency of interest by filtering the signal with a bandpass filter. This produces a signal that is largely sinusoidal. Next, to produce purely positive values, the signal is rectified by squaring the signal or by computing its absolute value. Finally, the adjacent peaks are smoothed together via integration or low-pass filtering. The effects of each of these steps are illustrated in figure 7.7. Although the smoothed signal (fig. 7.7D) tracks the magnitude envelope of the frequency of interest, the resulting instantaneous magnitude estimate will be slightly delayed due to the smoothing step. When multiple-frequency band tracking is required, it is typically preferable to use an FFT- or AR-based method rather than using multiple bandpass filters and computing the band power of each output.

Fast Fourier Transform
The FFT is an efficient implementation of the discrete Fourier transform, which is the discrete-time equivalent of the continuous Fourier transform already discussed in this chapter. The FFT represents the frequency spectrum of a digital signal with a frequency resolution of sample-rate/FFT-points, where the FFT-point is a selectable scalar that must be greater or equal to the length of the digital signal and is typically chosen as a base 2 value for computational efficiency. Because of its simplicity and effectiveness, the FFT often serves as the baseline method to which other spectral analysis methods are compared.

The FFT takes an *N*-sample digital signal and produces *N* frequency samples uniformly spaced over a frequency range

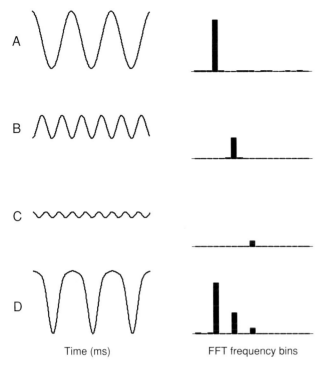

Figure 7.8 Fast Fourier transform. Four time-domain digital signals are shown on the left (shown as continuous signals for illustration purposes). The four corresponding FFT magnitude spectra are shown on the right. The time and frequency plots have the same respective amplitude scale. The leftmost FFT bin is centered on 0 Hz, and the rightmost is centered on sampling rate/2. Signals A, B, and C are harmonically related sinusoids (i.e., integer multiple frequencies of signal A) that sum to produce the nonsinusoidal periodic signal D. Because the FFT is a linear transform, the same holds for the magnitude spectra. Although the FFT phase is not shown, notice that the phase of the sinusoids has an important role in the shape of signal D in the time domain (i.e., shifting the phase of A, B, or C will alter the shape of D).

of ±sampling rate/2, thus making it a one-to-one transformation that incurs no loss of information. These frequency-domain samples are often referred to as *frequency bins* and are the digital equivalent of the results of a continuous Fourier transform, with the frequency resolution specified. The FFT will produce complex values that can be converted to magnitude and phase as shown in equations 7.3a and 7.3b. The FFT spectrum of a real signal has symmetry such that only half of the bins are unique, from zero to +sampling rate/2. These positive bins are shown in figure 7.8 for several sinusoids that comprise the periodic waveform in the bottom row. The bins from zero to −sampling rate/2 are the mirror image of the positive bins. Therefore, for an *N*-sample real signal, there are *N*/2 unique frequency bins from zero to sampling rate/2. Knowing this fact allows one to apply and interpret the FFT even without a firm grasp of the complex mathematics associated with the notion of "negative frequencies."

Finer frequency sampling can be achieved by appending *M* zeros to the *N*-sample signal, producing (*M* + *N*)/2 bins from zero to the sampling rate/2. This is known as *zero padding*. Zero padding does not actually increase the spectral resolution since no additional signal information is being included in the computation, but it does provide an interpolated spectrum with different bin frequencies.

Because *N*-sample signal blocks may section the signal abruptly to create false discontinuities at the edges of the block, artificial ripples tend to be produced around the peaks of the spectrum. This can be mitigated by multiplying the block of samples by a tapering windowing function that tapers the samples at the edges of the sample block, thus reducing the ripples in the spectrum. Although this acts to smooth the spectral ripples, it also expands the width of the frequency peaks, and thus lowers overall spectral resolution. In many cases, this is a tolerable tradeoff for obtaining a smoother spectrum.

Note that it is also common to refer to the *power* spectrum rather than the *amplitude* spectrum. Recall that signal power is proportional to the squared signal amplitude. Each bin of the FFT magnitude spectrum tracks the sinusoidal amplitude of the signal at the corresponding frequency. A simple estimate of the power spectrum can be obtained by simply squaring the FFT magnitude. However, more robust FFT-based estimates can be obtained by using variants of the periodogram (Hayes 1996). Wolpaw and McFarland (1994), Pregenzer and Pfurtscheller (1999), and Kelly et al. (2005) provide examples of FFT-based methods applied to BCIs.

Autoregressive Modeling

Autoregressive (AR) modeling is an alternative to Fourier-based methods for computing the frequency spectrum of a signal. AR modeling assumes that the signal being modeled was generated by passing white noise through an infinite impulse response (IIR) filter. The specific weights of the IIR filter shape the white noise input to match the characteristics of the signal being modeled. *White noise* is essentially random noise that has the unique property of being completely uncorrelated when compared to any delayed version of itself. The specific IIR filter structure for AR modeling uses no delayed input terms and *p* delayed output terms. This structure allows efficient computation of the IIR filter weights. Because white noise has a completely flat power spectrum (i.e., the same power at all frequencies), the IIR filter weights are set so as to shape the spectrum to match the actual spectrum of the signal being analyzed. It has been posited that filtering a white-noise process with an AR filter is a suitable model for the generation of EEG, since EEG is essentially a mixture of spontaneously firing spatial sources (synapses and neurons), measured at different locations (i.e., electrode positions). This process can be approximated to a first order by filtering a white-noise process (effectively it assumes a linear generation model for the EEG with constant excitation which, however, is unlikely to occur in the brain). In sum, the filter weights used for AR spectral analysis of EEG are based on the assumption that EEG is equivalent to filtering white noise with an IIR filter.

Because the IIR filter weights define the signal's spectrum, AR modeling can potentially achieve higher spectral resolution for shorter signal blocks than can the FFT. Short signal blocks are often necessary for BCI outputs such as cursor control in which frequent feature updates are essential. Additionally, the IIR filter structure accurately models spectra with sharp, distinct peaks, which are common for biosignals such as EEG. Hayes (1996) discusses the theory and various approaches for computing the IIR weights (i.e., AR model) from an observed signal. The estimated power spectrum can be computed from the IIR filter weights as follows:

$$\hat{P}_{AR}(\omega) = \frac{|b(0)|^2}{\left|1 + \sum_{k=1}^{p} a_p(k)e^{-jk\omega}\right|^2}$$

(7.10)

where $a_p(k)$ and $b(0)$ are the estimated IIR filter weights and p is the AR model order. In this case, frequency bins similar to the FFT can be defined by evaluating equation 7.10 at the frequencies of interest. Alternatively, since the relevant information is contained in the filter weights, it is also common to use the weights themselves as features.

The primary issue with AR modeling is that the accuracy of the spectral estimate is highly dependent on the selected model order (p). An insufficient model order tends to blur the spectrum, whereas an overly large order may create artificial peaks in the spectrum. One approach is to view the EEG as being comprised of 3–6 spectral peaks representing some combination of delta, theta, alpha, beta, and gamma waves (see chapter 13, in this volume). In this case each peak can be represented as a pair of the p poles (i.e., roots of the denominator in equation 7.10) of an AR model, which requires only a relatively low model order of 6–12. However, this reasoning fails to account for distinct spectrally adjacent or overlapping signals (such as mu-rhythm and visual alpha-rhythm activity) or for other narrow-band and/or wide-band activity (such as EOG and EMG) that may contaminate the signal. The complex nature of the EEG signal should be taken into account for accurate spectral estimation, and this often cannot be reliably accomplished with such small model orders. It should be noted that the model order is dependent on the spectral content of the signal and the sampling rate. For a given signal, the model order should be increased in proportion to an increased sampling rate. For scalp EEG sampled at 160 Hz, model orders of 10–20 are frequently prudent. On the other hand, a small model order may be adequate when only a few frequencies are of interest and when other aspects of the signal are eliminated by bandpass-filtering prior to AR spectral analysis. McFarland et al. (2008) discuss AR model-order selection for BCI applications.

The Burg Algorithm (Hayes 1996) is commonly used for estimating the weights in equation 7.10 because, unlike most other methods, it is guaranteed to produce a stable IIR model. It is also possible to generate a single AR model using multiple signals. This is known as *multivariate AR modeling*. Anderson et al. (1998), Pfurtscheller et al. (1998), Wolpaw and McFarland (2004), and Burke et al. (2005) apply various methods of AR modeling to BCI applications.

TIME-FREQUENCY FEATURES (WAVELETS)

Wavelet analysis solves one major drawback of conventional spectral-analysis techniques based on the power spectrum, that is, that the temporal and spectral resolution of the resulting estimates are highly dependent on the selected segment length, model order, and other parameters. This is particularly a problem when the signal contains a wide range of relevant frequency components, each possessing temporally distinct amplitude modulation characteristics. For instance, for a given sample block length, the amplitude of a particular high-frequency component (with respect to the block length) has the potential to fluctuate significantly over each cycle within the sample block. In contrast, the amplitude of a lower-frequency component will not do so because a smaller number of cycles occur within the sample block. For a given sample block, the FFT and AR methods produce only one frequency bin that represents these fluctuations at the respective frequency. By observing this bin in isolation, it is not possible to determine when a pulse at that particular frequency occurs within the sampling block. *Wavelet analysis* solves this problem by producing a time-frequency representation of the signal. However, as predicted by Heisenberg's uncertainty principle, there is always a time/frequency resolution trade-off in signal processing: it is impossible to precisely determine the instantaneous frequency and time of occurrence of an event. This means that longer time windows will produce spectral estimates having higher frequency resolution, while shorter time windows will produce estimates having lower frequency resolution.

The output of the FFT can be realized from a set of parallel bandpass filters (a so-called *filter bank*), with each filter centered at uniform frequency intervals. In contrast, *wavelet analysis* designs a filter bank to achieve an improved time-frequency resolution. In wavelet analysis a characteristic time-limited pulse shape, called the *mother wavelet*, is used to construct a template for each temporal FIR bandpass filter in the filter bank. Typically, mother wavelets tend to be oscillatory in nature, and thus have a bandpass magnitude response. Each template filter in the filter bank is correlated with the signal of interest. The output of a given template filter will have a comparatively large magnitude when it overlaps with a portion of the signal that is similar to the template filter. This filtering process is repeated multiple times in parallel via the filter bank, using the same template shape for each filter but stretching or compressing it by different factors or *scales* for the different filters in the bank. Since each scaled mother wavelet filter has a unique temporal length and represents a unique oscillation-frequency characteristic, each filter output represents a unique time-frequency content of the signal. This scheme results in a more effective, nonuniform time-frequency tiling (i.e., resolution of adjacent time-frequency bins) compared to the FFT because changes in high-frequency characteristics can be identified over shorter time intervals than with the segment length used by the FFT. This time-frequency tiling and corresponding mother-wavelet scaling are illustrated in figure 7.9.

There is a wide variety of mother wavelets, and each has specific time-frequency characteristics and mathematical properties. In addition, application-specific mother wavelets can be developed if general pulse characteristics are known or desired. Moreover, different sets of scaling and shifting factors can be applied, and relationships existing among these factors can be used for computation of a wavelet transform. Just as the FFT provides an efficient computation of the Fourier Transform for digital signals, the *discrete wavelet transform* (DWT) provides an efficient computation of the wavelet transform using specific scale and shift factors that minimize redundancy in the

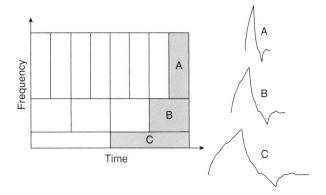

Figure 7.9 The diagram on the left indicates the time-frequency tiling (i.e., resolution of adjacent time-frequency bins) achieved by a wavelet analysis. Note that the higher-frequency content of a signal is computed over shorter time intervals (A), and the lower-frequency content is computed over longer time intervals (C). The time-domain waveforms on the right represent different scales of an example mother wavelet that could be used to compute the wavelet coefficient for the corresponding time-frequency tile.

time-frequency representation. Graimann et al. (2004), Bostanov (2004), and Qin and He (2005) apply wavelet analysis to various BCI paradigms. Mallot (2008) provides the theoretical details of wavelets.

SIMILARITY FEATURES
Phase Locking Value

Brain activity that occurs synchronously (i.e., in the same phase) across multiple channels can be relevant to BCI applications. The *phase locking value* (PLV) is a measurement of the level of phase coupling that occurs between two signals occupying the same narrow frequency range. This is a useful approach for quantifying the phase relationship between signals from two different EEG electrodes. First, both of the signals are filtered using a narrow bandpass filter. Then, the instantaneous phase difference between the filtered signals is computed either by using the Hilbert Transform (Proakis and Manolakis 2007) or the phase information provided by the FFT. Because the instantaneous phase difference tends to vary over time, the values must be averaged to determine the consistency of phase coupling between the signals. However, because phase is circular (i.e., 0 radians is equivalent to 2π radians), phase cannot be averaged directly. Instead, each phase-difference observation is converted into a vector having a magnitude equal to one (represented here as a complex exponential). The vectors are summed and divided by the number of observations as follows:

$$\theta(t) = \theta_{signal1}(t) - \theta_{signal2}(t)$$
(7.11)

$$PLV = \left| \frac{1}{N} \sum_{t=1}^{N} e^{j\theta(t)} \right|$$
(7.12)

Equation 7.11 represents the instantaneous phase difference between the two bandpass-filtered signals. In equation 7.12, the magnitude of the resultant vector represents the PLV. When

all of the individual vectors in the sum have the same instantaneous phase, the vectors all point in the same direction and the resultant sum will equal one. The closer the PLV is to 1, the more consistent the phase difference between the signals (i.e., they are phase locked with each other.) When the instantaneous phase difference is random with a uniform distribution, the PLV will be near zero, indicating that the signals are not phase coupled in the frequency band examined. Gysels and Celka (2004), Brunner et al. (2006), and Wei et al. (2007) apply the PLV in BCI applications.

Coherence

Whereas the PLV measures the phase relationship between two narrow-band signals, *coherence* measures the correlation between the *amplitudes* of two narrow-band signals. In this case, the "narrow bands" are selected from among the spectral bins of an FFT or other spectral-estimation method. The power spectrum of the signals, $S_{xx}(f)$, is used rather than the amplitude spectrum. $S_{xx}(f)$ is equivalent to the squared Fourier transform of the signals. $S_{xy}(f)$ is an average of several individual estimates of the cross spectrum between signals x and y. The coherence between these signals is determined as follows:

$$\gamma_{xy}^2(\omega) = \frac{\left| S_{xy}(\omega) \right|^2}{S_{xx}(\omega) S_{yy}(\omega)}$$
(7.13)

The amplitude of $\gamma_{xy}^2(\omega)$ will have a value ranging between 0 (if there is no coherence) and 1 (if there is perfect coherence). It should be noted that a sufficiently large number of observations is necessary to accurately estimate coherence. Thus, coherence is not likely to be useful as a feature for online BCI operation.

Mahalanobis Distance

Features can be defined by measuring the similarity between certain signal features and predetermined baseline or archetypal distribution(s) of these features. The *Euclidian distance* (the familiar "straight line" distance between two points in space) is one possible similarity feature that can be used to compare a feature vector to a baseline feature vector. When the potential exists for the features comprising the feature vector to be correlated, the *Mahalanobis distance* (D_M) is preferred because it accounts for the covariance among features and is scale invariant:

$$D_M(x) = \sqrt{(x-\mu)^T \Sigma^{-1} (x-\mu)}$$
(7.14)

where x is the multivariate feature observation and Σ and μ are the covariance matrix and the mean of the archetypal distribution, respectively. Example Euclidean and Mahalanobis distance contours from the mean of a two-dimensional feature space are illustrated in figure 7.10. In this figure, features 1 and 2 are correlated, and observations along the equal-Euclidean-distance contour (in blue) clearly do not have a consistent relationship with the joint distribution of the features, in contrast to the Mahalanobis contour (in red). Essentially, feature-vector observations that exist on equal probability contours of the

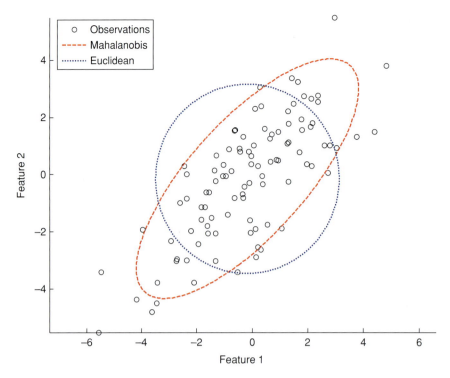

Figure 7.10 *Example of equidistant Mahalanobis (red) and Euclidean (blue) contours from the mean of a two-dimensional feature distribution having correlated features. The Mahalanobis contour captures the covariance of the features, but the Euclidian contour does not.*

joint probability-density function defined by the archetypal features have an equal Mahalanobis distance from the mean of the distribution and thus have an equal probability of belonging to the archetypal distribution.

THIRD STEP: FEATURE CONDITIONING

The distributions and the relationships among the features can have a significant effect on the performance of the translation algorithm that follows feature extraction. These effects depend on the characteristics of the particular translation algorithm. This section reviews common methods of *feature-conditioning* (*post-processing*) that can improve the performance of particular translation algorithms.

NORMALIZATION

In signal conditioning, *signal normalization* is commonly accomplished by subtracting the signal mean and scaling the signal amplitude to have unit variance (i.e., variance equal to 1). Features can also be normalized. *Feature normalization* is advantageous when the features comprising a feature vector display differences in their means or dynamic ranges that are not relevant to their BCI usage. For example, the derivation of feature weights for a multiple-regression algorithm can be very sensitive to differing feature magnitudes. Features of greater magnitude will tend to dominate the results, even if their greater magnitude has no bearing on their usefulness. Furthermore, translation algorithms tend to perform better when the features comprising the feature vector have similar dynamic ranges. If feature dynamic ranges differ substantially, the algorithm may be biased by being more sensitive to some features than to others. Nevertheless, normalization should be

used with caution and only in clearly appropriate situations, because it does discard interchannel information that could conceivably be relevant to the particular BCI application.

LOG-NORMAL TRANSFORMS

Some feature-translation algorithms, such as Fisher's Linear Discriminant (see chapter 8, in this volume), achieve optimum results when the input features have Gaussian distributions. Input features often are not natively Gaussian-distributed. For example, a feature defined as the magnitude of an FFT amplitude bin will likely not have a Gaussian or symmetric distribution since the lower range of the feature is bounded by zero and the upper range is unbounded. Moreover, the power of the EEG frequency spectrum is inversely proportional to frequency. In many cases unimodal non-Gaussian distributed features can be effectively shaped to be more Gaussian by applying a monotonically increasing nonlinear transformation. A monotonically increasing transformation guarantees that the transformed feature values will have the same ordering as the original values with different spacing between the values.

Although specialized transforms can be derived for shaping known feature distributions into more Gaussian distributions, the simple log-normal transform shown below has proved effective for transforming a variety of general unimodal distributions to be more Gaussian:

$$y = \log x$$

(7.15)

This transform is especially effective for EEG because it compensates for the decrease in power with increasing frequency and thus creates a more symmetric distribution.

FEATURE SMOOTHING

For some feature-extraction methods and applications, the resulting features may exhibit undesirable fluctuations over short periods. Although these may or may not be an artifact of the processing, they can potentially disrupt the feedback to the user that is a key aspect of BCI operation. Whatever their origins, these fluctuations can be suppressed by applying a simple median filter or low-pass filter that is based on the frequency of the fluctuations. Note that a causal low-pass filter will introduce some delay to the signal. This may result in some brain responses being followed by a transient rebound effect in the features that reflect the response. This rebound can be used to reinforce detection of the response, but it can also be suppressed with a properly designed digital filter.

PCA AND ICA

When the extracted features are highly correlated, principal component analysis (PCA) and independent component analysis (ICA) can be applied to decorrelate the features, and/or reduce the dimensionality of the feature vector. Effectively reducing the dimensionality of the feature vector can greatly simplify the training and effectiveness of the translation algorithm, particularly when few observations are available for training the translation algorithm (see chapter 8, in this volume). Use of PCA and ICA in the feature domain is identical to their use for the raw signal samples, except that for the feature domain, matrix X is comprised of feature observations rather than signal samples.

EXTRACTING FEATURES FROM SPIKE TRAINS

Up to this point we have focused on extracting features from continuously varying signals, such as those recorded by EEG, ECoG, and local field potentials (LFPs). Each of these signals (as well as, indirectly, those recorded by MEG, fMRI, fNIRS, and PET) is a complex reflection of the activity of *many* different synaptic and neuronal sources. At the same time, neurons communicate by producing discrete impulses (i.e., the *action potentials* or *spikes* described in chapter 2) at specific time instances. This neuronal activity produces a very different type of signal, the *spike train*, which reflects the activity of a *single neuron*. The final section of this chapter summarizes the feature-extraction methods commonly applied to spike trains.

By present understanding, the action potential (or neuronal spike) is the fundamental electrical event responsible for the transfer of information among neurons in the brain. In contrast to EEG, ECoG, or other continuously varying signals that reflect the activity of many neurons and synapses, each spike train reflects the activity of one particular neuron. Whenever the neuron's internal state and its concurrent synaptic inputs combine to achieve a specific voltage threshold, the neuron produces a spike. Thus, a spike train reveals very specific information: it tells when a specific neuron fires. At the same time, it reveals relatively little about what is going on in the network(s) to which that one neuron belongs. In contrast, EEG signals tell us about what large populations of neurons are

doing and yet little about specific neurons. Spike trains are *microscale* brain activity (see chapter 2, in this volume) and are recorded by microelectrodes within the brain (as are LFPs). In contrast, EEG recorded from the scalp and ECoG recorded on the brain surface are, respectively, *macroscale* and *mesoscale* (see chapter 3, in this volume) brain activity. The timing of the spike (i.e., when it occurs in time) is important and is usually measured with a resolution of 1 msec.

THE STRUCTURE OF SPIKE TRAINS

The key information in EEG, ECoG, or LFP activity is the continuous fluctuation of voltage over time. In contrast, the key information in spike trains is the time at which each spike occurs (see chapter 2, in this volume). In most spike-recording situations relevant to BCI applications, we assume that all the spikes produced by a given neuron are the same. Signals like this, that is, signals that carry information only in the time at which a discrete event occurs, are called *point processes* (Snyder 1975). Due to the great difference between continuous signals like EEG and those comprised of point processes like spike trains, the methods used to extract information from them differ. To discuss spike-train analysis, we start by introducing some terminology and the mathematical models of spike trains from which features are defined.

Because we assume that all spikes produced by a given neuron are identical, and that key information in a spike train resides in the timing of spikes, it is reasonable to model a spike train as a sequence of identical, instantaneous mathematical functions, each of which represents an individual spike. These functions are intended to represent the spike's timing information without regard to the spurious amplitude fluctuations that are common in actual spike recordings. Thus, a spike train can be mathematically modeled as a train of theoretical spikes termed *delta functions*, $s(t) = \sum_{i=1}^{n} \delta(t - t_i)$, where $\delta(t)$ is a delta function and intuitively has unit area only when $t = t_i$, and is zero otherwise. More precisely, the delta function extracts the value of any function at the time the argument of $\delta(t)$ is zero, or $x(t_i) = \int x(t)\delta(t - t_i)dt$ for arbitrary $x(t)$, where the limits of the integral are over the domain of $x(t)$ (McClellan et al. 2003). This is equivalent to the signal sampling process discussed in the *Sampling* section of this chapter, where $x(t)$ represents the signal. However, in this case, the delta functions are not used to sample a continuous analog signal; instead, they are used as a mathematical representation of a spike train.

Perhaps the most widely used feature of a spike train is the *firing rate*, which measures the number of events per unit time (Dayan and Abbott 2001). This property can be captured in different features. The *spike-count rate* is the number (n) of spikes in a given time interval T, or $V = n/T = 1/T \int s(t)dt$. If one substitutes the definition of the delta function in $s(t)$, one sees indeed that the value of the integral is just the number of spikes in $[0, T]$. The problem is that neurons tend to change their firing rate over time, so it is also necessary to calculate the time-dependent firing rate. However, we need a value of T large enough to give a reliable assessment of the rate; if the neuronal firing rate changes very fast compared with this value, it is difficult to obtain an accurate description of the change in rate. Thus, it is often necessary to compromise in choosing the parameters (e.g., the value of T) used to extract features related to firing rate.

The severity of the necessary compromise can be eased by acquiring more data. Let us assume that a researcher repeatedly stimulates the same neuron, collects the data for each stimulus, and then aligns the data with respect to the stimulus. In each trial, the spike-count average can be computed, perhaps with a $T_1 < T$, and then averaged over the trials. This is called the *trial average*, denoted here by $< r >$. With a sufficient number of trials, T_1 can be decreased to a rather small value (i.e., ΔT). Now we can define the firing rate as $r(t) = 1 / \Delta T \int_{t}^{t + \Delta T} < s(\tau) > d\tau$. This method of estimating the firing rate is called the *Peristimulus Time Histogram* (PSTH) (Dayan and Abbott 2001), and it provides better temporal resolution than the spike count rate over a given time window.

Looking closely at the definition of r, it is clear that it actually counts the number of spikes during a prespecified time interval. The advantage of focusing on the number of spikes per time window is that we now have integer numbers that resemble the continuous-amplitude time series of the EEG. The experimenter must select the time interval that makes sense for the experiment (e.g., it might vary from 10 to 100 msec), and this will constrain the time resolution of the analysis. In sum, extracting features from spike trains is not, after all, very different from extracting features from continuous signals. The same methods discussed in this chapter for continuous signals (e.g., autocorrelation functions, filters, FFTs, etc.) can also be applied to spike trains that have been binned into intervals. However, this approach does sacrifice the information contained in the exact times of individual spikes; if we believe that this information is important (e.g., for a BCI application), then we need to employ a different set of methods for extracting features from spike trains. We now look at some of these methods.

THE POISSON PROCESS

The simplest model for the timing of the individual spikes in a spike train is a *Poisson process* (Papoulis 1965). In a Poisson process, we define a time interval [0, T] and assume we have n points to place within the time interval. The question then is: what is the probability of getting k of these n points within a given sub-interval t_0 of [0, T]? This is clearly a random experiment governed by probability laws. Assuming that the placement of each point is independent of the placement of all the others, and that each point has a probability p of being placed in the interval ($p = t_0 / T$), and probability ($q = 1 - p$) of being placed outside this interval, the probability of k points falling in t_0 is the binomial distribution:

$$P\{k\} = \binom{n}{k} p^k q^{n-k}.$$

(7.15)

Using very large limits for n and a very small interval, we obtain:

$$P\{k\} = e^{-\lambda t_0} \frac{(\lambda t_0)^k}{k!}.$$

(7.16)

where $\lambda = n/T$. If the interval t_0 becomes infinitesimal and we are interested only in the probability that a single point lands in the infinitesimal interval t_0 (which becomes just a point t in the line), we can ignore the exponential and obtain $P\{k=1\} = \lambda$. λ is called the rate (or *intensity*), and it measures the density of points in a *macroscopic* interval.

To go from points in the line to spike trains, we define a random process as an index set of random variables over time. Specifically, let $z(t) = \sum_i \delta(t - t_i)$. If the values of t_i are random variables specified by the binomial distribution law given above in equation 7.15, this random process is called a *Poisson process*. What is interesting in the Poisson process is that both the mean and the autocorrelation function are completely specified by λ:

$$E\{z(t)\} = \lambda$$

(7.17)

$$R(t_1, t_2) = \lambda^2 + \lambda \delta(t_1 - t_2)$$

(7.18)

If we idealize a spike as a delta function, and assume that spikes occur randomly according to the statistics described above, then the spike train becomes a realization of a Poisson process.

Another consequence of the descriptive power of λ is that we can ignore where the actual spikes are and just describe spike trains more roughly, but also more compactly, by their intensity value λ. This gives rise to the two major types of processing methods for spike trains (Sanchez and Principe 2007): the timing methods in which the actual spike times matter; and the rate methods in which just the λ matters. In general, λ may also be a function of time [i.e., $\lambda(t)$], which makes the process an inhomogeneous Poisson process (Dayan and Abbott 2001).

EXTRACTING FEATURES FROM SPIKE TIMES

SINGLE-CHANNEL SPIKE TRAINS

The first step in analyzing spike trains is to describe them by the firing rate (also called the *intensity* or *rate function*). In order to apply Poisson-process models, two important decisions must be made: the size of the time window (or interval), and how to smooth the integer values over time. There are four basic methods to estimate the intensity function: windows (binning); kernels; nonparametric regression; and a newly introduced reproducing-kernel Hilbert space method (Paiva et al. 2009). The first two of these are discussed here; the last two are more complex and will not be addressed here (see Paiva et al. 2009 for their description).

For simple *binning*, the firing rate over each time interval is estimated to be constant with a value proportional to the number of spikes within the interval. A more elaborate estimate can be achieved by using a *kernel* or *kernel function*, which is simply a mathematical function that is centered on each spike. The amplitudes of the overlapping kernel functions in a spike train are then summed to estimate the intensity function. Figure 7.11 shows an example of a spike train (A) and its reconstruction using rectangular windows (B), a Gaussian

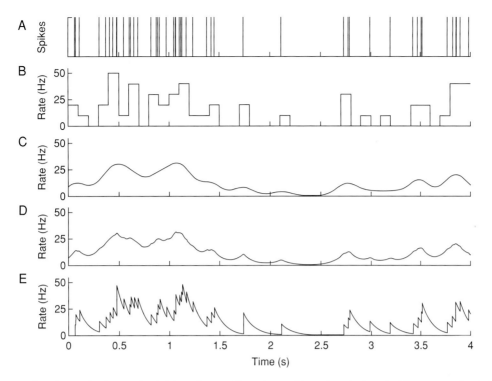

Figure 7.11 *Reconstruction of a spike train by three methods: (A) a spike train; (B) resolution of the spike train shown in A by a rectangular window; (C) resolution by Gaussian kernels; (D) resolution by Laplacian kernels; (E) resolution by an exponential function.*

kernel (C), a Laplacian kernel (D), and an exponential function (E). These are expressed, respectively, as:

Rectangular
$$\kappa_R(x) = \begin{cases} 1 & |x| < a \\ 0 & |x| \geq a \end{cases}$$
(7.19)

Gaussian
$$\kappa_G(x) = \exp\left(\frac{-x^2}{2\sigma^2}\right)$$
(7.20)

Laplacian
$$\kappa_L(x) = \exp\left(\frac{-|x|}{\tau}\right)$$
(7.21)

Exponential
$$\kappa_E(x) = \exp\left(\frac{-x}{\tau}\right)u(x)$$
(7.22)

The firing rate at each point in time can be estimated from the graphs in figure 7.11, but it is important to remember that there is an intrinsic limitation to the resolution in all reconstructions due to the binning (i.e., the window length or, in exponential functions, the denominator, called the *kernel bandwidth*).

In analyzing spike trains from sensory cortex, characterizing the cause of the spike is often important; in this case the *spike-triggered average* (STA) is used. In contrast, in analyzing spike trains from motor cortex, describing the consequences of a spike is frequently the objective; in this case, the *tuning curve* (see chapter 2) is used (this is sometimes useful for sensori-cortex neurons as well).

Spike-Triggered Average

The STA estimates the mean value of a stimulus over the time before a spike occurs. Several stimuli are presented, and they are aligned with the occurrence of the spike. This is expressed as:

$$S_A(\tau) = \left\langle \frac{1}{n}\sum_{i=1}^{n} x(t_i - \tau) \right\rangle$$
(7.23)

where the spike is assumed to occur at t_i and $x(t)$ is the input stimulus (Dayan and Abbott 2001). The STA can reveal the stimulus waveform that tends to precede the generation of the action potential and can indicate the length of the stimulus history that is relevant.

Tuning Curves

It is sometimes important to characterize neural response when some property of the stimulus changes (e.g., in visual cortex, during the observation of the rotation of a bright line). If the neuron is processing information from the stimulus, its firing rate will change when the stimulus changes. One can therefore count the number of spikes during the presentation of the stimulus at each angle and then create a curve as a function of the parameter (angle in this case) (Georgopoulos et al. 1986). The Gaussian tuning curve can be constructed as:

$$T(\theta) = r_{max}\exp\left(-1/2\left(\frac{\theta - \theta_{max}}{\sigma}\right)^2\right)$$
(7.24)

where r_{max} is the largest firing rate observed θ_{max}, is the maximal angle used (normally negative and positive), and σ is the width of the Gaussian (T is measured in Hz).

A very similar strategy can be used for motor control, but in this case, the external consequences of spike firing are of interest. For example, the experimental subject might be engaged in reaching a target in a center-out task (normally with the hand) to different points arranged in a circle. The neuronal firing rate is estimated for each one of the directions in the circle using the relationship:

$$T(\theta) = \left| r_0 + (r_{max} - r_0)\cos(\theta - \theta_{max}) \right|$$

(7.25)

where r_0 is the mean firing rate. The absolute value is used here to preserve the interpretation of firing rate even when $T(\theta)$, measured in Hz, is negative.

The metric for evaluating the tuning property of a neuron is called the *tuning depth*, defined as the difference between the maximum and minimum values in the neural tuning curve $T(\theta)$, normalized by the standard deviation of the firing rate, std(r) (Paiva et al. 2009).

$$tuning\ depth = \frac{r_{max} - r_{min}}{std(r)}$$

(7.26)

The tuning depth is normalized between 0 and 1 for uniformity. However, the normalization loses the relative scale between the tuning depth of different neurons when it is necessary to compare different neurons with different rates. Figure 7.12 shows the tuning depth of two motor cortex neurons.

The tuning curve is the basis of the *population vector algorithm* proposed by Georgopoulos et al. (1986) (see chapter 2, this volume) to show that motor-cortex neurons are sensitive to all the possible directions in space. The population vector algorithm can therefore be used as a generative model for BCIs since the movement direction can be predicted from the preferred direction vectors of all neurons active at each time step, with the active neurons appropriately weighted according

to each neuron's tuning curve. The BCIs reported by Taylor et al. (2002) and Velliste et al. (2008) were based on this idea. The basic algorithm was further improved using a state model within a Bayesian formulation (Schwartz et al. 2001; Wu et al. 2006; Brockwell et al. 2004).

PAIRWISE SPIKE-TRAIN ANALYSIS
Features Reflecting Similarity between Spike Trains

It is sometimes relevant to quantify the similarity between two spike trains. This is analogous to the comparison between two continuous signals using cross-correlation (Eliasmith and Anderson 2003). The problem is that spikes are delta functions, so the cross multiplication most probably yields zero unless spikes occur at precisely the same time in each train (i.e., they overlap). This difficulty can be avoided if a kernel is applied to the spikes; use of a kernel essentially applies a linear filter to the spike train. The most commonly used kernel is the exponential kernel, $h(t)=\exp(-t/\tau)u(t)$, where $u(t)$ is the Heaviside function (zero for negative time, 1 for positive time) and τ controls the decay rate of the exponential. Other functions can be used, but this decaying exponential is a good example that allows for on-line operation because it is causal.

The spike train $s_i(t) = \sum_{m=1}^{N_i} \delta(t - t_m^i)$ is filtered by $h(t)$ to yield $y_i(t) = \sum_{m=1}^{N_i} h(t - t_m^i)$. We select a second spike train $s_j(t)$ and filter it by the same filter to obtain $y_j(t) = \sum_{m=1}^{N_j} h(t - t_m^j)$ where the spike times t_j (and possibly the number of spikes N_j) are different. The cross-correlation between the two spike trains $y_i(t)$ and $y_j(t)$ is defined (Dayan and Abbott 2001) as:

$$C_{i,j}(\tau) = \int y_i(t) y_j(t - \tau) dt$$

(7.27)

This cross-correlation function is obtained by shifting one of the filtered spike trains in time. It measures the similarity between the two spike trains at different time shifts (i.e., different *lags*). The time of the $C_{i,j}(\tau)$ peak shows the lag at which the two spike trains are most similar.

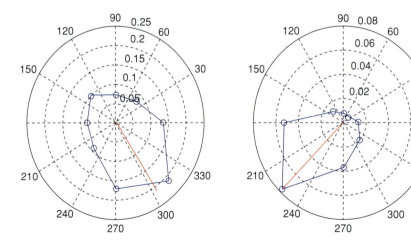

Figure 7.12 The tuning curves for two motor-cortex neurons (at left and right). The tuning curve for each neuron is shown in blue. Each point in each tuning curve is estimated in 45° sectors centered at the point. The tuning curves display the sensitivity of the neuron to movement in each direction of the space. In this example, measured with respect to the subject position, the left neuron is tuned to movement segments at 300°, and the right neuron to movement segments at 230°. The red line in each plot represents that neuron's preferred direction (see chapter 2). (Data from Principe laboratory.)

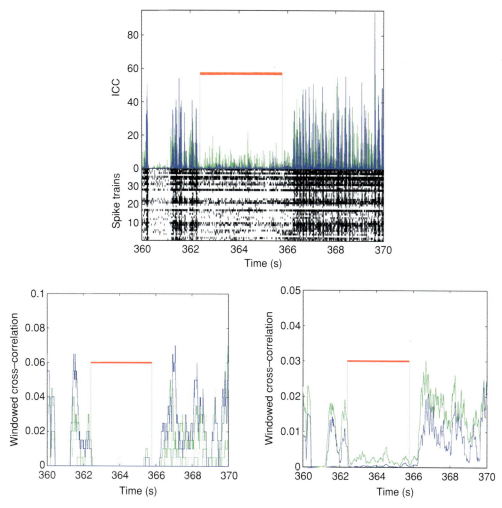

Figure 7.13 Comparison of kernel cross-correlation and the normal windowed cross-correlation functions. (Top) Kernel cross-correlation intraclass correlation coefficient (ICC) and the spike trains (i.e., raster plots) of 34 motor-cortex neurons. (Bottom) Standard windowed cross-correlation functions for two different strategies. (Bottom left) A 200-msec sliding window with 1-msec increment for one pair of neurons. (Bottom right) Same as the cross-correlation with kernels but spatially averaged across channel pairs. The data were collected from rat motor cortex (blue is right cortex, green is left cortex). The red segment represents the time period during which the animal is pressing the lever. The kernel cross-correlation (Top) shows both high- and low-frequency variations, but the high-frequency variation is much less evident in the conventional cross-correlations (Bottom). (Data from Principe laboratory.)

Figure 7.13 compares the results of applying a kernel cross-correlation (top panel) and normal windowed cross-correlation functions (bottom panels) to microelectrode-array data collected from the motor cortex of a rodent during a lever-press task. Thirty-four neurons were used for this analysis. In the top panel, pairwise correlations were computed using equation 7.27 where $h(t)$ is a first-order low-pass filter with a $t = 1$ msec time constant; these were averaged over all pairs of neurons for the same lever press. The figure shows that the similarity among the neural firings is lost during lever pressing (indicated by the red bar), and increases back to its baseline after the lever press. Figure 7.13 (bottom) presents the results for the cross-correlation at zero lag using the rate method discussed in this chapter's section *The Structure of Spike Trains*. The data are based on a sliding window of 200 msec, over spikes binned with a 1-msec rectangular window, on a selected pair of channels (visually judged to have high correlation with the lever-pressing task) (fig. 7.13, bottom left), as well as averaged over all neurons (fig. 7.13, bottom right). As expected,

much of the temporal resolution in the fine structure of the spike firing is lost (e.g., the high-frequency changes in spike activity) with this analysis, but it is nevertheless clear that spike-train correlations decrease markedly during lever press.

As a special case, we can perform the same operation on a single filtered spike train to calculate its autocorrelation:

$$C_{i,i}(\tau) = \int y_i(t) y_i(t - \tau) dt$$

(7.28)

This autocorrelation function measures the similarity in the structure of the spike train over different time lags. It is very useful in detecting periodicities in spike trains.

Features Reflecting Differences between Spike Trains

It is sometimes important to measure *dissimilarity* among spike trains. Dissimilarity is important in using firing patterns to distinguish among different classes of neurons. The actual number of different classes of neurons is often not known, which makes it impractical to try to classify spike trains into different classes. Nevertheless, *clustering* can still explore the structure of the responses.

Clustering is the division of the data into subgroups such that the elements of a subgroup are more similar among themselves than they are to the other members of the dataset. The definition of a proper dissimilarity metric (called here a *distance* for simplicity) is critical for accurate clustering. The most widely used spike-train distances are:

- the van Rossum distance (van Rossum 2001)
- the Cauchy-Schwarz distance (Paiva et al. 2009)
- the Victor-Purpura distance (Victor and Purpura 1997)

The *van Rossum distance* extends to spike trains the concept of Euclidean distance. Thus, it maps a full spike train to a point. The distance between two spike trains S_i and S_j is defined as:

$$d_{vR}(S_i, S_j) = \frac{1}{\tau} \int \left(y_i(t) - y_j(t)^2 \right) dt$$

(7.29)

Thus, small distances are obtained when the spike-train time structures are similar.

The *Cauchy-Schwarz (CS) distance* metric is the inner product distance between pairs of vectors (the cosine of the angle between the vectors). This metric can be generalized using the Cauchy-Schwarz inequality, yielding

$$d_{CS}(g_i, g_j) = -\log \frac{\vec{g}_i \cdot \vec{g}_j}{\|\vec{g}_i\| \|\vec{g}_j\|}$$

(7.30)

where g_i and g_j are vectors representing two spike trains. To apply this equation to spikes, one normally applies to spike-time differences a filter with an impulse response that is a Gaussian function, to obtain:

$$d_{CS}(S_i, S_j) = -\log \frac{\sum_{m=1}^{N_i} \sum_{n=1}^{N_j} \exp\left[\frac{-(t_m^i - t_n^j)^2}{2\sigma^2} \right]}{\sqrt{\left(\sum_{m=1}^{N_i} \sum_{m=1}^{N_i} \exp\left[\frac{-(t_m^i - t_m^i)^2}{2\sigma^2} \right] \right) \left(\sum_{n=1}^{N_j} \sum_{n=1}^{N_j} \exp\left[\frac{-(t_n^j - t_n^j)^2}{2\sigma^2} \right] \right)}}$$

(7.31)

The *Victor-Purpura distance* evaluates the minimum cost of transforming one spike train into the other by using three basic operations: spike insertion, spike deletion, and spike movement. This approach operates on the spike trains without the filter. To implement this, let us define the cost of moving a spike at t_m to t_n as $q|t_m - t_n|$, where q is a parameter that sets the time scale of the analysis, and is chosen such that at the end we will get a distance measure (i.e., a metric that obeys the property of distances). The cost of deleting or inserting a spike is set to one. Let us define

$$K_q(t_m^i, t_n^j) = \min\{q | t_m^i - t_n^j |, 2\} = \begin{cases} q | t_m^i - t_n^j | & | t_m^i - t_n^j | < 2/q \\ 2 & otherwise \end{cases}$$

(7.32)

The Victor Purpura distance between spike trains S_i and S_j is defined as

$$d_{VP}(S_i, S_j) = \min_{C(S_i \leftrightarrow S_j)} \sum_l K(t_{C_i[l]}^i, t_{C_j[l]}^j)$$

(7.33)

where the minimization is between the set of all unitary operations $c[l]$ that transform S_i into S_j.

SUMMARY

Signals recorded from the brain typically contain substantial noise and extraneous information that often interfere with detecting and measuring those features of the signals that are useful for BCI applications, that is, that reflect the intent of the user. Thus, before the signals can be translated into outputs, the useful features of the signals must be extracted and presented to the translation algorithm in an appropriate format. This chapter reviews the full range of the standard methods used to extract features from brain signals. These include methods appropriate for continuous signals such as EEG (e.g., spatial and temporal filtering, template matching, spectral analysis) as well as methods appropriate for signals reflecting point processes such as single-neuron activity (e.g., firing rate, spike-triggered averaging, tuning curves, measures of spike-train similarity or dissimilarity). In general, the most desirable methods are those that are theoretically motivated and biologically realistic and that have been found to perform well in actual real-time BCI applications. For successful BCI operation, feature extraction must be followed by a translation algorithm that is appropriate to the features extracted, to the application, and to the user. Translation algorithms will be the subject of the next chapter.

REFERENCES

Anderson CW, Stolz EA, and Shamsunder S. 1990 Multivariate autoregressive models for classification of spontaneous electroencephalographic signals during mental tasks. *IEEE Trans. Biomed. Eng.* 45 277–286.

Bashashati A, Fatourechi M, Ward RK, and Birch GE. 2007 A survey of signal processing algorithms in brain–computer interfaces based on electrical brain signals. *J. Neural Eng.* 4 (2) R32–R57.

Blankertz B, Müller KR, Krusienski DJ, Schalk G, Wolpaw JR, Schlogl A, Pfurtscheller G, Millán JR, Schroder M, and Birbaumer N. 2006 The BCI competition: III. Validating alternative approaches to actual BCI problems. *IEEE Trans. Neural Syst. Rehabil. Eng.* 14 153–159

Bostanov V 2004 BCI competition 2003–data sets Ib and IIb: feature extraction from event-related brain potentials with the continuous wavelet transform and the t-value scalogram *IEEE Trans. Biomed. Eng.* 51 1057–1061.

Brockwell AE, Rojas AL, and Kass RE. 2004 Recursive Bayesian decoding of motor cortical signals by particle filtering. *J. Neurophysiol.* 91 1899–1907.

Brunner C, Scherer R, Graimann B, Supp G, Pfurtscheller G. 2006 Online control of a brain–computer interface using phase synchronization. *IEEE Trans. Biomed. Eng.* 53 (12) 2501–2506.

Burke DP, Kelly SP, de Chazal P, Reilly RB, and Finucane C. 2005 A parametric feature extraction and classification strategy for brain–computer interfacing, *IEEE Trans. Neural Syst. Rehabil. Eng.* 13 12–17.

Dayan P, and Abbott L. 2001 *Theoretical Neuroscience*, Cambridge, MA: MIT Press.

Dien J, Spencer K, and Donchin E. 2003 Localization of the event related potential novelty response as defined by principal components analysis. *Cognit. Brain Res.* 17 637–650.

Dornhege G, Blankertz B, Krauledat M, Losch F, Curio GK, and Müller KR. 2006 Combined optimization of spatial and temporal filters for improving brain-computer interfacing. *IEEE Trans. Biomed. Eng.* 53 (11) 2274–2281.

Eliasmith C, and Anderson C. 2003 *Neural Engineering*, Cambridge, MA: MIT Press.

Farwell LA, and Donchin E. 1988 Talking off the top of your head: Towards a mental prosthesis utilizing event-related brain potentials. *Electroencephalogr. Clin. Neurophysiol. 80* 510–523.

Freeman W. 1975 *Mass Activation in the Nervous System*, Englewood Cliffs, NJ: Prentice Hall.

Garrett D, Peterson DA, Anderson CW, and Thaut MH. 2003 Comparison of linear, nonlinear, and feature selection methods for EEG signal *IEEE Trans. Neural Syst. Rehabil. Eng. 11* 141–144.

Georgopoulos A., A. Schwartz, R. Kettner, 1986 Neural population coding of movement direction, *Science 233* 1416–1419.

Goncharova II, McFarland DJ, Vaughan TM, and Wolpaw JR. 2003 EMG contamination of EEG: spectral and topographical characteristics *Clin. Neurophysiol. 114* 1580–1593.

Graimann B, Huggins JE, Levine SP, and Pfurtscheller G. 2004 Toward a direct brain interface based on human subdural recordings and wavelet-packet analysis. *IEEE Trans. Biomed. Eng. 51* 954–962.

Gysels E, and Celka P. 2004 Phase synchronization for the recognition of mental tasks in a brain–computer interface. *IEEE Trans. Neural Syst. Rehabil. Eng. 12* 406–415.

Hayes MH, 1996 *Statistical Digital Signal Processing and Modeling*. New York: John Wiley & Sons.

Hyvärinen A. 1999 Survey on independent component analysis. *Neural Comput. Surv. 2* 94–128.

Kelly SP, Lalor EC, Finucane C, McDarby G, and Reilly RB 2005 Visual spatial attention control in an independent brain–computer interface. *IEEE Trans. Biomed. Eng. 52* 1588–1596.

Krusienski DJ, Schalk G, McFarland DJ, and Wolpaw JR, 2007 A mu-rhythm matched filter for continuous control of a brain-computer interface. *IEEE Trans. Biomed. Eng. 54* 273–280.

Lemm S, Blankertz B, Curio G, and Müller KR. 2005 Spatio-spectral filters for improving the classification of single trial EEG. *IEEE Trans. Biomed. Eng. 52* 1541–1548.

Lyons RG. 2004 *Understanding Digital Signal Processing*, Englewood Cliffs, NJ: Prentice Hall.

Makeig S, Enghoff S, Jung T-P, and Sejnowski TJ. 2000 A natural basis for efficient brain-actuated control. *IEEE Trans. Rehabil. Eng. 8* 208–211.

Mallat, SG. 2008 *A Wavelet Tour of Signal Processing*. Orlando, FL: Academic Press.

McClellan J, Schafer R, and Yoder M. 2003 *Signal Processing First*. Upper Saddle River, NJ: Pearson.

McFarland DJ, Anderson CW, Müller KR, Schlogl A, and Krusienski DJ. 2006 BCI meeting 2005—Workshop on BCI signal processing: feature extraction and translation. *IEEE Trans. Neural Syst. Rehabil. Eng. 14* 135–138.

McFarland DJ, McCane LM, David SV, and Wolpaw JR. 1997 Spatial filter selection for EEG-based communication *Electroencephalogr. Clin. Neurophysiol. 103* 386–394.

McFarland DJ, and Wolpaw JR. 2008 Sensorimotor rhythm-based brain–computer interface (BCI): Model order selection for autoregressive spectral analysis. *J. Neural Eng. 5* 155–162.

Müller-Gerking J, Pfurtscheller G, and Flyvbjerg H, 1999 Designing optimal spatial filters for single-trial EEG classification in a movement task. *Clin. Neurophysiol. 110* (5) 787–798.

Paiva A, Park I, and Principe J. 2009 A spike train framework for spike train signal processing, *Neural Comput. 21* (3) 424–449.

Papoulis A. 1965 *Probability, Random Variables and Stochastic Processes*. New York: McGraw-Hill.

Pfurtscheller G, Neuper C, Schlogl A, and Lugger K. 1998 Separability of EEG signals recorded during right and left motor imagery using adaptive autoregressive parameters. *IEEE Trans. Rehabil. Eng. 6* 316–325.

Pregenzer M, and Pfurtscheller G. 1999 Frequency component selection for an EEG-based brain to computer interface. *IEEE Trans. Rehabil. Eng. 7* 413–419.

Proakis JG, and Manolakis DG, 2007 *Digital Signal Processing—Principles, Algorithms and Applications*. New York: Macmillan.

Qin L, and He B. 2005 A wavelet-based time-frequency analysis approach for classification of motor imagery for brain–computer interface applications. *J. Neural Eng. 2* 65–72.

Rieke F, Warland D, van Steveninick RdR, and Bialek W. 1997 *Spikes: Exploring the Neural Code*. Cambridge, MA: MIT Press.

Sanchez J, and Principe J. 2007 *Brain Machine Interface Engineering*. San Rafael, CA: Morgan & Claypool.

Schwartz AB, Taylor DM, and Tillery SIH. 2001 Extraction algorithms for cortical control of arm prosthetics. *Curr. Opin. Neurobiol. 11* (6) 701–708.

Serby H, Yom-Tov E, and Inbar GF 2005 An improved P300-based brain–computer interface. *IEEE Trans. Neural Syst. Rehabil. Eng. 13* 89–98.

Snyder DL. 1975 *Random Point Process in Time and Space*. New York: John Wiley & Sons.

Taylor DM, Tillery SIH, and Schwartz AB. 2002 Direct cortical control of 3D neuroprosthetic devices. *Science 296* 1829–1832.

van Rossum MCW. 2001 A novel spike distance. *Neural Comp. 13* (4) 751–764.

Velliste M, Perel S, Chance Spalding M, Whitford AS, and Schwartz AB, 2008 Cortical control of a prosthetic arm for self-feeding, *Nature 453* 1098–1101.

Victor JD, and Purpura KP. 1997 Metric-space analysis of spike trains: Theory, algorithms, & application. *Network: Comp. Neural Syst. 8* 127–164.

Wang Y, Príncipe J, Paiva A, and Sanchez J. 2009 Sequential Monte Carlo estimation of point processes on kinematics from neural spiking activity for brain machine interfaces. *Neural Comput. 21* (10) 2894–2930.

Wei Q, Wang Y, Gao X, and Gao S, 2007 Amplitude and phase coupling measures for feature extraction in an EEG-based brain-computer interface. *J. Neural Eng. 4* 120–129.

Wolpaw JR, and McFarland DJ. 1994 Multichannel EEG-based brain–computer communication. *Electroencephalogr. Clin. Neurophysiol. 90* 444–449.

Wolpaw JR, and McFarland DJ. 2004 Control of a two-dimensional movement signal by a noninvasive brain–computer interface in humans. *Proc. Natl Acad. Sci. USA. 101* 17849–17854.

Wu W, Gao Y, Bienenstock E, Donoghue JP, and Black MJ. 2006 Bayesian population decoding of motor cortical activity using a Kalman filter. *Neural Comput. 18* 80–118.

8 | BCI SIGNAL PROCESSING: FEATURE TRANSLATION

DENNIS J. McFARLAND AND DEAN J. KRUSIENSKI

The preceding chapter of this volume describes common methods for extracting features from brain signals for BCIs. Ideally, these features would be in a form that could directly communicate the user's intent. However, because the features represent indirect measurements of the user's intent, they must be *translated* into appropriate device commands that convey that intent. This is accomplished using a *translation algorithm*. The core of a translation algorithm is a *model*, which is a mathematical procedure typically comprised of a mathematical equation, set of equations, and/or mapping mechanism such as a lookup table. The model accepts the feature vector (i.e., the set of features) at a given time instant as its input and processes the feature vector to output a set of commands that the application device can recognize. For instance, an amplitude in a specific electroencephalographic (EEG) frequency band might be translated into a binary 0 or 1 that produces an "off" or "on" command, respectively, for a light switch. A more complex application might require that a set of features be translated into three-dimensional spatial coordinates that are used to update the position of a robotic arm.

The data used to develop a model may be just a few observations of a few features or many observations of many features. In either case the goal of the model is to describe the relationship between these features and the user's intent in a form that is simpler than the data that are actually measured. The value of such a description is that it can be used to convert future observations to appropriate output (i.e., it can be *generalized* to new data). For example, the relationship between two variables, X and Y, can be described by a simple linear function:

$$Y = bX + a \qquad (8.1)$$

where b is the slope of the linear function and a is the intercept on the y-axis. If this equation is used as a model for a BCI, X is the feature vector (e.g., EEG features extracted by methods such as those described in chapter 7) and Y is the vector of commands sent to an output device (e.g., movements of a cursor). As discussed later in this chapter, the values of b and a are parameters of the model that can be defined by a variety of different methods.

The relationship between X and Y defined by the model is usually not a perfect description of the relationship between the actual values of the features and the output commands

intended by the BCI user. Nevertheless, a model such as a simple linear equation may often provide a very good description of the relationship. If there are many observations, then the model provides a much more compact representation of the data than a simple enumeration of the original data. This may come at the expense of a certain degree of accuracy in the values of Y. Most important for BCI systems, the model allows generalization from past observations to future observations. Given a new observation of X (e.g., an EEG feature vector), the model provides a prediction of Y (e.g., the three-dimensional robotic arm movement intended by the user).

Because a model essentially comprises one or more equations, the individual features of the feature vector can be considered to be the independent variables of the equations. The dependent variable(s) of the equation(s) are the command(s) that are transmitted to the output device. Models often include initially undefined constants that act on the features such as scaling factors, exponential terms, summation bounds, and data window lengths (e.g., b and a in eq. 8.1). These constants are referred to as the *model parameters*. For simple linear models, which are often simply the sum of scaled features and a constant, the scale factors (i.e., the parameters that the features are multiplied by) are often referred to as *feature weights* or *coefficients*. Certain models, such as artificial neural networks, do not model feature extraction and translation as distinct, cascaded stages. Instead, these types of models may accept the raw EEG data as input, and then output the corresponding device commands without producing an intermediate, explicit feature-extraction stage.

The model parameters are commonly selected, or *trained* (also referred to as *learned* or *parameterized*) by using a set of training data. Each unit of training data (i.e., each observation) consists of a *feature vector* (or *training sample*) and its correct (i.e., intended) output (or *training label*). Through an iterative procedure, called *supervised learning*, the parameters are repeatedly adjusted until the model translates the feature vectors into output commands that are as accurate as possible (i.e., as close as possible to the correct output commands).

The accuracy of the model is evaluated with an *objective function* (also called a *cost function* or a *fitness function*). For instance, a common objective function is the mean-squared error (i.e., difference) between the model output and the correct output: the smaller this error, the more accurate the model. During the supervised learning process, the feature vectors (i.e., the training samples) are processed by the model with some initial parameters (selected randomly or using a priori information), the objective function then compares the model outputs to the correct outputs (i.e., the training labels), and the model parameters are then updated based on the objective function; finally, the process is repeated until stopping criteria are satisfied (e.g., the mean-squared error is minimized).

The fact that BCIs operate in real time places demands on the modeling of BCI data that are not typical of many other areas of neuroscience research. It is not sufficient to develop through post-hoc analysis a model that applies well to a given body of previously acquired data. Instead, the crucial requirement is that the model must apply to new data as well, that is, it must *generalize*. Its ability to generalize is tested (or *validated*) using an independent set of observations called *testing data*. Each unit of testing data (i.e., each observation) consists of a feature vector (i.e, *testing sample*) and its correct (i.e., intended) output (or *testing label*). Testing data are used to validate the model after its parameters have been fixed via training. In this validation, the testing data are processed by the model, and the model outputs are compared to the corresponding testing labels by using the same objective function employed for model training or some other measure of model accuracy. This model validation process is essential for evaluating how well a given model generalizes to new observations. However, some models and training procedures are prone to *overfitting*, in which the parameterized model is tuned so precisely to the training data that subtle differences between the training data and the test data prevent it from modeling the testing data accurately.

This chapter discusses the kinds of translation algorithms most frequently used in BCIs. It is meant to serve as a balanced introduction to the range of algorithms applicable to BCIs. Most algorithms in the BCI literature are based on, or closely related to, the algorithms presented in this chapter. Like the previous chapter, this chapter assumes that the reader has college-level linear algebra and calculus, minimal signal processing or machine-learning background, and basic knowledge gained from previous chapters.

The chapter is divided into four sections. The first section considers the factors important in selecting a model and provides an overview of the models used in BCI translation algorithms. As noted above, *the model is the core component of any translation algorithm*. The second and third sections discuss the two other components of a translation algorithm: selection of the features included in the model, and parameterization of the model. The final section describes methods for evaluating translation algorithms.

SELECTING A MODEL

Selecting an appropriate model is the key to developing a successful translation algorithm. Assuming that the input features contain the relevant information regarding the user's intent, the chosen model will determine how quickly and accurately

that intent is conveyed to the BCI output device (i.e., the application device). The processes of model selection and parameterization involve decisions based on the requirements of the BCI application as well as the nature and amount of data available for model development and optimization. For example, some applications only require a binary choice, whereas others require continuous highly accurate control in several dimensions. Simple models suitable for binary choice may not be able to provide accurate complex output commands. On the other hand, complex models that can provide such commands may encounter difficulty in generalizing well to new data.

A wide variety of models are available for use in BCI translation algorithms (McFarland, Anderson et al., 2006; Lotte et al., 2007; Principe and McFarland, 2008), and the list continues to increase. Indeed, the universe of possible models is infinite (Kieseppa, 2001). We focus in this chapter on simple representative examples of commonly used models, we illustrate how they work, and we consider the factors important in selecting and using them.

GENERAL PRINCIPLES

DISCRIMINANT MODELS AND REGRESSION MODELS

Models fall into two classes according to whether their outputs are *discrete* categories or *continuous* dimensions. Specifically, models are either *discriminant functions* (also called *classification functions*) or *regression functions* (McFarland and Wolpaw, 2005). Examples of simple discriminant and regression functions are illustrated in figure 8.1. A discriminant function translates the observations (i.e., the feature vectors) into discrete categories of output (e.g., specific letters). A regression function translates the observations into a continuous variable (e.g., cursor movement). For the two-target (i.e., two possible outputs) case illustrated in figure 8.1, both kinds of models require that a single function be parameterized. However, for the five-target case (i.e., with five possible outputs), the discriminant model requires that four functions be parameterized, while the regression model still requires that only a single function be parameterized. Discriminant functions are particularly useful in BCIs that produce simple "yes/no" or "target/nontarget" outputs (e.g., P300-based BCIs [Donchin et al., 2000; see chapter 12, in this volume]), whereas regression functions are well suited for BCIs that must provide continuously graded outputs in one or more dimensions (e.g., BCIs that produce cursor movements in two dimensions [Wolpaw and McFarland, 2004; see chapter 13, in this volume]).

For simplicity, the examples used in this section are discriminant functions (i.e., they have discrete, categorical outputs). Nevertheless, it is important to note that all the model types discussed here can also serve as regression functions that provide continuous outputs.

VARIATIONS IN THE DATA

As described above, model parameters are normally based on a body of previous observations (i.e., training data). This method assumes that future data will be similar to the training data and thus that the parameterized model will continue to

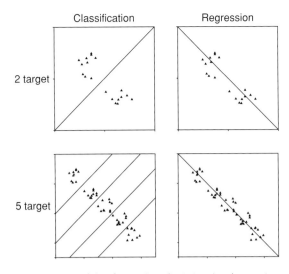

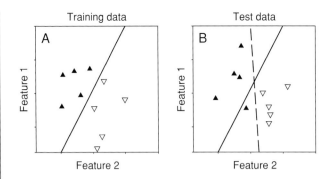

Figure 8.1 Comparison of classification (i.e., discriminant) and regression models. The diagonal lines are specific functions. For the two-target (i.e., two possible outputs) case, both models require only one function to separate the different outputs. However, for the five-target case (i.e., five possible outputs), the classification model requires four functions, whereas the regression approach still requires only a single function.

Figure 8.2 A simple linear discriminant (i.e., classifier) applied to training (A) and test (B) data sets. The feature vector has two features, and the discriminant function has two possible outputs (e.g., yes and no), represented by upward-pointing solid triangles and downward-pointing open triangles, respectively. (The features were produced by combining the output of a random-number generator with a constant that differed for the two outputs.) (A) The discriminant function based on the training data (solid line) perfectly classifies the training data. (B) The discriminant function based on the training data (solid line) does a good but not perfect job of classifying the test data. A discriminant function based on the test data (dashed line) does a perfect job, but because it is derived by post-hoc analysis, it could not have been used in actual online BCI operation.

work well (i.e., that it will generalize to new observations). However, biological data in general, and brain signals especially, normally display considerable apparently spontaneous (or chance) variation over time. Such chance variation is a problem for all models, particularly those used in BCIs, which must operate effectively using new data.

Figure 8.2 illustrates the problem with an example of a simple discriminant model (known as *Fisher's linear discriminant* [Fisher, 1936]) that uses two features and produces two possible outputs, represented by upward-pointing solid triangles and downward-pointing open triangles, respectively. The data (i.e., the observations) and the discriminant model are plotted in feature space. Figure 8.2A shows a small training data set of ten observations and a discriminant model that has been parameterized from the training data using a least-squares objective function (see below). The model works perfectly on the training data; it translates every observation into its correct output. Figure 8.2B shows this same model applied to a new test data set. In this case it performs well but not perfectly: one of the ten new observations is not correctly translated. The model might be reparameterized with these new observations (i.e., the dashed line), but it would be likely to again encounter a decrease in performance when applied to a newer set of test data. This example illustrates the fact that there is usually some drop in performance when a parameterized model is applied, or generalized, to new data. Nevertheless, successful model generalization is a crucial requirement for BCIs, since their online operation must always use new data.

The problem of chance variation may be reduced by using large sets of training data (in contrast to the very small set used in figure 8.2). The generalizability of models tends to increase as the number of observations in the training data set increases. At the same time, although models with more parameters (i.e., degrees of freedom) often provide a closer fit

to the training data, generalizability tends to decrease as the number of parameters in the model increases. Hence the choice of the number of parameters to include in the model often involves a trade-off between minimizing the model's error and maximizing its generalizability. Thus, the amount of training data available is an important factor in determining a model's complexity.

Another problem arises when the statistics of the data change over time. The data can be described by simple statistics, such as the average values (i.e., means) and variabilities of each feature. Feature variability is usually measured as *variance*, which is the average value of the square of the difference between each sample (i.e., observation) of the feature and the mean value of the feature. The data can also be described in terms of the relationships among the different features (e.g., the linear relationship or *covariance* between two features). One or more of these measures may change during BCI operation. Changes may occur as the user tires over the course of a day, as he or she acquires BCI experience and adopts new strategies, as a disease such as ALS progresses, or for a variety of other reasons. When such changes in the data statistics occur, the data are said to be *nonstationary*.

Figure 8.3 illustrates the impact of nonstationarity. As figure 8.3A shows, a parameterized model works very well with its training data. However, as figure 8.3B shows, it does not work well with a set of test data because the means and covariances of the data have changed. No amount of data in the original training set could have resulted in good generalizability since the statistics of the data have changed. Rather, it is necessary to have a translation algorithm that evolves, or *adapts*, as the data change. Given changing statistics, it is desirable to use adaptive algorithms. Although adaptation to changes in the mean of the data is relatively easy to accomplish, adaptation to changes in data covariances is more difficult.

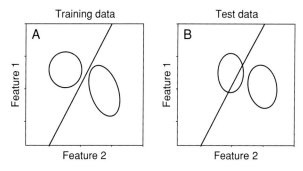

Training data   Test data

Feature 1 ← A   Feature 1 ← B

Feature 2   Feature 2

Figure 8.3 A simple linear discriminant applied to training (A) and test (B) data sets that have different statistics (i.e., mean and standard deviation). In this example the observations corresponding to the two possible outputs (e.g., yes and no) are represented by ellipses rather than shown as individual observations. The center and shape of each ellipse represent the mean and covariance, respectively, of the observations corresponding to each output. The discriminant function (solid line) in A separates the two outputs very well. In B, however, the data statistics have changed, and the original discriminant function is no longer effective. (Based on Vidaurre et al., 2006.)

In addition to the adaptive capability built into the translation algorithm, the BCI user can also be conceptualized as an adaptive entity: the user learns to use the BCI system (and usually improves performance). Consequently, BCI operation can be viewed as the interaction of two adaptive controllers, the BCI user and the BCI system (Wolpaw et al., 2002). Figure 8.4 shows three alternative concepts of the adaptation associated with BCI operation. In Figure 8.4A the user is assumed to provide signal features that do not change over time. The BCI is expected to adapt to these features through *machine learning*, a process in which the translation algorithm gradually improves the accuracy of its model by minimizing (or maximizing) an objective function (Blankertz et al., 2003). In contrast, in Figure 8.4B the translation algorithm does not change, and the user is expected to adapt the signal features to the algorithm through an operant-conditioning process (Birbaumer et al., 2003). This process is driven by reinforcement: when the user adapts the features appropriately, the BCI produces the output that the user intends. Figure 8.4C combines the adaptations of both 4A and 4B: both the user and the BCI system adapt so that BCI operation depends on the appropriate interaction of two dynamic processes (Wolpaw et al., 2002; Taylor et al., 2002). The user and system co-adapt as the user learns and the system adapts to the changing statistics of the user's signals. These ongoing changes further complicate the task of selecting a model and parameterizing it so that it generalizes well to new data.

SUPERVISED AND UNSUPERVISED LEARNING

Another issue in the design of BCI translation algorithms concerns whether or not the parameterization of the model algorithm is supervised. The discriminant model illustrated in figures 8.2 and 8.3 is parameterized through *supervised learning*, that is, by using a training data set in which the correct outputs are known (i.e., the outputs are labeled). However, sometimes labeled training data are not available. In this case, models can be parameterized using *unsupervised learning* techniques (Schalk et al., 2008).

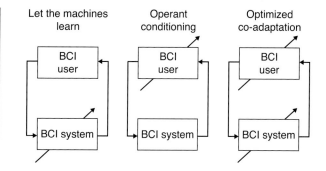

Let the machines learn   Operant conditioning   Optimized co-adaptation

BCI user   BCI user   BCI user

BCI system   BCI system   BCI system

Figure 8.4 Three concepts of BCI operation. The arrows through the user and/or the BCI system indicate that they adapt to improve and maintain the correlation between the user's intent and the BCI's output.

Up to the present, most BCI translation algorithms have relied mainly on supervised learning to parameterize their models. In real-life operation, however, BCIs do not usually have labeled training data; that is, they do not have perfect knowledge of the correct outputs (i.e., of what the user intends). The most common solution is to have periodic *calibration* sessions in which the BCI tells the user ahead of time what the correct outputs are. For example, *copy-spelling* is typically used to calibrate P300-based BCIs (e.g., Krusienski et al., 2008; see chapter 12, in this volume). Alternative solutions are possible. For example, if a BCI application includes an error correction option (e.g., a backspace command), the BCI might assume that whatever was selected and not corrected was, in fact, the user's intent.

COMMON FAMILIES OF MODELS

LINEAR LEAST-SQUARES DISCRIMINANT FUNCTIONS (CLASSIFICATION)

The *linear least-squares discriminant* (or *classification*) function is rooted in classical statistics and is one of the simplest and most commonly used models (Fisher, 1936). The general form of a linear model is given by:

$$Y = b_1 X_1 + b_2 X_2 \ldots b_n x_n + a \tag{8.2}$$

where Y is the predicted value (i.e., the BCI output), $b_1 \ldots b_n$ are weights (i.e., parameters) to be determined, a is a constant (i.e., another parameter) to be determined, and $X_1 .. X_n$ are the features used to predict Y.

Figure 8.5 illustrates a simple linear discriminant based on least-squares criteria. It uses two features, X_1 and X_2, to distinguish between two possible outputs (or classes), Y. Figure 8.5A illustrates the process. Using the available data, a linear function with the form of equation 8.2 is derived; it predicts the value of Y from the corresponding values of X_1 and X_2. In figure 8.5B, the values of X_1 and X_2 for which the predicted value of Y is 0 are indicated by the solid line (i.e., the *discriminant function*). This line separates the two classes, which will produce two different outputs.

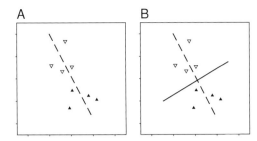

Figure 8.5 *A simple least-squares linear discriminant function is used to separate a set of observations into two possible BCI outputs (or classes). The axes are the two predictor variables (X_1 and X_2), and Y is a binary variable (the BCI output) that can have values of +1 or –1 (represented by open and filled triangles, respectively). The left panel illustrates the function that predicts class membership (i.e., the function $Y' = b_1 X_1 + b_2 X_2 + a$). The predicted value Y' is a continuous variable that goes from positive to negative. The dashed line in Panel A indicates the direction along which the predicted value of Y' changes from more positive (upper left) to more negative (lower right). The right panel shows the discriminant function (solid line), which is perpendicular to the function that predicts class membership and indicates the values of X_1 and X_2 for which the prediction is that $Y'=0$. Thus, this discriminant line separates the data into the two possible BCI outputs or classes (the Y = +1 and the Y = –1 class).*

In practice, the linear discriminant function can be obtained by solving the *normal* equation, which is given by:

$$b = (X'X)^{-1} X'Y \qquad (8.3)$$

where b is the vector of coefficients for the discriminant function, Y is the vector of class memberships, and X is an n by k matrix of features that predicts class membership. The n rows of X represent the individual observations and the k columns represent the individual features. The product, $X'X$, represents the covariance between features. The $()^{-1}$ operation indicates matrix inversion, and the $X'Y$ product represents the cross-product between X and Y (i.e., the covariance between class membership and features). This formula, written in matrix notation, provides a solution to several kinds of least-squares problems including both discriminant analysis and multiple regression. It is similar in form to the univariate formula for the slope of a straight line and can be solved by a direct computation.

We now consider how the discriminant function would be applied by a simple BCI, the P300-based matrix speller (e.g., Donchin et al., 2000; see chapter 12). The BCI user watches a matrix of letters as its rows or columns flash rapidly in succession and EEG is recorded. The user is asked to perform a copy-spelling task in order to provide a labeled set of training data. The problem is to make a classifier that can discriminate between the user's EEG response to the target (i.e., the letter to be spelled) and his/her responses to nontargets (i.e., all the other letters). Our prior knowledge of the target identity allows us to assign correct values to Y, the vector of class memberships (e.g., +1 and –1 for targets and nontargets, respectively). The specific features in the EEG (i.e., the voltages at specific electrodes and times) are the elements of the X matrix. By solving for the $b_1 \ldots b_n$ values in equation 8.2, we produce a discriminant

function that allows us to use the feature values associated with each letter to determine whether the letter is the target or a nontarget: the letter is the target if equation 8.2 yields a value of Y that is greater than 0. Assuming that this parameterized function generalizes well to new data, the user can now employ the BCI to spell whatever he or she wishes.

BAYESIAN CLASSIFIERS

The *Bayesian approach* to statistics uses the concept of *maximum likelihood* to combine prior knowledge with newly acquired knowledge to produce a *posterior probability* (Bickel and Levina, 2004). It produces the model parameters that are most likely to be correct based on the available data. For example, for a BCI that uses one feature, the first step is to assign each value of the feature to one of a limited number of categories (e.g., discrete ranges of EEG voltages). Then these category assignments are used to compute the probability of each possible class membership (i.e., the probability that each possible BCI output is the user's intended output). This is accomplished by means of Bayes's theorem:

$$P(Y \mid X) = \frac{P(Y)P(X \mid Y)}{P(X)}$$

$$(8.4)$$

where Y is the event (i.e., a specific BCI output) and X is the category of the feature. The notation $P(Y|X)$ indicates the probability of Y given X. Bayes's theorem states that predicting Y from X is computed by multiplying the prior probability of Y by the probability of X given Y, and then dividing by the probability of X. This simple relationship forms the basis for Bayesian statistics.

There are many ways in which this approach can be applied. Perhaps the simplest is the *naive Bayesian classifier* which makes the simplifying assumption that the features are independent. Thus,

$$P(Y \mid X_1, X_2, \ldots X_n) = \frac{P(Y)P(X_1 \mid Y)P(X_2 \mid Y)\ldots P(X_n \mid Y)}{P(X_1)P(X_1)\ldots P(X_n)}$$

$$(8.5)$$

where X_1, X_2, and X_n are the first, second, and nth features. Simply stated, the naive Bayesian classifier states that the prediction of Y given X_1, X_2, and X_n is computed by multiplying the prior probability of Y and each probability of X_i given Y, and then dividing by the product of the probabilities of X_1, X_2, $\ldots X_n$. The classifier then computes the posterior probability of all possible Ys and picks the one with the greatest likelihood.

The naive Bayesian classifier is a very straightforward and intuitive method for designing a classifier from training features. Whereas the Bayesian approach allows many degrees of complexity (e.g., Bayesian networks [Shenoy and Rao, 2005]), the naive Bayesian classifier serves as a useful contrast to the classical least-squares discriminant function (Fisher, 1936). As noted above, the naive Bayesian classifier considers the features in isolation from each other, whereas the least-squares discriminant considers the variances and covariances of the features. Thus, the naive Bayesian classifier is much simpler, and it performs very well in some situations, even when the features are not truly independent as assumed for the model. It has proved successful even when there are many features and very little training data (Bickel and Levina, 2004). This is typically the case at the start of BCI usage when there are as yet not enough observations to provide a good estimate of the covariance matrix. To summarize, the naive Bayesian approach provides a means of incorporating prior information into the discriminant. However, this approach does not deal with issues that arise due to correlations between the features (i.e., the problem of colinearity).

When the features are correlated, it is often the case that prediction is improved by giving more weight to features that have unique covariance with class membership. EEG features are frequently correlated with each other due to effects such as volume conduction. A case of correlated features is illustrated in figure 8.6, where the relationships between and among variables are indicated with Venn diagrams. The circles represent the variance of each variable and the overlap between circles represents their covariance. X_1, X_2, and X_3 are three features and Y is the BCI output. The intersection between X_1 and Y is about 30% of their areas, whereas the intersection between Y and X_2 is about 40% of their areas (i.e., the r^2 values for X_1 and X_2 are 0.30 and 0.40, respectively, where r^2 is the proportion of the total variance in the output Y that is accounted for by X_1 or X_2). Thus, X_2 is a better predictor of Y than X_1 is. X_3 also has about 40% overlap with Y, but it shares most of this with X_2. The unique correlation of X_2 or X_3 with Y is only about 10%, whereas the unique correlation of X_1 with Y is 30%. A model such as the naive Bayesian classifier, which assumes that the features are independent, would give greater weight to X_2 and X_3 than to X_1. In contrast, a model that takes covariance into account would give X_1 more weight than either X_2 or X_3.

Figure 8.7 illustrates a case where two features correlate but only one of them, X_1, predicts the BCI output, Y. Nevertheless, the overlap between X_2 and X_1 can remove some of the prediction error in X_1. In this case, X_2 is a *suppressor variable* (Friedman and Wall, 2005). The naive Bayesian model would not give a large weight to X_2 since it does not independently predict Y. In contrast, the least-squares discriminant function

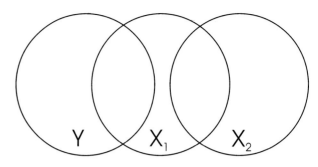

Figure 8.7 *Illustration of a suppressor variable. Feature X_1 overlaps with the BCI output Y, and feature X_2 overlaps with X_1, but X_2 does not overlap with Y. If X_2 is included in the model it serves as a suppressor variable that improves the usefulness of X_1 by eliminating some of the noise that it introduces.*

would give X_2 a weight of opposite sign to X_1, allowing it to subtract part of the X_1 prediction error.

McFarland, Anderson, et al. (2006) describe a case of a suppressor variable with a P300-based BCI. Given two features from electrode Cz, one at 0 msec and one at 240 msec after the stimulus, the 0-msec feature did not predict the correct output, but the 240-msec did. However, combining the 0-msec and 240-msec features in the model greatly improved prediction over that produced by the 240-msec feature alone. It is likely that inclusion of the 0-msec feature provided noise cancellation (i.e., it provided a baseline correction that removed slow drifts in the EEG signal).

A comparison of the linear least-squares discriminant with the naive Bayesian classifier illustrates the types of trade-offs that need to be considered in selecting among general families of models. The naive Bayesian classifier is simple and works well with a few training observations and a large number of features. However, when enough observations are available to accurately estimate the covariance matrix, the linear least-squares discriminant, which considers the relationships among the features, may perform better.

SUPPORT VECTOR MACHINES

Our first two families of models solve the problem of discriminating among different classes (i.e., different BCI outputs) by direct computations from the data (i.e., the features). In modern *machine-learning* approaches, computer algorithms gradually improve their performance by minimizing (or maximizing) some parameter of a model by iteration. One example of this approach is the support vector machine, illustrated in figure 8.8. The support vector machine selects specific observations at the border between two classes and uses these to define the upper and lower margins (i.e., the dotted lines) of a region that separates the classes. This acts to maximize the separation between the classes in order to produce greater generalizability. In figure 8.8, the circles and triangles are observations corresponding to the two classes, respectively. The solid circles are two of the support vectors. As such, they define the hyperplane that is the upper margin. Similarly, the solid triangle is the support vector that defines the lower margin. Thus, the support vector machine selects actual observations from the data set to define margins in feature space that separate the

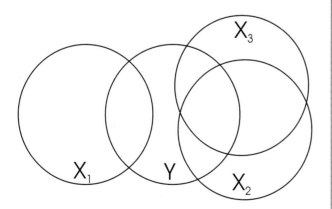

Figure 8.6 *Correlations among features (X_1, X_2, X_3), and between these features and the BCI output (Y). The variance of each variable is represented by a circle, and the covariance between any two variables is represented by the overlap of their circles. Note that the unique correlation X_1 with Y is greater than that of X_2 or X_3 with Y. This is because X_2 and X_3 share much of their overlap with Y.*

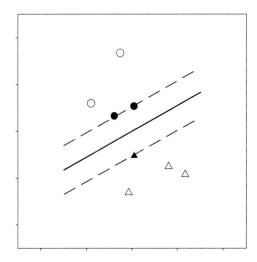

Figure 8.8 *A support vector machine generates a hyperplane (solid line) that defines the border between the observations belonging to two different classes (i.e., BCI outputs) shown as circles and triangles. The support vectors are the solid symbols. They define the upper and lower margins (dashed lines) of the region between the classes. The hyperplane (solid line) that separates the two classes is placed midway between the margins.*

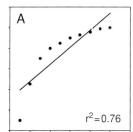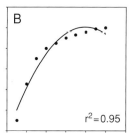

Figure 8.9 *Linear and quadratic regressions. In A, the data are fit with a linear function given by Y= bX + a. In B, the data are fit with a quadratic function given by Y= b_1X^2 + b_2X + a. The average distance between the line and the points is much smaller in B, and thus the r^2 value is much higher.*

data into different classes. New observations are classified according to whether they fall above or below the solid line midway between the two margins.

The support vector machine minimizes an objective function through a series of iterations. This function includes two components. The first component consists of the Euclidian distances between the observations in each class and the separating hyperplane. Observations that are on the correct side of the margin do not contribute to this component. The second component of the objective function is the Euclidian distance between the margins. Thus, the support vector machine must select observations from the data set that simultaneously minimize these two components of the objective function. A parameter in the model allows the relative influence of these two components to be tuned to the data type. Proponents of the support vector machine suggest that this algorithm can be trained with relatively few observations, that it generalizes well due to the presence of the margins, and that it is relatively insensitive to outliers (Parra et al., 2005).

NONLINEAR MODELS

The discussion so far has focused on linear methods for separating observations (i.e., feature vectors) into their correct classes (i.e., BCI outputs). However, linear methods may not always be effective (Müller et al., 2003). A variety of methods exist for addressing the problem of nonlinearity. One approach is to transform the data by some means that makes them more suitable for linear analysis. This is illustrated in figure 8.9. In figure 8.9A, the data are fit with a straight line. The proportion of the total variation in the data that is accounted for by the line (i.e., a linear model) is 0.76 (i.e., r^2). In figure 8.9B, the data are fit with a second-order equation (i.e., a quadratic model). For the quadratic model, r^2 is 0.95 indicating that the quadratic function fits the data better. In the linear case, the sole predictor of Y is X. In the quadratic case, the predictors of Y are X and

X^2; by projecting the single X into a two-dimensional space (i.e., X and X^2), the prediction has been improved. Although this is a simple linearizing projection, many other more complex projections are possible. Similar projections of the data can be used with either discriminant or regression functions.

Modern machine-learning algorithms make extensive use of projections of data into higher-dimensional feature space as a method of linearizing nonlinear problems. These are often referred to as *kernel* methods. A wide variety of kernels have been devised. Some of these, such as the Gaussian kernel, permit the construction of class-separating hyperplanes with very irregular shapes.

An alternative approach to nonlinearity is to use artificial neural networks (Müller et al., 2003). Artificial neural networks are simplified models of biological neural networks. Their primary purpose is not to simulate or replicate actual biological neural networks or brain activity. Rather, they are developed in the expectation that they will allow the powerful decision-making capabilities of biological neuronal networks to be applied to a variety of classification problems. Thus, for a BCI, the network input consists of the feature vectors, and its output consists of the commands sent to the application.

Artificial neural networks are comprised of individual units called *neurons*. In their basic form, illustrated in figure 8.10A, these neurons consist of a summing node, which sums all the inputs to the neuron, and a subsequent activation function, which produces the output. The activation function transforms the product of the summing node and can take any form. Threshold-type activation functions (i.e., functions that produce a binary, or Yes/No output) are common for classification applications. Each neuron can be envisioned as a simple classification unit. A neural network is formed by interconnecting individual neurons in a parallel and cascaded fashion, which combines the output of the individual neurons to form complex decision boundaries. Each neuron uses a decision hyperplane to convert a weighted sum of its inputs into an output. Its threshold activation function determines which side of the hyperplane the sum falls on; this defines the neuron's output. Neural networks typically have hidden layers of neurons (fig. 8.10B) that form unions between these decision boundaries and thereby demarcate unique regions corresponding to the different possible outputs of the network. Thus, through

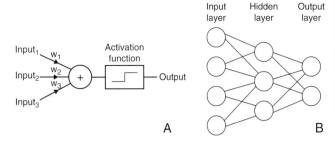

Input₁ w₁
Input₂ w₂ + → Activation function → Output
Input₃ w₃

Input layer Hidden layer Output layer

A   B

Figure 8.10 (A) An individual unit (or neuron) of a neural network. The three inputs on the left are weighted and summed. If the result reaches the threshold of the activation function, the unit produces an output. (B) A neural network classifier. The three layers of units (from left to right) are an input layer, a hidden layer, and an output layer. These are connected in sequence by connections that have variable weights. During training, these weights are adjusted using back propagation to minimize the difference between the network's actual output and its correct output.

training (i.e., iterative adjustments in the summing node and threshold function of each neuron), the hyperplanes produced by each neuron in the network partition the feature space to define the decision boundaries that represent each possible output.

Neural networks can vary widely in numbers of units, numbers of layers, and neuron interconnections. Figure 8.10B illustrates a simple feed-forward network that has four inputs and two outputs. These represent, for example, four brain signal features and two possible BCI commands. During network training, the network processes a set of labeled training data (i.e., feature vectors for which the correct output is known). After each observation is processed, the output of the network is compared to the correct output label to define the error (i.e., the difference between the actual output and the correct output). Then, the summing nodes of each neuron are slightly adjusted (or *updated*) so as to reduce the error. This updating process proceeds backward through the network from the output layer to the input layer, and thus it is called *backpropagation*. As training progresses through the labeled training data, the error in the network output diminishes.

A neural network with sufficient neurons is, in theory, capable of approximating any function. As a result, neural networks can be used to deal with non-linear aspects of BCI feature-translation problems. However, because the neural-network structures can become complex and each individual weight must be trained, the training process may be lengthy and require a large amount of labeled training data. Furthermore, satisfactory solutions are not always guaranteed because of practical limits on training algorithms and data sets.

As noted above, for the sake of simplicity, the model examples discussed in this section have all been discriminant functions (i.e., they have discrete, categorical outputs). However, each of these types of model can also be designed to produce a *continuous output*, and thus serve as a *regression function*. For example, equation 8.3 can produce coefficients for a discriminant function or for a regression function, depending on whether the vector of Y values is discrete or continuous. Similarly, both Bayesian models and support vector machines can be discriminant or regression functions, and neural networks can produce discrete or continuous outputs.

SELECTING FEATURES FOR A MODEL

In any BCI, the two parts of signal processing (i.e., feature extraction and feature translation) must work together well. Thus, the choice of the feature type (e.g., evoked-potential amplitude, power in a frequency band, single-neuron firing rates) and the choice of the model type (e.g., linear discriminant, Bayesian classifier, support-vector machine, etc.) necessarily affect each other. For example, if the feature type is P300 amplitude, a two-class classification algorithm may be most appropriate. In contrast, if the feature type is mu-rhythm power, a linear regression might be the sensible choice. Once the choices of feature type and model type have been made, the next steps are to determine the specific features to be used and the parameters to be applied to these features. These two steps can be taken in sequence (i.e., first feature selection and then parameter selection), or in one combined operation. This and the next sections of the chapter consider commonly used feature-selection and parameterization methods.

Since recordings from the brain often produce a large number of signals, some means of feature selection (i.e., discarding features that do not positively contribute to model accuracy) or dimension reduction (i.e., preprocessing the existing features in a way that eliminates irrelevant feature dimensions) is generally needed. As noted earlier there is a trade-off between better output accuracy for training data when more features are used and better generalization to new data when fewer features are used. The calculation of parameter values is always subject to error; these errors accumulate as the number of features, and therefore the number of parameters, increases. In contrast, parameter errors decrease as the amount of training data increases. Thus, the amount of data available for training the function is an important factor in deciding how many features to use. Simpler models (i.e., models using fewer features) will typically generalize better to new data and may be easier to implement within the constraints of real-time online operation. Furthermore, fewer features may make the resulting model easier to understand and thereby facilitate efforts to develop further improvements.

There are two basic approaches to selecting a subset of features from a larger collection of features. The first is to apply a *heuristic*, a simple rule based on common sense or experience. A very simple example of a heuristic would be to select only the upper 10% of the features based on their individual abilities to predict the correct output. The second approach is to include in the parameter-calculation process a *regularization* step, in which a constraint is placed on the parameters. An example of regularization would be to place a limit on the sum of the absolute values of the feature weights. These approaches restrict the number and/or weights of the features used in the model.

A simple heuristic that selects those features best able to predict the correct output when considered individually may not identify the optimal feature set since, as discussed above, correlations between the features may complicate matters. Generally, features that make unique contributions to output prediction are more useful. In addition, some features that do not predict the output themselves may be valuable because they suppress error in other features.

Ideally, a search for the optimal subset of features will consider all possible combinations. However, this ideal approach is often impractical due to the large number of features available. One alternative is to use a *stepwise heuristic*. A *forward stepwise selection* starts with the best individual feature (i.e., the feature that gives the best prediction when used by itself) and considers each of the remaining features in a pair-wise combination with this best feature. The optimal pair is selected on the basis of some criterion, and then this process is repeated with that pair being combined with each of the remaining features. Alternatively, a *backward selection* procedure starts with all of the features in the model and eliminates the one that contributes least to the prediction accuracy of the model. This process is then repeated with the remaining set of features. It is also possible to combine forward and backward procedures. Whichever method is used, there must be some stopping rule to determine at what point in the process the best model has been selected. The stopping rule is generally based on some criterion variable (such as r^2 or the percent of outputs correctly predicted). For example, the feature selection process might continue until the change in r^2 with each new iteration is no longer significant.

A regularization approach to feature selection might apply a penalty term to the feature weights during the step in which parameter values are determined (see below). An example of this approach is Lasso regression (Tibshirani, 1996). Applied to a least-squares regression model, this method limits the sum of the absolute values of the feature weights to a specific value. As described by Tibshirani (1996), this method may be applied so that many features receive weights of 0, which effectively eliminates them from the model. Because this method of regularization incorporates feature selection into the parameterization process, it is referred to as an *embedded technique*.

PARAMETERIZING A MODEL

After selection of a model and the specific features to be included in it, the next step is to assign specific values to the parameters of the model. This step is generally referred to as *parameter estimation* in recognition of the probable difference between the parameters calculated from the training data and the ideal parameters for new data. It recognizes that there is almost always some error in parameterization.

Parameters can be estimated in a number of ways. For a linear least-squares regression model, the parameters (i.e., feature weights and constants) can be computed directly by solving equation 8.2. Alternatively, they can be estimated by any of several *iterative optimization algorithms* (e.g., Press et al., 2007). These algorithms generate an approximate solution and then refine it in repeated cycles until acceptable accuracy is obtained. This approach has the advantage that it can also be applied to nonlinear functions (e.g., support-vector regression). However, iterative optimization algorithms are more computationally intense than direct solutions and do not guarantee a solution (i.e., they may never reach the desired degree of accuracy).

The parameterization process should also consider the time frame of the training data (i.e., how much training data

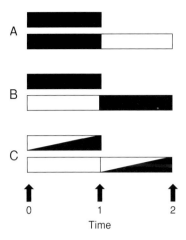

Figure 8.11 *Three possible data-windowing methods. The training data available at any given time are represented by the rectangles. The training data actually used for parameterization are represented by the filled areas. (A) The parameters are determined at Time 1 from the Time 0–1 data and are never changed. (B) The parameters are determined at Time 1 using the Time 0–1 data and are redetermined at Time 2 using the Time 1–2 data. (C) The parameters are determined as in B except that recent data are given more weight. In contrast to the static window method in A, the sliding window methods in B and C can track the changing statistics of the data.*

should be used). This time frame is referred to as the *data window*. Long data windows can provide more accurate parameter estimates. However, short time windows are more responsive to changes (i.e., nonstationarity) in the data. According to the static concept of BCI operation presented in figure 8.4A, the best approach would be to use as much data as possible since this should produce more accurate parameter estimates. However, according to the often more realistic coadaptive concept presented in figure 8.4C, the data window should be shorter so as allow the parameters to track the changes in the statistics of the data.

Figure 8.11 illustrates several possible data-windowing schemes. In figure 8.11A, the parameters are estimated from the data obtained between Times 0 and 1, and then are never changed. In figure 8.11B, the parameters are estimated at Time 1 using the Time 0–1 data and re-estimated at Time 2 using the Time 1–2 data. In figure 8.11AC, the parameters are estimated as in 8.11B, except that recent data are given more weight. In contrast to the scheme of figure 8.11A, those of figures 8.11B and C can track the changing statistics of the data.

If the statistics of the data do not change over time (i.e., the data are stationary) then the static data window illustrated in figure 8.11A makes sense. However, the sliding window technique of 8.11B or C is more appropriate if the data are nonstationary. This might be the case, for example, if the user's brain signals change as a function of time of day or if the user gradually adapts to the BCI more effectively over time. Any BCI translation algorithm could use this sliding window technique by periodically changing the training data used for parameterization. A smaller data window allows more accuracy in tracking changes in the data, whereas a longer data window provides more stable estimates of parameter values. Thus, there is a trade-off between tracking accuracy and stability.

The method illustrated in figure 8.11C also uses a sliding window, but in this case more recent data are given more influence in determining the parameters. The simplest example of this approach is the least-means squares (LMS) algorithm (Haykin, 1996). The LMS can be used to update the parameters of a linear function (e.g., eq. 8.1). To do this, the current parameter values are used to make a prediction of the next value of $Y(t)$. If $Y'(t)$ is the predicted value, the prediction error $e(t)$ is given by:

$$e(t) = Y(t) - Y'(t) \tag{8.6}$$

and each parameter in the vector of parameters is updated according to:

$$b(t+1) = b(t) + l \cdot e(t) \cdot X(t) \tag{8.7}$$

where $b(t+1)$ is the parameter vector at time $t+1$, l is a learning-rate parameter that controls the rate of adaptation, and $X(t)$ is the current feature vector. By this update, each parameter is changed a small amount in a direction that reduces the error on the current trial. As a consequence, this method should slowly converge on the best values for the parameters. An update occurs with each new observation, and the algorithm needs only to remember the parameters produced by the last update. With a properly selected learning rate, the LMS algorithm will track the least-squares solution for the parameters. This algorithm is related to the back propagation algorithm discussed earlier. The primary difference between them is the nature of the model they use to parameterize.

The use of the LMS algorithm just discussed is an example of *supervised learning*. Knowledge of the correct outcome is used to adaptively estimate model parameters. This is possible, for example, when labeled training data have been collected during a calibration session in which the BCI user is asked to produce certain outputs. However, in subsequent BCI use, the user's actual intent is not known by the BCI. As discussed by McFarland, Krusienski et al. (2006), estimating some model parameters does require labeled training data, whereas estimating others does not. For example, it is possible to estimate the mean and variance of the features without knowledge of the user's intent. For a BCI cursor-movement application, this information can be used to normalize the output of the translation algorithm in order to maintain constant cursor speed and minimize directional bias. On the other hand, determining the optimal feature weights requires knowledge of the user's intent.

The LMS algorithm is the simplest and one of the most widely used adaptive parameterization methods. More complex adaptive methods (e.g., the recursive least squares [RLS] and the related Kalman filter) have also been used to parameterize models in BCI translation algorithms (e.g., Black and Donoghue, 2007).

Adaptive parameterization methods such as the LMS and Kalman filter operate well when the error surface (i.e., the relationship of the output error to the feature vector and the labeled output) is relatively simple. In situations in which the error surface is complex, an adaptive method may converge on a local error minimum and miss a much lower error minimum

located elsewhere on the surface. Alternative optimization methods such as evolutionary algorithms (e.g., genetic algorithms and particle swarm optimization) are designed to avoid such suboptimal local minima and thus may provide superior parameterization in complex situations (Krusienski and Jenkins, 2005).

EVALUATING TRANSLATION ALGORITHMS

MEASURING PERFORMANCE

The performance of BCI systems in general, and BCI translation algorithms in particular, can be evaluated by comparing their actual outputs with the correct outputs (assuming, of course, that the correct outputs are known). A variety of evaluation measures are available (McFarland, Anderson, et al., 2006).

ACCURACY

The simplest evaluation method is measurement of the *accuracy* for a given application. For example, in a P300 matrix application, accuracy is the percent of total selections that are correct. Although accuracy is a straightforward measure, it has limitations that, depending on the BCI design and application, may necessitate additional or alternative measures.

In some applications, different kinds or degrees of errors are possible and may have very different consequences. For example, in moving a cursor to select a particular icon, an error could be failing to reach the icon, or it could be moving to another (incorrect) icon. The first error simply wastes time, whereas the second requires that a mistake be corrected.

Or, in the more graphic example summarized in table 8.1, suppose a user is in a BCI-driven wheelchair that can either move forward or stay in place. If the BCI correctly recognizes the user's intent, whether it is to move forward (a *true positive* [TP] output) or to stay in place (a *true negative* [TN] output), everything is fine. If the BCI fails to recognize the user's intent, its error can be an error of omission, a *false negative* (FN) or an error of commission, a *false positive* (FP). In a FN error, the user wants to move forward and the wheelchair stays in place. The result is that the user loses time and may become frustrated. In a FP error, the user wants to stay in place and the wheelchair moves forward. The result may be disastrous: if the wheelchair is facing a busy street or the edge of a cliff the user may be injured or killed. A BCI-driven wheelchair that makes numerous FN errors and no FP errors is clearly preferable to one that makes no FN errors and a few FP errors. Thus, in this

TABLE 8.1 Possible outcomes for a BCI-driven wheelchair

USER INTENT	ACTION	
	WHEELCHAIR STAYS IN PLACE (N)	WHEELCHAIR MOVES FORWARD (P)
Move forward (P)	Error: User stays in place (FN)	Correct (TP)
Stay in place (N)	Correct (TN)	Error: User may fall off a cliff (FP)

example, accuracy alone is clearly not an adequate measure of BCI performance.

A set of four measures is often used to assess performance in a P/N selection of this kind. Expressed in terms of the four possible outcomes described above, these measures are:

- Sensitivity (TP rate or Hit rate) = TP/(TP + FN)

- Selectivity (also called positive predictive value or precision) = TP/(TP + FP)

- Specificity (also called negative predictive value) = TN/(TN + FN)

- Accuracy = (TP + TN)/(TP + TN + FP + FN)

Depending on the nature of the P and N outputs, one or another of these measures may be most critical. Thus, in the example shown in table 8.1, in which a FP might be catastrophic, it is most important that selectivity be as close to 1.0 as possible. Accuracy alone is not an adequate measure of performance.

Accuracy has other limitations as well. Two different translation algorithms may have identical accuracies, but one of these algorithms may need much less time to produce each output; accuracy alone does not capture this important performance difference. Furthermore, accuracy alone does not capture the consistency of performance. For example, an algorithm for which accuracy averages 90% but varies from day to day or hour to hour from 40% to 100% may be less useful than an algorithm with a stable accuracy of 80%.

A particularly troublesome problem with accuracy arises in trying to compare performances when the number of possible choices is not constant. For example, it is not immediately clear whether an accuracy of 90% for two possible outputs is better or worse than an accuracy of 75% for four possible outputs. Making this determination may be important in configuring an application for a particular translation algorithm.

Although most BCIs to date use synchronous operating protocols (see chapter 10, in this volume) in which the BCI always knows when the person wants to use it, the most natural and flexible BCIs would use asynchronous protocols, in which the BCI itself recognizes when the person wants to use it (see chapter 10 for full discussion of this issue). Asynchronous protocols introduce the possibility of errors related to the BCI's need to recognize when the person wants to use it: in a false negative error, the system fails to recognize the person's desire to use the BCI; in a false positive error, the system begins producing BCI outputs when the person does not want to do so.

Finally, although accuracy can assess the performance of a BCI that produces a succession of discrete output commands, it may not be suitable for evaluating BCIs that produce continuous outputs, such as cursor movements.

ASSESSING CONTINUOUS OUTPUTS

The performance of a BCI that produces a continuous output can be evaluated with a continuous metric. The squared difference between the actual output and the correct output at each point in time (i.e., the *prediction error*) is frequently used for this purpose. If all the squared prediction errors are summed, then the resulting statistic is χ^2 (i.e., chi-squared). The χ^2 statistic represents the variance in the output that is due to *BCI error*. This value is often normalized by dividing by the total variance in the output, giving the proportion of the total variance due to error, or $1 - r^2$. The proportion of the variance in the output that is accounted for by the model is then r^2. These statistics can be used to summarize goodness-of-fit for both discrete and continuous data.

Error is often quantified in the engineering field in terms of root-mean-squared error (RMS). This metric is the square root of the average squared error (i.e., difference between actual and correct outputs). It is similar to measures used in statistics in that it is based on the squared difference between predicted and observed results.

If one simply added up all of the prediction errors made by a BCI, the sum would tend to be zero since positive errors would tend to cancel out negative errors. This can be avoided by summing their absolute values (i.e., ignoring their sign) or by summing their squared values. Historically, squared differences have been used because they are more tractable with traditional (i.e., precomputer) methods. However, modern computer technology has removed previous practical limitations on computations. As a result, modern machine-learning algorithms (e.g., support vector machines [see above]) often assess error as an absolute (i.e., Euclidean) difference between actual and correct output.

MINIMIZING ERROR VERSUS MINIMIZING COMPLEXITY

All other things being equal, the translation algorithm that produces the lowest prediction error should be used. However, as noted earlier, there are other important considerations, such as level of simplicity. Simpler models may generalize better to new data or may be easier to implement in real-time operation. Model complexity is usually evaluated in terms of the number of parameters that must be estimated. Often models with more parameters can achieve lower prediction error, at least on training data. Hence, there is often some trade-off between error and complexity. One objective method for selecting the optimal model is to minimize Akaike's information criterion (AIC) (Akaike, 1974), which is a weighted combination of prediction error and model complexity. Akaike's criteria can be expressed in terms of r^2 as:

$$AIC = 2k + n \ln(1 - r^2)/n \qquad (8.8)$$

where k is the number of parameters in the model and n is the sample size (e.g., the size of the training set). Thus, AIC decreases as the prediction error and/or the number of parameters decreases. The optimal trade-off between error and complexity is not clear. The uncertainty concerns how to determine the relative importance of error versus simplicity. A variety of alternatives have been proposed (see Stoica and Selen, 2004, for review).

In evaluating performance, it is usually more informative to compare different translation algorithms rather than to evaluate single algorithms in isolation. When one asks whether a translation algorithm does a good job of producing the correct output, the answer depends in large part on what other alternatives exist. As an example, a common use of AIC is to compare models of different complexity and select the one with the lowest value. In this way, an optimum combination of accuracy and complexity might be obtained.

BIT RATE AS A MEASURE OF BCI PERFORMANCE

Wolpaw et al. (2002) suggested evaluating BCI performance using *bit rate*. Bit rate, or *information transfer rate*, is the standard method for measuring communication and control systems. It is the amount of information communicated per unit time. Based on Shannon and Weaver (1964) and summarized very well in Pierce (1980), this measure incorporates both speed and accuracy in a single value. Bit rate has been most commonly applied to assess the performance of an entire BCI system, rather than its translation algorithm in isolation. Appropriately applied, it can be a very valuable measure. Inappropriately applied, it can provide results that are misleading or irrelevant.

Figure 8.12 shows the relationship between accuracy and bit rate for different numbers of possible selections. Bit rate is shown both as bits/trial (i.e., bits/selection), and as bits/min when 12 selections are made per minute (e.g., a reasonable rate for a P300-based BCI). For example, the bit rate of a BCI that has a 10% error rate with two choices is equal to that of a BCI that selects among four choices with a 35% error rate. This

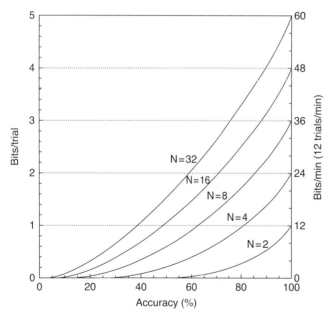

Figure 8.12 *Information transfer rate in bits/trial (i.e., bits/selection) and in bits/ min (for 12 trials/min) when the number of possible outputs (i.e., N) is 2, 4, 8, 16, or 32. As derived from Pierce (1980) (and based on Shannon and Weaver, 1964), if a trial has N possible outputs, if each output has the same probability of being the one that the user desires, if the probability (P) that the desired output will actually be produced is always the same, and if each of the other (i.e., undesired) outputs has the same probability of selection, that is, (1 − P)/(N − 1), then bit rate, or bits/trial (B), is: B = log$_2$N + Plog$_2$P + (1 − P) log$_2$[(1 − P)/(N − 1)]. For each N, bit rate is shown only for accuracy ≥100/N (i.e., ≥chance). (From Wolpaw et al., 2002)*

figure provides an objective answer to a question posed earlier in this section: an error rate of 10% with two choices is worse than an error rate of 25% with four choices.

The great importance of accuracy, illustrated in figure 8.12, is often not fully appreciated in BCI research. With two choices, 90% accuracy is literally twice as good as 80%, and only half as good as 100%. Bit rate provides an objective measure for measuring improvement in a BCI translation algorithm and for comparing different algorithms. It can also help select among different applications (Wolpaw et al., 2002). Other measures based on Shannon's theory (Shannon and Weaver, 1964; Pierce, 1980), such as mutual information (Schlogl et al., 2002), are also useful.

At the same time, in using bit rate to assess BCI performance, it is important to realize that this measure can be applied to a given application in different ways, and the resulting values for bit rate may differ greatly (even by orders of magnitude) (Luce, 2003). For example, in a cursor-movement application, bit rate might be calculated for the trajectory of cursor movement or simply for the resulting output selection. The former method may produce much higher bit rates than the latter because the information needed to specify a trajectory is usually much greater than that needed to select among a limited number of outputs. The difference may be further accentuated if the analysis focuses only on the early part of the movement (e.g., the first 0.5 sec) and thus uses a very small denominator for calculating bits/time.

In general, in applying bit rate to assess BCI performance, two principles should be observed. First, the numerator (i.e., the information) should be the information in the final output of the given application, not the information in some part of the process that leads to the output. For example, in a cursor movement application, the information in a trial is defined by the number of possible outputs, not by the details of the movement. Second, the denominator (i.e., the time) should be the total time needed for an output, not the time occupied by some limited segment of the process that leads to the output. For example, in a P300 matrix application, the time is the total time from the beginning of one selection (i.e., trial) to the beginning of the next. In sum, if bit rate is to be most useful in evaluating BCI performance, it should be applied in a way that approximates as closely as possible the actual performance of the BCI for its user.

There is probably no single evaluation measure (not even bit rate) that is sufficient for all BCI applications. For example, in terms of bit rate, a BCI transmits information if its error rate is less that 1-(1/N), where N is the number of possible outputs. Thus, a P300-based 6 × 6 matrix BCI application, which has 36 possible outputs, transmits information as long as it makes errors on less that 1-(1/36) (i.e., <97.2%) of the selections. However, in reality, this application is of practical value only if its error rate is much lower, that is, 30% or less (Sellers et al., 2006). If the error rate is higher, the frequent need for correction (e.g., backspacing in a spelling application) renders the system unacceptably slow. Nevertheless, measures such as bit rate and r^2 are extremely useful in comparing different BCI translation algorithms, and they are essential for providing benchmarks for the iterative processes of developing and optimizing new alternatives.

THE GOLD STANDARD: ONLINE EVALUATION

BCI systems operate in real time. The user and the BCI system must interact effectively to ensure that the user's intent is accomplished. The user must produce brain signals that the BCI can interpret, the BCI must translate these signals into outputs, and the user must be informed of these outputs in a timely fashion so that he or she can continue to generate signals that embody the desired intent. As a result, the ultimate test of any BCI translation algorithm is how it performs in actual real-time operation. In engineering terms, this is called *closed-loop performance*: the BCI user is continually aware of the consequences of BCI operation and can therefore adjust the brain signals to ensure that the correct intent continues to be accomplished. Real-time performance is the ultimate test of the ability of a translation algorithm to generalize to new data. The real-time environment ensures that training and test data are independent. Thus, effectiveness in real-time, closed-loop performance is the gold standard for evaluating BCI translation algorithms. Although closed-loop performance is the ideal method for comparing alternative algorithms, it is often difficult to implement direct comparisons, particularly when many different algorithms or different variations of a single algorithm need to be compared.

The impact of closed-loop performance on the user (and the BCI if it too adapts) may be complex and may develop gradually over prolonged performance. Individual users typically differ widely in their initial characteristics and/or in their subsequent adaptations during closed-loop performance. In addition, the consequences of closed-loop experience with a given algorithm make it very difficult to adequately compare several different algorithms in a single person. As a result, closed-loop evaluation is extremely time consuming and labor intensive, and it is generally only practical after the set of possible algorithms has been winnowed down to a small number of particularly promising alternatives.

Thus, for a given BCI application, the process of evaluating different models and different methods for selecting their features and determining their parameters typically begins with paradigms simpler than closed-loop operation, paradigms that facilitate the comparison of large numbers of alternatives. The common feature of these paradigms is that they do not evaluate the consequences of providing the output of the BCI to the user in real time; that is, they do not involve closed-loop operation. Rather they employ offline analyses of BCI data already acquired.

The most effective BCI research will usually incorporate both offline and online evaluations. Offline evaluations can be used to identify a small number of particularly promising alternatives, which can then be submitted to online closed-loop testing (e.g., Krusienski et al., 2008; McFarland and Wolpaw, 2005). By identifying the best of these few alternatives, the online results may lead to a new series of offline evaluations comparing different versions of this algorithm, and the new offline results may in turn lead to new online studies. This iterative offline/online research process may prove particularly effective in optimizing BCI function. Up the present however, this coordinated research design has been relatively rare in BCI research.

Finally, it should be noted that, although the online evaluations that do occur usually involve normal volunteers for reasons of practicality, the BCI users most appropriate for these studies are the people for whom the particular BCI application is intended. The many different neuromuscular disorders that create the need for BCI-based communication and control may themselves affect a user's interactions with a BCI system, and thus the performance of the translation algorithm.

THE WORKHORSE OF BCI RESEARCH: OFFLINE EVALUATION

Offline evaluations have clear limitations. Most important, they cannot evaluate the impact of differences among algorithms in the ongoing feedback they provide during online closed-loop operation. Thus, they cannot address how well a particular algorithm enables and encourages the continual adaptations of user to system and system to user that are frequently essential for stable and effective BCI performance.

Offline evaluations may also have additional limitations specific to particular BCI applications. For example, a BCI action in which the user moves a cursor to a desired icon on a screen typically ends when an icon is reached. As a result, the time necessary is a function not only of the user's brain signals but also of the algorithm that translates those signals into cursor movement. Thus, if an offline evaluation applies a new algorithm to brain signals that were gathered during online operation with a different algorithm, the stored data may not be sufficient, that is, the brain signals may run out before the new algorithm brings the cursor to an icon.

Nevertheless, when applied appropriately, and when used mainly to guide selection of particularly promising algorithms for subsequent online testing, offline evaluations are extremely valuable, indeed essential, in BCI research and development.

ALTERNATIVE PARADIGMS FOR OFFLINE EVALUATIONS

Three kinds of paradigms are commonly used for offline evaluations in BCI research. Two of these collect brain signals during open-loop performance and then, in offline analyses, compare the effectiveness of different algorithms in producing the appropriate output.

In the first type of paradigm, BCI users simply engage in cognitive operations such as mental arithmetic or mental rotation of a geometric figure without feedback of any kind, and brain signals are recorded while they do so. (Many common psychophysiological experiments provide data of this kind.) The goal is then to devise a translation algorithm that can determine from the brain signals which operation the person was engaged in. (Often the evaluation stops at this point and does not proceed to online real-time experiments in which the subject uses these cognitive operations to produce specific BCI outputs in closed-loop BCI operation.)

In the second type, brain signals are recorded while subjects are using the BCI, but the subjects are told what outputs to produce and are not given feedback as to the outputs actually produced. The resulting signals are analyzed offline with the different candidate algorithms, and the results are compared. The algorithms giving the best results (i.e., the closest match between correct output and actual output) may then be compared in online closed-loop performance.

The third kind of offline paradigm collects data during closed-loop operation with a particular translation algorithm and then in offline analyses compares the performance of a set of candidate algorithms. This paradigm is most appropriate when ongoing user adaptation is minimal (e.g., in a P300-based BCI) or when the candidate algorithms to be compared do not differ greatly from each other. For example, Krusienski et al. (2006) used data from a P300-based matrix speller to compare the performance of five methods: Fisher's linear discriminant; stepwise discriminant analysis; a linear support vector machine; a support vector machine with a Gaussian kernel; and Pearson's correlation of univariate features. Although performance did not differ markedly among these techniques, Fisher's linear discriminant and stepwise discriminant analysis produced the best overall results.

CROSS-VALIDATION IN OFFLINE EVALUATIONS

The primary goal in developing a new BCI translation algorithm is an algorithm that performs well with new brain signals as well as with those used to develop the algorithm. That is, the algorithm must generalize well to future data. Thus, its performance should be evaluated using data different from those used to define and parameterize it. This process is called *cross-validation*.

In the simplest cross-validation scheme, the data are divided into a training set and a test set. The training set is used to parameterize the algorithm, and then the test set is used to evaluate its performance. This method works well when there is a large amount of data available. Ideally, the training set should include enough data to avoid over-fitting (see above), and the test set should have enough data to get an accurate estimate of performance. Often, however, the data are limited. Thus, it is common to use a resampling scheme such as *K-fold cross-validation*. In *K*-fold cross-validation, the data set is divided into *K* partitions. Each of the *K* subsamples is used once as the test set while the remaining *K* – 1 samples are used for training; that is, each subsample provides one *fold* of the cross-validation. The results for the *K* folds are then averaged to yield the final cross-validation performance of the algorithm. Other methods are also possible. For example, in the *bagging* method (Li et al., 2010), training and test sets are created by repeated random sampling of the entire body of data (i.e., partitions are created by sampling the data with no restriction on how often a given sample is used).

EVALUATING SPECIFIC ASPECTS OF TRANSLATION ALGORITHMS

The examples given in preceding sections illustrate the complexities involved in comparing algorithms that may differ in a variety of ways (e.g., type and number of features used, model type, amount of training data, parameterization method, etc.). What is most apparent is that it is not possible to arrive at simple conclusions about which algorithms are best. Multiple factors (e.g., the amount of training data available) affect how different algorithms perform relative to each other. Although it is probably safe to say that more complex models usually require more training data, further research is needed to determine how specific aspects of different model families interact with the characteristics (e.g., amounts, stationarity) of the training and test data.

EVALUATING DIFFERENT MODELS

In comparing different models for use in translation algorithms, it is often important to consider which differences between models are most relevant and to what extent these differences can be changed. For example, an investigator may observe a difference in performance between a Fisher's linear discriminant model and a support vector machine that uses Gaussian kernels. This difference could be due to several factors, such as the fact that the support vector machine uses the kernel function to deal with nonlinearities. However, a kernel function can also be used with Fisher's linear discriminant (Müller et al., 2001), and this might markedly change the performance difference between the models. Similarly, a regularization parameter, which is implicit in a support vector machine, can also be used by a Fisher's discriminant. Thus it should be possible to determine what specific aspects of these two algorithms account for differences in their performances.

Lotte et al. (2007) reviewed the literature on BCI classification algorithms. They noted that either regression or classification algorithms can be used but that classification algorithms were the most popular approach. Thus, it was the one they reviewed. They concluded that support vector machines generally performed well and attributed this to their use of regularization (see *Feature Selection* section above). They also discussed the need for systematic comparisons of classifiers within the same context. It should be noted that most of the work that they reviewed involved offline data analyses.

CONSIDERING THE AMOUNT OF TRAINING DATA

A number of studies have found that the relative performance of different model classes can vary with the amount of data available for training. For example, Vidaurre et al. (2007) used spectral features from data collected while subjects imagined left- or right-hand movements to compare linear, quadratic, and regularized discriminant functions in regard to their accuracy in determining for each trial which movement the subject was imagining. They found that the results of the comparison depended on the amount of data used for training the functions. With a small amount of data available for training, the linear discriminant function performed best. With more data available for training, the three functions performed similarly. Besserve et al. (2007) also examined the effect of the amount of data available for training a translation algorithm. They used spectral features from EEG data collected while subjects performed a visuomotor tracking task to reproduce the track. They compared three models: a linear discriminant; a support vector machine; and a *k*-nearest-neighbor algorithm. With large sets of training data, the three algorithms performed similarly as more features were included in the models. However, with smaller data sets, the performance of the linear discriminant function declined more sharply than those of the other two models as additional features were added. The very different conclusions these two studies reach as to the value of linear discriminant functions illustrate the inconsistencies in the literature and the complexities involved in selecting methods for specific purposes.

EVALUATING FEATURE SELECTION

Several offline studies have evaluated the feature-selection process. Millán et al. (2002) used spectral EEG features from data collected while the subject imagined motor movements. They showed that selecting only the most relevant features improved performance. Krusienski et al. (2008) used data from a P300-based BCI matrix-selection application to examine the effects of including various subsets of electrodes in a stepwise linear discriminant analysis. They found that larger numbers of electrodes could improve performance and they identified a set of eight electrodes that was extremely effective. Krusienski et al. (2008) went on to validate this offline result in online testing and thus showed that, in this example at least, offline results did generalize to online closed-loop performance.

McFarland and Wolpaw (2005) reported offline analyses exploring the effects of feature selection in a BCI application that used spectral features of EEG sensorimotor rhythms to control cursor movements. They found that a small subset of features chosen by stepwise regression produced r^2 values nearly as large as those produced by the entire feature set. They then showed that these results did generalize to online closed-loop performance.

Overall, these studies indicate that careful attention to selecting (from among the many features usually available) only those features most relevant to the specific BCI application helps to achieve translation algorithms that are simpler and perform better in online closed-loop operation.

EVALUATING ADAPTIVE ALGORITHMS

Several groups have explored the use of adaptive BCI translation algorithms. Their studies show that adaptation is beneficial and suggest which aspects of translation are most worthwhile to adapt. The superiority of adaptive algorithms is not surprising, since numerous factors can contribute to non-stationarities in the data. These factors include: technical factors such as variations in electrode placement or impedance; general user factors such as warm-up and fatigue and spontaneous variations; and application-specific user factors such as learning. Shenoy et al. (2006) showed that the statistics of the data may change between calibration and online control. To calibrate a linear discriminant algorithm, they asked subjects to engage in several motor-imagery tasks in response to visual stimuli and extracted features from the EEG data by a common spatial patterns analysis. They then used the algorithm online to move a cursor in a two-target application and found that the statistics of the data were different for calibration and online operation. They showed that performance was improved by using any of several simple adaptive procedures to update the parameters of the algorithm. It was not necessary to modify feature selection. They discussed factors likely to cause

differences between the calibration data and the online data, such as the greater demand for visual processing during online operation. The change in the data between calibration and online performance further emphasizes the importance of online closed-loop testing.

Linear regression algorithms are frequently employed in BCIs that use features derived from cortical single-neuron activity (e.g., neuronal firing rates [Serruya et al., 2002; Taylor et al., 2002]). Wu and Hatsopoulos (2008) examined single-neuron data offline from monkeys that had been operantly conditioned to perform a target-pursuit application. They showed that an adaptive Kalman filter was more accurate than stationary algorithms in predicting arm position, and they suggested that this reflects the fact that the motor system changes over time.

In an online study, Vidaurre et al. (2006) evaluated the effects of algorithm adaptation on performance of a two-target cursor-movement application controlled by spectral features of EEG recorded over sensorimotor cortex. They found that adaptive algorithms performed better than static algorithms. Furthermore, continuous adaptation was superior to periodic (i.e., between sessions) adaptation. They suggest that adaptive algorithms are particularly useful for training inexperienced BCI users, who often produce less stable patterns of brain activity.

At the same time, it is likely that adaptation is more important for some BCIs than for others. For example, learning effects appear to be much more prominent in BCIs that use sensorimotor rhythms than in those that use P300 responses. Thus, adaptive algorithms, especially those capable of continuous ongoing adaptation, are likely to be more valuable for sensorimotor rhythm-based BCIs.

DATA COMPETITIONS

The BCI research community has invested considerable effort in facilitating offline evaluations and comparisons of alternative BCI translation algorithms. In this vein, several data competitions have been organized (Sajda et al., 2003; Blankertz et al., 2004; Blankertz et al., 2006), with entries submitted by researchers from around the world. In these competitions several data sets, each consisting of data collected with a variety of closed-loop or open-loop paradigms (e.g., P300-based BCI data, sensorimotor rhythm-based BCI data, self-paced tapping data), are provided to the research community. Typically, a portion of each set is training data, and is provided with labels as to the correct BCI outputs, while the rest of the set comprises test data for which the correct outputs are not provided. The task of the contestants is to determine the correct outputs for the test data. Their performances in doing this determine the results of each competition.

In assessing the results of these competitions, Blankertz et al. (2004) noted that some entries had accuracy near chance on the test data, suggesting that their methods, although perhaps performing well with training data, did not generalize well to the test data. In contrast, other entries produced excellent results for the test data. Blankertz et al. (2006) also found that most of the competition winners employed linear methods (e.g.,

Fisher's linear discriminant or linear support vector machine). They also noted that several winning algorithms incorporated both time-domain and frequency domain measures.

Although these data competitions provide useful suggestions for algorithm improvements, it is still difficult to assess the relative merits of the approaches employed because, while the results depend in part on the algorithms employed, they also depend on how well the algorithms were implemented. In addition, since the entries differed in multiple respects (e.g., different preprocessing and signal extraction methods as well as different translation algorithms), the contribution of each difference to the superiority of one entry over another is often not clear. Moreover, since most of the BCI competition data sets have been rather small, the differences among the most successful entries have often not been statistically significant. Finally, because these competitions necessarily involve only offline evaluations, their results still require online closed-loop testing to establish their validity.

SUMMARY

A BCI translation algorithm uses features extracted from brain signals to produce device commands that convey the user's intent. The core component of an effective translation algorithm is an appropriate *model*. A model is a mathematical abstraction of the relationship between independent variables (i.e., brain signal features) and dependent variables (i.e., the user's intent as expressed by the BCI outputs). Depending on the BCI application, the model may produce discrete categorical outputs (i.e., classification) or continuous output along one or more dimensions (i.e., regression). Models may take many forms and may be simple or complex. The two other components of a translation algorithm are the method for *selecting the features* used by the model and the method for *determining the model's parameters* (e.g., the weights applied to the features).

The primary goal in developing a translation algorithm is to maximize its ability to generalize to new data, since BCIs must operate online in real time. Success in post-hoc data analysis, although helpful in developing an algorithm, is not sufficient. As an overall principle, generalizability increases as the amount of data used for parameterization increases, and it decreases as the number of features (and thus the number of parameters) increases. At the same time, changes over time in the brain signal features (e.g., due to spontaneous variations, learning, technical factors) may prompt the development and use of adaptive translation algorithms (e.g., algorithms that reparameterize their models periodically).

Linear models such as Fisher's discriminant analysis and multiple regression have been used in BCIs for some time. More recently, alternative approaches such as Bayesian methods and support vector machines have also become popular. Many trade-offs must be considered in selecting from among these general families of models, as well as in selecting features for and parameterizing a particular model. Complex models sometimes fit existing data better than simple models, but they may not generalize as well to new data. Limiting the model to only the most relevant signal features often improves its ability to generalize.

BCI development relies heavily on offline analyses of data gathered during BCI operation or during a wide variety of open-loop psychophysiological studies. These analyses can be extremely useful in comparing different models, different feature selection methods, and different parameterization methods. In this work, it is imperative to test alternative algorithms on data sets different from those used to parameterize them (i.e., it is necessary to cross-validate them).

At the same time, however, offline analysis cannot establish how well an algorithm will perform in actual online closed-loop operation, because it cannot reproduce the unpredictable ongoing interactions between the new algorithm and the BCI user. Thus, once offline analyses have identified the most promising algorithms, these algorithms should be assessed in actual online closed-loop evaluations. Whereas online studies of normal volunteers are useful and are often most practical, the BCI users most appropriate for these studies are the people with severe disabilities for whom BCI applications are primarily intended. Thus, they should be included whenever possible.

REFERENCES

Akaike, H. (1974) A new look at statistical model identification. *IEEE Transactions on Automation and Control, 19*, 716–723.

Besserve, M., Jerbi, K., Laurent, F., Baillet, S., Martinerie, J., and Garnero, L. (2007) Classification methods for ongoing EEG and MEG signals. *Biological Research, 40*, 415–437.

Bickel, P., and Levina, E. (2004) Some theory for Fisher's linear discriminant function, "naive Bayes," and some alternatives when there are many more variables than observations. *Bernoulli, 10*, 989–1010.

Birbaumer, N, Hinterberger, T., Kübler, A., and Newman, N. (2003) The thought-translation device: Neurobehavioral mechanisms and clinical outcomes. *IEEE Transactions on Neural Systems and Rehabilitation Engineering, 11*, 120–123.

Black, M J, and Donoghue, J.P. (2007) Probabilistic modeling and decoding neural population activity in motor cortex. In G. Dornhege, J. R. Millán, T. Hinterberger, D. J. McFarland, and K.-R. Müller (Eds.) *Toward Brain-Computer Interfacing*, Cambridge, MA: MIT Press, 147–159.

Blankertz, B., Dornege, G., Schafer, C., Krepki, R., Kohlmorgen, J., Müller, K-R., Kunzmann, V., Losch, F., and Curio, G. (2003) Boosting bit rates and error detection for the classification of fast-paced motor commands based on single-trial EEG analysis. *IEEE Transactions on Rehabilitation Engineering, 11*, 100–104.

Blankertz, B., Müller, K.-R., Curio, G., Vaughan, T.M., Schalk, G., Wolpaw, J.R., Schlogl, A., Neuper, C., Pfurtscheller, G., Hinterberger, T., Schroder, M., and Birbaumer, N. (2004) The BCI competition 2003: Progress and perspectives in detection and discrimination of EEG single trials. *IEEE Transactions on Biomedical Engineering, 51*, 1044–1051.

Blankertz, B., Müller, K.-R., Krusienski, D., Schalk, G., Wolpaw, J.R., Schlogl, A., Pfurtscheller, G., Millan, J., Schroder, M., and Birbaumer, N. (2006) The BCI competition III: Validating alternative approaches to actual BCI problems. *IEEE Transactions on Neural Systems and Rehabilitation Engineering, 14*, 153–159.

Donchin, E., Spencer, K.M., and Wijesinghe, R. (2000) The mental prosthesis: Assessing the speed of a P300-based brain-computer interface. *IEEE Transactions on Neural Systems and Rehabilitation Engineering, 8*, 174–179.

Fisher, R.A. (1936) The use of multiple measurements in taxonomic problems. *Annals of Eugenics, 7*, 179–188.

Friedman, L., and Wall, M. (2005) Graphical views of suppression and multicollinearity in multiple linear regression. *American Statistician, 59*, 127–136.

Haykin, S. (1996) *Adaptive Filter Theory*, Upper Saddle River, NJ: Prentice-Hall.

Kieseppa, I.A. (2001) Statistical model selection criteria and the philosophical problem of underdetermination. *British Journal of the Philosophy of Science, 52*, 761–794.

Krusienski, D.J., and Jenkins, W.K. (2005) Design and performance of adaptive systems based on structured stochastic optimization strategies. *IEEE Circuits and Systems Magazine, 5*, 8–20.

Krusienski, D., Sellers, E.W., Cabestaing, F., Bayoudh, S., McFarland, D.J., Vaughan, T.M., and Wolpaw, J.R. (2006) A comparison of classification techniques for the P300 speller. *Journal of Neural Engineering, 3*, 299–305.

Krusienski, D.J., Sellers, E.W., McFarland, D.J., Vaughan, T.M., and Wolpaw, J.R. (2008) Toward enhanced P300 speller performance, *Journal of Neuroscience Methods, 167*, 15–21.

Li, Y., Kambara, H., Koike, Y., and Sugiyama, M. (2010) Application of covariance shift adaptation techniques in brain-computer interfaces. *IEEE Transactions on Biomedical Engineering, 57*, 1318–1324.

Lotte, F., Congedo, M., Leuyer, A., Lmarche, F., and Arnaldi, B. (2007) A review of classification algorithms for EEG-based brain-computer interfaces, *Journal of Neural Engineering, 4*, 1–13.

Luce, R.D. (2003) Whatever happened to information theory in psychology, *Review of General Psychology, 7*, 183–188.

McFarland, D.J., Anderson, C.W., Müller, K.R., Schlogl, A., and Krusienski, D.J. (2006) BCI meeting 2005—Workshop on BCI signal processing: Feature extraction and translation. *IEEE Transactions on Neural Systems and Rehabilitation Engineering, 14*, 135–138.

McFarland, D.J., Krusienski, D.J., and Wolpaw, J.R. (2006) Brain-computer interface signal processing at the Wadsworth Center: Mu and sensorimotor beta rhythms. *Progress in Brain Research, 159*, 411–419.

McFarland, D.J., and Wolpaw, J.R. (2005) Sensorimotor rhythm-based brain-computer interface (BCI): Feature selection by regression improves performance. *IEEE Transactions on Neural Systems and Rehabilitation Engineering, 14*, 372–379.

Millán, J. del R., Franze, M., Mourino, J., Cincotti, F., and Babiloni, F. (2002) Relevant features for the classification of spontaneous motor-related tasks. *Biological Cybernetics, 86*, 89–05.

Müller, K.-R., Anderson, C.W., and Birch, G.E. (2003) Linear and nonlinear methods for brain-computer interfaces. *IEEE Transactions on Neural Systems and Rehabilitation Engineering, 11*, 165–169.

Müller, K.-R., Mika, S., Ratsch, G., Tsuda, K., and Scholkopf, B. (2001) An introduction to kernal-based learning algorithms. *IEEE Neural Networks, 12*, 181–201.

Parra, L.C., Spence, C.D., Gerson, A.D., and Sajda, P. (2005) Recipes for the linear analysis of EEG. *Neuroimage 28*, 326–341.

Pierce, J.R. (1980) *An Introduction to Information Theory*. New York: Dover Press.

Press, W.H., Teukolsky, S.A., Vetterling, W.T., and Flannery, B.P. (2007) *Numerical Recipes: The Art of Scientific Computing*. 3rd ed. New York: Cambridge University Press.

Principe, J.C., and McFarland, D.J. (2008) BMI/BCI modeling and signal processing. In: TW Berger, JK Chapin, DJ McFarland, JC Principe, WV Soussou, DM Taylor and PA Tresco (Eds.) *Brain-computer interfaces: An international assessment of research and development trends*. Berlin: Springer 47–64.

Sajda, P., Gerson, A., Müller, K-R., Blankertz, B., and Parra, L. (2003) A data analysis competition to evaluate machine learning algorithms for use in brain-computer interfaces. *IEEE Transactions on Neural Systems and Rehabilitation Engineering, 11*, 184–185.

Schalk, G., Leuthardt, E.C., Brunner, P., Ojemann, J.G., Gerhardt, L.A., and Wolpaw, J.R. (2008) Real-time detection of event-related brain activity. *NeuroImage, 43*, 245–249.

Schlogl, A., Neuper, C., and Pfurtscheller, G. (2002) Estimating the mutual information of an EEG-based brain-computer interface. *Biomedizinische Technik, 47*, 3–8.

Sellers, E.W., Krusienski, D.J., McFarland, D.J., Vaughan, T.M., and Wolpaw, J.R. (2006) A P300 event-related potential brain-computer interface (BCI): The effects of matrix size and inter stimulus interval on performance. *Biological Psychology, 73*, 242–252.

Serruya, M.D., Hatsopoulos, N.G., Paminski, L., Fellows, M.R., and Donoghue, J.P., (2002) Instant neural control of a movement signal. *Nature, 416*, 1411–1142.

Shannon, C.E., and Weaver, W. (1964) *The Mathematical Theory of Communication*. Urbana, IL: University of Illinois Press.

Shenoy, P., Krauledat, M., Blankertz, B., Rao, R.P., and Müller, K-R. (2006) Towards adaptive classification for BCI. *Journal of Neural Engineering, 3*, 13–23.

Shenoy, P., and Rao, R.P.N. (2005) Dynamic bayesian networks for brain-computer interfaces. In L. K. Saul, Y. Weiss, and L. Bottou (Eds.). *Advances in Neural Information Processing Systems*, Vol. 17. Cambridge, MA: MIT Press, 1265–1272.

Stoica, P., and Selen, Y. (2004) Model order selection: A review of information criterion rules. *IEEE Signal Processing Magazine 21(4)*, 36–47.

Taylor, D.M., Tilery, S.I.H., and Schwartz, A.B. (2002) Direct cortical control of 3D neuroprosthetic devices. *Science, 296*, 1829–1832.

Tibshirani, R. (1996) Regression shrinkage and selection via the Lasso. *Journal of the Royal Statistical Society, Series B, 58*, 267–288.

Vidaurre, C., Scherer, R., Cabeza, R., Schlogl, A., and Pfurtscheller, G. (2007) Study of discriminant analysis applied to motor imagery bipolar data. *Medical and Biological Engineering and Computing, 45*, 61–68.

Vidaurre, C., Schlogl, A., Cabeza, R., Scherer, R., and Pfurtscheller, G. (2006) A fully on-line adaptive BCI. *IEEE Transactions on Biomedical Engineering, 53*, 1214–1219.

Wolpaw, J.R., Birbaumer, N., McFarland, D.J., Pfurtscheller, G., and Vaughan, T.M. (2002) Brain-computer interfaces for communication and control. *Clinical Neurophysioogy, 113*, 767–791.

Wolpaw, JR and McFarland, DJ. (2004) Control of a two-dimensional movement signal by a noninvasive brain-computer interface in humans. *Proceedings of the National Academy of Sciences, 101*, 17849–17854.

Wu, W., and Hatosopoulos, N.G. (2008) Real-time decoding of nonstationary neural activity in motor cortex. *IEEE Transactions on Neural Systems and Rehabilitation Engineering, 16*, 213–222.

9 | BCI HARDWARE AND SOFTWARE

J. ADAM WILSON, CHRISTOPH GUGER, AND GERWIN SCHALK

Hardware and software are critically important in implementing brain-computer interfaces (BCIs) and in ensuring that they function effectively in real time. Indeed, the recent advent and wide availability of powerful, inexpensive hardware and software are some of the principal factors responsible for the recent explosive growth in BCI research and development. BCI hardware provides the physical means through which brain signals are acquired, digitized, stored, and analyzed. It typically includes the sensors that detect brain activity, an amplifier with an analog-to-digital converter, a computer that processes the digitized signals, and the cables that connect these components to one another. BCI software controls the storage and analysis of the digitized signals and their conversion into outputs that achieve the user's intent.

Effective development of BCI hardware and software presents some challenges that are often not present in the development of other technologies. For example, since it is as yet unclear which sensor modalities, which brain signals, and which processing methods are optimal for any given BCI application, it is necessary to evaluate and compare the efficacy of many different sensors, brain signals, and processing methods. At the same time, there is little commercial interest in exploring these issues since the target BCI-user population is relatively small. In many ways this situation mirrors that of the early days of computer technology, a time that was characterized by small market opportunities and little technical standardization. Success in such early stages of development hinges on the capacity to quickly evaluate and compare many different promising options. As a result, a crucial function of BCI technology is to ensure not only that a given BCI system can be implemented but also that this implementation can be accomplished rapidly and efficiently. In other words, it is essential to optimize the processes that transform new BCI designs into functioning implementations.

Such process optimizations may be achieved with widely available and widely applicable sets of clearly defined technical specifications and the tools based on those specifications. For example, in early computer development, the introduction of the RS-232 standard for serial connectivity, and connectors based on that standard, removed the need to develop a new communication protocol for every new printer or other device, thereby greatly facilitating the subsequent development and use of all kinds of input/output devices. Similarly, use of appropriate sets of specifications and tools for hardware and software should also be useful in BCI development, particularly as development of new BCI systems becomes progressively more complex.

To work successfully, such sets of specifications and tools must satisfy two criteria. First, they need to be applicable to a well-defined and large set of needs. For example, specifications of a unique electrode configuration that are applicable to only a very small range of needs would likely find only limited use. In contrast, specifications for connectors (e.g., for implanted devices or EEG caps) could be used for a wide range of BCI applications, and thus wide adoption is more likely. Second, such technical specifications need to be accompanied by a number of implementations that can be readily used. For the example of the connector specifications, these implementations may be physical connectors in different shapes and sizes, adapters for other common connectors, and so forth. For BCI software, technical specifications should be accompanied by a set of software implementations that realize the technical specifications. In addition to these two criteria, the technical specifications and their implementations must be properly communicated to the engineers who build the BCI systems.

This chapter discusses the key components of the hardware and software currently used in BCI research and design, and it describes evaluation procedures that can help ensure that research BCI systems perform as desired. (Other BCI systems, such as those used for commercial purposes, will likely incorporate a closed system consisting of a digital signal processing [DSP] chip, a field-programmable gate array [FPGA], or other fixed solutions tightly integrated with the amplifier and device output or display [Brunner et al., 2011].) The chapter is divided into three major sections. The first section covers BCI hardware and describes the sensors that detect brain signals, the components that amplify and digitize these signals, the interface hardware that connects different components, and the client hardware that runs BCI software. The second section covers BCI software and describes: the data acquisition components that record, digitize, and store brain signals; the signal-analysis components that extract signal features that represent the user's intent and that translate these features into commands that embody the user's intent; the output components that realize that intent; and the operating protocol that determines the configuration, parameterization, and timing of operation. This section also presents important principles for designing BCI software and lists software tools currently used for BCI research. Finally, a section on evaluation procedures describes the components of the timing characteristics of a

BCI system and the procedures to evaluate them, with representative results.

HARDWARE

SENSORS

Sensors detect physiological signals and transform them into voltages that can be amplified and digitized for processing by a computer so that they can ultimately provide useful output signals. Most BCI systems use electrophysiological sensors (e.g., electroencephalographic [EEG] electrodes, electrocorticographic [ECoG] electrode grids, or micro-, needle, or wire electrodes). BCIs can also use sensors that detect magnetic or metabolic signals, (e.g., magnetoencephalography [MEG] (Mellinger et al., 2007), functional near-infrared spectroscopy [fNIRS], or functional magnetic resonance imaging [fMRI]). Because most current BCIs use electrophysiological signals, the discussion presented here focuses primarily on electrophysiological techniques. Methods using nonelectrical sensors are discussed in chapters 4 and 18 as well as in chapter 3 of this volume (MEG).

In all electrophysiological techniques, electrodes detect the electrical voltage generated by neuronal activity and pass it to the amplification unit. Although the different types of electrodes share similar operating principles in serving this function, their design (e.g., size, material, geometry) usually depends on the recording location (e.g., the scalp, the cortical surface, or within the cortex) and the application for which they are used. Figure 9.1 shows four types of sensors. For EEG

recordings (fig. 9.1A), the electrodes are placed on the scalp and are not in direct electrical contact with the conductive tissue, so conductive electrode gel is usually applied between the electrode and the skin (although "dry electrodes," not using gels, are currently under development [e.g., (Popescu et al., 2007; Taheri et al., 1994)]). Other sensors, such as ECoG electrodes (fig. 9.1B) or microelectrodes (figs. 9.1C and D), are in direct electrical contact with conductive tissue and thus do not require conductive gels. Figure 9.2 shows the locations of EEG, ECoG, and intracortical electrodes.

Sensors do not measure the electrical potential at a single electrode but, rather, the potential difference between two electrodes (see chapters 3 and 6, this volume). Different electrode configurations (or *montages*) are used depending on the electrode type and location and on the kind of information to be obtained from the recording. The two most commonly used configurations are called *monopolar* and *bipolar* montages (although as explained in chapter 3, all recordings of voltage are, strictly speaking, bipolar since they necessarily measure a potential difference between two locations). In a *bipolar* montage, the signal recorded from each electrode is the potential difference between it and another electrode placed over a different brain area. In this case both electrodes are usually sensitive to brain activity, that is, both are considered to be *signal* electrodes. In contrast, in a *monopolar* montage, the signal recorded from each electrode is the potential difference between it and a designated *reference* (or *common*) electrode, which is most often placed at some distance from the brain. The reference electrode is usually considered to be neutral

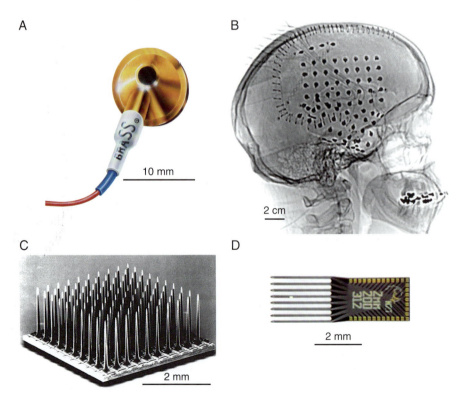

A

B

C

D

10 mm

2 cm

2 mm

2 mm

Figure 9.1 *(A) A single EEG electrode (image courtesy of Grass Technologies, West Warwick, RI) (B) X-ray showing two implanted subdural Ad-Tech ECoG electrode grids and a short strip of 4 electrodes (Ad-Tech, Racine, WI). (C) The Utah/Cyberkinetics microelectrode array (Maynard et al., 1997). (D) One configuration of the Michigan microelectrode array (Kipke et al., 2003).*

(i.e., largely insensitive to brain activity) (see chapter 6 of this volume for full discussion of this complex issue). (An example of a nonneutral reference is the mastoid in an EEG experiment that involves activity in auditory cortices [which are located near the mastoid].) Thus, in a bipolar montage every signal electrode is referenced to another signal electrode. In contrast, in a monopolar montage, every signal electrode is referenced to a neutral electrode. These configurations can be used whether one is acquiring signals by EEG, ECoG, or microelectrode recording. (It should be noted that, in traditional EEG parlance, signal and reference electrodes were often referred to as *active* and *inactive* electrodes. However, at present the term *active* is generally used as defined later in this chapter, and *inactive* has largely disappeared.)

ELECTROENCEPHALOGRAPHY
Introduction to EEG

The most common method for recording brain signals in humans is electroencephalography (EEG), which is noninvasive, safe, and relatively inexpensive. EEG is recorded with electrodes placed on the scalp. It is the summation of the electrical activity of thousands to many millions of synapses, neurons, and axons in the underlying brain, particularly the cortex, that produces detectable scalp voltages, as described in chapter 3 (Fisch and Spehlmann, 1999). Many factors influence the overall quality of the signal, including the strengths of the sources and their distances from the electrodes, the locations of the electrodes on the scalp, the electrical impedances of the electrodes and of the tissues between them and the sources, and the recording montage. It is estimated that at least 6 cm^2 of synchronized cortical activity is required to generate a reliably detected scalp potential (Nunez and Srinivasan, 2006). Chapters 3 and 6 in this volume discuss the basic principles of EEG recording in detail. Here, we review the types of EEG electrode types, their electrical characteristics, and their placement.

EEG Electrode Design

As discussed in chapter 6, EEG electrodes can be made of different metal or metal/metal-salt combinations; the choice of metal can have a significant impact on the type and quality of recordings. The most commonly used EEG electrodes are made of gold, tin, or silver/silver-chloride (Ag/AgCl) (fig. 9.1A). Gold and tin electrodes are maintenance-free and have a good frequency response for most EEG purposes. For recording EEG signals that include frequencies below 0.1 Hz, Ag/AgCl electrodes provide superior results. In order to reduce large offset (i.e., DC) potentials, all electrodes connected to the same amplifier should use the same material. Nonetheless, even when identical materials are used, small offset potentials can be accentuated by movement artifacts, as described later in this chapter.

EEG electrodes can be *passive* or *active*. *Passive electrodes* are simply metal disks (made of either tin, silver, silver/silver chloride, or gold-plated silver) that are connected to an amplifier by a cable. A good electrode-scalp interface is critical for obtaining good recordings. This is achieved by cleaning or lightly abrading the skin and using conducting gels at the interface between the scalp and the electrode to allow current to travel from the scalp to the sensor and then along the cable to the amplifier. Since the amplitude of brain signals is small, they are susceptible to contamination by movements of the cable and by environmental electromagnetic noise such as power-line interference. Thus, it is often important to shield, shorten, and stabilize the cable. Passive electrodes are relatively inexpensive and are used in the vast majority of clinical and research EEG recordings.

In contrast, *active electrodes* contain a preamplifier with a 1–10× gain built inside the electrode. Although this added component itself adds some noise (because the input impedance and the signals are larger), it also makes the electrode considerably less sensitive to such factors as environmental noise and cable movements. Consequently, active electrodes can perform well in environments with higher environmental noise or higher electrode-skin impedance. Like passive electrodes, active electrodes require gel at the interface between the scalp and the electrode.

The gels used with EEG electrodes are necessary but not ideal for long-term recording because they usually dry out and stop functioning after some time. Thus, a number of research groups are trying to develop *dry electrodes*, i.e., electrodes that do not require gel. Although these efforts have produced encouraging results indicating the feasibility of dry electrodes (e.g., Fonseca et al., 2007; Luo and Sullivan, 2010; Popescu et al., 2007; see also chapter 6, in this volume), there is at present no robust and widely available dry electrode for EEG recording. Researchers are also investigating water-based electrodes, which will simplify EEG setup and clean-up (Volosyak et al., 2010).

The impedance of the skin-electrode junction is called the *electrode impedance*. It is the opposition to alternating current and is measured in units of ohms (Ω). This impedance between the scalp and the electrode is one of the most important factors determining the quality and stability of EEG recordings. The conducting electrode gel placed between the electrode and the scalp decreases the impedance and allows current to travel more easily from the scalp to the sensor. Impedance is measured between two electrodes placed on the scalp. That is, for so-called *monopolar recordings*, it may be measured between the so-called *signal electrode* and the so-called *reference electrode*, between a pair of signal electrodes (for so-called *bipolar* recordings), or between one signal electrode and all the others. The impedance is frequency dependent. The specific frequency used to define the impedance of a system varies from one manufacturer to another but is typically in the range of around 20 Hz. The impedance depends on the surface area of the electrodes, the condition and preparation of the skin, the properties of the gel, and the amount of time that has lapsed since electrode placement. Sometimes the skin is slightly abraded (e.g., with an abrasive electrode paste or a blunt needle) to decrease impedance. Electrode gels containing NaCl in concentrations of 5–10% can also help in reducing impedance. For good EEG recording, the impedance should be below 5000 Ω (Fisch and Spehlmann, 1999).

EEG Electrode Placement and Signal Characteristics

The maintenance of secure and stable electrode placement on the scalp is one of the most critical requirements in

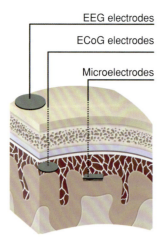

EEG electrodes
ECoG electrodes
Microelectrodes

Figure 9.2 Different BCI recording modalities. EEG electrodes, ECoG electrodes, and intracortical microelectrodes are placed in different locations. (Modified from Leuthardt et al., 2006b.)

EEG recording. Along with high impedance, unstable placement is one of the most common causes of poor or artifact-laden EEG recordings. Many research and clinical groups use commercially available electrode caps (e.g., Electro-Cap International, Eaton, OH; g.tec, Graz, Austria), which allow for fast and accurately positioned placement of the electrodes. Most caps use the standard International 10–20 system of electrode placement (see chapter 6 and Klem et al., 1999) or an extended version of that system (Oostenveld and Praamstra, 2001; Sharbrough et al., 1991). Many caps come with built-in electrodes at fixed locations, as shown in figure 9.3, right, but have the disadvantage of the inflexibility of the montage and the difficulty of replacing an electrode in case of failure. Other caps (fig. 9.3, left) have many locations into which the individual electrodes must be screwed. The advantage of these caps is that many different montages can be implemented, individual electrodes can be easily replaced in the event of failure, and electrode height can be adjusted as needed to reduce impedance; on the other hand, each electrode must be inserted or removed independently, and the wires must be brought together and properly handled so as to minimize environmental noise and movement artifacts.

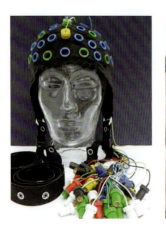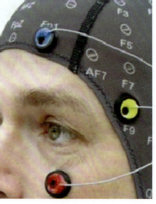

Figure 9.3 (Right) Electrode cap with built-in electrodes giving a specific montage. (Left) Electrode cap with many sites for individual screwed-in electrodes.

EEG signals typically have an amplitude of 10–20 µV, a spatial resolution on the scale of centimeters, and a bandwidth of 0–70 Hz (i.e., they record signals in this frequency range). These relatively poor signal characteristics are the result of volume conduction through the tissue between the brain and the electrode. As the EEG signals pass through the dura, fluids, skull, and skin, the signals spread and blur. Furthermore, the tissue acts as a low-pass filter, attenuating fast high-frequency components of the signal. Therefore, EEG can provide information only about the electrical activity of the brain over large, highly synchronous areas.

ELECTROCORTICOGRAM
Introduction to ECoG

The electrocorticogram (ECoG) is recorded from electrodes that are surgically implanted below the skull. The electrodes are placed either above the dura (i.e., *epidural*) or below the dura (i.e., *subdural*). Because placement of the electrodes requires surgery, ECoG recording in humans is typically accomplished by recording from patients who have such electrodes implanted for short periods (up to 1–2 weeks) for clinical-evaluation reasons. These are usually people who are under evaluation for surgery for epilepsy or tumor abatement and who are interested in participating in a research protocol. Since this population is limited, many fewer subjects are available for BCI studies with ECoG than with EEG.

ECoG Electrode Design

ECoG electrodes used in humans are typically made of platinum, silver, or stainless steel and are available in strip or grid configurations (e.g., 64 electrodes arranged in an 8 × 8 array; see fig. 9.1B) (see chapter 15 of this volume). The electrodes in the array are embedded into a thin and flexible silastic sheet. Each exposed recording site is generally about 2–3 mm in diameter, with interelectrode distances of 5–10 mm. Each individual electrode connects to a ribbon cable that is several feet long and connects to the amplifier and digitizer. Several research groups have begun to build ECoG recording arrays using photolithographic procedures with highly flexible, biocompatible substrates such as polyimide, and electrode sites with materials such as platinum (Kim et al., 2007; Rubehn et al., 2009). Although these new designs have provided very encouraging results in animal studies, they are not yet approved for use in humans. Since ECoG arrays include many different electrode configurations that are chosen based on the clinical needs of each individual patient, there is little standardization among the configurations used for ECoG BCI studies.

ECoG Electrode Placement Signal Characteristics

Since ECoG electrodes are implanted in humans for clinical purposes (e.g., for localizing seizure foci and functional mapping in patients with epilepsy [Crone et al., 1998] or for continuous stimulation for patients with chronic intractable pain [Stadler et al., 2010; Tsubokawa et al., 1991]), the clinical goals for the patient, not the research goals, must always be the highest priority. Despite the resulting disadvantages, ECoG recording has many advantages. First, compared to EEG sensors, ECoG recording sensors are located closer to the sources of the brain signals recorded. Second, ECoG signals have amplitudes that are higher than those recorded with EEG (e.g., a maximum of 50–100 µV for ECoG, compared to 10–20 µV for EEG [Leuthardt et al., 2004b]). Third, spatial resolution is on the scale of millimeters, versus the cm scale used for EEG (Freeman et al., 2000; Slutzky et al., 2010). Finally, ECoG can record a frequency bandwidth up to at least 250 Hz (Leuthardt et al., 2004a) compared to EEG's bandwidth maximum of about 70 Hz. It is these superior characteristics that explain the use of ECoG in preoperative evaluation for brain surgery. At the same time, they have facilitated investigations in BCI research and other areas.

ECoG is typically recorded in a monopolar configuration; signals are referenced to an electrode located either over a functionally silent area of cortex or placed subdermally (i.e., under the skin but outside the skull). Because ECoG signals have relatively large amplitudes and are recorded inside the skull, they are not very susceptible to noise from sources outside the brain when the electrodes have a good ground electrode. Moreover, as in EEG recordings, the reference electrode should be placed in an area in which voltage is not modulated by the experimental conditions.

INTRACORTICAL RECORDING

Introduction to Intracortical Recording

Microelectrodes surgically implanted within the brain are used to record extracellular neuronal action potentials (spikes) or local field potentials (LFPs). These microelectrodes (figs. 9.1 and 9.2) consist of an exposed conductive metallic area placed on an insulated substrate; both the electrode metal and the insulated structure can vary based on the fabrication method and experimental application. With a few notable exceptions (e.g., Hochberg et al., 2006; Kennedy et al., 2004), BCI studies with this recording technology have been limited to animals (i.e., mainly rodents and monkeys). As described in detail in chapter 5, microelectrodes can be fabricated by different procedures and in different configurations: individual microwires with a distant reference; twisted wires that produce a tetrode configuration (Harris et al., 2000); silicon micromachined arrays such as the Utah array (Nordhausen et al., 1996) (fig. 9.1C), MEMS-based silicon arrays such as the Michigan electrode array (Wise et al., 1970) (fig. 9.1D); and the cone electrode, in which a standard wire electrode is placed inside a hollow glass cone, into which cortical neurites grow (Kennedy, 1989). The Utah array and Michigan electrodes have become widely used for chronic intracortical recordings. Each electrode system has an array of electrodes that varies in geometry, dimension, and electrode count. The Utah array is designed as a "bed-of-needles," in which the recording sites are placed in a 10 × 10 flat plane, and generally record at a single depth in cortex (see fig. 9.1C). Each electrode needle is typically 1.2 mm long, with an exposed surface of 50 µm, and approximately 400 µm between adjacent needles. Conversely, the Michigan electrode has recording sites placed at different depths on one or more probes, allowing recordings in three dimensions. The Michigan electrode array typically has at least 16 electrode sites and can have more than 64. The site spacing and diameters vary depending on the application (e.g., whether spikes or LFPs are being recorded).

Intracortical Electrode Design. A wide range of materials are used for the electrode sites and for the electrode support

structure. Microwire arrays are commonly made of stainless steel or tungsten. The Utah array uses Teflon™-insulated platinum-iridium wires soldered to a silicon micromachined base. The Michigan electrode array consists of a silicon-substrate base with gold leads and iridium recording sites deposited by photolithography. Cone electrodes use an insulated gold wire placed in a hollow glass cone.

Due to the small dimensions of their exposed recording areas, microelectrodes have very high impedances—hundreds of kilohms to several megohms. Thus, the signals are usually amplified by a preamplifier located as close as possible to the electrode prior to transmission to the main amplifier. This reduces environmental noise from the signal (e.g., 60- or 50-Hz power-line noise and movement artifacts), since the brain signal is amplified before the noise is introduced.

Intracortical Signal Characteristics

Two of the most important limitations of microelectrode recordings are the technical demands imposed by the recording and processing from many sites at high bandwidth (e.g., 25–50 kHz) and the difficulties of establishing and maintaining recordings from individual neurons over longer periods.

In the recording of action potentials the quality of the recording is typically assessed by the signal-to-noise ratio (SNR) (see chapter 7 in this volume), which is the ratio of the signal amplitude (i.e., the peak-to-peak amplitude of an action potential) to the noise amplitude (i.e., the background noise). An acceptable standard deviation of the background noise may be 10–20 µV, whereas desired action-potential amplitudes are on the order of 100 µV or more.

AMPLIFIERS

Brain signals have relatively small amplitudes (e.g., 10–20 µV for EEG; 50–100 µV for ECoG, 1 µV for evoked potentials). Thus, after they are detected by an electrode, and before they can be used by a computer in a BCI application, they must first be *amplified* (and perhaps filtered) and *digitized*. Signal amplification, and (depending on the system design) signal digitization, are accomplished by the *biosignal amplifier*.

The biosignal amplifier must amplify the source signal without distortion, and it must suppress noise as much as possible. Amplifiers have either analog outputs or an integrated analog-to-digital conversion (ADC) unit. When an amplifier is used for recordings in humans, it must be safe and properly approved for human use. This is particularly important when invasive recording methods are used (e.g., in the case of ECoG and intracortical recordings), since the electrodes make direct contact with brain tissue and must be electrically isolated from any power sources.

AMPLIFIER DESIGN

Biosignal amplifiers used for neural recordings are instrumentation amplifiers. They are differential amplifiers (i.e., measuring a potential difference) and have high-impedance input buffers and a high common-mode rejection ratio (CMMR). The CMMR is the measure of how well a differential amplifier rejects a common signal present on both input leads.

A *channel* consists of a pair of electrodes, and the amplifier measures the difference in potential between those two electrodes. Ideally, the amplifier should augment only those signals that differ between the two input electrodes, and it should attenuate or eliminate the signal components that are common to both signals. The CMRR is typically between 60 and 110 dB (i.e., between 99.9% and 99.9997% of a potential that is common to the two electrodes is eliminated). Additional electronics applied to individual electrodes before the instrumentation amplifier (e.g., a preamplifier or other filtering) may introduce different gains on each channel, and therefore reduce the CMRR of the amplifier.

For EEG recording with 128 electrodes on the scalp, an amplifier with 128 *channels* contains 128 inputs for the electrodes, as well as an input for the so-called reference electrode and an input for the ground. For BCIs, amplifiers with fewer channels (e.g., 8 or 16) can be used quite effectively. A typical instrumentation amplifier is shown in figure 9.4. This amplifier includes a buffering stage and an amplification stage. The buffering stage consists of a high-impedance input buffer that uses a voltage follower circuit for each signal input. Because this high impedance allows only an insignificant amount of current to flow into the amplifier, it prevents a high-resistance source from being loaded down (i.e., dissipated) (Clark and Webster, 1995). The amplification stage, which follows buffering, amplifies the difference between the two input signals. The equation for the differential gain of this amplifier is given by:

$$V_0 = \left(1 + \frac{2R_1}{R_g}\right)\frac{R_s}{R_2}(V_2 - V_1)$$

(9.1)

In EEG recordings, electrodes are typically placed on the scalp with 2.5–10 cm between adjacent electrodes, and the ground electrode is usually placed elsewhere on the head (e.g., on the forehead or the mastoid behind the ear). A typical montage is shown in figure 9.4. All EEG recordings measure the *difference* in potential between two electrodes. As already noted, the convention is to call EEG recording *monopolar* when an electrode potential is compared to that of a so-called reference electrode that is placed at an electrically distant location, and to call EEG *bipolar* when an electrode potential is compared to that of any one of the other so-called signal electrodes on the head (see chapters 3 and 6 in this volume). In either case, each *channel* consists of a pair of electrodes, and the amplifier measures the difference in potential between them. Typically, for bipolar recording, EEG amplitude is 5–20 μV depending on the scalp location, interelectrode distance, and the underlying brain activity. Bipolar recordings are less sensitive to widespread noise and other artifacts and are more sensitive to localized brain activity.

In so-called monopolar recordings, all the channels of the amplifier use as their negative input a common, or reference, electrode that is often placed on the ear lobe or mastoid (fig. 9.5). The other electrodes are connected to the positive inputs of the amplifier channels. As in the bipolar montage, the ground electrode is usually located on the head. Monopolar EEG recordings typically have amplitudes up to 50 μV. Monopolar recordings are more sensitive to broadly distributed EEG activity as well as to widespread noise and other artifacts and are less sensitive to localized brain activity. Nevertheless, monopolar recording has a significant advantage: because all the channels use the same reference, the

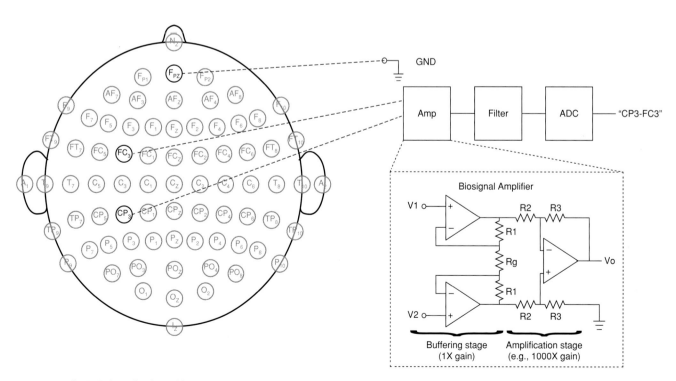

Figure 9.4 *Bipolar EEG channel with amplifier. In this example, the potential difference between electrodes CP3 and FC3 combine to make channel (CP3-FC3). Electrode FPz is used as the ground. The differential amplifier circuit is also shown.*

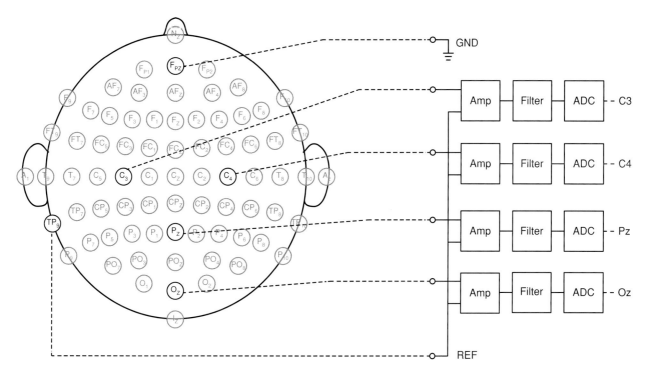

Figure 9.5 Electrode montage for monopolar EEG recording. In this example, the electrodes C3, C4, Pz, and Oz are all referenced to a mastoid electrode (TP9). Electrode FPz is used as the ground. Refer to figure 9–4 for the amplifier circuit.

digitized signals can be used to reconstruct with software any desired montage. By this means it is possible to focus on EEG components with particular spatial-distribution characteristics (e.g., McFarland et al., 1997) (see chapter 7 of this volume for discussion of spatial filtering).

In most cases, EEG amplifiers can also be used to record ECoG signals, which have characteristics similar to those of EEG in terms of bandwidth, amplitude, and impedance (all within about one order of magnitude of EEG). However, there are a few important differences. First, ECoG signals, particularly those used for BCIs, contain high-frequency information (e.g., 70–250 Hz) not seen in EEG recordings, which typically have a low-pass cutoff (see chapter 7) of around 70 Hz or lower. Therefore, the amplifier filtering must allow high-frequency signals to pass through unattenuated. Second, the anti-aliasing filter (see chapter 7) must have a higher low-pass cutoff and the sampling rate must be high enough to record high-frequency signals.

Amplifier designs for intracortical recordings also have specific requirements. First, very high sampling rates are required by the ADC (>25 kHz), so an appropriate anti-aliasing filter must be incorporated. Second, the type of signal being recorded may affect the required filtering. For example, single-unit recordings typically remove all low-frequency signals (e.g., less than 300 Hz), in order to retain only the spike waveforms. Because the electrode arrays used for single-unit recordings can also record LFPs, the amplifier must be designed specifically for the type of recorded signal and the application. However, it is also possible to record the wideband signal, and then perform digital filtering later in software.

AMPLIFIER REQUIREMENTS

The amplifier input impedance should be much higher than the electrode impedance (i.e., the impedance of the electrode-scalp interface). If it is not, the signal will be significantly attenuated. EEG or ECoG electrode impedance is normally in the range of 0.10–20 kΩ (at 1 kHz). The amplifier input impedance should be at least 100 times larger than this (i.e., at least several megohms). The amplifier input impedance should be correspondingly higher for electrodes that have higher impedances, such as microelectrodes for recording from individual neurons. In such cases preamplifiers with very high input impedances are often used; the buffering stage in the differential amplifier shown in figure 9.4 satisfies this requirement.

An important consideration in choosing an amplification system is the number of channels required. This is determined in part by the type of signal to be recorded and processed. For example, eight or fewer channels may be sufficient for EEG components such as slow waves or P300 evoked responses that have low spatial frequencies (Birbaumer et al., 2000; Guger et al., 2003; Krusienski et al., 2006; Pfurtscheller et al, 1997). The number of channels needed also helps determine the signal-analysis methods that should be used. For example, algorithms that integrate information from different cortical sites (e.g., common spatial patterns [CSP]) require more channels (Guger et al., 2000; McFarland and J. R. Wolpaw, 2003; Ramoser et al., 2000). ECoG and neuronal recordings often use 16 to several hundred channels (Campbell et al., 1989; Leuthardt et al., 2004a; Rousche et al., 2001). Many modern amplification systems provide many channels and high per-channel sampling rates (e.g., systems made by such vendors as Plexon, g.tec, Tucker-Davis Technologies, and Alpha-Omega). At the same time, the amplitude resolution and dynamic range of the ADC can have a significant effect on the bandwidth of the signals recorded. For example, ADCs with 16-bit resolution are often unable to accurately record DC potentials. In contrast, ADCs with 24-bit resolution have a sufficient input range to prevent saturation when presented with large DC potentials, while they still maintain the resolution for recording small and fast potential changes. As a result, most 16-bit ADCs have a high-pass filter applied prior to digitization to remove the DC offset potential. Therefore, BCIs that use low-frequency waves should consider whether or not a 16-bit ADC is appropriate.

ANALOG-TO-DIGITAL CONVERSION

The signals that are recorded from the brain are analog signals, and are normally converted to digital signals before any further processing. This analog to digital conversion is called *digitization. Digitization* is performed by an analog-to-digital converter (ADC). An ADC digitizes signals from each electrode many times per second; this is called the sampling rate. For example, an ADC with a sampling rate of 256 Hz acquires 256 samples per second, or one sample every 1/256th of a second (i.e., one every 4 msec). As discussed in chapter 7, to accurately acquire and reconstruct the information present in the signal, the sampling frequency must meet the requirements of the *Nyquist* criterion, that is, it must be at least two times larger than the highest frequency occurring in the signal. If the Nyquist criterion is not satisfied, that is, if the signal contains frequency components higher than half the sampling rate, then the digital signal will be distorted by *aliasing* (see chapter 7). When aliasing occurs, digitized signals with frequencies that are higher than half the sampling rate masquerade as signals of lower frequency. It is then impossible, in the digital version of the signal, to distinguish between an aliased signal and an actual low-frequency signal. In practice, the sampling rate should be several times higher than the signal of interest, since the anti-aliasing filter (next section) is not perfect and does not completely eliminate higher-frequency signals.

FILTERING

Biological signals typically contain a large range of frequencies. Thus, it is necessary either to digitize them at a very high sampling rate or to remove nonessential higher-frequency information with an *anti-aliasing* filter prior to digitization. For example, since scalp-recorded EEG signals are largely limited to frequencies below 100 Hz, higher-frequency activity in EEG recordings is mainly non-EEG noise (such as electromyographic [EMG] activity). This unwanted activity can be removed by applying an anti-aliasing filter with a *corner frequency* (see below) of 100 Hz to the signal prior to digitization. The signal can then be safely digitized with a relatively modest sampling rate of at least 200 Hz. In contrast, neuronal action potentials contain relevant information at frequencies up to several kilohertz; thus, the filter frequency range and sampling rate need to be much higher for neuronal action potentials than for EEG. In sum, the choice of digitization parameters is determined by the kind of signals being recorded and the frequency-sensitivity characteristics of the sensor that records them (e.g., EEG electrodes, ECoG electrodes, or microelectrodes).

In addition to anti-aliasing filters, amplification systems may incorporate additional analog filters that limit signal content to specific frequency ranges. Analog filters can be constructed using resistors, capacitors, and inductors, but because of the physical size of inductors, most amplifiers use filters with only resistors and capacitors. These are called *RC filters*. RC filters make it possible to block some frequencies (e.g., frequencies that contain noise) while allowing others to pass. It is relatively simple to construct them in different configurations and with different resistors and capacitors that together determine the particular frequencies that are blocked. The two possible types of RC filter are called *low-pass* and *high-pass* filters. As the names suggest, *low-pass* filters allow low frequencies to pass while blocking higher frequencies; in contrast, *high-pass* filters allow high frequencies to pass while blocking lower frequencies (e.g., the direct current [DC] component of the signal). Low-pass and high-pass filters can also be combined to create what are called *bandpass* filters. When low-pass and high-pass filters are combined to eliminate a narrow frequency band, they create what are called *notch* filters. In contrast to *bandpass* filters, which let a range of frequencies pass, notch filters block a range of frequencies and are often used to suppress interference from 50-Hz or 60-Hz power lines.

It is important to select an analog filter (e.g., Bessel, Butterworth, or Chebychev designs) with characteristics appropriate for the signal and the application. Analog filters are characterized by their *order*, their *corner frequencies*, and their *phase* (Thomas et al., 2004). A filter's *order* is the number of stages of the filter (i.e., the number of times the filter is applied in succession). A filter's *corner frequency* is the transition frequency between the passed and blocked range: it is the frequency at which the signal amplitude is attenuated by 3 dB compared to the peak amplitude (i.e., it is reduced to 29.3% of the peak amplitude). A filter's *phase* specifies the frequency-dependent time displacements it produces (i.e., how much it delays a component of a specific frequency). A higher filter order is more effective in suppressing unwanted frequencies but produces larger phase shifts in the signal. Filters with high orders can also be unstable.

For several reasons it is often advantageous to use analog filters prior to digitization instead of applying the digital filters after digitization. First, analog filters are required to prevent aliasing (i.e., a digital filter cannot be applied to a digital signal to remove aliasing because aliasing occurs in the digitization process). Second, digital filters may become unstable due to the rounding errors of the digital processor. On the other hand, digital filters do not eliminate the original signal (i.e., it is always possible to go back to the original unfiltered digitized data), whereas analog filters (which are incorporated into the amplification system) do not permit going back to the original unfiltered data (i.e., the only data available are the filtered data). Furthermore, it is easy to apply a variety of different digital filters to the same data and compare the results. Like analog filters, digital filters can be characterized by their order, corner

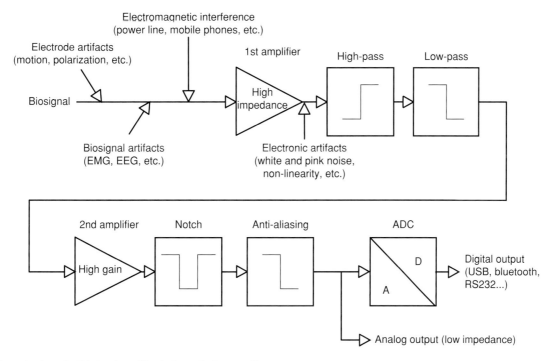

Figure 9.6 *Schematic of a typical biosignal amplifier design and relevant artifacts.*

frequencies, phase, and type (e.g., Butterworth or Chebychev). Figure 9.6 shows a typical biosignal amplifier design with its analog filters.

DIGITIZATION

Once analog signals are appropriately amplified and filtered, they are digitized by the ADC. The choice of the sampling rate depends largely on the kind of brain signals being recorded. EEG signals are often acquired with a sampling frequency of 256 Hz. Typically, analog filtering between 0.5 and 100 Hz (Guger et al., 2001) is applied, although particular brain signals may require other filtering ranges. For example, slow-wave recordings require a high-pass filter with a very low corner frequency (e.g., 0.01 Hz) (Birbaumer et al., 2000). P300-based systems may use a 0.1–30 Hz bandpass filter (Sellers et al., 2006). ECoG recordings are often filtered with a bandpass filter of about 0.5–500 Hz and then digitized with a sampling frequency of 1000 Hz (Leuthardt et al., 2004a). Neuronal action potential (spike) recordings are typically filtered with a bandpass of 100 Hz to 6 kHz, and digitized at about 40 kHz (Zhang et al., 1998), because spikes typically have durations of <1 msec.

In addition to using an appropriate ADC sampling rate, it is extremely important to ensure that the voltage range and resolution of the ADC are appropriate for the signal being digitized. Most ADCs digitize signals using 16-bit, 24-bit, or 32-bit resolution over some input range (e.g., ± 250 mV). The smallest signal change that the ADC can detect is dependent on the resolution and the input range:

$$V_{res} = \frac{V_{range}}{2^N}$$

(9.2)

where V_{res} is the resolution, V_{range} is the input voltage range, and N is the number of bits. For example, a 24-bit amplifier with an input range of ± 250 mV can detect signal changes as small as (i.e., has a resolution of) $500\,\text{mV}/2^{24} = 0.03\mu\text{V}$, whereas a 16-bit amplifier with the same input range has a resolution of $500\,\text{mV}/2^{16} = 7.6\mu\text{V}$. Conversely, a 16-bit ADC with a resolution of 0.03 μV would have an input range of only 1.95 mV, whereas a 32-bit ADC with a resolution of 0.03 μV could handle an input range of over 127 V. Therefore, an ADC with at least 24-bit resolution is needed to record signals that include large slow potentials or DC potentials. It is also important to note that the theoretical resolution of an ADC can be smaller than its actual resolution, because the ADC itself can introduce noise to the signal, and hence the smallest bits are not always a reliable representation of the signal.

Brain signals recorded with many channels (i.e., many electrodes) yield a spatial representation of the brain activity. If brain signals from different channels contribute to an analysis (as is the case with many BCI analysis techniques), all the channels should be digitized simultaneously. However, if the digitization system contains only one ADC that digitizes signals from different channels in succession, the samples from different channels are acquired at different times. Several solutions to this problem are possible: (1) using an amplifier with simultaneous sample-and-hold, which holds multiple analog values until the digitizer is ready to read the sample; (2) sampling at a very high rate so that the discrepancies in sample times among channels are very small; (3) using a separate ADC for each channel and synchronizing their sampling; (4) interpolating between the successive samples from each channel to derive the expected values from all channels at specific time points (e.g., McFarland et al., 1997). When multiple amplification systems are used, the problem of non-simultaneous sampling is greatly exacerbated unless the systems are synchronized.

ARTIFACTS

Electrical signals recorded from the brain (and EEG signals in particular) have small amplitudes and thus, despite all precautions, remain highly susceptible to various forms of contamination (fig. 9.6). As discussed in chapter 7, recordings can be contaminated by biological artifacts (e.g., EMG activity, ECG activity, EOG activity), electrode or connector artifacts (e.g., *electrode pops* [i.e., unstable tissue contact], movement potentials, DC offsets), electromagnetic interference (e.g., capacitive or inductive coupling with power lines), and noise inherent to the amplifier and the digitization process. Each artifact can affect the biosignals differently over different frequency ranges. For example, for low-frequency EEG recordings (e.g., <30 Hz), it may be more important to eliminate wideband EMG artifact (which can distort the entire signal) and less important to eliminate 60-Hz noise.

Nevertheless, external electrical sources, especially 50- or 60-Hz alternating current (AC) power lines, are often major sources of artifacts. Thus, it is important to maximize the distance of the subject from electronic devices and power cords, and it may be necessary to use additional shielding around the subject to reduce noise artifacts. This problem may be particularly difficult in hospital settings or in the homes of people with severe disabilities due to the frequent nearby presence of equipment such as ventilators. Artifacts can also come from magnetic fields. Since this type of artifact depends on the physical separation between the wires that connect the two electrodes of each channel to the amplifier, these wires are often twisted together to reduce the space between them and thereby reduce artifacts induced by magnetic fields.

Electrode movements can also produce artifacts by changing the DC offset voltage produced by the metal-electrolyte and the electrolyte-skin junctions. For example, stainless-steel electrodes, which have a high electrode impedance, can generate high DC voltages (from the mV range up to the V range) that can be larger than the brain signals themselves (e.g., EEG is usually 5–20 µV at the amplifier input). DC offsets can be reduced by ensuring that all electrodes are of the same material and that the same gel is always used. This avoids the polarization

between electrodes that can introduce a large DC offset potential. (The same principle of always using the same material holds true for any recordings within the brain that use a reference [e.g., a skull screw].) At the same time, if a DC voltage is stable and does not saturate the amplifier, it is often not a significant problem. However, if a DC voltage does saturate the amplifier or if it varies over time, it can be a severe problem. Such variations are often produced by electrode movements that affect the electrical properties of the electrode-tissue interface.

Electrode movements can be minimized in several ways. silver/silver chloride electrodes are nonpolarizable and thus have less motion artifact than polarizable electrodes (e.g., platinum) (Bronzino, 2006). In general, the designs and integration of the EEG electrodes, their cables, and the electrode caps are all important in minimizing instability at the metal-gel and gel-skin junction. Movement at the gel-metal junction can be reduced by having the electrode contact only the gel and not the skin itself. Movement at the gel-skin junction can be reduced by preparing the skin with abrasive gel to achieve optimal impedance and by ensuring that the electrode is tightly fixed in place (e.g., with collodion or a tight cap). In the case of active electrodes the gel can be used without abrasion. It is also worthwhile to minimize the possible movement of the cables that connect the electrodes to the amplifier (e.g., by taping or otherwise anchoring them to the chair or bed), and to make the cap, electrodes, and electrode wires as light in weight as possible. For all recording methods (EEG, ECoG, intracortical recordings), flexible wires are important to reduce the danger of traction on the electrodes. Electrode platforms now under development will include on-chip filtering, amplification, and digitization, and wireless transmission that can reduce or remove many of these concerns.

HARDWARE INTERFACES

After digitization, brain signals are communicated to a host device, most commonly a personal computer, through a hardware interface. The most common interfaces are listed in table 9.1. Even a Bluetooth™ transmitter is not completely wireless, since it requires connections between the electrode array and the amplifier and ADC. Its advantage is that it does not tether the user to a computer and allows freer movement.

TABLE 9.1 Commonly used hardware interfaces and their properties

INTERFACE	DATA RATE (MB/SEC)	EASE OF USE	AVAILABILITY	# CONNECTED DEVICES	DISTANCE FROM COMPUTER (M)
RS232	0.25	++	+	1	<1
Bluetooth 2.0	0.26	++	++	8	<100
USB 2.0	60	+++	+++	127	<10
PCIe 2.0	500/lane	++	+	1–4	<1
Firewire 800	100	++	+	63	<10
Ethernet	25–250	++	+++	NA	<1000

INTERFACE PROTOCOLS

RS232 was one of the first standardized transmission protocols. Computer serial ports use the RS232 protocol for serial binary data transmission. It is robust and easy to use, but its low data transmission rate (or *bandwidth*) limits it to transmitting relatively few channels and at low rates. Although the electrical definition of the RS232 interface is standardized, there are several different RS232 connectors available.

Bluetooth™ is a wireless protocol for transmitting data over distances of less than 100 m. The mobility provided by this wireless protocol is a big advantage for biosignal recordings because subjects can move freely with the recording device. However, such wireless or mobile systems entail high power consumption. With current technology, devices can be designed to work for several days without recharging. Up to eight Bluetooth™ devices can be connected wirelessly to a single computer simultaneously. However, the bandwidth is shared among the devices so that the maximum data rate is divided by the number of devices.

USB is a serial bus standard for connecting devices to a host computer. The USB protocol has recently become the de-facto standard communication protocol for most new devices, replacing other serial and parallel port devices. USB 2.0 provides a much higher bandwidth than Bluetooth™ or RS232 and therefore allows more data to be transferred (e.g., higher sampling rates and/or more channels). The main advantage of USB is that it is standard in nearly all new computers including laptops. However, if multiple devices are connected to the same USB hub (a single hub with multiple ports), the bandwidth is shared among all devices, thus lowering overall bandwidth for each device.

Firewire is a serial bus interface standard for high-speed communications that is often used by computers. It is currently one of the fastest interfaces and has many of the same properties as the USB protocol. It has some additional technical advantages. For example, Firewire devices can be connected sequentially to allow for multiple devices on a single hub. The new Firewire 800 protocol is 66% faster than the USB 2.0 protocol, but it is not as widespread as the USB standard.

Peripheral component interconnect (PCI) is a bus standard for internal connection of hardware components, such as a data-acquisition (DAQ) board. PCI provides very high data-transfer rates compared to USB, with varying degrees of digital resolution (e.g., 16, 24, or 32 bits), depending on the board. New PCI Express interfaces provide even higher data-transfer rates; this increases the number of channels and/or the sampling rates per channel that are possible. The primary disadvantage of PCI is that the PCI card must be installed internally within the PC. This means that only desktops and laptops that have PCI slots (most laptops do not) can be used and that the PC needs to be turned off to install the PCI card. As a result, PCI-based systems are not as portable as systems that use the interfaces described above.

Ethernet is a network interface that is available on most computers. It is capable of very high data-transfer rates. A disadvantage of ethernet is that most computers have only one ethernet port.

To compare the different interfaces described above, it is useful to compare their transmission capabilities. An RS232-based interface with a 115-kBit/sec bandwidth allows transmission of 11 channels of 16 bits/sample data (plus one start and stop bit per byte) at 512 Hz/channel. This might be sufficient for EEG or limited ECoG recordings but not for spikes. A single USB 2.0-based interface port is capable of transmitting up to 26 channels of 32 bits/sample data at 38.4 kHz/channel, with guaranteed bandwidth and retransmission if an error occurs. Finally, a PCI Express 2.0 card is capable of transmitting 8 GB/sec when using 16 lanes (500 MB/lane), and it can thereby potentially transmit thousands of channels of 32-bit/sample data at 40 kHz/channel. Thus, for applications that require high sampling rates and many channels, PCI Express interfaces may be the only possible choice.

TRANSMISSION PRINCIPLES

With any of these types of interface, digital data are typically transferred from the data-acquisition device to the computer in *blocks*. The smallest possible block size is one sample, in which only one sample *per channel* is transmitted at each time step. For example, if 64 channels are recorded, each block would contain a total of 64 samples. However, for the computer software receiving the data, there is usually a significant computational cost involved in acquiring each block of data, no matter how large or small it is. This cost often makes it impractical to use blocks that contain only one sample per channel, particularly with high sampling rates. For this reason, most devices transfer data in larger blocks (e.g., 30 samples per channel). For example, if 64-channel data are collected in 30-msec blocks with a sampling rate of 1000 Hz, 1920 samples (64 channels × 30 samples) are transmitted in each block. If the sampling rate is 500 Hz, 960 samples are transmitted in each block (64 channels × 15 samples).

CLIENT HARDWARE

Biosignals are detected by the electrodes and transmitted to the amplifier and ADC, where they are filtered and digitized, respectively. The filtered and digitized data are transmitted to client hardware (e.g., a PC or dedicated microcontroller). The client hardware handles several tasks: it controls data acquisition; it stores the data from the ADC; it processes data to extract brain-signal features and to translate them into output commands; and it sends the output commands to the application device. Depending on the the BCI's purpose, there are several options for the client hardware (see table 9.2). The selection depends on the demands of the planned usage, specifically those regarding portability, computational power, and whether or not a standardized operating system (e.g., Microsoft Windows) with compatible drivers is required. We briefly consider the selection of client hardware for a variety of applications.

For clinical EEG and ECoG BCI applications, it is important to have complete BCI systems that are reliable and easy to operate and that have an adequate sampling rate and number of channels. In these situations, a portable and wearable data-acquisition device that can be mounted on a wheelchair or beside the patient may be particularly desirable. Although pocket PCs are highly portable, can be switched on rapidly,

TABLE 9.2 The different client hardware options and their characteristics

	PRICE	INTERFACES AVAILABLE	PERFORMANCE	SCREEN	PORTABILITY
Laptops	–	++	++	+	+
Netbook	+++	+/–	–	–	++
PC	+/–	+++	+++	+++	–
Pocket PC	+/–	–	–	–	+++

and can also be easily mounted, they are limited in processing capabilities and screen size. Since BCI research and development often address questions that require more channels, higher sampling rates, and more demanding real-time analyses, it is often essential to use powerful, highly flexible BCI systems. Conventional laptops and PCs are typically more capable of satisfying the need for many channels, high sampling rates, and high interface bandwidth.

Spike recordings using microelectrodes arrays typically require much higher sampling frequencies than EEG/ECoG recordings. Thus, they require very high digitization capabilities and data-transmission rates. A highly capable PC workstation or dedicated hardware is often the solution adopted in this situation.

Finally, in accord with the definition of a BCI used throughout this book, it should be noted that the application hardware itself (e.g., wheelchair, robotic arm, etc.) is not part of the BCI per se. That is, the BCI is responsible for the tasks of acquiring brain signals and processing them to generate output commands. These commands are then implemented by the application which may (e.g., as in a speller) or may not (e.g., as with a robotic arm) be physically housed in the computer that performs the other functions (e.g., signal processing) of the BCI.

FUTURE DIRECTIONS

Future hardware development that would have a major impact on improving BCI systems includes improvements to sensor technologies. For EEG electrodes it is desirable that electrodes can be rapidly applied and that they can function robustly without gel. Development of practical and robust dry electrodes will be a major step in achieving these goals (see chapter 6 of this volume). For ECoG, one can expect development of highly flexible ECoG arrays with very high channel counts and high spatial resolution (see chapter 15 of this volume). For implantable microelectrode arrays, one can expect further miniaturization that increases spatial resolution and decreases damage to brain tissue caused by chronic implantation (see chapter 5 of this volume).

SOFTWARE

COMPONENTS OF BCI IMPLEMENTATION

While the components of BCI hardware provide the technical capability to acquire signals from the brain, to analyze them, and to produce real-time outputs, it is the BCI *software* that determines and coordinates what actually happens. BCI *software* contains four key components:

- *Data acquisition*, which amplifies, digitizes, transmits, and stores brain signals

- *Signal analysis*, which extracts signal features that represent the user's intent and translates these features into commands that embody the user's intent

- *Output*, which uses these commands to control an output device (e.g., a cursor, an environmental controller, a wheelchair) and which provides feedback to the user about the results of the output

- An *operating protocol*, which configures and parameterizes the acquisition, analysis, and output components and determines the onset, offset, and timing of operation.

In *data acquisition*, brain signals are recorded, stored, and made available for analysis. The parameters that describe this data acquisition include. the number of signal channels that are acquired; the signal sampling rate; and the block size (i.e., the number of signal samples that are transferred to the signal processing module in each batch of data). Different BCIs vary substantially with regard to these parameters. For example, a BCI for a P300-based clinical application may require acquisition of 8 channels at a sampling rate of 256 Hz per channel; a BCI for ECoG research may require acquisition of 128 channels at a sampling rate of 1000 Hz per channel; and a BCI that uses a microelectrode array to record from single neurons may require acquisition of more than 128 channels at 40 kHz per channel. Many hardware vendors offer software that can acquire and store brain signals using hardware made by that vendor (e.g., Neuroscan, EGI, BrainProducts, Plexon, Tucker-Davis, or Ripple).

In *signal analysis*, signals acquired from the brain are transferred into output device commands. This process has two stages. As described in chapters 7 and 8, the first stage is *feature extraction,* which involves the extraction of specific brain-signal features that reflect the intent of the user. The second stage is *translation* in which those features are converted into device commands. These two stages are realized using a number of mathematical operations, such as frequency analyses or spike sorting (for feature extraction), and linear or nonlinear algorithms (for translation). These two stages can be realized using software products that address specific requirements or that can be adapted to a variety of different needs. Several manufacturers offer software that can extract features (e.g., the firing rate) from neuronal activity (e.g., Tucker-Davis, Cyberkinetics, or Plexon). More general software, capable of many different analyses, includes Matlab™ (which is the de-facto standard for signal analysis in a wide range of domains), LabView™, or the open-source languages Octave (which is mostly compatible with Matlab) or Python with its numerical analysis packages.

The *output* component of the software controls the output device and conveys appropriate information (i.e., *feedback*) about that output to the user. For some applications the output and the feedback are identical (e.g., a BCI spelling application that puts its output on a screen in front of the user, or a robotic arm the movements of which can be seen by the user). In other applications the output and feedback are different (e.g., an environmental control application in which the output is a command for room-temperature change, and the feedback is an indication of the change that appears on the user's screen). All BCIs require some sort of feedback on performance to achieve and maintain optimal performance. Several capable commercial software programs can provide feedback via visual or auditory stimuli (e.g., E-prime, Presentation, Inquisit, DirectRT, STIM, Cambridge Research VSG, or Superlab). In some of these packages, the stimuli can be dependent on external input and thus could be used to provide feedback in a BCI.

The *operating protocol*, discussed in chapter 10 of this volume, defines the configuration and parameterization of the data acquisition, signal analysis, and output components and determines the onset, offset, and timing of operation. Thus, the operating protocol ties the function of these three individual components together and ensures that the BCI functions effectively.

DESIGN PRINCIPLES FOR R&D BCI SOFTWARE

The four key components of the BCI software can be realized using a large variety of technical approaches. In selecting among these approaches to build the most useful BCI software, particularly in the present early stage of BCI research and development, three criteria must be met:

- The software must satisfy the technical requirements of real-time operation. It must encompass the full range of sampling and update rates, have sufficient speed of analysis, and have low and reliable output latency.

- The software should allow the efficient implementation of a broad range of BCI designs and should facilitate subsequent modifications. That is, it should be able to accommodate different types of brain signals, signal analyses, and outputs.

- The software should readily accommodate different hardware components and different operating systems.

SATISFYING THE TECHNICAL REQUIREMENTS FOR A BCI SYSTEM

This first criterion is itself often very challenging. An effective BCI must acquire signals from the brain, analyze these signals to produce output commands, and produce the output (and associated feedback), and it must do all this in real time with minimal delays and stable timing. Software that is optimized for any one of these three steps, such as the programs mentioned above (e.g., E-prime, etc.), may not be able to interact effectively with the other steps in a timely fashion. For example, analysis of brain signals during stimulus presentation requires that the timing of stimulus presentation is known with respect to the timing of data acquisition. Existing experimental protocols that integrate signal acquisition with stimulus presentation often configure stimulus presentation software to output the timing of stimulus presentation (e.g., to the parallel port) and then record that output signal along with the brain signals. Although this approach allows for accurate association of stimulus timing with brain signal samples, it is substantially limited in the complexity of the paradigms it can support. There are several reasons for this. First, each type of event that needs to be registered in this way requires its own signal channel (which may reduce the number of brain-signal channels that can be recorded, if enough synchronous digital input channels are not available). Second, the hardware that accomplishes this requires making new cable connections, and so forth. Third, there is no record in the data file about the nature of the events on the different event channels (which impedes offline interpretation).

ACCOMMODATING MANY DESIGNS AND SUBSEQUENT MODIFICATIONS

The second criterion is that the software should be able to implement any specific BCI design and to accommodate subsequent modifications needed. Later modification should be relatively easy and should not require extensive reprogramming. This is particularly important for BCI studies with humans since these studies often involve many different kinds of studies by many different researchers at many different locations. Nevertheless, this principle has generally not received the attention it deserves. Successful adherence to this requirement depends mainly on the BCI software framework's architecture (i.e., the flexibility and capacities of the software's different components and their interactions), which must be general enough to accommodate changes in key parameters of the system. For example, BCI software should not limit a BCI system to a specific number of signal channels, to a specific sampling rate, or to specific signal-analysis methods. Although software with such limitations may perform effectively in specific configurations, a desired change in the configuration may necessitate extensive reprogramming of the entire system. It is often difficult or impossible to assess the flexibility of a given BCI system by simply evaluating its performance in a specific configuration.

The third criterion is that the software should readily accommodate different hardware components and different operating systems. This makes it possible and practical for a BCI system's data collection and data analysis, as well as its further development, to be performed by different personnel in different locations with potentially different hardware. System or experimental development may be performed in one laboratory using a particular brand of data acquisition hardware, whereas data collection may be performed in a different laboratory using different hardware. Unfortunately, this principle is also rarely considered.

Moreover, the data stored during online operation should be readily available for analysis by other research groups. It is an all-too-common practice for data to be stored in a format specific to a particular study and for essential details of the study to be stored elsewhere (e.g., notebooks, clinical databases, etc.). This practice hinders or prevents analyses by others as part of collaborative projects. In contrast, when data and associated parameters are stored in a standard format they can be easily accessed and evaluated by many different investigators. Thus, BCI software that stores all online data and associated parameters in a standardized format can greatly facilitate BCI research and development and can also contribute to the efficient and effective oversight of clinical applications.

In summary, BCI software must first and foremost implement a system that, from a technical perspective, functions properly. In addition, since most research environments involve different people, a variety of experiments, and sometimes multiple locations (i.e., in BCI research programs rather than isolated BCI research projects), it is also critical to build such BCI implementations using a software architecture that can accommodate the differing parameters of different BCI paradigms and that can facilitate the interaction and collaboration of different people. Creating a system with these demanding characteristics from scratch is complex, difficult, and thus costly, irrespective of what language or software environment (e.g., C++ or Matlab™) is used for the implementation. Thus, as an overall approach, it is desirable to build BCI systems using general-purpose BCI software that appropriately addresses these requirements and that also solves the issues of complexity, difficulty, and cost associated with system development.

OVERVIEW OF GENERAL-PURPOSE BCI RESEARCH SOFTWARE

In the earliest days of BCI development, all laboratories wrote their own software to handle the specific needs of their respective BCI applications. Typically, there was little capacity for the products of one group's efforts (e.g., their software and hardware) to satisfy another group's needs. Based on the considerations described above, it became clear that this was a needlessly inefficient approach and that it would be beneficial to try to develop a general-purpose BCI software platform that could implement many different BCI designs, a platform that could accommodate a wide variety of brain signals, processing methods, output types, hardware components, operating systems, and so forth. The goal was to enable researchers to make changes in their BCI systems easily and without extensive reprogramming.

Such general-purpose BCI software platforms have been developed. These platforms include:

- a Matlab/Simulink-based system (Guger et al., 2001) that has recently been commercialized as g.BCIsys (http://www.gtec.at/products/g.BCIsys/bci.htm) and intendiX (http://www.intendix.com/)

- a flexible brain-computer interface described by Bayliss (2001)

- the BF++ framework (Bianchi et al., 2003) (http://www.brainterface.com)

- xBCI (http://xbci.sourceforge.net)

- rtsBCI, which is a Matlab/Simulink-based system that is part of the BioSig package (Schlögl et al., 2004) (http://biosig.sf.net)

- Pyff, a platform-independent framework to develop BCI feedback applications in Python (Venthur and Blankertz, 2008)

- Real-Time Messaging Architecture (RTMA) (Velliste et al., 2009)

- OpenViBE (Renard et al., 2007)

- BCI2000 (Schalk et al., 2004; Mellinger et al., 2007; Schalk, 2009; Schalk and Mellinger, 2010; Wilson and Schalk, 2010)

Of these systems, the only openly available platforms that have been used in laboratories beyond those that developed them are OpenViBE and BCI2000. Development of these two systems is supported by dedicated funding. Thus, these two projects have the impetus and resources to continue to develop, maintain, and disseminate the software. Both OpenViBE and BCI2000 represent general-purpose BCI software platforms that can also be used for other data acquisition, stimulus presentation, and brain-monitoring applications. Both platforms are based on a modular design that is implemented in C++.

OpenViBE can use 10 different data-acquisition devices. Current realizations support EEG-based one- or two-dimensional BCIs using motor imagery, a P300-based speller, and real-time visualization of brain activity in two or three dimensions. OpenViBE's functions are documented for users as well as developers on a project wiki. A number of published studies have used OpenViBE (e.g., Lécuyer et al., 2008; Lotte et al., 2010). OpenViBE is available under the LGPL license at http://openvibe.inria.fr.

BCI2000 can use more than 18 different data-acquisition devices and can synchronize them with signals from a variety of other input devices (e.g., joystick, mouse, keyboard,

Nintendo Wii controller, Tobii™ eye trackers). It currently supports BCIs that use EEG signals (e.g., P300, sensorimotor rhythms, slow cortical potentials), ECoG signals, or local field potentials, and has a basic capability to support BCIs that use spikes. Current realizations support three-dimensional cursor movements, a P300 speller, and a sequential menu-based speller. It can also provide programmable auditory-visual stimulation. BCI2000 also comes with a certification procedure to document system timing of any BCI2000 configuration (Wilson et al., 2010). BCI2000 and its use are described in tutorials and references targeted at users and developers on a project wiki and also in a book (Schalk and Mellinger, 2010). BCI2000 is available free of charge for research and educational purposes at http://www.bci2000.org.

BCI2000 is based on a general model that consists of four interconnected modules:

- source (data acquisition and storage)
- signal processing
- application
- operator interface

These modules communicate using a generic protocol based on TCP/IP, and they can therefore be written using any programming language on any operating system. The communication between and among the modules uses this generic protocol to transmit all information needed for operation. Thus, the protocol does not need to be changed if a module is changed. The distinctive property of this structure is that changes may be made in one or more of the modules without necessitating changes to the other modules or to the rules by which they interact with one another. In addition, the modules are interchangeable (e.g., any signal acquisition module can be used with any signal processing module without requiring any additional programming or configuration). This allows new acquisition systems, algorithms, and applications to be developed quickly and integrated into the BCI2000 framework without the need to worry about re-implementing previously existing modules.

BCI2000 has had and continues to have a substantial impact on BCI research. By the end of 2010, it had been acquired by more than 600 laboratories around the world. It has provided the basis for studies reported in more than 150 peer-reviewed publications that describe BCIs based on EEG, ECoG, and MEG recordings. For example, it has been used to demonstrate cursor control using: EEG (McFarland et al., 2008a, 2008b, 2010; J. R. Wolpaw and McFarland, 2004); ECoG (Blakely et al., 2009; Felton et al., 2007; Leuthardt et al., 2004a; Leuthardt et al., 2006a; Miller et al., 2010; Schalk et al., 2008c; Wilson et al., 2006); and MEG signals (Mellinger et al., 2007). It was used for control of a humanoid robot by a noninvasive BCI (Bell et al., 2008) and for exploring the BCI usage of P300 evoked potentials (Furdea et al., 2009; Kübler et al., 2009; Nijboer et al., 2008; Sellers et al., 2006, 2010; Townsend et al., 2010; Vaughan et al., 2006) and steady-state visual evoked potentials (SSVEP) (Allison et al., 2008). It has been used in a BCI based on high-resolution EEG techniques (Cincotti et al.,

2008a) and for BCI control of assistive technologies (Cincotti et al., 2008b). BCI2000 has also provided the basis for the first extensive clinical evaluations of BCI technology for the needs of people with severe motor disabilities (Kübler et al., 2005; Nijboer et al., 2008; Vaughan et al., 2006) and the first application of BCI technology to functional restoration in people after strokes (Buch et al., 2008; Daly et al., 2009; Wisneski et al., 2008). Finally, several studies have used BCI2000 for purposes other than online BCI control (e.g., mapping of cortical function using ECoG [Brunner et al., 2009; Kubánek et al., 2009; Leuthardt et al., 2007; Miller et al., 2007a, 2007b; Schalk et al., 2007, 2008a, 2008b]); the optimization of BCI signal processing routines [Cabrera and Dremstrup, 2008; Royer and He, 2009; Yamawaki et al., 2006]).

In summary, general-purpose BCI software has been effective in implementing functioning BCI systems, in reducing the complexity, time, and cost of setting up and maintaining those BCI systems, and in enabling multisite studies using multiple acquisition systems and computers.

Although it is able to satisfy the requirements of BCI research and development programs, general-purpose BCI software may become superfluous, even cumbersome, in the future when specific BCI designs are validated and finalized for clinical use. When this time comes, it may be optimal to implement a dedicated BCI software system specifically for each particular purpose. Even in these cases, however, it may be advantageous to retain such properties as the modularity of components that are liable to be changed in the future; this should facilitate the implementation of future modifications and expansions as well as the continual oversight of system function.

EVALUATING BCI HARDWARE AND SOFTWARE

Timing performance is the technical metric of greatest interest in evaluating the ability of BCI hardware and software to support an effective BCI system. To work properly, BCI systems must perform a sequence of tasks that are properly timed and coordinated. Without proper timing, the BCI will perform poorly or will fail entirely. The tasks that must be properly timed include acquisition of the brain signals, storage of these signals so that they can be processed in blocks, their analysis (i.e., extracting features and translating them) to produce output commands, and implementation of these commands by the application. Moreover, these must be accomplished in a closed-loop manner by providing feedback of task performance to the user. In addition, these steps must be properly coordinated in real time and they must occur on time. All the tasks of the BCI that connect the user's brain signals to the output device must be accomplished quickly with little or no variation (*jitter*) in timing. Thus, in evaluating BCI hardware and software, *timing* considerations are critical. The timing characteristics of a BCI system, and thus its suitability for specific applications, depend on its individual hardware and software components and on the manner in which these components interact. The principles involved in assessing a BCI's timing are reviewed here (and presented in more detail in Wilson and Schalk, 2010).

TIMING CHARACTERISTICS OF A REPRESENTATIVE BCI SYSTEM

LATENCY OVERVIEW

The operation of any BCI can generally be seen as occurring in three stages: data acquisition; data processing; and output. All three stages might be controlled by a single program (e.g., a single Matlab script or C-language program). Alternatively, they might be controlled by multiple independent programs that interact with each other via a defined communication protocol (e.g., a network-aware protocol like BCI2000 or OpenViBe). By whichever means these three steps are constructed, each step requires time and thus entails delay *latencies*. If these latencies are too long or too unpredictable, they can interfere with, or entirely prevent, effective real-time operation of the BCI system.

Figure 9.7 shows the timeline of events in the operation of a typical BCI system. It shows the progression of three blocks of data (blocks N1, N2, and N3) from the arrival of the brain signals at the amplifier, to production of the BCI output, to the execution of the BCI's command by the application, with the times of each successive event marked.

Let us examine the progress of the first block data, N1. During the period from t_{-2} to t_{-1}, data are collected, and the ADC amplifies, digitizes, and stores the data in a hardware buffer where it waits to be transmitted to the PC. The first sample collected in the block of data stays in the buffer for the duration of the block (e.g., 30 msec) while it waits for the rest of the data in the block to be collected, amplified, digitized, and stored in the buffer. In the figure this process is illustrated in the box labeled "ADC." We will call this period the *sample block duration*. Sample block durations are typically several tens of milliseconds long. A 30-msec data block acquired, for example, at a sampling rate of 1000 Hz would contain 30 samples per channel. At t_{-1}, the digitized data block (block N1) is ready to be transmitted to the PC. From t_{-1} to t_0 (the box labeled "DT" for data transfer), the data are transmitted to the BCI's PC; this transmission is completed at t_0. Thus, at t_0, the data block N1 has been stored in PC memory (RAM) and is ready to be processed. From t_0 to t_1 (the box labeled "SP" for signal processing), the data are processed and translated into a command that is sent to the application device at t_1. From t_1 to t_2, the command is processed by the application device, which executes the command at t_2.

Figure 9.7 also shows the onset and duration of the progression of the next two sets of data (blocks N2 and N3). Note that the progression of block N2 is offset from block N1's progression by the time period represented by t_{-2} to t_{-1}; thus, while the N1 block reaches application output at t_2, block N2 reaches output at t_6. If the sample block duration is 30 msec, block N2's output occurs 30 msec after N1's.

The *latency* is the period of time represented by the difference in two time points. For example, the signal-processing latency is t_1 minus t_0. The magnitude and variability of each latency depend on the system parameters, as well as on the capacities of the hardware and software. Effective BCI operation requires that these latency magnitudes and variabilities fall within acceptable limits. To understand these latencies better, we now examine them in more detail.

ADC LATENCY

The time period for acquisition of data for a sample block is fixed by the BCI protocol. The amplification, digitization,

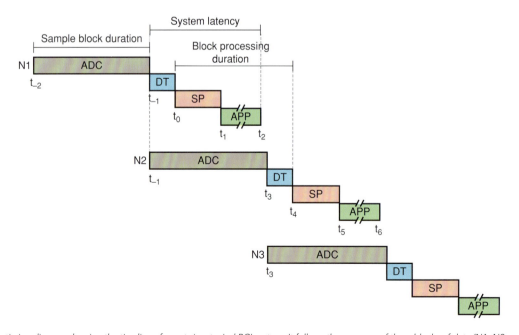

Figure 9.7 System timing diagram showing the timeline of events in a typical BCI system. It follows the progress of three blocks of data (N1, N2, and N3) from the amplifier input to the BCI's application device. Abbreviations: ADC, analog-to-digital converter; DT, data transfer; SP, signal processing; APP, application. The times (t) that define the latencies of each successive event are marked.

and storage of the data typically have latencies of <1 μsec and are often in the range of 10 nsec; they are therefore negligible on the scale of the acquisition duration of a single sample (i.e., at a sampling rate of 25 kHz one sample is acquired every 40 μsec). The exact latency depends on the type of converter used (e.g., flash, successive-approximation, sample-and-hold, counter, or tracking ADC, each of which has a different digitization method, speed, and precision [Tompkins, 1993]). Note that because data are always transmitted in blocks containing a certain number of samples, the last sample acquired for a data block will spend only a minimum time in hardware and software buffers, whereas the samples acquired earliest will spend a longer time (approximately t_{-2} to t_{-1}) in the buffers.

DATA-TRANSFER LATENCY

The *data-transfer latency*, L_{DT} is the latency between the time at which all the data in the block have been acquired, amplified, digitized, and stored in the buffer (t_{-1} for N1) and the time at which the data are acquired by the PC software to be available to the PC software for processing. In figure 9.7, for the N1 block, this is the time from t_{-1} to t_0. Using the times defined in figure 9.7:

$$Data\ Transfer\ Latency = L_{DT} = t_0 - t_{-1} \qquad (9.3)$$

For amplifiers connected via bandwidth-limited serial interfaces, the transmission latency may have a measurable impact on amplifier latency. When using USB 2.0 or PCI card connections, transmission latency (t_{-1} to t_0) may generally be neglected, as illustrated by the following example. If we assume acquisition of 16 channels of 24-bit (3-byte) data and transmission of blocks of eight samples, each block corresponds to 384 bytes of data. At USB 2.0 speed (i.e., a maximum transmission rate of 60 MB/sec), these data should take approximately 6.4 μsec to transfer, which is less than the duration of a single sample's acquisition. On the other hand, if the configuration is changed to 64 channels and a block duration of 100-msec and is sampled at 4800 Hz (equal to 92,160 bytes), the transmission time will be approximately 1.5 msec, assuming that transmission starts instantaneously and without interruption. Because this is on the time scale of events during the BCI task, it may be important to take this latency into account.

SIGNAL-PROCESSING LATENCY

The *signal-processing latency*, L_{SP} is defined as the total time required for the data to be processed, that is, for the signal features to be extracted and translated into an output command. From figure 9.7, this is the time from t_0 to t_1):

$$Processing\ Latency = L_{SP} = t_1 - t_0 \qquad (9.4)$$

The signal-processing latency depends on the complexity of the processing and on CPU speed. For example, the processing for a cursor-movement application might extract the power spectrum from every data block, whereas the processing for a matrix-selection application might extract evoked potential amplitude. The computational demands of these different feature extractions may differ considerably. The number of channels that need to be processed will, of course, also affect

processing time. These factors will help determine the minimum acceptable capacities of the processing hardware and software. The system must be able to process each block at least as fast as it is acquired and amplified, digitized, and stored by the ADC, that is, by the time the next block is ready for processing. Thus, the time from t_0 to t_{+1} must be shorter than the time from t_{-2} to t_{-1}. Otherwise, the BCI will lag progressively further behind (i.e., the time elapsed between brain signal input and device output will get longer and longer over time), and BCI performance will degrade.

APPLICATION-OUTPUT LATENCY

The *application-output latency*, L_{App}, is defined as the delay from the time at which the BCI command is issued to the time at which the application device implements this command. From figure 9.7, this is the time from t_1 to t_2:

$$Application\ Output\ Latency = L_{App} = t_2 - t_1 \qquad (9.5)$$

The application latency is determined by a number of factors that depend largely on the nature of the application's output. For example, if the output is cursor movement on a video screen, its latency is affected by the speed of the graphics card, the type of monitor (e.g., cathode-ray tube [CRT] or liquid crystal display [LCD]), and the monitor resolution and refresh rate. If the output is the movement of a robotic arm, the application output latency depends on the response time of the robot and the distance to be moved.

SYSTEM LATENCY

The *system latency* is defined as the *minimum* time interval between brain signal input to the ADC and the related change that this causes in the application output. Recalling that the last sample in block N1 is collected just before or at t_{-1}, the system latency is the time from t_{-1} to t_2. It can be calculated as the sum of data-transfer, signal-processing, and application latencies:

$$System\ Latency = (t_2 - t_{-1}) \qquad (9.6)$$

The system latency *jitter* is the standard deviation of the system latencies in a given test and provides a measure of the variability in overall system timing.

BLOCK PROCESSING DURATION

The *block processing duration* is the time interval between successive blocks of data that have been transmitted to the PC for processing. As figure 9.7 shows, N1's data are presented to the PC at t_0, whereas N2's data are presented to the PC at t_4. Thus:

$$Block\ Processing\ Duration = (t_4 - t_0) \qquad (9.7)$$

Ideally, the block processing duration should be identical to the sample block duration. However, inconsistencies in operating-system timing may interrupt and delay data transfer and/or signal processing, causing the time period between data blocks to be different from the expected block duration. (This introduces a *jitter*; see below.) The *block processing jitter* is the standard deviation of equation (9.7) for all block durations in a single test.

The block processing duration is the primary indicator of the system's ability to perform real-time signal processing in a BCI paradigm. The block processing duration must be no longer than the sample block duration. If the time required to process a block of data is longer than the time to acquire the data, the system will still be processing block *N*1 when block *N*2 is ready to be transferred for signal processing. In a closed-loop system, this means that the application output and feedback are progressively delayed. This quickly produces performance degradation. If this is the case, adjustments must be made (e.g., the signal-processing algorithms need to be optimized to increase performance, or a more powerful signal-processing computer system must be used, or the task itself must be modified).

TIMING JITTER

All of the latencies described in this chapter have some variability. This variability is called *jitter*. *Jitter* is defined as the standard deviation of the measured latencies. The jitter is essentially a measure of the timing consistency of each system component. For example, the output latency may have a mean of 10 msec but a jitter of 8 msec, which indicates that there is much variability in the time required to update the output. Jitter can potentially have significant effects on the user's BCI performance, particularly with stimulus-evoked BCIs such as the P300 speller in which the evoked-response signal processing depends on the precise timing of the stimulus delivery.

Furthermore, jitter that occurs early in the BCI system chain of events will affect all later components as well. For example, a large data transfer jitter will propagate through the signal-processing and application components and will increase the variability of output timing.

The sources of jitter depend on the hardware, software, and operating system used. For example, BCIs running on the Microsoft Windows operating system must compete with other system services (e.g., antivirus programs, email programs, interactions with hardware, and other background programs). At any time, Windows may decide that another process has a higher priority than the BCI program and therefore allow the other process to finish before BCI processing can begin. This problem can be mitigated by disabling services and other programs in Windows, by increasing the task priority of the BCI program, or by using a real-time operating system such as some versions of Linux. (However, many hardware drivers are available only for Windows operating systems, in which case Windows is the only option.)

The timing definitions described here apply to any BCI system. All systems that record and process brain-signal data and generate a device command will have some latency between acquisition of the brain signals and the corresponding action executed by the application device. This is true regardless of the nature of the brain signals (e.g., EEG, ECoG, or neuronal action potentials) or the choice of output device (e.g., a robotic arm, computer cursor, or a spelling application).

REPRESENTATIVE RESULTS

In this section we describe the timing characteristics of a representative test BCI system in terms of the latencies defined

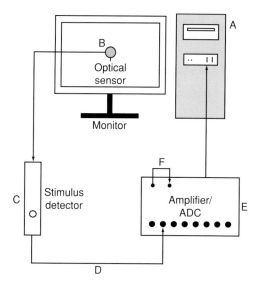

Figure 9.8 *Components of the test BCI validation system: (A) computer running BCI2000; (B) monitor and optical sensor; (C) stimulus detection trigger box; (D) TTL outputs from trigger box to amplifier; (E) amplifier; (F) amplifier digital output to digital input.*

above, and address factors that have substantial effects on timing performance. This representative system uses a g.USBamp amplifier/digitizer and a g.TRIGbox stimulus-detection box (both from g.tec Guger Technologies, Graz, Austria) and the BCI2000 software platform (Schalk et al., 2000). BCI2000 is executed on an 8-core, 2.8-GHz Mac Pro with 6 GB RAM and an NVIDIA 8800 GTX graphics card. We tested the system performance with two different operating systems, Microsoft Windows XP SP3 and Windows Vista SP1, and two different monitors, a CRT monitor with a refresh rate of 100 Hz and an LCD monitor with a refresh rate of 60 Hz.

Figure 9.8 shows this test BCI system and the timing evaluation system. The system was controlled by BCI2000 running on a PC (seen in fig. 9.8A). It repeatedly presented (not shown in the figure) a white rectangular stimulus on a black background. The optical sensor (B in fig. 9.8) was placed over the area of the monitor where the stimulus appeared. The sensor provided input to the stimulus detection box (C in fig. 9.8). The threshold levels were set so that changes in video luminescence were properly detected. When the detection box detected a stimulus, it generated a 250-mV pulse that was recorded by the amplifier (E). (It is also possible to generate a 5-V pulse, which can be recorded on a synchronous digital input channel.) This allowed accurate measurement of the timing of the stimulus. The data transfer latency was measured by using the digital input and output lines; immediately following the acquisition of a data block, the digital output line was pulsed and recorded on a digital input line (F). This pulse appeared in the next data block after a period of time equal to the block duration latency, since the next block was already being amplified, digitized, and stored while the current block was being transmitted to the PC.

Figure 9.9 shows the system latency components during a cursor movement task as a function of the sampling rate and

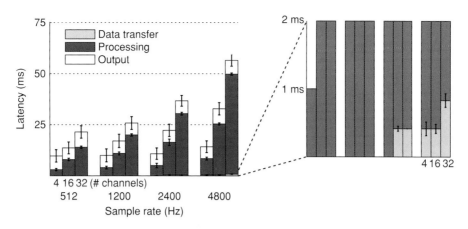

Figure 9.9 *System latency components for different BCI configurations running on Windows XP. The three segments of each bar are the contributions of the three latencies (i.e., data transfer, processing, and output) to the system latency, which is the total height of each bar. Each group of three bars contains results for 4, 16, and 32 channels; the four groups of bars represent four different sample rates (i.e., 512, 1200, 2400, and 4800 Hz). In the inset, the latencies are expanded to make the relatively short duration of the data-transfer latency visible. This duration is less than the time for a single sample unless large amounts of data are transferred (i.e., with high sampling rates and channel counts).*

the number of channels. Each latency result is described in detail here.

DATA-TRANSFER LATENCY

The data-transfer latency (light gray bars in fig. 9.9) varied with the amount of data transmitted (fig. 9.9, inset panel at right): when data with more channels or a higher sampling rate were acquired, more time was required to transmit the data over the USB 2.0 connection. Nevertheless, this delay was insignificant compared to the latencies for processing and output; it was less than 1 msec even for 32 channels sampled at 4800 Hz. Because the data-transfer latency was measured by analyzing the digitized signals, the resolution of the reported values was dependent on the sampling rate. Specifically, sampling rates of 512, 1200, 2400, and 4800 Hz correspond to a timing resolution of 1.95 msec, 0.83 msec, 0.42 msec, and 0.21 msec, respectively. These values are smaller than acquisition of a single sample at the given rate. As the figure shows, the processing latency (dark gray bars) accounted for most of the overall latency and varied with the amount of data processed.

SIGNAL-PROCESSING LATENCY

The signal-processing latency was significantly ($p < 0.001$, ANOVA) influenced by the sampling rate and number of channels. This is expected, since the signal-processing procedure for the cursor-movement task involves performing a common-average reference for the entire data block and then calculating the power spectrum of every channel. Therefore, larger sample rates or channel counts produced a corresponding increase in the amount of time required to process the data. This would be the case for any signal-processing algorithm.

It is important to understand how the algorithmic complexity relates to the amount of data processed. That is, it is usually not reasonable to expect that there will be a linear relationship between the amount of data to be processed and the time required to process the data. For example, a simple matrix-matrix multiplication, as is done when computing a spatial filter involving combinations of all channels, increases as a *power of three* with the number of elements. Thus, doubling the number of channels will increase the processing time by (2^3) (i.e., by 8 times). Therefore, it is critical to consider the computer's ability to process even small increases in the amount of data resulting from more channels or a higher sample rate.

OUTPUT LATENCY

In contrast to the signal-processing latency, the *video-output latency* did not depend on the number of channels, sampling rate, or task ($p = 0.67$). The mean video-output latency on the MacPro Windows XP system using a CRT monitor with a refresh rate of 100 Hz was 5.06 ± 3.13 msec. The minimum and maximum output latencies were 1.33 msec and 11.33 msec, respectively. Because the current implementations of the BCI2000 feedback protocols are not synchronized to the refresh rate of the monitor, the video output latency values could range from 0 msec (i.e., when the output command was issued precisely at the monitor refresh) to the inverse of the refresh rate (i.e., when the output command was issued immediately following a refresh). The latency could be as much as 10 msec at a refresh rate of 100 Hz. The experimental results corresponded closely to this: 1/(11.33 msec – 1.33 msec) equals 100 Hz. The minimum output latency (1.33 msec) should then correspond to the latency of the system (operating system and video card) in processing a graphics command and sending it to the monitor.

As described, all tests were replicated using an LCD monitor. In this case, the mean video output latency was 15.22 ± 5.31 msec, with a range of 7.29 to 27.16 msec. The maximum possible refresh rate for this monitor was 60 Hz. (The mean value is larger for the LCD monitor due to the *on* time for liquid crystals, which is the amount of time required for the crystals to reconfigure and let light pass through when a current is applied [Stewart, 2006].) The performances of the CRT and LCD monitors are compared in figure 9.10 which shows that the CRT monitor almost always produces

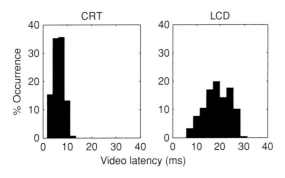

Figure 9.10 Comparison of BCI2000 video output latencies for CRT and LCD monitors, for all tests.

substantially smaller output latencies with less variation among latencies.

Thus, the timing properties of the monitor are important to consider when designing a BCI system, and the type of monitor selected can have a significant impact on the performance of the BCI. An LCD monitor, although weighing less and being more accessible, may not have acceptable performance for all BCI applications due to its inherent variability in timing. However, LCD monitor technology is progressing at a fast pace, and newer monitors are available with 120-Hz refresh rates and response times of <1 msec.

OPERATING SYSTEM

In addition to the tests described above, all tests were replicated on the same Mac Pro system using Windows Vista Enterprise instead of Windows XP in order to determine the effect that the operating system has on the tasks using otherwise identical hardware and the CRT monitor. There were no significant measurable differences in the ADC latency or signal-processing latency between Windows XP and Windows Vista for any task, sampling rate, or number of channels ($p > 0.5$).

However, the video-output latencies for Windows Vista were significantly larger than those for Windows XP ($p < 0.001$) (fig. 9.11). The mean video-output latency for Windows Vista was 20.26 ± 7.56 msec (with a range from 6.12 msec to 42.39 msec) compared to 5.72 ± 1.62 msec (with a range of 1.33 msec to 11.33 msec) with Windows XP. Figure 9.11 shows

the distributions of video-output latencies for Windows XP and Windows Vista on the Mac Pro. The data suggest that the timing of stimulus presentation using Vista, at least with this particular hardware and driver configuration, may be inadequate for many BCI applications. It is usually impossible to observe such timing inconsistencies with the naked eye. The BCI system running on Windows Vista did not appear to have different timing characteristics (e.g., stimulus presentation timing) compared to the Windows XP system. Nevertheless, our analysis showed that the timing on the Windows Vista system was far more variable (Wilson and Schalk, 2010). Thus, unless the actual stimulus delivery time is measured and taken into account by the BCI, this more variable timing might impair the performance of BCI systems that depend on precise stimulus timing, such as those based on P300 evoked potentials.

This consideration of BCI timing characteristics and our evaluation of a representative BCI reveal that choices regarding the system's monitor and the operating system can have a substantial effect on the timing performance of the BCI system. In particular, using Windows Vista and/or an LCD monitor may reduce the performance of the BCI system due to increased latencies and jitter in stimulus presentation and due to loss of the tight temporal relationship between timing of stimulus presentation and timing of data acquisition. In summary, determination of the timing of each new system configuration is very important in evaluating and comparing BCI system software and hardware.

SUMMARY

This chapter discusses the key components of the hardware and software currently used in BCI development and describes evaluation procedures that can help ensure that BCI systems perform as desired. The section on hardware describes the different types of sensors that detect brain signals, the components that amplify and digitize these signals, the interface hardware that connects different components, and the client hardware that runs BCI software. These descriptions indicate that the engineering principles behind BCI hardware are relatively well understood so that the selection and configuration of BCI hardware can be accomplished by appropriately applying and integrating current understanding of analog and digital electronics.

The section on software describes the different components of BCI software: data acquisition components that record, digitize, and store brain signals; signal analysis components that extract signal features that represent the user's intent and that translate these features into commands that embody the user's intent; output components that control the application that realizes that intent; and the operating protocol that determines the configuration, parameterization, timing, and oversight of operation. This section also describes important principles for designing BCI software and lists currently used software tools for BCI research. As is the case for implementation of hardware, the implementation of BCI software follows well-established principles of software design.

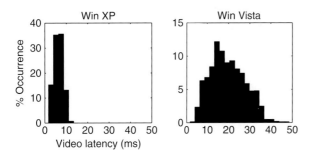

Figure 9.11 Comparison of video output latencies for Windows XP and Windows Vista.

The section on procedures to evaluate hardware and software describes the components of the timing characteristics of a BCI system, procedures to evaluate them, and representative results. These descriptions indicate that assessment of timing characteristics is an important issue in BCI development and that satisfactory results can be achieved with careful implementation.

In summary, development of BCI hardware and software is an ongoing endeavor. Its challenges are caused mainly by the simple fact that the level of standardization in both hardware and software is not very high despite ongoing efforts in both areas. An additional major issue is the need for sensors that can acquire brain signals with high fidelity, reliability, and robustness. It is anticipated that these hardware challenges can be successfully addressed and that further software improvements will make significant contributions to the success of future BCIs.

REFERENCES

Allison, B. Z., D. J. McFarland, G. Schalk, S. D. Zheng, M. M. Jackson, and J. R. Wolpaw. Towards an independent brain-computer interface using steady state visual evoked potentials. *Clin Neurophysiol*, 119(2):399–408, 2008.

Bayliss, J. D. *A Flexible Brain-Computer Interface*. PhD thesis, University of Rochester, Rochester, NY, 2001.

Bell, C. J., P. Shenoy, R. Chalodhorn, and R. P. Rao. Control of a humanoid robot by a noninvasive brain-computer interface in humans. *J Neural Eng*, 5(2):214–220, 2008.

Bianchi, L., F. Babiloni, F. Cincotti, S. Salinari, and M. G. Marciani. Introducing BF++: A C++ framework for cognitive bio-feedback systems design. *Meth Inform Med*, 42(1):102–110, 2003.

Birbaumer, N., A. Kübler, N. Ghanayim, T. Hinterberger, J. Perelmouter, J. Kaiser, I. Iversen, B. Kotchoubey, N. Neumann, and H. Flor. The thought translation device (TTD) for completely paralyzed patients. *IEEE Trans Rehabil Eng*, 8(2):190–193, 2000.

Blakely, T., K. J. Miller, S. P. Zanos, R. P. Rao, and J. G. Ojemann. Robust, long-term control of an electrocorticographic brain-computer interface with fixed parameters. *Neurosurg Focus*, 27(1), 2009. See, http://thejns.org/toc/foc/27/1.

Bronzino, J. D. *The Biomedical Engineering Handbook*. Boca Raton, FL: CRC Press, 2006.

Brunner, P., A. L. Ritaccio, T. M. Lynch, J. F. Emrich, J. A. Wilson, J. C. Williams, E. J. Aarnoutse, N. F. Ramsey, E. C. Leuthardt, H. Bischof, and G. Schalk. A practical procedure for real-time functional mapping of eloquent cortex using electrocorticographic signals in humans. *Epilepsy Behav*, 2009.

Brunner, P., Bianchi, L., Guger, C., Cincotti, F., and G. Schalk. Current trends in hardware and software for brain-computer interfaces (BCIs). *J Neural Eng*, 8(2):025001, 2011.

Buch, E., C. Weber, L. G. Cohen, C. Braun, M. A. Dimyan, T. Ard, J. Mellinger, A. Caria, S. Soekadar, A. Fourkas, and N. Birbaumer. Think to move: a neuromagnetic brain-computer interface (BCI) system for chronic stroke. *Stroke*, 39(3):910–917, 2008.

Cabrera, A. F., and K. Dremstrup. Auditory and spatial navigation imagery in brain-computer interface using optimized wavelets. *J Neurosci Methods*, 174(1):135–146, 2008.

Campbell, P. K., R. A. Normann, K. W. Horch, and S. S. Stensaas. A chronic intracortical electrode array: preliminary results. *J Biomed Mater Res*, 23(A2 Suppl):245–259, 1989.

Cincotti, F., D. Mattia, F. Aloise, S. Bufalari, L. Astolfi, F. De Vico Fallani, A. Tocci, L. Bianchi, M. G. Marciani, S. Gao, J. Millán, and F. Babiloni. High-resolution EEG techniques for brain-computer interface applications. *J Neurosci Methods*, 167(1):31–42, 2008.

Cincotti, F., D. Mattia, F. Aloise, S. Bufalari, G. Schalk, G. Oriolo, A. Cherubini, M. G. Marciani, and F. Babiloni. Non-invasive brain-computer interface system: towards its application as assistive technology. *Brain Res Bull*, 75(6):796–803, 2008.

Clark, J., and J. Webster. *Medical Instrumentation: Application and Design*. New York: Wiley, 1995.

Crone, N. E., D. L. Miglioretti, B. Gordon, J. M. Sieracki, M. T. Wilson, S. Uematsu, and R. P. Lesser. Functional mapping of human sensorimotor cortex with electrocorticographic spectral analysis. i. alpha and beta event-related desynchronization. *Brain*, 121(Pt 12):2271–2299, 1998.

Daly, J. J., R. Cheng, J. Rogers, K. Litinas, K. Hrovat, and M. Dohring. Feasibility of a new application of noninvasive Brain Computer Interface (BCI): a case study of training for recovery of volitional motor control after stroke. *J Neurol Phys Ther*, 33(4):203–211, 2009.

Felton, E. A., J. A. Wilson, J. C. Williams, and P. C. Garell. Electrocorticographically controlled brain-computer interfaces using motor and sensory imagery in patients with temporary subdural electrode implants. Report of four cases. *J Neurosurg*, 106(3):495–500, 2007.

Fisch B. J., and R. Spehlmann. *Fisch and Spehlmann's EEG Primer: Basic Principles of Digital and Analog EEG*. Amsterdam: Elsevier Science Health Science Division, 1999.

Fonseca, C., J. P. Silva Cunha, R. E. Martins, V. M. Ferreira, J. P. Marques de Sá, M. A. Barbosa, and A. Martins da Silva. A novel dry active electrode for EEG recording. *IEEE Trans Biomed Eng*, 54(1):162–165, 2007.

Freeman, W. J., L. J. Rogers, M. D. Holmes, and D. L. Silbergeld. Spatial spectral analysis of human electrocorticograms including the alpha and gamma bands. *J Neurosci Methods*, 95(2):111–121, 2000.

Furdea, A., S. Halder, D. J. Krusienski, D. Bross, F. Nijboer, N. Birbaumer, and A. Kübler. An auditory oddball (P300) spelling system for brain-computer interfaces. *Psychophysiology*, 46(3):617–625, 2009.

Guger, C., G. Edlinger, W. Harkam, I. Niedermayer, and G. Pfurtscheller. How many people are able to operate an EEG-based brain-computer interface (BCI)? *IEEE Trans Neural Syst Rehabil Eng*, 11(2):145–147, 2003.

Guger, C., H. Ramoser, and G. Pfurtscheller. Real-time EEG analysis with subject-specific spatial patterns for a brain-computer interface (BCI). *IEEE Trans Rehabil Eng*, 8(4):447–456, 2000.

Guger, C., A. Schlögl, C. Neuper, D. Walterspacher, T. Strein, and G. Pfurtscheller. Rapid prototyping of an EEG-based brain-computer interface (BCI). *IEEE Trans Neur Syst Rehabil Eng*, 9(1):49–58, 2001.

Harris, K. D., D. A. Henze, J. Csicsvari, H. Hirase, and G. Buzsáki. Accuracy of tetrode spike separation as determined by simultaneous intracellular and extracellular measurements. *J Neurophysiol*, 84(1):401–414, 2000.

Hochberg, L. R., M. D. Serruya, G. M. Friehs, J. A. Mukand, M. Saleh, A. H. Caplan, A. Branner, D. Chen, R. D. Penn, and J. P. Donoghue. Neuronal ensemble control of prosthetic devices by a human with tetraplegia. *Nature*, 442(7099):164–171, 2006.

Kennedy, P., D. Andreasen, P. Ehirim, B. King, T. Kirby, H. Mao, and M. Moore. Using human extra-cortical local field potentials to control a switch. *J Neural Eng*, 1:72, 2004.

Kennedy, P. R. The cone electrode: a long-term electrode that records from neurites grown onto its recording surface. *J Neurosci Methods*, 29(3):181–193, 1989.

Kim, J., J. A. Wilson, and J. C. Williams. A cortical recording platform utilizing microECoG electrode arrays. *Conf Proc IEEE Eng Med Biol Soc*, 2007:5353–5357, 2007.

Kipke, D. R., R. J. Vetter, J. C. Williams, and J. F. Hetke. Silicon-substrate intracortical microelectrode arrays for long-term recording of neuronal spike activity in cerebral cortex. *IEEE Trans Neural Syst Rehabil Eng*, 11(2):151–155, 2003.

Klem, G., H. Lüders, H. Jasper, and C. Elger. The ten-twenty electrode system of the International Federation. The International Federation of Clinical Neurophysiology. *Electroencephalogr Clin Neurophysiol*, 52:3, 1999.

Krusienski, D., F. Cabestaing, D. McFarland, and J. Wolpaw. A comparison of classification techniques for the P300 speller. *J Neural Eng*, 3(4):299–305, 2006.

Kubánek, J., K. J. Miller, J. G. Ojemann, J. R. Wolpaw, and G. Schalk. Decoding flexion of individual fingers using electrocorticographic signals in humans. *J Neural Eng*, 6(6), 2009.

Kübler, A., A. Furdea, S. Halder, E. M. Hammer, F. Nijboer, and B. Kotchoubey. A brain-computer interface controlled auditory event-related potential (P300) spelling system for locked-in patients. *Ann N Y Acad Sci*, 1157:90–100, 2009.

Kübler, A., F. Nijboer, J. Mellinger, T. M. Vaughan, H. Pawelzik, G. Schalk, D. J. McFarland, N. Birbaumer, and J. R. Wolpaw. Patients with ALS can use sensorimotor rhythms to operate a brain-computer interface. *Neurology*, 64(10):1775–1777, 2005.

Lécuyer, A., Lotte, F., Reilly, R., Leeb, R., Hirose, M., and Slater. M. Brain-computer interfaces, virtual reality, and videogames. *IEEE Computer*, 41:66–72, 2008.

Leuthardt, E., K. Miller, N. Anderson, G. Schalk, J. Dowling, J. Miller, D. Moran, and J. Ojemann. Electrocorticographic frequency alteration mapping: a clinical technique for mapping the motor cortex. *Neurosurgery*, 60:260–270; discussion 270–1, 2007.

Leuthardt, E., K. Miller, G. Schalk, R. Rao, and J. Ojemann. Electrocorticography-based brain computer interface–the Seattle experience. *IEEE Trans Neural Syst Rehabil Eng*, 14:194–198, 2006.

Leuthardt, E. C., G. Schalk, D. Moran, and J. G. Ojemann. The emerging world of motor neuroprosthetics: a neurosurgical perspective. *Neurosurgery*, 59(1):1–14, 2006.

Leuthardt, E. C., G. Schalk, J. R. Wolpaw, J. G. Ojemann, and D. W. Moran. A brain-computer interface using electrocorticographic signals in humans. *J Neural Eng*, 1(2):63–71, 2004.

Lotte, F., Van Langhenhove, A., Lamarche, F., Ernest, T., Renard, Y., Arnaldi, B., and Lécuyer, A. Exploring large virtual environments by thoughts using a brain-computer interface based on motor imagery and high-level commands. *Presence: teleoperators and virtual environments*, 19(1):54–70, 2010.

Luo, A., and T. J. Sullivan. A user-friendly SSVEP-based brain-computer interface using a time-domain classifier. *J Neural Eng*, 7(2):26010, 2010.

Maynard, E., C. Nordhausen, and R. Normann. The Utah intracortical electrode array: a recording structure for potential brain-computer interfaces. *Electroencephalogr Clin Neurophysiol*, 102(3):228–239, 1997.

McFarland, D., W. Sarnacki, and J. Wolpaw. Electroencephalographic (EEG) control of three-dimensional movement. *Society for Neuroscience Abstracts Online* http://www.abstractsonline.com/Plan/ViewAbstract.aspx?sKey=fa317e68-3331-4f94-b0d9-6fa70986f1e4&cKey=cd433551-1b3f-48f0-9fd0-3de3d157ae87&mKey={AFEA068D-D012-4520-8E42-10E4D1AF7944}, 2008.

McFarland, D. J., D. J. Krusienski, W. A. Sarnacki, and J. R. Wolpaw. Emulation of computer mouse control with a noninvasive brain-computer interface. *J Neural Eng*, 5(2):101–110, 2008.

McFarland, D. J., L. M. McCane, S. V. David, and J. R. Wolpaw. Spatial filter selection for EEG-based communication. *Electroenceph Clin Neurophysiol*, 103(3):386–394, 1997.

McFarland, D. J., W. A. Sarnacki, and J. R. Wolpaw. Electroencephalographic (EEG) control of three-dimensional movement. *J Neural Eng*, 7(3):036007, 2010.

McFarland, D. J. and J. R. Wolpaw. EEG-based communication and control: speed-accuracy relationships. *Appl Psychophysiol Biofeedback*, 28(3):217–231, 2003.

Mellinger, J., G. Schalk, C. Braun, H. Preissl, W. Rosenstiel, N. Birbaumer, and A. Kübler. An MEG-based brain-computer interface (BCI). *Neuroimage*, 36(3):581–593, 2007.

Miller, K. J., M. Dennijs, P. Shenoy, J. W. Miller, R. P. Rao, and J. G. Ojemann. Real-time functional brain mapping using electrocorticography. *Neuroimage*, 37(2):504–507, 2007.

Miller, K., E. Leuthardt, G. Schalk, R. Rao, N. Anderson, D. Moran, J. Miller, and J. Ojemann. Spectral changes in cortical surface potentials during motor movement. *J Neurosci*, 27:2424–2432, 2007.

Miller, K. J., G. Schalk, E. E. Fetz, M. den Nijs, J. G. Ojemann, and R. P. Rao. Cortical activity during motor execution, motor imagery, and imagery-based online feedback. *Proc Natl Acad Sci USA*, 107(9):4430–4435, 2010.

Nijboer, F., E. W. Sellers, J. Mellinger, M. A. Jordan, T. Matuz, A. Furdea, S. Halder, U. Mochty, D. J. Krusienski, T. M. Vaughan, J. R. Wolpaw, N. Birbaumer, and A. Kübler. A P300-based brain-computer interface for people with amyotrophic lateral sclerosis. *Clin Neurophysiol*, 119(8):1909–1916, 2008.

Nordhausen, C. T., E. M. Maynard, and R. A. Normann. Single unit recording capabilities of a 100 microelectrode array. *Brain Res*, 726(1–2):129–140, 1996.

Nunez, P., and R. Srinivasan. *Electric Fields of the Brain: The Neurophysics of EEG*. New York: Oxford University Press, 2006.

Oostenveld, R., and P. Praamstra. The five percent electrode system for high-resolution EEG and ERP measurements. *Clin Neurophysiol*, 112(4):713–719, 2001.

Pfurtscheller, G., C. Neuper, D. Flotzinger, and M. Pregenzer. EEG-based discrimination between imagination of right and left hand movement. *Electroencephalogr Clin Neurophysiol*, 103(6):642–651, 1997.

Popescu, F., S. Fazli, Y. Badower, B. Blankertz, and K.-R. Müller. Single trial classification of motor imagination using 6 dry EEG electrodes. *PLoS One*, 2(7):e637, 2007.

Ramoser, H., J. Müller-Gerking, and G. Pfurtscheller. Optimal spatial filtering of single trial EEG during imagined hand movement. *IEEE Trans Rehabil Eng*, 8(4):441–446, 2000.

Renard, Y., G. Gibert, M. Congedo, F. Lotte, E. Maby, B. Hennion, O. Bertrand, and A. Lecuyer. OpenViBE: an open-source software platform to easily design, test and use Brain-Computer Interfaces. In *Autumn school: From neural code to brain/machine interfaces*, http://www.mitpressjournals.org/doi/abs/10.1162/pres.19.1.35, 2007.

Rousche, P. J., D. S. Pellinen, D. P. J. Pivin, J. C. Williams, R. J. Vetter, and D. R. Kipke. Flexible polyimide-based intracortical electrode arrays with bioactive capability. *IEEE Trans Biomed Eng*, 48(3):361–371, 2001.

Royer, A. S., and B. He. Goal selection versus process control in a brain-computer interface based on sensorimotor rhythms. *J Neural Eng*, 6(1):16005, 2009.

Rubehn, B., C. Bosman, R. Oostenveld, P. Fries, and T. Stieglitz. A MEMS-based flexible multichannel ECoG-electrode array. *J Neural Eng*, 6:036003, 2009.

Schalk, G. Effective brain-computer interfacing using BCI2000. *Conf Proc IEEE Eng Med Biol Soc*, 5498–5501, 2009.

Schalk, G., P. Brunner, L. A. Gerhardt, H. Bischof, and J. R. Wolpaw. Brain-computer interfaces (BCIs): detection instead of classification. *J Neurosci Methods*, 167(1):51–62, 2008.

Schalk, G., J. Kubánek, K. J. Miller, N. R. Anderson, E. C. Leuthardt, J. G. Ojemann, D. Limbrick, D. Moran, L. A. Gerhardt, and J. R. Wolpaw. Decoding two-dimensional movement trajectories using electrocorticographic signals in humans. *J Neural Eng*, 4(3):264–275, 2007.

Schalk, G., E. C. Leuthardt, P. Brunner, J. G. Ojemann, L. A. Gerhardt, and J. R. Wolpaw. Real-time detection of event-related brain activity. *Neuroimage*, 43(2):245–249, 2008.

Schalk, G., D. McFarland, T. Hinterberger, N. Birbaumer, and J. Wolpaw. BCI2000: A general-purpose brain-computer interface (BCI) system. *IEEE Trans Biomed Eng*, 51:1034–1043, 2004.

Schalk, G., and J. Mellinger. *A Practical Guide to Brain-Computer Interfacing with BCI2000*. Springer, 2010.

Schalk, G., K. J. Miller, N. R. Anderson, J. A. Wilson, M. D. Smyth, J. G. Ojemann, D. W. Moran, J. R. Wolpaw, and E. C. Leuthardt. Two-dimensional movement control using electrocorticographic signals in humans. *J Neural Eng*, 5(1):75–84, 2008.

Schlögl, A., G. Müller, R. Scherer, and G. Pfurtscheller. BioSig—an open source software package for biomedical signal processing. *2nd Open ECG Workshop*, Berlin, Germany, 2004.

Sellers, E. W., A. Kübler, and E. Donchin. Brain-computer interface research at the University of South Florida Cognitive Psychophysiology Laboratory: the P300 Speller. *IEEE Trans Neural Syst Rehabil Eng*, 14(2):221–224, 2006.

Sellers, E. W., T. M. Vaughan, and J. R. Wolpaw. A brain-computer interface for long-term independent home use. *Amyotroph Lateral Scler*, 11(5):449–55, 2010.

Sharbrough, F., G. Chatrian, R. Lesser, H. Luders, M. Nuwer, and T. Picton. American electroencephalographic society guidelines for standard electrode position nomenclature. *Electroenceph Clin Neurophysiol*, 8:200–202, 1991.

Slutzky, M. W., L. R. Jordan, T. Krieg, M. Chen, D. J. Mogul, and L. E. Miller. Optimal spacing of surface electrode arrays for brain-machine interface applications. *J Neural Eng*, 7(2):26004, 2010.

Stadler, J. A. 3rd, D. J. Ellens, and J. M. Rosenow. Deep brain stimulation and motor cortical stimulation for neuropathic pain. *Curr Pain Headache Rep*, 15(1):8–13, 2010.

Stewart, N. Millisecond accuracy video display using OpenGL under Linux. *Behav Res Methods*, 38(1):142–145, 2006.

Taheri, B. A., R. T. Knight, and R. L. Smith. A dry electrode for EEG recording. *Electroencephalogr Clin Neurophysiol*, 90(5):376–383, 1994.

Thomas, R., A. Rosa, and G. Toussaint. *The Analysis and Design of Linear Circuits*. New York: Wiley, 2004.

Tompkins, W. *Biomedical Digital Signal Processing: C-Language Examples and Laboratory Experiments for the IBM PC*. Upper Saddle River, NJ: Prentice-Hall, 1993.

Townsend, G., B. K. LaPallo, C. B. Boulay, D. J. Krusienski, G. E. Frye, C. K. Hauser, N. E. Schwartz, T. M. Vaughan, J. R. Wolpaw, and E. W. Sellers. A novel p300-based brain-computer interface stimulus presentation paradigm: moving beyond rows and columns. *Clin Neurophysiol*, 121(7):1109–1120, 2010.

Tsubokawa, T., Y. Katayama, T. Yamamoto, T. Hirayama, and S. Koyama. Chronic motor cortex stimulation for the treatment of central pain. *Acta Neurochir Suppl (Wien)*, 52:137–139, 1991.

Vaughan, T. M., D. J. McFarland, G. Schalk, W. A. Sarnacki, D. J. Krusienski, E. W. Sellers, and J. R. Wolpaw. The Wadsworth BCI research and development program: at home with BCI. *IEEE Trans Neural Syst Rehabil Eng*, 14(2):229–233, 2006.

Velliste, M., J. Brumberg, S. Perel, M. Fraser, M. Spalding, A. Whitford, A. McMorland, E. Wright, F. Guenther, P. Kennedy, and A. Schwartz. Modular software architecture for neural prosthetic control. In *Program No. 895.1*.

2009 Neuroscience Meeting Planner. Chicago: Society for Neuroscience, 2009.

Venthur, B., and B. Blankertz. A platform-independent open-source feedback framework for BCI systems. In *Proceedings of the 4th International Brain-Computer Interface Workshop and Training Course*. Graz, Austria: Verlag der Technischen Universität Graz, 2008.

Volosyak, I., Valbuena, D., Malechka, T., Peuscher, J., A. Gräser. Brain-computer interface using water-based electrodes. *J Neural Eng*, 7:066007, 2010.

Wilson, J., E. Felton, P. Garell, G. Schalk, and J. Williams. ECoG factors underlying multimodal control of a brain-computer interface. *IEEE Trans Neural Syst Rehabil Eng*, 14:246–250, 2006.

Wilson, J., J. Mellinger, G. Schalk, and J. Williams. A procedure for measuring latencies in brain-computer interfaces. *IEEE Trans Biomed Eng*, 57(7):1785–97, 2010.

Wilson, J., and G. Schalk. Using BCI2000 for HCI-centered BCI research. In D. Tan and A. Nijholt (Eds.), *Brain-Computer Interfaces*. Springer, 2010.

Wise, K. D., J. B. Angell, and A. Starr. An integrated-circuit approach to extracellular microelectrodes. *IEEE Trans Biomed Eng*, 17(3):238–247, 1970.

Wisneski, K. J., N. Anderson, G. Schalk, M. Smyth, D. Moran, and E. C. Leuthardt. Unique cortical physiology associated with ipsilateral hand movements and neuroprosthetic implications. *Stroke*, 39(12):3351–3359, 2008.

Wolpaw, J. R., and D. J. McFarland. Control of a two-dimensional movement signal by a noninvasive brain-computer interface in humans. *Proc Natl Acad Sci USA*, 101(51):17849–17854, 2004.

Yamawaki, N., C. Wilke, Z. Liu, and B. He. An enhanced time-frequency-spatial approach for motor imagery classification. *IEEE Trans Neural Syst Rehabil Eng*, 14(2):250–254, 2006.

Zhang, K., I. Ginzburg, B. McNaughton, and T. Sejnowski. Interpreting neuronal population activity by reconstruction: unified framework with application to hippocampal place cells. *J Neurophysiol*, 79(2):1017–1044, 1998.

10 | BCI OPERATING PROTOCOLS

STEVEN G. MASON, BRENDAN Z. ALLISON, AND JONATHAN R. WOLPAW

Previous chapters in this section describe BCI operation from signal acquisition, through feature extraction and translation, to output commands, and the hardware and software that produce it. BCIs do not operate in isolation; they operate in the world, that is, in an environment. Their environment has three essential elements: the BCI user; the BCI application; and, usually, external support for the BCI. Just as the individual steps of BCI operation (i.e., signal acquisition, feature extraction, etc.) interact with each other according to a protocol (see chapter 9, this volume), each BCI interacts with its environment according to a protocol. This protocol, specifying how the BCI relates to its environment, is called the BCI's *operating protocol.*

A BCI operating protocol has four key elements. Each can be stated as a question:

- Who initiates BCI operation: the BCI or the user?

- Who parameterizes the feature extraction and translation process: the BCI or its external support?

- Does the BCI tell its application what to do or how to do it?

- Does the BCI try to recognize its own errors or is this left entirely to the user or the application?

Taken together, the answers to these questions comprise a BCI's operating protocol.

This chapter addresses each of these questions in turn. Each question has two possible answers, and each answer defines a particular class of BCI operating protocols. Although specific BCI protocols may bridge classes (e.g., some aspects of parameterization might be handled by the BCI and others by external support), these questions and their answers provide a framework for understanding operating protocols. The chapter describes the characteristics, advantages, and disadvantages of each protocol class, and it provides illustrative examples from among existing or conceivable BCIs. It concludes with a discussion of the specialized operating protocols needed for user training and for research.

THE KEY ELEMENTS OF THE BCI OPERATING PROTOCOL

HOW IS BCI OPERATION INITIATED?

As is true for anyone who can engage in a particular intentional action, a BCI user is sometimes actively using the BCI (e.g., using it to communicate with someone) and is at other times not using the BCI (e.g., is doing something else, sleeping, daydreaming, etc.):

- The state of active BCI use is referred to as *intentional control.*

- The state of other activities is referred to as *no intentional control,* or more simply, *no control.*

By this terminology, a person is using the BCI during *intentional control* and not using the BCI during *no control* (Mason et al. 2007; Mason and Birch 2005).

Ideally, BCI use should be as easy and convenient as a person's muscle-based actions. That is, the person should be able to operate the BCI in a self-paced mode, in which the BCI is readily available, and in which the user can perform *intentional control* whenever s/he desires (Mason et al. 2006). To allow such user-paced operation, a BCI must be able to differentiate reliably between the user's *no-control* state and the user's *intentional-control* state. This is a difficult requirement. It is difficult because a wide range of brain activity signals might correspond to *no control,* and the BCI must be able to recognize all of them as indicating the no-control state. If the BCI is unable to accurately distinguish between *no control* and *intentional control,* brain activity during *no control* will sometimes be translated into unintended actions. This problem of sending an unintended message or command has been called the "Midas Touch Problem," after the greedy king who wished that everything he touched would turn to gold, then accidentally turned his daughter into gold (Moore 2003). For many BCI applications, even a small number of such false-positive errors could make BCI use very frustrating and possibly impractical. For other BCI applications, it could even be hazardous: if, for example, the BCI controlled a motorized wheelchair on the sidewalk next to a busy city street.

At present, BCI operating protocols address the need to avoid unintended actions during a no-control state in one of two ways: through *synchronous* protocols that limit BCI actions to times when the user can safely be assumed to be in the intentional-control state; and, alternatively, through *self-paced* (or *asynchronous*) protocols that are able to distinguish satisfactorily between the no-control state and the intentional-control state.

SYNCHRONOUS PROTOCOLS

A *synchronous protocol* limits the times during which the BCI will actually convert the user's brain activity into action (Mason and Birch 2005; Müller-Putz et al. 2006). One kind of

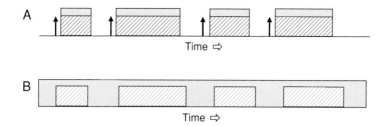

Figure 10.1 *(A) A synchronous operating protocol. Shading indicates the times when the BCI is available for control, and hatching indicates the times when the BCI expects the user to be providing control commands. The arrows indicate the cues provided by the BCI prior to the onset of the BCI usage periods. (B) A self-paced (also called asynchronous) operating protocol. The continuous shading indicates that the BCI is always available to the user. The hatched rectangles indicate periods of intentional control that are initiated by the user and recognized by the BCI. The time periods between hatching are periods of no control.*

synchronous protocol gives the user a specific sensory stimulus and analyzes the brain activity that occurs during a fixed period immediately afterward. The BCI converts brain signals into output only during that poststimulus period. In this way, the protocol limits and specifies the times when the BCI will convert brain activity into action. Alternatively, the protocol might provide cues, such as a "get-ready" indicator to inform the user of an impending period of expected *intentional control*. Synchronous BCI operation is depicted in figure 10.1A.

One common type of synchronous BCI is a P300 speller discussed in detail in chapter 12, this volume. The user views a matrix containing letters and/or other items. Each row or column of the matrix flashes in succession, and the subject notes (e.g., counts) each flash that contains the letter that s/he wants to communicate. The resulting brain activity can be used to identify which row and column contain the desired letter and thus allows the user to spell with brain activity (Farwell and Donchin 1988; Sellers et al. 2006; Vaughan et al. 2006; Jin et al. 2010). This BCI is *synchronous* because the output is based on the user's responses to stimuli (i.e., flashes) presented on a schedule determined by the BCI.

In a second type of synchronous BCI, users spell by imagining different types of movements. Brain-imaging techniques can determine which kind of movement imagery a person is performing. For example, users might think about moving the left hand, right hand, feet, or other areas and thereby direct a cursor or arrow to select a particular letter (Wolpaw et al. 2003; Scherer et al. 2004; Pfurtscheller et al. 2006; Müller et al. 2008). Such a BCI is synchronous because users must imagine the movements at specific times. One drawback to these synchronous protocols is that the BCI *expects* intentional control when it gives the prompt, and if the user does not respond with appropriate brain activity during the specified period, the result may be an undesired action. The two synchronous BCI approaches described above typically do not even consider the possibility that the user does not intend to use the BCI at the specified time. Hence, such BCIs will always identify one of the possible items as the target (or will identify a direction for cursor movement, etc.), which will of course be a mistake if the user does not intend any control. In addition, the user may find that a synchronous protocol, in which the BCI specifies the times of operation, is awkward and unnatural for many real-world tasks.

SELF-PACED PROTOCOLS

The alternative to a synchronous protocol is a *self-paced* protocol (also referred to as an *asynchronous* protocol). A *self-paced* protocol distinguishes between no-control and intentional-control states. This mode of operation is depicted in figure 10.1B. It allows a person to use the BCI whenever s/he desires. Self-paced protocols can yield more natural and dynamic interactions between the user and BCI, but they are much more challenging to develop. Initial efforts to develop reliable self-paced protocols have had some success, but they are not yet suitable for general use outside the laboratory.

Self-paced steady-state visual evoked potential-based (SSVEP-based) BCI designs have been described in several studies (Trejo et al. 2006; Allison et al. 2010). To produce a BCI output, the user focuses on one of a set of rapidly flickering lights each of which represents a different possible output. Whenever the BCI detects a significant increase in EEG activity at the same frequency as one of the flickering targets, it implements the command associated with that target. Thus, users can move a cursor to spell, select numbers, or perform other tasks by focusing on a target whenever they wish. If the user is doing something other than using the BCI and is not attending to any of the flickering targets, then there is no increase in the activity associated with any of the targets, and the BCI does not produce outputs. (See chapter 14 for further discussion of such SSVEP-based BCIs.)

Self-paced BCIs can rely on motor imagery as well. Some BCIs allow users to navigate through a virtual environment (Leeb et al. 2007; Scherer et al. 2008) by imagining movements at any time. If the BCI detects the EEG activity associated with one of several specific mental tasks (such as imagining left-hand movement), then that activity is translated into a particular command.

COMBINED SYNCHRONOUS AND SELF-PACED PROTOCOLS

It is certainly also possible to design BCIs that combine self-paced and synchronous protocols. For example, the BCI might remain in an inactive standby mode until the user produces a specific sequence of sensorimotor rhythm amplitudes (or some other brain activity) that rarely if ever occurs by chance and that can serve as a reliable self-paced key to activate the BCI. The activated BCI might then operate under a synchronous protocol to support intentional control until the user produces another (or the same) self-paced key to return the BCI to the standby mode.

For example, one recently developed system allows users to turn an SSVEP BCI on or off by imagining foot movement (Pfurtscheller et al. 2010). Other types of such *semisynchronous* BCIs might facilitate more flexible operation. They might use contextual cues to interpret user requests and thus allow users to perform different tasks with the same signal. For example, if a user imagines foot movement while playing a virtual soccer game, the system might perform different actions based on the game state. The avatar might run forward if the ball is far away, or kick the ball if it is nearby, or the BCI might switch to a strictly synchronous mode for a special action such as a penalty kick. BCIs that combine users' commands with other relevant information to produce appropriate outputs should become increasingly common and capable as BCIs are integrated with ambient intelligence and context-aware systems (Allison 2009; Millán et al. 2010).

CURRENT USE OF SYNCHRONOUS AND SELF-PACED PROTOCOLS

At present, the realization of reliable, fully self-paced BCI protocols remains one of the most difficult and important problems confronting the development of BCIs that are suitable for widespread use outside the laboratory. Until such protocols are further developed and validated in online testing, synchronous protocols can certainly serve in simple BCI communication systems for people who cannot use conventional (i.e., muscle-based) assistive communication devices (e.g., Vaughan et al. 2006; Kübler and Birbaumer 2008; Nijboer et al. 2010; Sellers et al. 2010).

HOW IS THE FEATURE-EXTRACTION AND TRANSLATION PROCESS PARAMETERIZED?

In the feature extraction and translation operations, the BCI extracts specific features from the brain signals and uses them as independent variables in calculations that produce dependent variables (i.e., the commands that go to the application). The *parameters* of these operations specify how often they occur, which features are extracted, how they are extracted, and the forms and constants of the equations that translate the extracted features into the dependent variables. Appropriate parameter selection, or parameterization, is obviously essential for effective BCI performance. Parameters vary widely among BCIs as a function of signal type and of the methods used for feature extraction and translation. Nevertheless, BCI operating protocols can be broadly grouped into two categories:

- preparameterized protocols
- self-parameterized protocols.

PREPARAMETERIZED PROTOCOLS

Preparameterized BCI protocols use fixed parameters that have been selected for the BCI. For example, a BCI might be parameterized from the results of an initial session in which the user is asked to imagine a specific set of actions. Analysis of the brain signals associated with the imagined actions can yield an optimal set of parameters for translating the user's brain activity into the specific application commands linked to the specific imagined actions (Pfurtscheller et al. 2006; Trejo et al. 2006; Müller et al. 2008). These protocols are most suited for limited single-time BCI studies in which a single prestudy parameterization is sufficient (Allison et al. 2010). In contrast, in real-life use, it would be typical for a BCI to be used repeatedly over many days or more, and it is thus likely that periodic repetitions of the preparameterization procedure would be needed (Nijboer et al. 2010). On the other hand, some BCI systems can function well for prolonged periods with the same set of parameters (Sellers et al. 2006).

SELF-PARAMETERIZED PROTOCOLS

Self-parameterized (also called *adaptive*) BCI protocols select and modify their own parameters. They might do this through periodic automated procedures. For example, a P300 BCI used for word-processing could periodically conduct a brief automated copy-spelling session in which the user is given a number of letters (i.e., target letters) to select from a matrix. Analysis of the responses evoked by target versus nontarget letters would yield an updated set of parameters for translating the user's brain activity into letter selection. Alternatively, a BCI might incorporate continuing parameter updating into its standard operation. For example, a sensorimotor rhythm (SMR)-based BCI might continually adjust the constants in the equations that convert SMR amplitudes into cursor movements by making simple assumptions about average intent over past movements (e.g., that, on the average, the user intended to move right as often as s/he intended to move left).

Because self-parameterized BCI protocols can adjust (at least in theory, see chapter 8, this volume) to spontaneous and adaptive changes in the user's brain signals, they are generally preferable in BCIs for everyday use. They will undoubtedly become more common as BCI research and development evolve. During this transition time, many, indeed most, protocols are and will continue to be partially self-parameterized in that they select and/or update some parameters on their own and receive the remainder from elsewhere (e.g., from procedures conducted by technical support personnel or researchers). For example, in the SMR-based BCI system described in Wolpaw and McFarland (2004), the features used are selected by the experimenters while the weights assigned to those features are continually updated by the BCI itself. In a recent long-term study of SMR-based and P300-based BCI usage, key parameters were updated automatically, and, in addition, some parameters were modified as needed by the experimenters (Nijboer et al. 2010).

DOES THE BCI TELL ITS APPLICATION WHAT TO DO OR HOW TO DO IT?

After recording brain signals, a BCI performs two operations. First, it extracts signal features such as the power in specific frequency bands or the firing rates of specific neurons. Then, it translates these features into commands that operate an application (also called a device) such as a word-processing program, an environmental control unit, a wheelchair, or a neuroprosthesis. Although all BCIs extract signal features and translate them into commands, their operating protocols fall into two classes in terms of the nature of the commands that they produce (Wolpaw 2007). These two classes are described and illustrated in chapter 1 of this volume (see also fig. 1.6) and include:

- goal-selection protocols
- process-control protocols

GOAL-SELECTION PROTOCOLS

In a *goal-selection* (or simply *selection*) protocol (also referred to as a *discrete-control* protocol), signal features are translated into specific commands selected from among a finite set of possible commands: "type the letter E"; "turn the TV to channel 3"; "pick up the apple"; and so forth. Thus, in a goal-selection protocol, each feature-translation operation produces a different command chosen from among a defined set of discrete commands.

P300-based and SSVEP-based BCIs (see chapters 13 and 15, this volume) illustrate how synchronous or asynchronous BCIs can rely on goal-selection protocols. In both examples, the user can select among a set of different goal-selection commands by attending to one item out of a set of choices.

PROCESS-CONTROL PROTOCOLS

In a *process-control* (or simply *process*) protocol (also referred to as a *continuous-control* or *kinematic-control* protocol), signal features are translated into commands that produce the next step in a process (e.g., movement of a cursor or a wheelchair, progressive opening and closing of a robotic hand, change in the force exerted by a neuroprosthesis, etc.). In a process-control protocol, each feature-translation operation produces the next step in an ongoing process (e.g., the next movement of a cursor on a computer screen). For example, the self-paced BCIs mentioned above (Leeb et al. 2007; Scherer et al. 2008), which enable users to move through a virtual environment via imagined movement, rely on process control. So do many other BCIs, including other SMR-based BCIs, single neuron-based BCIs, and even some P300-based BCIs (e.g., Hochberg et al. 2006; Citi et al. 2008; McFarland et al. 2010).

COMPARISON OF GOAL-SELECTION AND PROCESS-CONTROL PROTOCOLS

The question of how the BCI converts the user's intention into action—by either a goal-selection protocol or a process-control protocol—focuses exclusively on the nature of the command that results from the feature translation. From that command onward, a BCI could serve many different applications in many different ways. For example, a goal-selection protocol, which is commonly used for applications such as word-processing, could also be used to drive a wheelchair if the set of commands included: "go to the kitchen"; "go to the TV"; and so forth. Conversely, a process-control protocol, which is commonly used to move a cursor, could operate a TV if the process moved the cursor to reach icons that then executed actions such as "turn TV on," "select channel 10," and so forth.

Furthermore, a particular BCI application might switch back and forth between process-control and goal-selection protocols. Thus, a BCI mouse-control application, in which a process-control protocol moves the cursor to an icon, might then switch to a goal-selection protocol to decide whether to select (i.e., click on) that icon or continue on to another icon (e.g., McFarland et al. 2008). For example, Cherubini et al. (2008) describe a BCI system that can allow commands in three modes: single-step, semi-autonomous, or autonomous. In the single-step mode, the robot moves a fixed short distance with each movement command, whereas in the semi-autonomous mode, each movement command causes the robot to move a graded distance in one direction, avoiding obstacles through artificial intelligence. These first two modes are process-control protocols. In contrast, in the third mode, the autonomous mode, each command selects a target from among a set of targets in a defined environment, and the robot then moves to the target. This mode is a goal-selection protocol. As noted at the beginning of this chapter, chapter 11 discusses applications to which either or both of these two classes of operating protocols (goal-selection and process-control) might be applied.

HOW ARE TRANSLATION ERRORS HANDLED?

For a communication or control interface, an error is a failure to recognize the user's intent. All such interfaces face the problem of errors, and BCIs are no exception. A BCI might mistakenly recognize "Yes" as "No," "Type an A" as "Type a B," or "Stay in place" as "Go forward." Furthermore, a BCI that uses a self-paced operating protocol might commit false-positive or false-negative errors by mistaking the no-control state for the intentional-control state or vice versa. That is, the BCI might produce output when the user does not intend to use the BCI, or it might not produce output when the user does intend to use the BCI. (The former is analogous to a smartphone with a touch screen sensing a touch when no touch has occurred.)

In their present early stage of development, BCIs are particularly prone to translation errors. The importance of such errors and the measures taken to eliminate them or minimize their impact vary widely across BCIs and their applications. In word-processing applications, for example, misspellings may be tolerated or easily fixed. On the other hand, in prosthesis or wheelchair control applications, movement errors may have severe consequences. Nevertheless, even for an application as safe as word-processing, too many errors can make the BCI very inefficient, unacceptably frustrating, or even entirely useless.

The need to minimize errors often leads to slower performance. In P300-based goal-selection protocols, for example, it is possible to reduce errors by increasing the number of stimulus sequences per selection, but performance will consequently be slower. To reduce errors for SMR-based process-control protocols, the length of the data segment used to determine each step (e.g., each cursor movement) may be increased or the size of each step may be decreased, but again performance will be slower. Thus, the benefits of measures that reduce errors must be weighed against the concomitant slowing of performance. In fact, users themselves often have preferences in this regard, with some preferring fast error-ridden performance and others preferring slow but accurate performance.

BCI operating protocols handle errors in one of two ways:

- through *error-blind* protocols
- through *error-detection* protocols

ERROR-BLIND PROTOCOLS

In *error-blind* protocols, the BCI operation does not include any provision for detecting or correcting errors. Most current BCI operating protocols fall into this category. These error-blind protocols do not themselves recognize errors, nor do they incorporate any measures for dealing with them. Although they may consider the likelihood of errors in defining parameters such as the number of stimulus sequences per selection (e.g., Jin et al. 2010), they do not include any procedures for detecting or eliminating errors during BCI use. Rather, they simply identify the user's intent through their feature extraction and translation procedures and send the (hopefully correct) result to the application.

In these error-blind protocols, error recognition and correction is left to the *user* and/or to the *application*. For example, in a word-processing application, the user may recognize mistakes and correct them by backspacing. Or a wheelchair-movement application might recognize a wall (or a drop-off) ahead and therefore ignore a "Move forward" command from the BCI. In both of these examples, the BCI operating protocol is not responsible for detecting or addressing the error. In the first example, the user does this, and in the second example, the application does.

ERROR-DETECTION PROTOCOLS

In *error-detection* protocols, the BCI operation includes specific measures for avoiding, detecting, and/or correcting errors. BCIs that use error-detection protocols are at present confined primarily to laboratory settings. These BCIs use the person's brain signals not only to recognize intent but also to detect errors. They may, for example, recognize from the brain signals that are evoked by the *execution* of a command whether or not that command was an error (Schalk et al. 2000; Parra et al. 2003; Buttfield et al. 2006; Ferrez and Millán 2008). Or, they might recognize from signal features *simultaneous* with those used to recognize intent that an error is occurring (Bayliss et al. 2004). Or, perhaps even better, they might use particular signal features to predict errors ahead of time and then take appropriate measures (such as not sending the fallacious intent to the application). For example, Makeig and Jung (1996) showed that EEG measures could predict up to 10 sec ahead of time when sonar operators were more likely to make errors (see other examples in chapter 23, this volume). Although BCIs that incorporate error correction into their operating protocols are just beginning to be explored, their development is likely to become increasingly important as efforts to produce truly useful BCIs continue to advance.

OPERATING PROTOCOLS FOR USER TRAINING AND SYSTEM TESTING

The central purpose of BCI systems is to provide communication and control. BCI operating protocols are designed to serve this purpose. At the same time, special protocols are often needed for system parameterization and testing and for user training. The special protocols that serve these purposes typically have a distinctive feature: the intent of the user, and thus the *correct* output of the BCI, are established ahead of time and are known to the user, the operator/experimenter, and the BCI. Protocols of this kind can be called *directed-output* (or *supervised learning*) protocols, or simply *directed* protocols. They allow the actual output of the BCI to be directly compared to its correct output. Such protocols are often used to parameterize BCI systems. For example, the copy-spelling routines used to develop or update classifiers for P300-based BCI spelling applications are directed protocols (e.g., Sellers et al. 2006; Vaughan et al. 2006; Nijboer et al. 2010) (see chapter 12, this volume). Comparable routines can be used to parameterize SMR-based BCIs that rely on specific motor imagery (e.g., Scherer et al. 2004; Pfurtscheller et al. 2006; Müller et al. 2008) (see chapter 13, this volume) and SSVEP-based BCIs (e.g., Trejo et al. 2006) (see chapter 14, this volume).

Furthermore, directed protocols can guide the BCI user and/or the BCI system in their *adaptive* interactions that seek to improve the correspondence between the user's intent and the brain-signal features that the system extracts and translates into output. This guidance function has been particularly important in the development of SMR-based BCI control of multidimensional cursor movements (e.g., Wolpaw and McFarland 2004; McFarland et al. 2010) (see chapter 13, this volume).

Directed protocols are widely used in BCI research. Indeed, such protocols produce the data reported in most BCI studies. These protocols allow the success of different BCI designs, and of different modifications of specific designs, to be assessed and compared. Thus, they are essential tools in the development and validation of more effective systems (Müller-Putz et al. 2006; Pfurtscheller et al. 2006). Furthermore, a self-parameterized BCI protocol might reparameterize itself periodically by employing a directed-protocol subroutine.

At the same time, it is important to understand that directed protocols only approximate real-life protocols in which the user alone specifies the intent to be translated into device commands. Although the approximation is often close, this is not necessarily always true. One major concern is that the user's brain activity may be substantially different for directed and real-life protocols. This issue may reduce the confidence with which the results obtained with a directed protocol can be extrapolated to real-life BCI operation.

SUMMARY

A BCI operates in an environment that includes the BCI user, the BCI application, and, usually, external support for the BCI. It interacts with this environment according to an *operating protocol.* BCI operating protocols can be characterized in terms of four fundamental questions, each of which has two possible answers.

The first question is: How is BCI operation initiated? In *synchronous* protocols, the BCI initiates its own operation. In *self-paced* (or *asynchronous*) protocols, the user's brain signals initiate BCI operation. Synchronous protocols are simpler to develop. However, self-paced protocols may provide more natural and convenient communication and control. The BCI systems now being introduced into clinical use have synchronous protocols, whereas self-paced protocols are an area of increasing research interest.

The second question is: Into what does the BCI convert the user's brain signals? In a *goal-selection* protocol, each feature translation operation produces a command that is selected from among a finite set of possible commands (e.g., the letters of the alphabet). In a *process-control* protocol, each feature translation operation produces a command that is the next value in an ongoing process (e.g., the movement of a cursor).

The third question is: How is the feature-extraction and translation process parameterized? *Preparameterized* protocols use fixed parameters that have been provided to the BCI. *Self-parameterized* protocols select and modify their own parameters, either continually during the course of their normal operation or through periodic automated procedures. Although preparameterized protocols are simpler to develop, self-parameterized protocols are generally more suitable for long-term usage. Many current BCIs use protocols that are partially preparameterized and partially self-parameterized.

The fourth question is: How are errors handled? *Error-blind* protocols do not themselves recognize errors, nor do they incorporate any measures for dealing with them; error handling is left to the user and/or to the application. In contrast, *error-detection* protocols use the person's brain signals not only to recognize intent, but also to detect errors. Error-detection protocols are just beginning to be developed and they are likely to become increasingly important.

Finally, BCI training and testing rely heavily on special *directed* protocols in which the correct output is established ahead of time. These protocols are used to parameterize BCI systems, and they are essential for the laboratory development and optimization of better systems. They can also guide the BCI user and the BCI system in optimizing the BCI's recognition and implementation of the user's intent. At the same time, directed protocols may not provide perfect guidance to how BCIs will function in real-life operation when the user alone determines the correct output.

REFERENCES

Allison, B.Z. (2009). The I of BCIs: Next generation interfaces for brain – computer interface systems that adapt to individual users. In: Human-Computer Interaction: Novel Interaction Methods and Techniques, Jacko, J (Ed.), Springer-Verlag, Berlin Heidelberg, 558–568.

Allison, B. Z., T. Luth, D. Valbuena, A. Teymourian, I. Volosyak, and A. Graser. 2010. BCI demographics: how many (and what kinds of) people can use an SSVEP BCI? IEEE Trans Neural Syst Rehabil Eng. 18:107–116.

Bayliss, J. D., A. S. Inverso, and A. Tentler. 2004. Changing the P300 brain computer interface. CyberPsychology and Behavior 7:694–704.

Buttfield, A., P. W. Ferrez, and J. del R. Millán. 2006. Towards a robust BCI: error potentials and online learning. IEEE Trans Neural Syst Rehabil Eng. 14:164–168.

Cherubini, A., G. Oriolo, F. Macrí, F. Aloise, F. Cincotti, and D. Mattia. 2008. A multimode navigation system for an assistive robotics project. Auton Robots 25:383–404.

Citi L., R. Poli, C. Cinel, and F. Sepulveda. 2008. P300-based BCI mouse with genetically-optimized analogue control. IEEE Trans Neural Syst Rehabil Eng. 16:51–61.

Farwell, L. A., and E. Donchin. 1988. Talking off the top of your head: toward a mental prosthesis utilizing event-related brain potentials. Electroencephalogr Clin Neurophysiol 70:510–523.

Ferrez, P. W. and J. del R. Millán. 2008. Error-related EEG potentials generated during simulated brain-computer interaction. IEEE Trans Biomed Eng 55:923–929.

Hochberg, L. R., M. D. Serruya, G. H. Friehs, J. A. Mukand, M. Saleh, A. H. Kaplan, A. Branner, D. Chen, R. D. Penn, and J. R. Donoghue. 2006. Neuronal ensemble control of prosthetic devices by a human with tetraplegia. Nature 13(442):164–171.

Jin, J., B. Z. Allison, C. Brunner, B. Wang, X. Wang, J. Zhang, C. Neuper, and G. Pfurtscheller. 2010. P300 Chinese input system based on Bayesian LDA. Biomed Technik 55:5–18.

Kübler A., and N. Birbaumer. 2008. Brain-computer interfaces and communication in paralysis: extinction of goal directed thinking in completely paralysed patients? Clin Neurophysiol. 119:2658–2666.

Leeb, R., F. Lee, C. Keinrath, R. Scherer, H. Bischof, and G. Pfurtscheller. 2007. Brain-computer communication: motivation, aim, and impact of exploring a virtual apartment. IEEE Trans Neural Syst Rehabil Eng 15: 473–482.

Makeig, S., and T. P. Jung. 1996. Tonic, phasic, and transient EEG correlates of auditory awareness in drowsiness. Brain Res Cogn Brain Res. 4:15–25.

Mason, S. G., A. Bashashati, M. Fatourechi, K. F. Navarro, and G. E. Birch. 2007. A comprehensive survey of brain interface technology designs. Ann Biomed Eng 35:137–169.

Mason, S. G., and G. E. Birch. 2005. Temporal control paradigms for direct brain interfaces—rethinking the definition of asynchronous and synchronous. Paper presented at HCI International, at Las Vegas, NV.

Mason, S. G., J. Kronegg, J. E. Huggins, M. Fatourechi, and A. Schloegl. 2006. Evaluating the performance of self-paced brain computer interface technology. Available from http://www.bci-info.org//Research_Info/documents/articles/self_paced_tech_report-2006-05-19.pdf.

McFarland, D. J., Krusienski, D. J., Sarnacki, W. A., and Wolpaw, J. R. 2008. Emulation of computer mouse control with a noninvasive brain-computer interface. J Neural Eng, 5:101–110.

McFarland, D.J., Sarnacki, W.A. and Wolpaw, J.R. 2010. Electroencephalographic (EEG) control of three-dimensional movement. J Neural Eng, 11;7(3): 036007.

Millán, J. del R., R. Rupp, G. R. Müller-Putz, et al. 2010. Combining brain-computer interfaces and assistive technologies: State-of-the-Art and Challenges. Front Neurosci. 7(4):161.

Moore, M. M. 2003. Real-world applications for brain-computer interface technology. IEEE Trans Neural Syst Rehabil Eng. 11:162–165.

Müller, K. R., M. Tangermann, G. Dornhedge, M. Krauledat, G. Curio, and B. Blankertz. 2008. Machine learning for real-time single-trial EEG-analysis: from brain-computer interfacing to mental state monitoring. J Neurosci Methods 167:82–90.

Müller-Putz, G. R., R. Scherer, G. Pfurtscheller, and R. Rupp. 2006. Brain-computer interfaces for control of neuroprostheses: from synchronous to asynchronous mode of operation. Biomed Technik 51(2):57–63.

Nijboer F., N. Birbaumer, and A. Kübler. 2010. The influence of psychological state and motivation on brain-computer interface performance in patients with amyotrophic lateral sclerosis—a longitudinal study. Front Neurosci. 21(4):55.

Parra, L. C., C. D. Spence, A. D. Gerson, and P. Sajda. 2003. Response error correction—a demonstration of improved human-machine performance using real-time EEG monitoring. IEEE Trans Neural Syst Rehabil Eng. 11:173–177.

Pfurtscheller G., B. Z. Allison, C. Brunner, G. Bauernfeind, T. Solis-Escalante, R. Scherer, T. O. Zander, C. Mueller-Putz, C. Neuper, and N. Birbaumer. 2010. The hybrid BCI. Front Neurosci 4:42.

Pfurtscheller, G., G. R. Müller-Putz, A. Schögl, B. Graimann, R. Scherer, R. Leeb, C. Brunner, C. Keinrath, F. Lee, G. Townsend, C. Vidaurre, and C. Neuper. 2006. 15 years of BCI research at Graz University of Technology: current projects. IEEE Trans Neural Syst Rehabil Eng. 14:205–210.

Schalk, G., J. R. Wolpaw, D. J. McFarland, and G. Pfurtscheller. 2000. EEG-based communication: presence of an error potential. Electroencephalogr Clin Neurophysiol 111:2138–2144.

Scherer, R., F. Lee, A. Schlögl, R. Leeb, H. Bischof, and G. Pfurtscheller. 2008. Toward self-paced brain-computer communication: navigation through virtual worlds. IEEE Trans Biomed Eng 55:675–682.

Scherer, R., G. R. Müller, C. Neuper, B. Graimann, and G. Pfurtscheller. 2004. An asynchronously controlled EEG-based virtual keyboard: improvement of the spelling rate. IEEE Trans Biomed Eng 51:979–984.

Sellers, E. W., A. Kübler, and E. Donchin. 2006. Brain-computer interface research at the University of South Florida Cognitive Psychophysiology Laboratory: the P300 speller. IEEE Trans Neural Syst Rehabil Eng 14:221–224.

Sellers, E.W.,T.M. Vaughan, and J.R. Wolpaw. 2010. A brain-computer interface for long-term independent home use. Amyotrophic Lateral Sclerosis 11:449–455.

Trejo, L. J., R. Rosipal, and B. Matthews. 2006. Brain-computer interfaces for 1-D and 2-D cursor control: designs using volitional control of the EEG spectrum or steady-state visual evoked potentials. IEEE Trans Neural Syst Rehabil Eng. 14:225–229.

Vaughan, T. M., D. J. McFarland, G. Schalk, W. A. Sarnacki, D. J. Krusienski, E. W. Sellers, and J. R. Wolpaw. 2006. The Wadsworth BCI research and development program: at home with BCI. IEEE Trans Neural Syst Rehabil Eng. 14:229–233.

Wolpaw, J. R. 2007. Brain-computer interfaces as new brain output pathways. J Physiol 579:613–619.

Wolpaw, J. R. and D.J. McFarland. 2004. Control of a two-dimensional movement signal by a non-invasive brain-computer interface in humans. Proc Natl Acad Sci USA 101:17849–17854.

Wolpaw JR, McFarland DJ, Vaughan TM, Schalk G. 2003. The Wadsworth Center brain-computer interface (BCI) research and development program. IEEE Trans Neural Syst Rehabil Eng. 11:204–207.

11 | BCI APPLICATIONS

JANE E. HUGGINS AND DEBRA ZEITLIN

The ultimate practical goal of most brain-computer interfaces (BCIs) is to operate devices that provide communication or control capacities to people with severe disabilities. The device operated by a BCI is referred to as its *application*. The application is not part of the BCI. It receives the BCI's output commands, and it converts these commands into useful actions, thus making the BCI and the application together into a potentially powerful assistive device. Without a useful application, a BCI is an interesting research endeavor or conversation novelty of no practical value. Thus, a BCI's applications are crucial to its utility and to its subsequent clinical and commercial success.

Hypothetical BCI applications, as presented in science fiction books and films, range from living in alternate realities (e.g., *The Matrix,* Warner Bros. Pictures 1999), to enhancing human abilities (Gibson 1984), to becoming a spaceship (McCaffrey 1969). Even in the scientific literature BCI studies have sometimes looked toward goals of these types as eventual future applications (e.g., Vidal 1973). The appeal of BCIs as mainstream technologies, or at least as mainstream toys, is apparent from the appearance in the news and at trade shows of games or game controllers that claim brain signals as their control source (e.g., Heingartner 2009; Twist 2004; Snider 2009). Advertisements for these products may evoke images of using brain power to become super-human.

In reality, however, the limited capabilities that true BCIs can currently provide make them of interest mainly to people with significant physical impairments. Many people with disabilities already use *assistive technology* (AT) to provide accessible interfaces with commercial devices that were not designed with a disabled user in mind. For example, an AT can provide an alternative interface to an existing technology (e.g., a head-controlled computer mouse) or it can provide alternative methods of accomplishing a task (e.g., a wheelchair to provide mobility). By either means, an AT restores function to people with significant impairments by providing an alternative method for task completion. Successful BCIs could significantly extend the usefulness of AT and could allow it to serve people who cannot be adequately served by current AT devices, all of which depend in some measure on muscle control.

As BCI researchers develop BCIs for everyday use by people with physical impairments, they should seek the involvement of experts who are experienced in evaluating and meeting the needs of people with physical impairments. These experts include prospective BCI users with personal experience of disability, as well as medical or AT experts who provide AT technology to those who need it. The basic principles and clinical realities that have proven critical to development and dissemination of conventional (i.e., muscle-based) AT are equally relevant to BCI-based AT. Thus, they are emphasized throughout this chapter.

This chapter addresses BCI development and implementation as an exciting and potentially important new AT area. It has six major sections. The first section places BCIs in the context of AT and describes the target users. The second section examines the types of control schemes (i.e., goal selection versus process control) for BCI control of AT applications. The third section considers the kinds of AT applications that BCIs might operate. The fourth section discusses the most important factors involved in selecting and providing AT applications controlled by BCIs. The fifth section describes two basic approaches to configuring BCI-controlled AT applications (i.e., BCI/AT versus BCI+AT). Finally, the sixth section discusses approaches to performance optimization.

BCIs IN ASSISTIVE TECHNOLOGY AND THEIR POTENTIAL USERS

BCIs IN ASSISTIVE TECHNOLOGY

An assistive technology (AT) is a device or procedure that bridges the gap between the physical (or cognitive) abilities of people with impairments and a function that they want to perform. For example, a wheelchair provides mobility and improves function for people who are otherwise unable to move around in their homes or communities by themselves. Likewise, a communication device that produces spoken words can enable those who cannot speak to communicate with others, either face to face or by telephone.

AT typically uses a person's remaining functional abilities to replace lost or missing function. Thus, a manual wheelchair allows arm function to replace missing leg function, and a head-controlled computer mouse allows head movement to replace hand function for mouse operation. AT for cognitive impairments typically relies on the physical ability to take notes or to access lists of instructions to overcome memory or other cognitive limitations. Since BCIs do not require physical movement, they have been proposed mainly for people with severe physical rather than cognitive impairments. In the future BCIs might also prove useful to the much larger numbers of people with less significant impairments who would benefit from an additional interface option for accessing technology. For example, a person who operates a communication system using a switch activated by muscle activity may find a BCI useful for operating environmental control of lights, temperature, or an entertainment system. At this time, only one research group appears to be exploring the use of BCIs to help people with cognitive impairments (e.g., Hsiao et al. 2008; and see chapter 22 in this volume).

A BCI might be integrated with an application so that together they constitute a stand-alone AT device (referred to here as a *BCI/AT* device or system) that provides a specific function (e.g., speaking phrases through a voice simulator). Alternatively, a BCI might serve as a general-purpose or *plug-and-play* interface that replaces standard physical interfaces (e.g., a joystick or mouse) to operate existing AT applications (e.g., a power wheelchair, a computer cursor, or a robotic arm). Such general-purpose or plug-and-play systems will be referred to in this chapter as *BCI + AT* devices or systems to distinguish them from stand-alone *BCI/AT* systems. Whereas the stand-alone *BCI/AT* option is limited to a single application (which it may perform very well), the plug-and-play BCI + AT option has more versatility (but may or may not perform as well for each of its various possible applications).

Throughout the lengthy history of AT research and development, numerous AT devices have been created. Most of these can be easily configured to be controlled by muscle-based interfaces such as a switch, joystick, keyboard, or computer mouse. The interface selected is matched to the user's available abilities. For example, a wheelchair can be driven by a joystick, or by a keypad of small switches, or by a switch activated by breath control. Thus, AT can provide many useful functions to people who can produce even the simplest muscle activation. In contrast, BCIs are intended primarily for people who cannot produce such muscle actions or who cannot produce them consistently or reliably. If BCIs can provide the same standard outputs as switches, joysticks, keyboards, and computer mice, they can operate existing AT. A BCI with standard outputs that could replace a USB keyboard, USB mouse, joystick, or mechanical switch closure could be used to control many different devices. Table 11.1 lists some examples of existing AT devices that might be controlled by a plug-and-play BCI.

As BCIs move toward clinical use to directly benefit people with physical impairments, their development will benefit from the input of people trained in AT. AT development and implementation are areas of rehabilitation engineering that meld engineering and medical knowledge about disability. AT is a well-established component of patient care and has a lengthy history, a large literature, and a corps of trained personnel who can be of great use to BCI researchers. Working in conjunction with physicians, physical and occupational therapists, and speech-language pathologists, AT personnel have experience in evaluating the needs of and current abilities of people with disabilities and in determining their options for interfacing with technology. Thus, AT service providers can assist in designing BCIs to meet the needs of people with physical impairments, and they are well positioned to compare BCI performance with that of other options. The Rehabilitation Engineering and Assistive Technology Society of North America (RESNA), founded in 1981 (Cooper et al. 2007), provides a meeting ground for researchers and clinicians in this field and can be a good resource for BCI researchers and developers. Graduate degrees in AT are available from a number of institutions (www.resna.org; http://www.athenpro.org/node/124). Further information on the evaluation of the abilities of people with physical impairments, on the prescription of AT, and on comprehensive coverage of AT can be found in Cook and Hussey (2002).

POTENTIAL USERS OF BCI-OPERATED AT

PEOPLE WITH TOTAL, CLASSICAL, OR INCOMPLETE LOCKED-IN SYNDROME

The choice of interface to operate an AT depends on the abilities of the user. Interfaces for severely disabled users are usually driven by body motion, eye-blink, breath, myoelectric activity, eye gaze, or voice. These modes of device control all require some degree of muscle activation and usually some actual physical movement. Such conventional AT interface options are accessible to anyone who can reliably make one of these or similar muscular actions. Nevertheless, some people are unable to produce even the minimal muscle activations needed to control such conventional AT interfaces.

Given the limited capabilities of current BCIs, one logical group of potential BCI users consists of people who are unable to make any voluntary muscle activation and who thus may be described as having *total locked-in syndrome* (total LIS) (i.e., the inability to activate any muscle despite having adequate cognitive function [see chapter 19 in this volume]). However, it is difficult to assess whether individuals with total LIS retain adequate levels of higher cortical function and whether (and when) they are sufficiently alert to operate a BCI. Moreover, this profound level of immobility may make it difficult for these individuals to perceive a BCI display and may limit their ability to observe the output of a BCI's operation. Such difficulties have not yet been thoroughly addressed in research studies, and it is as yet unclear whether BCIs can be useful to people with total LIS. Furthermore, *total LIS* appears to be quite rare (although it may sometimes be misdiagnosed as coma).

Total LIS should be distinguished from the more common syndromes *classical LIS* and *incomplete LIS* (see chapter 19, this volume). *Classical LIS* is defined as total immobility, but with retention of vertical eye movements and blinking as well as EEG evidence of undisturbed cortical function (Bauer et al. 1979) (see chapter 19, this volume). In contrast to the case for people with total LIS, people with classical LIS can be assessed for cognitive capacity and alertness because they usually retain some limited communication ability (i.e., via eye movements). People with *incomplete LIS* retain remnants of voluntary movement, such as a finger twitch. Total LIS, classical LIS, and incomplete LIS may result from any of a number of disorders or events, including brainstem stroke, advanced amyotrophic lateral sclerosis (ALS) (Hayashi and Oppenheimer 2003), trauma (Bauer et al. 1979; Katz et al. 1992), tumor (Bauer et al. 1979), viral infection (Katz et al. 1992), or severe cerebral palsy (Neuper et al., 2003) (see chapter 19, this volume).

TABLE 11.1 Different types of AT devices that could be operated by a BCI using switch, USB-mouse, or USB keyboard interfacing; short examples of features and performance enhancement features are provided

DEVICE	AI CATEGORIES	SWITCH-TYPE BCI	MOUSE-TYPE BCI	KEYBOARD–TYPE BCI	FEATURE	PERFORMANCE ENHANCEMENT FEATURE
Vantage[1]	AAC*	C,P**	C,P		Pictorial based	Icon prediction
DynaWrite[2]	AAC	C,P		C,P	Text-based, stand-alone	Word prediction, macros
Imperium[3]	ECS	C			ECS nested menus	
Relax II[4]	ECS	C			ECS simple menu	
DynaVox Vmax[5], Prentke Romich ECO2,[6] Tobii C12[7]	AAC, ECS, CA	C	C		Comprehensive communication, computer access and environmental control systems with many input methods	Word/Icon prediction, stored text
Wivik[8]	CA	C,P	C,P	C,P	Speech output	Word prediction, macros
WordQ[9]	CA			C,P		Word prediction
DASHER[10]	CA	C	C,P		Unique time-dependent mouse-based text entry	Unique word prediction features
REACH Interface Author[11]	AAC, CA	C,P	C,P	C,P	Text based, computer based	Word prediction, Smart key prediction
Cowriter[12]	CA	P		P		Word prediction
PointSmart[13]	CA		P			Gravity effect
Assistive Mouse Adapter[14]	CA		P			Tremor reduction
Smart Mustang Motorized Wheelchair[15]	M	P				Line following and obstacle avoidance

[1] Prentke Romich Company, Wooster, OH.
[2] DynaVox Mayer-Johnson, Pittsburgh, PA.
[3] Tash, Inc, Richmond, VA.
[4] Tash, Inc, Richmond, VA.
[5] DynaVox Mayer-Johnson, Pittsburgh, PA.
[6] Prentke Romich Company, Wooster, OH.
[7] Tobii Technology AB, Danderyd, Sweden.
[8] Holland Bloorview Kids Rehabilitation Hospital; Toronto, Ontario, Canada.
[9] GoQ Software, Dover, NH.
[10] University of Cambridge, Cambridge, UK.
[11] Applied Human Factors, Inc., Helotes, TX.
[12] Don Johnston Incorporated, Volo, IL.
[13] Infogrip, Inc, Ventura, CA.
[14] Montrose Secam Limited, Iver, Bucks, UK.
[15] Smile Rehab Ltd, Newbury, Berkshire, UK.
* AT Categories: AAC—Augmentative and Alternative Communication; ECS—Environmental Control System; CA—Computer Access, M—Mobility (but note associated safety issues).
** "C" indicates appropriate for control by that type of BCI. "P" indicates the presence of potentially beneficial performance enhancement features.

PEOPLE WITH SOME RESIDUAL MOTOR FUNCTION

From the AT perspective, people with classical LIS or incomplete LIS are part of a larger population consisting of people who have lost all *useful* muscle function except for very limited and focal control (e.g., limited eye movements, slight twitches of a muscle, imprecise control of a head-pointing device). It is this population, people with very little remaining muscle function (and especially those whose remaining muscle function is unreliable or easily fatigued), who are potentially the greatest beneficiaries of current BCIs. At the same time, because these people do have some muscle function, BCIs may be competing with a considerable range of conventional muscle-based AT devices. Thus, although conventional AT cannot help people with total LIS, it is frequently able to help people who have minimal movement capability, including those with classical

LIS or incomplete LIS. For example, residual eye movements or tiny muscle twitches can be used to operate a switch. In fact, any trace movement can be used to communicate yes/no (either through technology or to an observant communication partner). A simple yes/no response can enable a surprisingly complex array of communication capabilities when combined either with technology that fulfills the same purpose or with a partner who presents options one at a time.

A low-technology but effective method of communication is *manual scan* using a communication board that includes letters, common sentences, and/or words. This technology requires a communication partner who points to each item on the board and waits for a yes/no response that may be given with minimal muscle movement (e.g., eye blink or change of gaze direction) to indicate what the user wants to communicate. The communication partner can speed communication by guessing at word or sentence completion and getting a yes/no confirmation on the guess. Although labor-intensive for the communication partner, this communication method has proven successful and has been used even for large projects (the best known being Jean-Dominique Bauby's writing of his book *The Diving Bell and the Butterfly* [Bauby 1997]). Such use of manual scan with a communication partner can enable communication, but the reliance on the communication partner may shape or direct the content of the communication. The user cannot communicate independently; rather, communication is the product of a duet involving user and partner, and the speed of communication will depend on the familiarity of the communication partners and the complexity of the topic. AT that replaces the need for a communication partner can provide independence in communication. The restoration of some measure of independence is often very important and highly desirable to people with very limited useful muscle control. (On the other hand, reducing or replacing the need for a communication partner also reduces the immediate social interaction of communication, which the user may also value.)

With appropriate conventional (i.e., muscle-based) AT, a selection can be made using any muscle contraction or physical movement of which the user is capable. Options from which a user selects can be presented as either visual or audio prompts. The number of functions that an AT user can control with even a single switch is manifold and is limited only by budget, by the user's tolerance for the complexity of the interface and the generally slow rate of control, and by the support system available for acquiring, customizing, and maintaining the technology. Communication rate can be increased by a predictive system that includes spelling and natural-language semantic prediction of word order. In addition, a communication system can speak aloud the user's selections. An AT controlled by a single switch can also operate an environmental-control system that allows the user to perform such tasks as turning on the radio or television, changing channels, and even adjusting the temperature in the room.

For people with advanced ALS, AT controlled by commercially available systems using eye gaze or a switch operated by residual muscle activity is currently able to provide communication, computer access, and control of the environment (e.g., Tobii C12, Tobii Technology AB, Danderyd, Sweden; ECO2

with ECOpoint, Prentke Romich Co., Wooster, OH; DynaVox EyeMax, DynaVox Mayer-Johnson, Pittsburgh, PA). Such systems can provide all these functions through touch-screen, switch-scanning, head-movement, or eye-gaze interfaces. For many people with advanced ALS, BCIs do not as yet provide enough additional function to be preferred over these other methods. However, BCIs should enable them to continue to communicate as their disease progresses and as their other (muscle-based) capabilities diminish. Indeed, some people with ALS have chosen to try a BCI and use it regularly in preparation for their anticipated eventual loss of muscle function.

For the small number of people with total LIS, BCIs may be the only option. However, for the much larger group of people who retain minimal muscle function (i.e., those who can use other AT), BCIs can serve as a useful alternative interface that may replace a muscle-based interface when muscles fatigue or become unreliable. Thus, BCIs will compete with other AT interfaces operated by muscle function. To compete successfully, they must provide significant added capability. It is expected that as research and development advance and generate more powerful, convenient, and robust BCI systems, these improved BCIs should become useful for the large number of people with severe disabilities who are now served by many different conventional AT interfaces.

THE IMPORTANCE OF A USER-ORIENTED APPROACH

For BCIs to compete successfully for users both now and in the future and to provide additional benefits beyond conventional AT, BCI researchers and developers must employ a user-oriented approach to system design. Ultimately, the choice between a muscle-based interface and a BCI will depend on the capabilities and priorities of individual users as well as on the speed, accuracy, and convenience that each type of interface provides.

USER-SELECTED GOALS
In all areas of life, people are generally most successful at, and most eager to engage in, the activities that they themselves want to do. Young children may excel at remembering the names of their favorite dinosaurs but cannot remember the names of the continents. Adults put off starting tedious projects. Likewise, people with physical impairments are more likely to use AT if the task that it enables is one that they value and desire. Indeed, one of the primary factors responsible for abandonment of AT is the lack of consideration of the user's desires during device (i.e., application) selection (Brown-Triolo 2002). In developing useful BCIs, we must be sure that they provide people with the applications they want in order to meet their own personal goals. People with physical impairments are as diverse as those without physical impairments, and their personalities, goals, and dreams are as varied. The uses to which they want to put an AT device, whether BCI-controlled or not, are often surprising and depend on personality, individual life experiences, and desires. Although the extent of disability is unavoidably a limiting factor, with sufficient motivation and support, many activities are available for

people with significant physical impairments. With appropriate AT, a person with tetraplegia since childhood may still pilot a sailboat, and someone with a double amputation of the lower limbs may still engage in downhill skiing.

A survey of 63 people with ALS showed that, among all areas of potential AT use, they placed highest priority on communication (Gruis et al., 2011). Thus, it is expected that many potential BCI users will value communication applications (e.g., interacting with people directly, reading and writing emails, accessing the internet, participating in telephone calls). They may want to have independent control of some form of entertainment (e.g., television, music, or books). Other users may most highly value activities such as maintaining current employment, or writing memoirs, books, or articles. For potential users whose life expectancy permits long-term goals, the focus may expand beyond basic computer access and control of the environment to include educational and vocational goals. Thus, BCIs and their AT applications should be aimed at serving these and other purposes important to their users, and they should be easily configurable to serve the particular goals of each user.

APPROPRIATE TRAINING AND SUPPORT STRUCTURE

Successful use of any AT depends on user acceptance. User acceptance must be accompanied by adequate user training and by the presence of an appropriate support structure. The importance of these factors is often not adequately appreciated. AT devices are frequently provided without any training in their use. For example, a wheelchair may simply be given to a person's spouse to take home without basic instructions in how the user gets in and out or navigates around obstacles. Sometimes expensive augmentative communication devices are provided or obtained without provision for training the intended user or caregiver in how to use the device or customize the vocabulary. In such cases, the devices may be used very little or not at all.

Although the nature of BCI technology makes the need for *user* training obvious, it may be less apparent that *caregivers* also need significant training. Caregivers are normally responsible for daily AT setup and routine maintenance, and this is equally true for BCI-operated AT. A user may have several caregivers who differ in their levels of technical competence and comfort. For an EEG-based BCI to be successful, the caregivers must have basic computer skills and be sufficiently trained and detail oriented to ensure that electrode placement and impedance are appropriate and that the electrodes are adequately cleaned on a regular basis. Without attention to such requirements, successful BCI use is not possible.

Most often, one or two caregivers or family members take the responsibility for setup and maintenance of an AT. Therefore, an individual's routine use of an AT device, whether operated by a conventional interface or by a BCI, can be affected by the caregivers' schedules. Caregiver turnover can also be an issue, because new caregivers must be trained whenever an old caregiver leaves. If a caregiver is unwilling or unable to perform the routine tasks and to troubleshoot any unexpected malfunctions, the caregiver can effectively prevent successful AT use by even the most eager user.

The support essential for use of AT extends beyond the physical tasks of setup and equipment maintenance. For face-to-face conversation, it is generally necessary to have willing conversation partners who will persevere in the face of the slow communication rates that BCI-controlled communication systems typically provide. Such systems will be used only if the user has good opportunities to talk, people to talk to, and things to talk about. Thus, family members, friends, and acquaintances may need to act as enablers who provide opportunities for use of BCI-controlled AT. Successful use of BCI-controlled AT therefore requires adequate training not only in the obvious areas of BCI setup, maintenance, and troubleshooting, but also in less obvious areas such as communication strategies and BCI usage opportunities. AT professionals experienced in the use of alternative and augmentative communication devices can be a great resource in designing, planning, and implementing such training so that the BCI succeeds in improving the user's quality of life.

CONSIDERATION OF USER ROUTINE AND PREFERENCES
Setup Time

If a BCI-controlled AT system is to be successfully adopted as an integral part of a person's communication and control strategy, its use must fit within the user's daily routine. While a 15–20 minute setup time may seem like a small price to pay for BCI use over many hours, this may be unacceptable in a routine that may already require up to two hours for basic daily activities such as bathing, dressing, toileting, taking medicines, acquiring nutrition (possibly through a feeding tube), transferring into a wheelchair, and adjusting the seating system for optimal comfort. For an EEG-based BCI, the ease with which the electrodes can be applied and removed will be a consideration, as will any BCI-related additional daily hygiene, such as washing electrode gel from the hair. For a person in a wheelchair or for someone who uses a ventilator, washing out the electrode gel may be a significant challenge, although a dry shampoo can facilitate this task. (The inconvenience of the electrode gel is one of the major reasons for the desirability of dry electrodes; see chapter 6, this volume.) Similarly, for BCIs that use implanted recording arrays, a requirement for daily calibration may constitute an impediment to user acceptance.

Fatigue may also be a factor for users with particular disorders (e.g., people with ALS who often need to rest after completing their morning routine); any need for additional rest may increase the perceived cost of BCI setup time. Thus, factors that can reduce BCI setup time may be of paramount importance to the successful integration of BCIs into people's daily lives.

Appearance

Acceptance of BCI technology may also depend on the BCI's appearance. The electrode caps currently used with EEG-based BCIs are obvious. Whereas some users with few other interface options may not be concerned about their appearance while using a BCI, others may still consider this an important issue. For people with less severe impairments who have a wider range of AT options available and who may lead less sequestered lives, BCI acceptance may depend in considerable part on their appearance when they are using the BCI.

Portability

BCI portability is another often overlooked factor that may be essential for clinical and commercial success. For some users, the ability to communicate outside the home may be exceedingly important. Accurate communication during medical appointments can be a matter of life and death. Participation in community activities such as religious services, family sporting events, or hobby clubs may be key factors in an individual's quality of life. BCI-based communication outside the confines of the controlled home environment presents additional challenges to BCI development because unpredictable environments can interfere with signal recording (e.g., electrical noise associated with power lines, elevators, automatic door openers, and many other devices that may produce recording artifacts; see chapter 7, this volume). As users come to rely on BCIs as an extension of themselves and as a primary means of communication, they will expect to be able to use their BCI systems wherever they go and with unfamiliar conversation partners. Thus, BCIs for use outside the home must be portable, must have a setup time short enough to enable setup after transport, and must be sufficiently robust to operate reliably in a wide variety of complex environments.

If BCIs are to move beyond the laboratory and become useful AT devices for people with significant motor impairments, they must serve each user's most important purposes, they must be adequately supported and easily integrated into the user's life, and they should be portable and robust enough to function in a variety of environments.

THE COST OF INADVERTENT ACTIVATIONS

Conventional AT interfaces for people who have extreme functional disabilities are particularly susceptible to inadvertent device activations (i.e., unintended outputs) because these interfaces are designed to detect very small movements or tiny physiological signals that are not typically used for device control. AT interfaces particularly likely to produce such inadvertent activations include pressure switches, accelerometers, and electromyographic (EMG) switches (activated by the electrical activity of a muscle). As discussed further in chapter 10, BCIs too must avoid inadvertent activations.

Inadvertent activations are an important issue because they are one of the most frequent causes for abandonment of AT devices. For example, so that they are able to call a nurse independently, hospital intensive-care patients may be given a switch that uses a small motor action such as wrinkling the forehead if no other voluntary movement is available. If the switch repeatedly calls the nurse when the patient does not intend to do so, the staff may decide to remove the device (and presumably check on the patient more frequently). In this case, although the patient might be able to learn to perform the forehead movements reliably enough to use the switch effectively, the device would be abandoned before this learning can take place. (This example also further illustrates the importance of

caregiver acceptance of an AT device.) Although the issue of inadvertent activations is of particular importance for BCIs, it is often overlooked, probably because the devices that most of us use in our everyday lives are not linked to such small movements and are therefore not as susceptible to inadvertent activations.

Each BCI application will have a particular cost associated with inadvertent activations. For some applications, the consequences are simply annoying or inconvenient (e.g, calling a nurse or caregiver unnecessarily) or frustrating (e.g, choosing incorrect letters in spelling). For other applications, inadvertent activations may place the user or others at risk (e.g, rolling a wheelchair down a staircase or into another person). Furthermore, users' sensitivity to inadvertent activations may depend on the situation. When actively using a BCI, the user recognizes personal involvement in errors that occur and may therefore have a relatively high tolerance for the occasional inadvertent output. In contrast, during *no-control* periods (see chapter 10) (especially those during which a sleep mode of some sort has been activated in the BCI), the user may be much less tolerant of inadvertent BCI output because such errors will be perceived as solely the fault of the BCI. Furthermore, such errors may entail an inordinate drain on time and energy for the user or a caregiver to undo their effects. Reliable avoidance of such errors may be a key factor in ensuring user (and caregiver) acceptance of BCI-controlled AT devices.

Avoiding inadvertent activation is particularly critical for a BCI, because the user is generally always in contact with the BCI once it is set up. Only a few BCI studies (e.g., Birch et al. 2003) have begun to explore this issue despite its high importance in practical settings. As discussed in detail in chapter 10, if the BCI uses an *asynchronous* operating protocol, it must determine from brain activity alone whether the user is intending control or is, instead, engaged in some other task (e.g., thinking, composing text, watching TV, sleeping, etc.).

Even for the synchronous BCIs now beginning to be provided to users, the problem of inadvertent activations remains. Solutions are cumbersome. For example, in use of a P300-based keyboard, one approach to minimizing inadvertent activation is for the user to activate a sleep-mode or pause function, during which the system recognizes that it should ignore signals. Once in this sleep mode, the only option available is to exit the sleep mode; this operation typically requires the user to activate the "restart" option twice in succession. A user who wishes to take only a short break to think of the next word to type may be frustrated by having to make three selections to do so (i.e., one to stop the BCI and two to restart it). Accurate automated recognition of a no-control state would be highly beneficial, especially since such states (e.g., brief daydreaming) may occur transiently even when a user is actively engaged in using the BCI.

CONTROL SCHEMES: MATCHING BCIs WITH APPLICATIONS

The function of a BCI application is to accomplish the user's intent (i.e., goal), whether it is to spell letters, to control the room environment, or to move objects with the hand of a robotic arm. In developing a BCI for use with a specific application, it is essential to ensure that the BCI is compatible with the application. A particular BCI should be matched with the application only after considering both the BCI's characteristics and capabilities (e.g., operating protocol and output type, system speed, accuracy, reliability) and those of the application (e.g., its degree of automation, the nature of the action it produces).

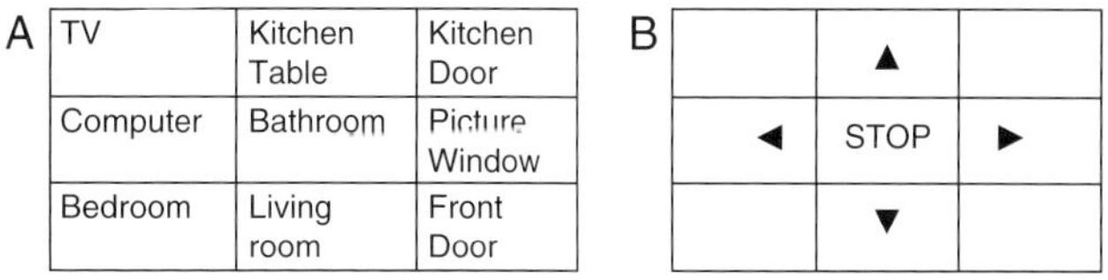

The application's operation has three principal elements:

- The *command* that the BCI provides to the application. This is the output of the BCI and the input to the application, and it can be either a *goal-selection* command or a *process-control* command.

- The *conversion* of the BCI's command(s) into the application's action. This conversion can be either *direct* or *indirect*.

- The *action* that the application produces. This is the output of the application and it accomplishes the user's goal. It can be either *discrete* or *continuous* or both.

The options for these elements, with their principal advantages and disadvantages, are discussed in this section. Appropriate matching of the BCI to the application is critical for ensuring that the application's action accomplishes the user's intent.

THE BCI'S COMMAND TO THE APPLICATION: GOAL SELECTION OR PROCESS CONTROL

The output of the BCI is a *command* that serves as the input to the application. This command is generally expressed as a specific voltage. This voltage might have a specific *set* of possible values (e.g., *–2, –1, 0, +1, +2*), or it might be capable of having any value within a specific *range* of values (e.g., *–5 to +5*). (It should be noted that all outputs provided by digital hardware are, technically, discrete values; however, their typically high-resolution [e.g., 16- or 32-bit] ensures that BCI commands can effectively assume any value.)

The command from the BCI to the application can be in the form of either *goal selection* or *process control* (see chapters 1 and 10 in this volume; see fig. 1.6, this volume). A *goal-selection* command simply tells the application what the user's goal is (e.g., a voltage of *–1*, or a voltage that falls between *0* and *–1*, might correspond to a particular goal, such as a specific desired location of the user's wheelchair). The application's task is then to perform the action that achieves the goal. In contrast, a *process-control* command does not tell the application what the goal is; rather, it tells the application what to do to achieve the goal (e.g., a specific voltage would correspond to a movement of the wheelchair in a specific direction). Figure 11.1 illustrates these two different kinds of BCI commands for an application that drives a wheelchair. Figure 11.1A shows nine possible wheelchair destinations, that is, nine possible goals. The BCI sends a goal-selection command that tells the

Figure 11.1 *Possible control interfaces for driving a wheelchair. (A) A goal-selection interface provides single selection destinations, but limited options. It relies on automation for safety and task completion. (B) A process-control interface provides directional control but requires multiple selections to reach a destination. It could incorporate automatic hazard detection for safety.*

application which destination to go to. Figure 11.1B shows five possible wheelchair directions (*Forward, Backward, Right, Left, Stop*). In this case, the BCI sends a series of process-control commands that step-by-step move the wheelchair to the desired destination.

From both the user's and BCI's perspective, goal selection is generally easier than process control because the achievement of the goal, which may involve complex high-speed interactions (e.g., fig. 1.6 in chapter 1), is handled by the application. Well-functioning goal selection can provide faster, more natural control. Indeed, as discussed in chapter 1 of this volume, goal selection may be more closely aligned to the way in which the nervous system normally behaves (i.e., motor control is normally distributed across multiple levels of the CNS rather than micromanaged by the cortex itself). However, goal selection may limit the flexibility and usefulness of the application (e.g., in fig. 11.1A, only nine destinations are possible). Furthermore, goal-selection may place high demands on the application device, which is expected to automate the accomplishment of the user's goal. For applications such as robotic arm control, or even wheelchair movement, sophisticated high-speed automation is important. Poor automation can frustrate the user, especially if the automation misses an obvious solution or is unable to adapt to different circumstances (e.g., an obstacle necessitating a different movement path). Poor automation can even be dangerous if it does not recognize important safety concerns (e.g., in piloting a wheelchair near a staircase).

From the application's perspective, process control is often easier than goal selection because the BCI tells it exactly what to do to achieve the user's goal. Process control may also be better able to accommodate a wider variety of goals and may adapt more easily to different situations or unexpected events (e.g., an obstacle in the way of a movement, a heavier object to be lifted). Process control may increase the flexibility of function and decrease the automation necessary in the application. On the other hand, it may also require considerably greater speed and complexity in the BCI's output, and thus it can place greater demands on both the user and the BCI. For example, process control of a robotic arm would require the user and the BCI to support the complex high-speed multijoint interactions that goal selection would otherwise delegate to the application. In practice, applications that combine goal-selection and process-control commands could be good options: goal selection commands could allow the application to handle basic components of an action, while process-control commands might be used to provide increased precision or adaptation to changing circumstances. For example, goal selection might move the hand of a robotic arm to a specific location, and process control might control the action the hand performs (e.g., button push, full hand grasp, thumb-finger pinch, finger point, etc.).

CONVERTING THE BCI'S COMMAND(S) INTO THE APPLICATION'S ACTION: DIRECT VERSUS INDIRECT

In accord with terminology developed in the AT literature, an application can convert the BCI's commands into the action that achieves the user's goal either *directly* or *indirectly* (Cook and Hussey 2002). In *direct selection*, a goal-selection command is converted into the action. In *indirect selection*, a series of *process-control commands* produces the action.

Figure 11.2A illustrates a *direct selection*. A P300-based BCI (see chapter 12, this volume) presents the letters of the alphabet in a matrix and enables the user to choose among them. The BCI command indicates to the application the letter chosen by the user, and the application simply displays that letter on the screen, adds it to a document in progress, and so forth. As illustrated here, direct selection can be fast and easy for the user and the BCI, and thus it is often preferable if it can encompass an adequate array of possible actions. On the other hand, for applications such as robotic arm control, direct selection may entail a high degree of automation in the application.

Figure 11.2B illustrates an *indirect selection*. To spell a letter, the user first chooses among three groups of letters, then among subgroups of the group chosen, and finally among the letters of the subgroup. Thus, the BCI sends *three* commands to the application for each letter that the application produces. Morse code is an example of indirect selection: a dot or a dash is itself meaningless, but three dots mean selection of the letter S and three dashes mean selection of the letter O. A P300-based BCI can also provide indirect selection when, for example, its matrix includes icons that lead to new matrices that provide the user with further options. When used appropriately, indirect selection can be very efficient and powerful. It can allow simple "yes/no" or "0/1" BCI output commands to produce a theoretically unlimited number of different actions. (In fact,

indirect selection methods such as Morse code have been shown to outperform more modern direct-selection methods such as text messaging [Henderson 2005].) On the other hand, for applications such as robotic-arm control, indirect selection places high demands on both the user and the BCI.

Direct and indirect selection may also be used in combination if a user desires more selections than can be provided with direct selection. Direct selection can allow quick access to the most frequent selections, whereas indirect selection can make less frequent selections available (e.g., by using matrix items that lead to submatrices). A cell phone provides a good example of combined direct and indirect selection. It has a keypad for direct selection of numbers (the most common selections), but also, with labels on specific numbers, provides indirect access to letters, punctuation, and symbols. Whereas direct-selection interfaces may make all the selections visible, thereby minimizing memory requirements, indirect selection often involves the additional cognitive load of recalling a code or a sequence of actions in order to perform the desired selection.

THE APPLICATION'S ACTION: DISCRETE AND/OR CONTINUOUS

The *action* is the final outcome of the user's expression of intent through the BCI and the application. This action can be *discrete* (e.g., selecting a letter), or *continuous* (e.g., wheelchair movement to a location), or both (e.g., continuous cursor movement followed by discrete icon selection). Both discrete and continuous actions can be produced by either goal-selection or process-control commands from the BCI. For example, a discrete letter selection might be produced by a P300-based BCI that gives a goal-selection command to choose a given matrix item, or by an SMR-based BCI that gives a series of process-control commands that move a cursor to the letter. A continuous wheelchair movement to a location might be produced by a P300-based BCI that gives a series of goal-selection commands (e.g., move forward one meter, turn 90 degrees to the right, etc.) that move the wheelchair to the location, or by an SMR-based BCI that gives a series of process-control commands (a succession of two-dimensional movements [i.e., $\Delta x_1 \Delta y_1$, $\Delta x_2 \Delta y_2$, etc.]) that move the wheelchair to the location.

CURRENT AND POTENTIAL AT APPLICATIONS OF BCIs

The potential applications of BCIs are limited only by the imagination. As BCI researchers develop BCIs to control various applications, it is essential that they keep in mind the purposes that the application serves for the users and the other AT options that are already available to them. If BCIs are to become widely accepted and used by large numbers of people, they will not be used in isolation but instead will be part of a suite of AT devices employed by people with a variety of abilities and impairments. Table 11.1 gives examples of some existing AT devices that could be controlled by a BCI. The applications

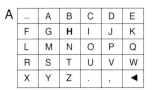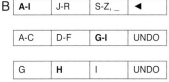

Figure 11.2 (A) A direct-selection interface by which the letter H can be selected with a single action. With this interface, the user must be able to accurately select one of 30 options. ◄ indicates a backspace selection. (B) An interface using indirect selection that requires three steps to select the letter H. Each row illustrates a single selection step offering four options. For the purpose of this illustration, the correct option is in boldface. The UNDO command would return the user to the previous selection step in case a mistake is made.

described in this section are within the realm of possibility with the current state of BCI performance or should be achievable in the foreseeable future. We will review the categories of BCI AT applications from two perspectives: that of the user and that of the developer of the technology.

THE USER'S PERSPECTIVE: FUNCTIONS THAT BCI APPLICATIONS COULD PROVIDE

From the user's perspective, BCI-controlled AT applications can be classified based on the functions that they support. These include primarily:

- communication
- mobility
- activities of daily living.

COMMUNICATION

Communication is usually the highest-priority need for people who have lost the ability to communicate. A person who is able to communicate can generate personal care, environmental control, mobility, and most other capabilities by asking others to perform these tasks on one's behalf. Thus, communication has generally been the first application to which BCIs have been put (e.g. Kuebler et al. 1999; Farwell and Donchin 1988; Kennedy et al. 2000; Wolpaw et al. 1998).

Among AT professionals, the term *augmentative and alternative communication* (AAC) is used for the special function of providing communication. AAC services are frequently provided by teams of AT professionals, including speech-language pathologists. Conferences devoted to AAC or organized by users of AAC meet nationally and internationally (e.g., http://www.aacinstitute.org/; http://www.isaac-online.org/en/home.shtml).

Communication encompasses not only standard verbal conversation but also preparation of written statements that can be delivered immediately or later through a text-to-speech device or as preprogrammed text. Communication can also occur through a sequence of symbols or pictures that have meaning to both communication partners. Communication software programs can increase the rate and efficiency of communication by using core vocabularies combined with automatic text-to-speech conversion, word prediction, prestored text, or semantic expansion of picture sequences into text or verbal statements. Thus, computer-based communication systems may speed the production of text, allow preparation of text for later delivery, or translate symbolic communication into text or speech. These capabilities are important since communication ability encompasses the ability to communicate not only with familiar partners but also with unfamiliar partners who may not understand the abbreviations or shortcuts known to familiar partners (Hidecker et al. 2008).

Because AAC professionals often recommend multiple modes of communication for those who need AAC services, BCIs might serve a useful communication role even if a user has other options for communication. Multimodal communication encompasses a range of communication modalities, from no technology to high technology, with each modality serving a particular purpose or being preferred under particular circumstances. For the current target population of BCI users, who have extremely significant disabilities, BCIs may constitute their only modality. However, many potential users still have a reliable way of signaling Yes/No with a familiar communication partner, and together with this partner, they might even be able to carry out letterboard-based communication. For these users the BCI can restore independent communication and/or enable more detailed and efficient communication on topics of the user's choice, as well as communication with unfamiliar or distant partners (e.g., via email). Moreover, a BCI-controlled AT application could be valuable to users of muscle-based AT applications when muscle fatigue occurs.

As with all AAC methods, the role that a BCI AAC application plays within the spectrum of a user's communication options will be affected by the time and energy associated with its setup and use. To take a non-BCI example, a person with quadriplegia may use writing sticks (essentially pencils attached to the hands) for short projects such as email, but may use a computer-based voice recognition system for longer projects. For short projects the loss in typing efficiency with the sticks is offset by avoiding the annoyance of donning the voice-input microphone headset and having to speak aloud each word and punctuation mark with minimal inflection. For longer projects the gain in speed provided by the voice input system justifies the time and energy needed for its setup and use. For the same reasons BCI methods that minimize setup time and maximize efficiency will achieve wider acceptance and more extensive use. Even then, they may still not be preferred for every situation.

MOBILITY

Mobility is a key factor in independence and therefore a function that is highly valued by many potential BCI users. In a survey of people with ALS conducted by Huggins et al. (2011), interest in BCI-based operation was high for all kinds of AT applications, but power-wheelchair operation tended to generate more interest than other noncommunication tasks (Huggins et al., 2011). Mobility encompasses several categories of abilities: the ability to adjust body position while sitting or lying down (e.g., for comfort, line of sight, pressure relief, respiration, or other aspects of health); the ability to move about within the living quarters; and the ability to leave the living quarters and travel in the community. The provision of wheelchairs, alternative seating options, and other body-positioning capacities is another specialty area within the field of AT (http://www.iss.pitt.edu).

Since AT devices for mobility can be operated by joystick, switch, or scanning controls, they could presumably also be operated by BCIs. Thus, BCIs might serve as interfaces to any of the systems that operate adjustable beds, seating systems, power wheelchairs, and adapted driving systems, and could thereby provide a range of mobility functions. Several projects for BCI control of wheelchairs are already underway (e.g., Galan et al. 2008; Leeb et al. 2007). However, whereas errors in communication may be undesirable and frustrating, errors in mobility control can be dangerous. The risks of errors while driving a motor vehicle or even a wheelchair are obvious. In addition, for a person with reduced respiratory capacity, fatal consequences could result simply from getting stuck in a completely horizontal position, thereby increasing respiratory load (Allen et al. 1985; Blair and Hickam 1955). Thus, safety considerations are paramount in any type of AT mobility application. In situations in which incorrect or inadvertent commands could pose dangers, BCI accuracy and reliability will be critically important. To help manage these risks, it will be important to incorporate appropriate safety technology such as sensors that detect and prevent unsafe conditions (e.g., as in obstacle-avoiding wheelchairs [Simpson 2005]). The use of many mobility applications will involve accommodations to the physical parameters of the device (e.g., size, weight), timing considerations based on movement speed, and consideration of the frequency and severity of hazards in the environment.

ACTIVITIES OF DAILY LIVING

Although communication is the primary function enabling self-determination, the ability to perform activities of daily living (ADLs) provides a measure of independence and correspondingly a feeling of not being a burden to others. Different cultures place different levels of importance on independence. Cultural background, interpersonal relationships, and personal experience help to determine the priority a particular user places on independence in ADLs and help to determine which ADLs are considered most important. ADLs encompass self-care tasks such as eating, dressing, and toileting, as well as many of the functions frequently included in the term *environmental control* (e.g., room temperature and lighting). The field of neuroprosthetics also includes ADL applications such as bowel and bladder control and restoration of sexual function (Hamid and Hayek 2008). The ability to independently perform a key set of ADLs (along with the ability to summon assistance in an emergency) can often enable people with severe disabilities to live independently, supported by external assistance only at strategic times during the day (e.g., for rising and retiring, meals, and medications).

Environmental-control tasks are frequently well suited to the modest information-transfer rates of current BCIs, since a small amount of information can often adjust the environment in ways that do not then need to be modified very often (e.g., temperature, lights). At the same time this means that suppression of inadvertent activations is extremely important. Although BCI users may be quite satisfied to spend two minutes selecting a TV channel, they will be dissatisfied if an unintended BCI output changes the channel in the middle of the dramatic climax of a show, and if it then requires two minutes to return to the desired channel. Several projects have tested BCI applications that provide functions related to ADLs, including: general environmental control (Karmali et al. 2000); exploring a virtual environment (Leeb et al. 2007); and controlling assistive robots (Cincotti et al. 2008). Other ADL tasks have not yet been implemented with BCIs, and some may not yet be realistic for BCIs. As BCI users come to rely on their BCI-controlled applications as tools for independent living

and for functioning without constant supervision, BCI reliability will be a key factor in ensuring acceptability and safety.

THE DEVELOPER'S PERSPECTIVE: TYPES OF AT APPLICATIONS THAT BCIs COULD CONTROL

Since BCIs are by definition interfaces, they might simply replace the muscle-based interfaces that traditionally control AT applications. Thus, it is also appropriate to classify BCI-controlled applications in the same way that applications operated by other AT interfaces are classified. From the technological perspective, possible BCI-controlled AT applications can thus be classified as:

- switch-activated AT
- computer access (typing and mouse emulation)
- robotics
- functional electrical stimulation (FES)
- prosthesis control

SWITCH-ACTIVATED AT

Simple two-state, or binary, switches (i.e., "on/off" or "Yes/No") are a powerful AT tool for enabling people with the most severe impairments. Such switches can either be momentary (producing only a short-duration output after a single activation) or latched (remaining on or off until activated again). An AT system operated by a single switch can provide access to numerous functions, limited only by the maximum length and complexity of the switching sequence that the user is willing to tolerate. In communication devices, single switches are most often used to operate AT with either scanning or coded access (Cook and Hussey 2002). In scanning, possible selections are presented or highlighted sequentially. When the selection desired by the user is offered, the user activates the switch and the selection is made. Choosing a selection can then result in generation of a spoken word or a sentence (for communication), turning on a light or TV (for environmental control), typing a character, word, or sentence (for computer access and communication), or choosing a seating system adjustment (for mobility). In some cases selections are grouped so that a sequence of selections is necessary to produce a desired output. For example, a user may first select a device (e.g., TV) and then select the command for the device (e.g., next channel). Directed scanning allows the user to employ multiple switches to steer the direction of the scan and then select the desired item. This is similar to using keyboard arrow keys and key repeats to select the desired cell in a spreadsheet. In addition, single switches can be used for coded access to computers, such as in Morse-code typing.

Most stand-alone environmental-control systems are designed for operation by one or two switches (with one switch moving between options and the other activating the chosen option). Several studies have described BCIs that produce switch function (e.g., Friedrich et al. 2009; Mason and Birch 2000; Graimann et al. 2003). Because switch-activated AT requires only one degree of freedom, it can leverage the limited control that current BCIs can provide. However, accurate performance in the no-control state is particularly important for switch-activated applications, since a single inadvertent activation can require many correct activations to cancel its effect.

COMPUTER ACCESS

Computers and internet connections have become the basis for many ADLs and communication tasks that were once performed through manual manipulation of objects. Computer access typically involves both text generation from a keyboard and cursor movements with a mouse. However, recognized accessibility guidelines suggest that computer programs should be fully functional using only the keyboard or only a mouse, so many commercial mainstream and AT computer programs now include keyboard shortcuts that eliminate the need for use of a mouse, as well as menus or shortcut buttons that eliminate the need for typing (e.g., an on-screen keyboard for text generation). Nevertheless, these features are not yet ubiquitous, so BCIs that can replace both keyboard and mouse functions are still needed.

Typing

Typing is one of the most common BCI applications and indeed was the first application for which the P300-based BCI was tested (Farwell and Donchin 1988). Typing is a form of communication, whether printed, presented to a communication partner via the computer screen, sent as an email, or converted to speech and spoken aloud. Thus, typing can be an AT application vital for enabling social interactions and gainful employment. BCI typing is most often implemented using P300-based BCIs, which now produce typing speeds of about five characters per minute (Furdea et al. 2009; Townsend et al. 2010; Donchin et al. 2000), and might be made faster with core vocabularies and predictive-spelling options. In addition to typing text, typing can also activate icons or menu items, pre-stored sequences of commands (macros), or prerecorded speech. BCIs have been interfaced with commercial word-prediction and typing programs (Vaughan et al. 2006; Thompson et al. 2009). Text generation has also been achieved with BCIs operated by sensorimotor rhythms (e.g., Vaughan et al. 2006; Pfurtscheller et al. 2006) or by slow cortical potentials (Kuebler et al. 1999).

Mouse Emulation

Mouse emulation provides the ability to produce cursor movements using technology other than a standard computer mouse. AT devices for mouse emulation include trackballs, head-, foot-, or voice-controlled mouse emulation devices, and keyboard- or switch-operated mouse emulations (e.g., the standard Windows™ accessibility feature, MouseKeys). In these AT devices, cursor movements are typically used to operate AT by selection of icons on a screen, with each icon producing a function such as typing a letter, speaking a sentence, turning on a light, or loading a different screen of options. Numerous studies have shown that cursor movements can be controlled by EEG-based BCIs (e.g., Trejo et al., 2006; McFarland et al., 2008; Wolpaw et al., 1991; Li et al., 2010), by intracortical BCIs (e.g., Kim et al. 2008; Kennedy et al. 2004), or by ECoG-based BCIs (e.g.,

Leuthardt et al. 2004). Although use of a mouse also generally requires a click action for icon selection, many AT devices can be configured so that they do not require a mouse click. Instead, the selection occurs when the cursor is held in one place (e.g., on the icon) for a configurable amount of time. This is called a *dwell feature*, and it can be implemented either within the AT or incorporated as a feature of the BCI itself. Although the mouse click operation (or a substitute operation like dwelling) is very important, only some BCI designs for cursor movement include this option (e.g., McFarland et al, 2008).

ROBOTICS

Robotics has long been considered a potential AT application. Although robotic arms can provide many desirable functions, they are rarely used because of questions of mounting location, appropriate controls, cost, and safety. Although commercial devices such as feeders or page-turners, which can be described as special-purpose robotics, are available for ADLs, the performance of these devices is typically poor. Current feeders need someone to cut food and set up the feeder, and they may still require that the user reach for the food with head and neck movements; in addition, multiple attempts may be necessary to pick up food and deliver it to the user's mouth. All in all, to date such devices have produced frustration but little gain in independence. Similarly, page-turners are notoriously poor at their intended task and are impaired by glossy or heavy papers or tight bookbindings and sometimes by factors such as high room humidity (which can make it harder to pick up pages). Electronic devices for reading text and accessing books are frequently recommended as a replacement for robotic page-turners. Other robotics applications, such as obstacle-avoiding wheelchairs (Simpson 2005) or robotic exoskeletons to enhance mobility (e.g., (Gordon et al. 2006; Fleischer et al. 2006) are under development. These applications may be good candidates for BCI operation, since a semi-autonomous robot could be directed even by the limited information transfer available from a BCI. Indeed, some projects combining BCI technology and semi-autonomous robotic applications are already under way (e.g., Iturrate et al. 2009; Cincotti et al. 2008).

FUNCTIONAL ELECTRICAL STIMULATION

Functional electrical stimulation (FES), also referred to as functional neuromuscular stimulation (FNS), has long been a target BCI application (see chapter 22, this volume). FES can restore movement to a paralyzed limb through direct stimulation of a person's muscles, nerves, or spinal cord. Although FES systems for hand-grasp, standing, and mobility, as well as for bladder and bowel control, have been reported (Mauritz and Peckham, 1987; Johnston et al. 2005), and several systems have received approval from the Food and Drug Administration (FDA) in the United States (Hamid and Hayek 2008), their success as clinical applications remains uncertain. Müller-Putz et al. (2005) have demonstrated BCI operation of an FES system.

One of the key difficulties for FES-enhanced standing and walking is the need to use a walker to assist balance. This makes the FES user's arms unavailable for other tasks. Thus, a BCI might provide a great advantage for the FES user by eliminating the need for hand-control of the FES. However, the fine gradations of control and the rapidity with which adjustments must be made to maintain balance may be beyond the capabilities of current BCIs. For such BCI applications, goal-selection control with some degree of automation may be advantageous.

PROSTHESIS CONTROL

Control of prosthetic limbs is another long-standing target application for BCIs. User acceptance of prosthetic limbs is a complex and poorly understood problem. A review of 25 years of studies on prosthesis use and abandonment (Biddiss and Chau 2007) shows that the mean rates of rejection of prosthetics are in the range of 23–45%. Although this might seemingly present an opportunity for BCI technology (i.e., BCIs might prove better), many of the factors responsible for prosthesis rejection (e.g., weight, durability, and lack of sensory feedback [Biddiss and Chau 2007]) would presumably not be eliminated simply by using BCI technology.

Nevertheless, BCIs could provide alternative control interfaces for a prosthesis. Because a prosthesis is viewed as an intimate extension of the user's body (Biddiss and Chau 2007), BCI success with a prosthesis will depend on the ability of the BCI and the prosthesis to provide responsive, precise control without requiring undue attention on the part of the user. Thus, to compete with current control systems, BCIs would probably need to provide several independent continuous control signals that a user could manipulate easily and rapidly. These BCIs would need to compete successfully with other innovative prosthesis-control technologies now appearing, such as a system that involves transplanting residual nerves to other muscles in order to enable myoelectric control (Kuiken et al. 2009).

SELECTING AT APPLICATIONS FOR BCI CONTROL

INVOLVEMENT OF AT PROFESSIONALS

Choosing a useful BCI AT application for a person with physical impairments is a complex task. In addition to the technical aspects of the application itself, there is a subtext of interpersonal, psychosocial, sociological, and disability-rights issues that must be considered for successful acceptance of an AT. AT prescription is ideally accomplished by a team of certified AT professionals working in conjunction with others such as physical therapists, occupational therapists, speech-language pathologists, social workers, clinical psychologists, and physicians. AT professionals are expert in navigating issues relating to the prescription of technology, and they know a great deal about commercially available AT. Their input can be extremely helpful in the process of choosing a BCI-controlled AT application that is appropriate for a given individual or group. As BCI-controlled AT applications for people with physical impairments are developed, BCI researchers can partner with AT professionals in order to benefit from the years of research and development underlying current AT expertise and practice. Such partnerships will increase the likelihood of acceptance of BCI-controlled AT applications. AT professionals can also guide BCI researchers to the existing AT technology that is appropriate for BCI operation or suggest features that will improve the performance and acceptance of BCI-controlled applications.

Partnership with AT professionals can also help with the interpretation of research results and with the acquisition of funding. Subtleties of language used in manuscripts or grant proposals can reveal a BCI researcher's unfamiliarity with his/her target users and hinder publication or funding. Some commonly used terms (e.g., "wheelchair-bound") are considered offensive in the disability community (and can provoke a scalding lecture on how the wheelchair enables the rider, who is not "bound" to it at all). Even terms such as research "subject" (instead of "participant" or "user") or "disabled person" (instead of "person with a physical impairment"), can be viewed negatively. In the disability, rehabilitation engineering, and other communities, the use of appropriate language that places the individual above all labels based on functional ability is generally considered a sign of experience and understanding of the practical needs of people with physical impairments. For some funding agencies, inappropriate terminology can raise serious questions about the adequacy of the researcher's background. Partnership with an AT professional can help to avoid these and other pitfalls.

INVOLVEMENT OF TARGET USERS

When selecting appropriate AT applications for use with BCIs, the most authoritative experts will be the potential users themselves. The principles of universal design and user-centered practice strongly support the involvement of target users throughout the technological design process, including during research and development (Preiser and Ostroff 2010). Since the target users are the consumers of AT applications, their opinions will significantly affect whether these applications are a success. Individuals with conditions that classify them as potential BCI users are experts on the experience of living with one specific set of impairments, and their involvement as part of the design team can provide invaluable insights. Thus, it is essential that their opinions and experiences be considered in the design and selection of AT applications controlled by BCIs. This issue is discussed in more detail in chapter 19 of this volume.

STAND-ALONE BCI/AT SYSTEMS VERSUS BCI+AT SYSTEMS

BCI researchers and developers can take either of two approaches in using a BCI to operate an AT application. The first approach creates a stand-alone *BCI/AT* system, that is, a BCI that is integrated with a *new* AT device. The second approach creates a BCI that operates one or more *existing* commercial AT devices. These are called general-purpose or *plug-and-play* BCIs. Plug-and-play BCIs and the AT devices they control are referred to in this chapter as *BCI+AT systems.*

Creating a stand-alone BCI/AT system requires a development approach that reinvents an AT functionality so that it can be integrated with a BCI. In this case, the new stand-alone BCI/AT system would usually replicate AT functionality that is already commercially available in AT devices used with conventional (i.e., muscle-based) control interfaces. (The exceptions are in a few areas such as robotic and FES devices that may not be commercially available.) Because it does not take advantage of the considerable effort and experience embodied in existing AT devices, the development of stand-alone BCI/AT systems is generally not cost-effective, wastes development resources, and often limits the functionality available to the users.

In contrast, when possible, combining a BCI with commercially available AT devices to create BCI+AT systems will usually be more expeditious because it reduces the development effort and may in fact increase the functionality of the resulting product. The BCI simply replaces the conventional muscle-based interfaces for which the AT devices were originally developed. Designing such plug-and-play BCIs to operate existing AT devices frees BCI developers to focus time and resources on creating the most accurate and reliable BCI possible and on increasing the range of AT devices that the BCI can operate.

Although there are many advantages to plug-and-play BCIs that operate commercial AT devices, there may be instances in which the performance of a stand-alone BCI/AT system is significantly better. The potential relative advantages and disadvantages of the two approaches should therefore be carefully considered. To be successful, BCIs must be cost-effective for AT users, AT providers, and BCI developers. For people with newly acquired disabilities who for the first time require AT and for whom a BCI is the most appropriate interface, the economy and desirability of a stand-alone BCI/AT system versus a plug-and-play BCI+AT that uses commercial AT will depend on their relative costs and available functionalities.

BCI+AT SYSTEMS

In a BCI+AT system, the BCI simply replaces a physical switch or computer keyboard or mouse. Thus, such plug-and-play BCIs could be truly interchangeable with conventional AT interfaces. This capability would increase the number of devices that BCIs could operate and the number of people who could benefit from them. It could expand the market for BCI technologies to include people with a wide range of disabilities. A BCI might be the only usable AT interface for people with movement insufficient to operate muscle-based AT interfaces. For people whose physical abilities fatigue quickly, it could increase the efficiency of AT operation or provide a back-up or alternative interface that could still be operated even when physical fatigue sets in. For people with conventional interface options or those using several different AT devices, a plug-and-play BCI could also provide a back-up or alternative interface. For people with progressive disabilities, it could enable them to use their AT devices even if their physical condition deteriorates to the point where muscle-based interfaces are no longer usable.

Not only would plug-and-play BCIs provide great functionality, they would also be more cost effective for people with disabilities and for AT service-delivery personnel. A BCI that could operate commercially available AT would allow people with progressive disabilities to continue to use familiar and functional AT devices as they switch to (or add) a BCI when their condition progresses and conventional (i.e., muscle-based) interfaces begin to fail. In this way, the time, money, and effort already invested in AT systems would not be lost as their disabilities progress; and the functions that the AT provides would be maintained despite deterioration of their physical abilities. Furthermore, AT service-delivery personnel would not have to be retrained for new BCI-specific applications (as they would for BCI/AT systems); the BCI would simply be an alternative method for accessing all the functionality of the already familiar AT devices. Thus, the plug-and-play approach could reduce the technical-support burdens on new BCI companies, allowing them to concentrate on the functionality of the BCI controller, and leaving the AT applications, and their service delivery and support, to companies already specializing in these areas. In summary, a strategic focus on plug-and-play BCIs could result in both lower cost and increased functionality for the BCIs that eventually come to market.

Plug-and-play BCIs need to be easily configurable to suit the differing requirements of a variety of commercial AT devices. The on-site AT or AAC professionals who would perform this configuration are generally experienced in designing AT communication screens to fit the needs of individual users. An easily configurable plug-and-play BCI could therefore give its users access to all the functionality of commercial AT devices. Given the wide range of available commercial AT devices, a well-designed plug-and-play BCI could provide considerably greater functionality than that practical (or perhaps even possible) with a stand-alone BCI/AT system.

A few examples of the use of BCIs to operate commercially available AT have been reported. The Environmental Control BCI (Karmali et al. 2000), a BCI specifically developed for environmental control functions, uses hardware modules from the commercially available ActiveHome X10 Home Automation System (X10.com, Seattle, WA, USA) to control a light, fan, and radio. (X10 modules are frequently used in AT environmental control systems because of their easy installation and low price.) In this system, the BCI sends instructions to the X10 modules through an X10-command line interface (Karmali et al. 2000) to provide access to X10 home-automation modules. Similarly, BCI control of the novel Dasher text-entry program (http://www.inference.phy.cam.ac.uk/dasher), which was originally designed for operation by a cursor or by switches, has been implemented (Felton et al. 2007) and analyzed in detail (Wills and MacKay 2006).

A P300-based BCI speller has been combined with a commercial word-prediction program (Vaughan et al. 2006; Sellers et al. 2010) that runs transparently with many commercial programs and writes directly into these programs. It provides word prediction as well as speech output (in the form of reading back each selection or the full text upon completion). Several people with advanced ALS have used or are now using this BCI application in their daily lives (Sellers et al., 2010; Vaughan et al., 2006). Each of these people has a different need and agenda for it. One has used the system independently up to 6-8 hours per day for several years to maintain employment as a research scientist, to communicate with caregivers and family, and to write and send emails. Another, who has no access to any other AT device, uses the BCI to communicate basic needs to her caregiver. A third, who still has slight facial muscle control that she uses to provide single-switch computer access, uses the BCI to write articles and poetry, and plans to make greater use of the BCI as her disease progresses still further and as the BCI's range of applications expands.

STAND-ALONE BCI/AT SYSTEMS

The primary justification for choosing a stand-alone BCI/AT system is that it might provide dramatic advantages in important aspects of performance (e.g., convenience, speed, or accuracy). For example, a person with weak eye movements may have difficulty shifting gaze and visual focus between two screens (i.e., the BCI screen and the screen of the AT device). A stand-alone BCI could address this problem by integrating the two displays into one screen. On the other hand, future plug-and-play BCIs could be designed to eliminate this problem by making the BCI display transparent and superimposing it on the AT display or by using a retinal projection method (i.e., projecting an image directly into the user's eye) to display them together (Takahashi and Hirooka 2008).

A fully integrated stand-alone BCI/AT might outperform a plug-and-play BCI by being able to use task-performance information for real-time adaptations of BCI operation. On the other hand, a plug-and-play BCI might also be able to do this. For example, a backspace or correction key could allow the user to indicate incorrect BCI performance and thus guide BCI adaptation. (In this case, a separate correction key might be used to correct the user's—as opposed to the BCI's—errors.)

A stand-alone BCI/AT system could use natural-language (i.e., conventional) spelling and semantic rules in the commands it sends to the AT. In contrast, with a plug-and-play BCI, this might not be desirable because the commercial AT device might routinely utilize normally unused sequences of letters and numbers for performance-enhancement shortcuts. Thus, in this case, the stand-alone system might be preferable. For all such considerations, the advantages of a stand-alone system would need to outweigh the performance-enhancement features provided by the commercial AT device.

In summary, plug-and-play BCIs that operate standard AT devices in BCI+AT systems are in general likely to be easier to develop than stand-alone BCI/AT systems, and they are likely to be as, or more, effective. For particular needs or in particular circumstances, however, stand-alone BCI/AT systems may have advantages in performance or convenience that justify the added effort and expense needed for their development.

OPTIMIZING BCI-CONTROLLED AT PERFORMANCE

The types of errors that occur with current BCIs mirror those that typically occur with conventional AT devices for people with physical impairments (e.g., inaccurate cursor movement trajectories, incorrect key selections, etc.). For this reason, BCI development can benefit from AT performance-enhancement devices or optimization features designed to compensate for physical impairments. (Indeed, another advantage of using plug-and-play BCIs to operate commercially available AT devices is that they can benefit from the extensive past efforts of AT developers to enhance performance.) For example, in AT devices for people who type slowly, word prediction is often used in conjunction with scanning, on-screen keyboards, or physical keyboards. Users start to type a word and then choose the completion of the word from a list. Although word prediction has been shown to save keystrokes, it does not necessarily produce an increased rate of text generation, because the mental load of searching the list and selecting the word may slow the generation of text. Koester and Levine (1998) examined this trade-off and concluded that word prediction is useful for people who type slowly. Since BCI typing is typically slow, word prediction is likely to be beneficial; it is, in fact, already being used for BCI typing by people with severe disabilities (Vaughan et al. 2006). Nevertheless, the possibility that the additional cognitive load required by word prediction might interfere with BCI operation warrants further examination.

Variants of word prediction may provide greater enhancement by reducing or changing the cognitive load. For example, the Smart Key™ function (Applied Human Factors, Inc., Helotes, TX) limits the active keys to those likely to be used next, thereby reducing the number of possible selections and the likelihood of unintentional selections. An override key is included to allow the user to type words unknown to the Smart Key™ function. By incorporating natural-language spelling rules into the text-production stream, the Smart Key™ function could improve the typing accuracy of a plug-and-play BCI by rejecting unintended characters (essentially canceling probable errors). Dasher and MinSpeak™ also provide performance-enhancement features for text entry or communication that could benefit BCI use.

AT experience suggests that cursor movement can also be enhanced. The Assistive Mouse Adapter (Montrose Secam Ltd, Iver, Bucks, UK) is a hardware device designed to reduce unintentional mouse movements caused by hand tremor. It filters the signal from the mouse to produce smoother on-screen cursor movement. Some devices such as the PointSmart (Infogrip, Inc, Ventura, CA) also add a gravity (i.e., attractive) effect near potential cursor targets to assist with target acquisition.

These and other AT performance-enhancement features have been designed to compensate for the limited accuracy of conventional (i.e., muscle-based) AT control interfaces. It is quite likely that they can also help compensate for the limited accuracy and modest speed of current BCIs. BCI researchers may save substantial time and effort and improve their results by learning from and incorporating these existing performance-enhancement features.

SUMMARY

The goal of most brain-computer interfaces (BCIs) is to operate assistive technology (AT) devices that provide communication or control capacities to people with severe disabilities. The AT device operated by a BCI is referred to as its *application*. Although the application itself is not part of the BCI, it is the means by which the BCI's commands are put into action. Thus, the BCI sends *commands* to the application, which converts them into useful *actions*. A BCI's applications are crucial to its utility and to its clinical and commercial success.

The successful development and dissemination of BCI-controlled AT applications require attention to the needs and desires of the people for whom they are intended, those with severe disabilities. AT professionals can provide crucial expertise in the capabilities and usage of currently available AT devices and should be closely involved in the application development process. Prospective BCI users and their caregivers should also be consulted throughout the development process, and they should receive appropriate training when BCI systems are deployed.

A BCI provides *goal-selection* or *process-control* commands to an AT device. The AT device converts these commands *directly* or *indirectly* into actions that are either *discrete* or *continuous*. Successful development of BCI-controlled applications depends on appropriate matching of the BCI command, the AT conversion process, and the AT action.

BCI-controlled AT applications can be realized in two ways. *Plug-and-play* BCIs (referred to in this chapter as BCI+AT systems) simply replace muscle-based interfaces in controlling existing AT devices. Alternatively, fully integrated *stand-alone BCI/AT* systems can also be developed. In general, the plug-and-play approach is likely to have major advantages: a wider variety of functions; less time and expense involved in development; and greater acceptance by and convenience for users, caregivers, and technical support personnel.

BCI+AT and BCI/AT systems could potentially help their users in three major areas: communication; mobility; and activities of daily living. The AT applications that BCIs might operate include: switch-activated devices; computer access; robotics; functional electrical stimulation; and prosthesis control.

Ultimate acceptance of BCI+AT and BCI/AT systems will be based not only on the speed, accuracy, and usefulness of their applications but also on key factors such as their avoidance of inadvertent actions during periods when the user is not intending to operate the system. The development of BCI-controlled AT applications can benefit substantially from methods used to enhance the performance of conventional muscle-based AT interfaces.

In summary, as the functionality provided by BCI-controlled AT expands, and as technological advances increase convenience and reduce prices, BCI-controlled AT application are likely to be incorporated into the lives of many people, including not only those with the most significant impairments, but many others as well.

REFERENCES

Internet Sites

AAC Demographic Information, <http://aac.unl.edu/AACdemog.html>.
International Society for Augmentative and Alternative Communication, <http://www.isaac-online.org/en/home.shtml>.

PointSmart Product Details - Infogrip, Inc., 2003 <http://www.infogrip.com/product_view.asp?RecordNumber−988>.
Prentke Romich Company. *How do I Scan Using a Single Switch?* (2007) <http://support.prentrom.com/article.php?id=271>.
RESNA. <http://resna.org/resnaresources/resources-education>, (2009a).
RESNA. *RESNA Homepage*, <www.resna.org>, (2009b).
RESNA. *RESNA: Certification*, <http://resna.org/certifications/certification-what-is-certification>, (2009c).
Smart Key Technology, 1997–2006)<http://www.ahf-net.com/smartkey.htm>.
Synopsis for the Matrix, http://www.imdb.com/title/tt0133093/synopsis, 1999.
Welcome to Montrose Secam Ltd, <http://www.montrosesecam.com/>. Welcome to the AAC Institute Website, *http://www.aacinstitute.org/index.html*.

Published References

Allen, S. M., B. Hunt, and M. Green. Fall in Vital Capacity with Posture, British Journal of Diseases of the Chest, vol. 79/no. 3, (1985), pp. 267–271.
Bauby, J.-D. *The Diving Bell and the Butterfly*, Anonymous Translator (1st U.S. ed.). New York: A.A. Knopf, distributed by Random House (1997).
Bauer, G., F. Gerstenbrand, and E. Rumpl. Varieties of the Locked-in Syndrome, *Journal of Neurology*, vol. 221/no. 2, (1979), pp. 77–91.
Biddiss, E. A., and T. T. Chau. Upper Limb Prosthesis Use and Abandonment: A Survey of the Last 25 Years, *Prosthetics and Orthotics International*, vol. 31/no. 3, (2007), pp. 236–257.
Birch, G. E., S. G. Mason, and J. F. Borisoff. Current Trends in Brain-Computer Interface Research at the Neil Squire Foundation, *IEEE Transactions on Neural Systems and Rehabilitation Engineering*, vol. 11/no. 2, (2003), pp. 123–126.
Blair, E., and J. B. Hickam. The Effect of Change in Body Position on Lung Volume and Intrapulmonary Gas Mixing in Normal Subjects, *The Journal of Clinical Investigation*, vol. 34/no. 3, (1955), pp. 383–389.
Brown-Triolo, D. L., Understanding the Person Behind the Technology, in Scherer, M. J. ed., *Assistive Technology: Matching Device and Consumer for Successful Rehabilitation*, Washington, DC: American Psychological Association, (2002), pp. 31–46.
Cincotti, F., D. Mattia, F. Aloise, S. Bufalari, G. Schalk, G. Oriolo, A. Cherubini, M. G. Marciani, and F. Babiloni. Non-Invasive Brain–Computer Interface System: Towards its Application as Assistive Technology, *Brain Research Bulletin*, vol. 75/no. 6, (2008), pp. 796–803.
Cook, A. M., and S. M. Hussey., *Assistive Technologies: Principles and Practice*, Anonymous Translator (2nd ed,) St. Louis: Mosby (2002).
Cooper, R. A., H. Ohnabe, and D. A. Hobson., *An Introduction to Rehabilitation Engineering*, Anonymous Translator. Boca Raton, FL: Taylor & Francis (2007).
Donchin, E, K. M. Spencer, R. Wijesinghe, The mental prosthesis: assessing the speed of a P300-based brain-computer interface. *IEEE Transactions on Neural Systems and Rehabilitation Engineering*, vol. 8/no. 2 (2000) pp. 174–179.
Farwell, L. A., and E. Donchin. Talking Off the Top of Your Head: Toward a Mental Prosthesis Utilizing Event-Related Brain Potentials, *Electroencephalography and Clinical Neurophysiology*, vol. 70/no. 6, (1988), pp. 510–523.
Felton, E. A., N. L. Lewis, S. A. Wills, R. G. Radwin, and J. C. Williams. Neural Signal Based Control of the Dasher Writing System, *CNE 07. 3rd International IEEE/EMBS Conference on Neural Engineering* (2007), pp. 366–370.
Fleischer, C., A. Wege, K. Kondak, and G. Hommel. Application of EMG Signals for Controlling Exoskeleton Robots, *Biomedizinische Technik. Biomedical Engineering*, vol. 51/no. 5–6, (2006), pp. 314–319.
Friedrich, E. V., D. J. McFarland, C. Neuper, T. M. Vaughan, P. Brunner and J. R. Wolpaw. A Scanning Protocol for a Sensorimotor Rhythm-Based Brain-Computer Interface, *Biological Psychology*, vol. 80/no. 2, (2009), pp. 169–175.
Furdea A, S. Halder, D.J. Krusienski, D. Bross, F. Nijboer, N. Birbaumer, and A. Kübler. An auditory oddball (P300) spelling system for brain-computer interfaces. *Psychophysiology*, vol. 46/no. 3, (2009), pp. 617–625.
Galan, F., M. Nuttin, E. Lew, P. W. Ferrez, G. Vanacker, J. Philips, and R. Millán J. del. A Brain-Actuated Wheelchair: Asynchronous and Non-Invasive Brain-Computer Interfaces for Continuous Control of Robots, *Clinical Neurophysiology*, vol. 119/no. 9, (2008), pp. 2159–2169.
Gibson, W., *Neuromancer*, Anonymous Translator, New York: Ace Books (1984).
Gordon, K. E., G. S. Sawicki, and D. P. Ferris. Mechanical Performance of Artificial Pneumatic Muscles to Power an Ankle-Foot Orthosis, *Journal of Biomechanics*, vol. 39/no. 10, (2006), pp. 1832–1841.
Graimann, B., J. E. Huggins, A. Schlogl, S. P. Levine, and G. Pfurtscheller. Detection of Movement-Related Desynchronization Patterns in Ongoing

Single-Channel Electrocorticogram, *IEEE Transactions on Neural Systems and Rehabilitation Engineering*, vol. 11/no. 3, (2003), pp. 276–281.

Gruis, K.L. P.A. Wren, and J.E. Huggins, "Amyotrophic lateral sclerosis patients' self-reported satisfaction with assistive technology," Muscle Nerve, vol. 43/no. 5 (2011), pp. 643–647.

Hamid, S., and R. Hayek. Role of Electrical Stimulation for Rehabilitation and Regeneration After Spinal Cord Injury: An Overview, *European Spine Journal*, vol. 17/no. 9, (2008), pp. 1256–1269.

Hayashi, H., and E. A. Oppenheimer. ALS Patients on TPPV: Totally Locked-in State, Neurologic Findings and Ethical Implications, *Neurology,* vol. 61/no. 1, (2003), pp. 135–137.

Heingartner, D. Loser: Mental Block, *IEEE Spectrum,* (2009), pp. 42–43.

Henderson, M. A Race to the Wire as Old Hand at Morse Code Beats Txt Msgrs, *The Times,* April 16, (2005).

Hidecker, M. J. C., N. Paneth, P. Rosenbaum, R. D. Kent, J. Lillie, B. Johnson, and K. Chester. Developing a Classification Tool of Functional Communication in Children with Cerebral Palsy, *Developmental Medicine & Child Neurology,* vol. 50/Suppl 4, (2008), p. 43.

Hsiao, M. C., D. Song, and T. W. Berger. Control Theory-Based Regulation of Hippocampal CA1 Nonlinear Dynamics,.*IEEE Engineering in Medicine and Biology Society.Conference,* vol. 2008 (2008), pp. 5535–5538.

Huggins, J.E., P.A. Wren, and K.L. Gruis, "What would brain-computer interface users want? Opinions and priorities of potential users with amyotroph lateral sclerosis," *Amyotroph Lateral Scler.,* 2011 (in press).

Iturrate, I., J. M. Antelis, A. Kübler, and J. Minguez. A Noninvasive Brain-Actuated Wheelchair Based on a P300 Neurophysiological Protocol and Automated Navigation, *IEEE Transactions on Robotics,* vol. 25/no. 3, (2009), pp. 614–627.

Johnston TE, Betz RR, Smith BT, Benda BJ, Mulcahey MJ, Davis R, Houdayer TP, Pontari MA, Barriskill A., and Creasey G. H. Implantable FES system for upright mobility and bladder and bowel function for individuals with spinal cord injury. *Spinal Cord* vol. 43/no. 12 (2005) pp. 713–723.

Karmali, F., M. Polak, and A. Kostov. Environmental Control by a Brain-Computer Interface, vol. 4/(2000), pp. 2990–2992.

Katz, R. T., A. J. Haig, B. B. Clark, and R. J. DiPaola. Long-Term Survival, Prognosis, and Life-Care Planning for 29 Patients with Chronic Locked-in Syndrome, *Arch.Phys.Med.Rehabil.,* vol. 73/no. 5, (1992), pp. 403–408.

Kennedy, P. R., R. A. Bakay, M. M. Moore, K. Adams, and J. Goldwaithe. Direct Control of a Computer from the Human Central Nervous System, *IEEE Transactions on Rehabilitation Engineering* vol. 8/no. 2, (2000), pp. 198–202.

Kennedy, P. R., M. T. Kirby, M. M. Moore, B. King, and A. Mallory. Computer Control Using Human Intracortical Local Field Potentials, *IEEE Transactions on Neural Systems and Rehabilitation Engineering* vol. 12/no. 3, (2004), pp. 339–344.

Kim, S. P., J. D. Simeral, L. R. Hochberg, J. P. Donoghue, and M.J. Black. Neural Control of Computer Cursor Velocity by Decoding Motor Cortical Spiking Activity in Humans with Tetraplegia, *Journal of Neural Engineering,* vol. 5/no. 4, (2008), pp. 455–476.

Koester, H. H., and S. P. Levine. Model Simulations of User Performance with Word-Prediction, *Augmentative and Alternative Communication,* vol. 14 (1998), pp. 25–35.

Kuebler, A., B. Kotchoubey, T. Hinterberger, N. Ghanayim, J. Perelmouter, M. Schauer, C. Fritsch, E. Taub, and N. Birbaumer. The Thought Translation Device: A Neurophysiological Approach to Communication in Total Motor Paralysis, *Experimental Brain Research.Experimentelle Hirnforschung. Experimentation Cerebrale,* vol. 124/no. 2, (1999), pp. 223–232.

Kuiken, T. A., G. Li, B. A. Lock, R. D. Lipschutz, L. A. Miller, K. A. Stubblefield, and K. B. Englehart. Targeted Muscle Reinnervation for Real-Time Myoelectric Control of Multifunction Artificial Arms, *JAMA.* vol. 301/no. 6, (2009), pp. 619–628.

Leeb, R., D. Friedman, G. R. Müller-Putz, R. Scherer, M. Slater, and G. Pfurtscheller. Self-Paced (Asynchronous) BCI Control of a Wheelchair in Virtual Environments: A Case Study with a Tetraplegic, *Computational Intelligence and Neuroscience,* (2007), pp. 79642.

Leeb, R., F. Lee, C. Keinrath, R. Scherer, H. Bischof, and G. Pfurtscheller. Brain-Computer Communication: Motivation, Aim, and Impact of Exploring a Virtual Apartment, *IEEE Transactions on Neural Systems and Rehabilitation Engineering* vol. 15/no. 4, (2007), pp. 473–482.

Leuthardt, E. C., G. Schalk, J. R. Wolpaw, J. G. Ojemann, and D. W. Moran. A Brain-Computer Interface Using Electrocorticographic Signals in Humans, *Journal of Neural Engineering,* vol. 1/no. 2, (2004), pp. 63–71.

Li, Y., J. Long, T. Yu, et al. 'An EEG-Based BCI System for 2-D Cursor Control by Combining Mu/Beta Rhythm and P300 Potential', IEEE Trans Biomed Eng, (2010).

Mason, S. G., and G. E. Birch. A Brain-Controlled Switch for Asynchronous Control Applications, *IEEE Transactions on Bio-Medical Engineering,* vol. 47/no. 10, (2000), pp. 1297–1307.

Mauritz, K. H., and H. P. Peckham. 'Restoration of Grasping Functions in Quadriplegic Patients by Functional Electrical Stimulation (FES)', International Journal of Rehabilitation Research.Internationale Zeitschrift Fur Rehabilitationsforschung.Revue Internationale De Recherches De Readaptation, vol. 10/no. 4, Suppl 5, (1987), pp. 57–61.

McCaffrey, A., *The Ship Who Sang,* Anonymous Translator, New York: Walker, 1969).

McFarland, D. J., D. J. Krusienski, W. A. Sarnacki, et al. 'Emulation of Computer Mouse Control with a Noninvasive Brain-Computer Interface', Journal of Neural Engineering, vol. 5/no. 2, (2008), pp. 101–110.

Müller-Putz, G. R., R. Scherer, G. Pfurtscheller, and R. Rupp. EEG-Based Neuroprosthesis Control: A Step Towards Clinical Practice, *Neuroscience Letters*, vol. 382/no. 1–2, (2005), pp. 169–174.

Neuper, C., G. R. Müller, A. Kübler, et al. 'Clinical Application of an EEG-Based Brain-Computer Interface: A Case Study in a Patient with Severe Motor Impairment', Clinical Neurophysiology : Official Journal of the International Federation of Clinical Neurophysiology, vol. 114/no. 3, (2003), pp. 399–409.

Pfurtscheller, G., G. R. Müller-Putz, A. Schlogl, B. Graimann, R. Scherer, R. Leeb, C. Brunner, C. Keinrath, F. Lee, G. Townsend, C. Vidaurre, and C. Neuper. 15 Years of BCI Research at Graz University of Technology: Current Projects, *IEEE Transactions on Neural Systems and Rehabilitation Engineering*, vol. 14/no. 2, (2006), pp. 205–210.

Preiser W.F.E., E. Ostroff, ,*Universal Design Handbook.* 2nd ed. New York: McGraw-Hill (2010).

Sellers, E. W., T. M. Vaughan, and J. R. Wolpaw. 'A Brain-Computer Interface for Long-Term Independent Home use', Amyotrophic Lateral Sclerosis: Official Publication of the World Federation of Neurology Research Group on Motor Neuron Diseases, vol. 11/no. 5, (2010), pp. 449–455.

Simpson, R. C. Smart Wheelchairs: A Literature Review, *Journal of Rehabilitation Research and Development,* vol. 42/no. 4, (2005), pp. 423–436.

Snider, M. Toy Trains 'Star Wars' Fans to use the Force, *USA Today,* Jan. 7, 2009.

Takahashi H, Hirooka S. Stereoscopic see-through retinal projection head-mounted display. *Proceedings of the SPIE - The International Society for Optical Engineering.* vol. 6803 (2008) pp. 68031N-1–8.

Thompson, D. E., J. J. Baker, W. A. Sarnacki, and J. E. Higgins. Plug-and-Play Brain-Computer Interface Keyboard Performance, *NER 09. 4th International IEEE/EMBS Conference on Neural Engineering,* (2009), pp. 433–435.

Townsend G, B. K. LaPallo, C. B. Boulay, D. J. Krusienski, G. E. Frye, C. K. Hauser, N. E. Schwartz, T. M. Vaughan, J. R. Wolpaw, and E. W. Seller. A novel P300-based brain-computer interface stimulus presentation paradigm: moving beyond rows and columns, *Clinical Neurophysiology.* vol. 121/no.7, (2010) pp. 1109–1120.

Trejo, L. J., R. Rosipal, and B. Matthews. 'Brain-Computer Interfaces for 1-D and 2-D Cursor Control: Designs using Volitional Control of the EEG Spectrum Or Steady-State Visual Evoked Potentials', IEEE Trans.Neural Syst.Rehabil.Eng., vol. 14/no. 2, (2006), pp. 225–229.

Twist, J. *BBC NEWS | Technology | Brain Waves Control Video Game,* (updated March 24, 2004, 2004) <http://news.bbc.co.uk/2/hi/technology/3485918.stm>.

Vaughan, T. M., D. J. McFarland, G. Schalk, W. A. Sarnacki, D. J. Krusienski. E. W. Sellers, and J. R. Wolpaw. The Wadsworth BCI Research and Development Program: At Home with BCI, *IEEE Transactions on Neural Systems and Rehabilitation Engineering,* vol. 14, no. 2, (2006), pp. 229–233.

Vidal, J. J. Toward Direct Brain-Computer Communication, *Annual Review of Biophysics and Bioengineering,* vol. 2 (1973), pp. 157–180.

Wills, S. A., and D. J. MacKay. DASHER—an Efficient Writing System for Brain-Computer Interfaces?, *IEEE Transactions on Neural Systems and Rehabilitation Engineering,* vol. 14/no. 2, (2006), pp. 244–246.

Wolpaw, J. R., D. J. McFarland, G. W. Neat, et al. 'An EEG-Based Brain-Computer Interface for Cursor Control', Electroencephalography and Clinical Neurophysiology, vol. 78/no. 3, (1991), pp. 252–259.

Wolpaw, J. R., H. Ramoser, D. J. McFarland, and G. Pfurtscheller. EEG-Based Communication: Improved Accuracy by Response Verification, *IEEE Transactions on Rehabilitation Engineering,* vol. 6/no. 3, (1998), pp. 326.

PART IV. | EXISTING BCIs

12 | BCIs THAT USE P300 EVENT-RELATED POTENTIALS

ERIC W. SELLERS, YAEL ARBEL, AND EMANUEL DONCHIN

vent-related brain potentials (ERPs) in the EEG are manifestations at the scalp of neural activity that is triggered by, and is involved in the processing of, specific events. The voltages that constitute the ERP are embedded within the general EEG activity recordable from the scalp and are usually quite small relative to the *ongoing* EEG. However, because the ERPs are time-locked to events, and follow a constant time course, they can be extracted by averaging multiple trials of eliciting events. The result is a series of positive and negative voltage deflections that are referred to as *components*. The successive components typically differ in their stimulus rate and amplitude dependence, their topographical distributions, and their relationships to the information-processing activities of the brain. The components that can be recorded over the first 150 msec following the eliciting event tend to reflect activity in the primary sensory systems, and their waveforms and scalp distributions vary with the modality of the eliciting stimuli. These are known as the *exogenous* components. Longer-latency components tend to reflect information-processing activity that is cognitive in nature and is thus less dependent on stimulus modality and more dependent on the significance of the eliciting event in the subject's concurrent tasks. They are usually referred to as *endogenous* components.

Both early (exogenous) and late (endogenous) components of visual evoked potentials (i.e., VEPs) have been used as signal features for BCIs. The design and operation of BCIs that use endogenous ERP components differ both in principle and practice from those of BCIs that use exogenous ERP components. This chapter focuses on BCIs that use P300, an endogenous ERP component. Chapter 14 discusses BCIs that use exogenous VEP components.

THE P300 ERP AND P300-BASED BCIs

The P300 is a positive deflection that occurs in the scalp-recorded EEG after a stimulus that is delivered under a specific set of circumstances. It was first described by Sutton et al. (1965) and has been widely studied since then to explore higher cortical functions in humans (for review see Bashore & Van der Molen, 1991; Donchin, 1981; Duncan et al., 2009; Fabiani et al., 1987; Polich, 2007; Pritchard, 1981). Although it often occurs at a latency of about 300 msec relative to the eliciting stimulus (hence the designation of P300), its latency may vary from 250 to 750 msec (Comerchero & Polich, 1999; Magliero

et al., 1984; McCarthy & Donchin, 1981; Polich, 2007). This variability in latency reflects the fact that the P300 is elicited by the decision, not necessarily conscious, that a rare event has occurred, and the decision latency can, and does, vary with the nature (e.g., the difficulty) of the decision (Kutas et al., 1977). The P300 is usually largest over central parietal scalp and attenuates gradually as distance from this area increases.

In 1988, P300 was first used as the basis for a BCI (Farwell & Donchin, 1988), and a steadily growing number of research groups are currently pursuing its BCI applications. Current P300-based BCIs allow users to select items displayed on a computer screen. Thus, while the process is very different, a P300-based BCI selection is essentially equivalent to a selection by a standard computer keyboard. Because P300-based BCIs are noninvasive, use hardware that is portable and inexpensive, and can provide reliable performance, they are essentially the only BCIs that are currently being used outside of the laboratory by severely disabled people for important purposes in their daily lives, such as communication and environmental control. Furthermore, many different laboratories are exploring possibilities for further increasing the capabilities and usefulness of P300-based BCIs.

This chapter discusses the nature of the P300, addresses the principles of its BCI usage, reviews the major areas of P300-based BCI research, summarizes current clinical usage of P300-based BCIs, and considers the prospects for their further development.

THE ODDBALL PARADIGM

The specific set of circumstances for eliciting the P300 ERP is known as the *Oddball Paradigm*. This paradigm has three essential attributes (Donchin & Coles, 1988):

- A subject is presented with a series of events (i.e., stimuli), each of which falls into one of two classes.
- The events that fall into one of the classes are less frequent than those that fall into the other class.
- The subject performs a task that requires classifying each event into one of the two classes.

The events that fall into the less-frequent class (i.e., the *oddball* events) elicit a P300. As long as an experimental design adopts the three attributes of the oddball paradigm, any stimulus and any classification task can elicit a P300.

It is important to note that, although the two classes are generally two different classes of stimuli, this is not a requirement. As shown by Sutton et al. (1967), a P300 can be elicited by an event that consists of the absence of a stimulus, if that absence satisfies the conditions of the oddball paradigm. That is, a P300 ERP is elicited by rare events that violate the subject's expectations.

Most P300 studies have used visual or auditory stimuli. Figure 12.1 illustrates a typical P300 experiment. The letters O and X flash on a video screen in a random order at a rate of one per second (i.e., the stimulus onset asynchrony). The X occurs infrequently (e.g., 20% of the flashes) and is thus the oddball stimulus, while the O occurs frequently (e.g., the other 80% of the flashes). The subject is asked to count the number of times one of the stimuli (e.g., X) occurs. Each time a stimulus occurs, a marker is placed in the data file to indicate the identity of the stimulus, X or O. Each stimulus is presented on the screen for 100 msec, and then the screen is blank for 900 msec (i.e., the interstimulus interval [ISI]) until the presentation of the next stimulus. Figure 12.1A shows the time course of the experimental events.

Figure 12.1B displays the ERPs elicited by the oddball stimulus at midline electrode locations Fz, Cz, and Pz of the 10–20 system (see fig. 12.2) for 800 msec after the stimulus. The three responses show a typical P300 scalp topography: the most prominent potential is a positive component occurring about 350 msec after the X stimulus; and it is largest at the Pz electrode and attenuates at more anterior and posterior locations. It should be noted that the results would be essentially the same even if the subject had been asked to count the frequent O stimuli rather than the rare X stimuli: P300 is always elicited by the rare events (i.e., the X stimuli in

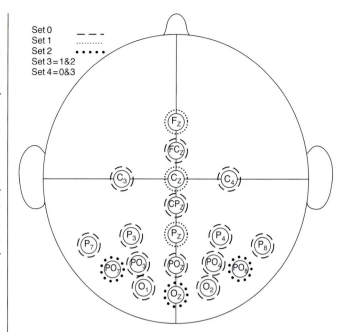

Figure 12.2 Electrode locations evaluated for use in a P300-based BCI by Krusienski et al. (2008). EEG was recorded from 64 electrodes. The sets of electrodes shown here (i.e., dashed, dotted, bold-dotted circles) were compared in regard to offline classification accuracy as described in the text.

this example) (Duncan-Johnson & Donchin, 1977). The next most salient components are the P100 and N200 components, which are considered to be exogenous components even though they can be modulated to some extent by attention (Heinze et al., 1994; Mangun, 1995; Mangun et al., 1993).

As noted, P300 latency may vary from 250 to 750 msec (Comerchero & Polich, 1999; Magliero, et al., 1984; McCarthy & Donchin, 1981; Polich, 2007). This variability is thought to reflect differences in the amounts of time it takes to classify

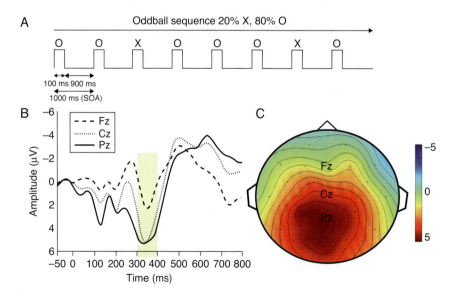

Figure 12.1 (A). Time course of rare (i.e., oddball) (X) and common (O) stimuli in a standard oddball protocol. (B) Average oddball ERPs from a subject for electrode locations Fz, Cz, and Pz, showing a progressively larger positive deflection from frontal, to central, to posterior sites. The convention used here shows positive amplitude down and negative amplitude up. (C) Topographical distribution of the average ERP amplitude 300–400 msec after the oddball stimulus. The large positive ERP component (i.e., P300) is maximum at Pz and is widely distributed over posterior-parietal regions.

different kinds of events. Kutas et al. (1977) demonstrated the relationship between the latency of the P300 and the difficulty of the classification task.

P300 ORIGIN AND FUNCTION

Some of the most compelling evidence related to the origin of the P300 has been provided by Knight and colleagues through studies in patients with brain lesions. Knight et al. (1989) showed that lesions in the temporal parietal junction abolished the auditory P300 at posterior scalp sites, even though the patients could still discriminate between the stimuli. In contrast, damage to lateral parietal cortex did not impair P300 generation. These results suggest that lateral parietal cortex is not critical in auditory P300 generation. Additional studies have extended these findings. In separate experiments using auditory, visual, or somatic stimuli, Knight and Scabini (1998) showed that prefrontal and lateral parietal lesions had no effect on P300 latency or amplitude. In contrast, temporoparietal junction lesions markedly reduced auditory and somatosensory P300s and reduced visual P300s. Soltani and Knight (2000) provide a comprehensive review of this important work.

Recently, studies that combine the high temporal resolution of EEG with the high topographical resolution of fMRI have provided some additional insight concerning the neural substrate of P300. In a standard auditory oddball task, Mulert et al. (2004) found the P300 to be accompanied by increased fMRI activity in the supplementary motor cortex, the anterior cingulate cortex, the temporoparietal junction, the insula, and the middle frontal gyrus. Furthermore, this fMRI activity was greater and occurred earlier in the right hemisphere than in the left hemisphere (Bledowski et al., 2004; Mulert et al., 2004). In patient studies involving intracranial recording, EEG, and fMRI, Linden (2005) implicated the inferior parietal lobule and the temporoparietal junction in P300 generation. In regard to the fMRI data (see chapter 4 in this volume), it should be noted that blood-flow-related activity measured over several seconds cannot be confidently attributed to an event (i.e., P300) that occurs somewhere in this period and lasts about 100 msec. Thus, fMRI results concerning the area(s) responsible for P300 generation must be interpreted cautiously.

The most comprehensive account of the functional role of P300 is called the *context-updating model* (Donchin, 1981; Donchin & Coles, 1988). Although this model does not make assumptions regarding the actual neural generators of P300, it proposes that the P300 reflects context-updating operations. According to the model, as stimuli are presented and evaluated, the degree to which the events are consistent with the current model of the context is assessed. When an event violates the expectations dictated by the model, and when the violation requires the model to be revised (i.e., *context updating*), a P300 is elicited. The model accounts for many of the salient characteristics of the P300 and is supported by a variety of behavioral and psychophysiological studies (e.g., (Adrover-Roig & Barcelo, 2010; Barcelo & Knight, 2007; Barcelo et al., 2007; Dien et al, 2003; Linden, 2005; Luu et al., 2007).

P300 AMPLITUDE AND STABILITY

The extensive studies of the past 45 years have defined the characteristics of the P300 in considerable detail. Here we focus on issues of particular importance to P300-based BCIs.

One issue particularly relevant for BCI usage comprises the factors that determine P300 amplitude. P300 amplitude is positively correlated with the time interval between events (i.e., stimuli). All other things being equal, longer interstimulus intervals result in higher amplitude P300s, at least up to intervals of about 8 sec (Polich, 1990; Polich & Bondurant, 1997). Whereas P300 amplitude in a standard oddball experiment is usually 10–20 μV, the P300s produced by BCI applications are usually 4–10 μV. This is presumably due to the rapid stimulus presentation rates used by P300-based BCIs and the resulting overlap of the ERPs to successive stimuli (Martens et al., 2009; Woldorff, 1993). P300 amplitude is also affected by moment-to-moment changes in the probability of the oddball stimulus (Donchin, 1981; Donchin & Isreal, 1980; Horst et al., 1980; Squires et al., 1977). For example, if, by chance, the oddball stimulus occurs two or more times in succession, P300 amplitude is reduced after the first oddball stimulus.

P300 amplitude is also affected by the sum total of the subject's concurrent activities. Thus, when a subject who is performing a task that elicits a P300 is asked to perform a secondary task at the same time, P300 amplitude decreases (Isreal, Chesney, et al., 1980; Isreal, Wickens, et al., 1980; Kramer et al., 1983; Sirevaag et al., 1989). Protocols may be designed that concurrently incorporate two different tasks and two different sets of stimuli and thereby elicit two different P300s. For example, Sirevaag et al. (1989) combined a joystick tracking task with an auditory discrimination task. As the relative difficulty of the two tasks was changed, and the attention each required changed correspondingly, the amplitudes of the two P300s also changed. As one task became more difficult and thus required more attention, the amplitude of its P300 increased, and the amplitude of the P300 associated with the other task decreased. These results and related studies show that attentional allocation and task difficulty affect P300 amplitude. They are relevant for P300-based BCIs since BCI users, in addition to simply watching for the desired stimuli (e.g., the letters they want to spell), are usually engaged in another task as well (e.g., planning the message being written with the BCI).

Another issue of particular importance for P300-based BCI applications is the extent to which P300 amplitude and latency change over time, both within an individual session and across days, weeks, months, and even years. In this area the available literature is mixed. Polich (1986) and Fabiani et al. (1987) showed robust test/retest correlations for peak amplitude and latency across sessions conducted within two weeks of one another. On the other hand, Kinoshita et al. (1996) found significant decreases in P300 amplitude when sessions were spread over several months. A number of studies have reported that P300 amplitude decreases during a session, and P300 latency can display cyclical variations over several hours (Lin & Polich, 1999; Pan et al., 2000; Ravden & Polich, 1999). To a considerable extent, much of the variability in P300 amplitude is due to latency variability (i.e., *latency jitter*). Kutas et al. (1977) showed that changes in P300 latency from trial to trial reduce the amplitude of the averaged P300 and that adjustment for this latency variability eliminates the apparent amplitude variability. Thus, studies that focus on P300 amplitude and do not adjust for latency variability may yield misleading results.

P300-BASED BCIs

The primary advantages of P300-based BCIs are that they are noninvasive, can be parameterized for a new user in a few minutes, require minimal user training, are usable by 90% of people (assuming ability to attend to the stimuli and to perform the classification task), can provide basic communication and control functions, and are relatively reliable. For these reasons, among present-day BCI systems, P300-based BCIs are the type most amenable to independent long-term home usage by people with severe disabilities. This section describes the initial P300-based BCI design and then reviews the ways in which this design has been modified and extended to improve or expand the communication and control it provides.

P300-based BCIs incorporate the three essential attributes of the oddball paradigm in a way that serves the needs of a communication and control system. Specifically:

- Stimuli representing possible BCI outputs are presented in a random order.

- The stimulus representing each possible output is presented rarely (e.g., with a probability of 1/[number of possible outputs]).

- The BCI user is asked to attend to the stimulus that represents the output he or she desires (i.e., the *target* stimulus)

With a BCI protocol that has these three essential attributes, the stimulus representing the desired BCI output (i.e., the target stimulus) becomes an oddball stimulus and thus elicits a P300 ERP.

THE ORIGINAL P300-BASED BCI STUDY

In 1988, Farwell and Donchin (Farwell & Donchin, 1988) described a P300-based spelling application, which they referred to as a *mental prosthesis*. Their hope was that people who were paralyzed could use it to communicate simple messages. In their first design, all the letters of the alphabet were presented one at a time on a video screen in a random order, and the subject was asked to note when the letter he or she wanted to select (i.e., the target letter) appeared. The target letter did elicit a P300. However, because the letters were presented at a rate of 1/sec, and multiple presentations of each letter had to be averaged to reliably detect the P300, several minutes were required for the subject to select just one letter. Thus, the design was modified to allow selections to be made more rapidly. In the new design, the subject viewed a 6 × 6 matrix of letters and other commands (fig. 12.3A). The stimulus

events were flashes of an entire row or column of the matrix. First the rows and then the columns flashed in random order at rates as high as 8/sec. At this rate, the six rows and six columns each flashed once in 1.5 sec. The BCI user was instructed to attend to a given letter and to keep a running mental count of the number of times that letter flashed. Farwell and Donchin (1988) did not ask the subject to foveate (i.e., look directly at) the target letter. They assumed that some BCI users might not be able to control gaze direction (e.g., due to ALS), and thus they relied instead on the evidence of Posner (1980) that attention can be focused away from the gaze fixation point.

It is important to emphasize that this BCI met the requirements of the oddball paradigm and capitalized on its properties. The subject was presented with a random sequence of events. The rare (or oddball) class included the flashes of the row and the column that contained the target letter, while the frequent class included the flashes of the other five rows and five columns. Farwell and Donchin (1988) predicted that only the two rare events would elicit detectable P300s and that once this row and column were identified, the target would be the letter at their intersection.

Figure 12.3B shows the time course of events in the operation of this BCI. Of particular interest is the fact that the rapid rate of stimulus presentation (e.g., every 125 msec) means that two or even three stimuli are delivered before a P300 to the first stimulus can occur. That is, the poststimulus EEG analysis epoch (originally 600 msec) for a given stimulus is still under way when the next several stimulus events occur. Thus, the analysis epoch for each stimulus overlaps those of the several preceding and the several succeeding stimuli. The impact of this overlap on P300 performance, and the measures that might be taken to reduce it (e.g., slower presentation rates), are addressed later in this chapter.

Using EEG recorded from a single electrode (Pz, referenced to linked ear electrodes) and a 600-msec post-stimulus analysis epoch, Farwell and Donchin (1988) compared four different classification algorithms: stepwise linear discriminant analysis (SWLDA); peak picking of amplitude in the 200- to 400-msec interval; the area under the curve in the same interval; and the covariance between the single trial data and a template representing the standard P300. It should be noted that SWLDA has been used since the 1960s for single trial detection of the P300 (Donchin, 1969; Donchin et al., 1970; Donchin & Herning, 1975; Horst & Donchin, 1980; Squires & Donchin, 1976). In this first P300-based BCI study, Farwell and Donchin (1988) found that the SWLDA and peak picking algorithms provided the highest accuracy in identifying the target stimulus (i.e., the item that the user wanted to select). They also found that accuracy was higher for a stimulus presentation rate of 4/sec than for a faster rate of 8/sec. As expected, more stimulus repetitions produced higher accuracy. Accuracy of 80% (with 2.8% [i.e., 1/36] expected by chance) required 20.9 sec per selection; and 95% accuracy required 26.0 sec. These two options gave selection rates of about 3.0 and 2.3 characters per minute, respectively.

This seminal study of 1988 demonstrated the feasibility of P300-based communication. It has since served as the starting point and the first benchmark for the many P300-based BCI studies that have followed.

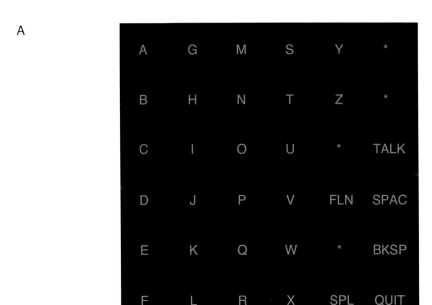

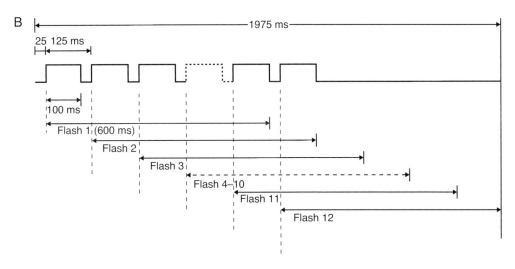

Figure 12.3 *(A) The 6 × 6 matrix of possible selections. (B) The time course for a series of 12 flashes with a stimulus onset asynchrony (i.e., time from beginning of one flash to the beginning of the next) of 125 msec. The six columns flashed in a random order and then the six rows flashed in a random order. The dashed flash line represents flashes 4-10. The 600-ms analysis epochs are indicated. (Modified from Farwell and Donchin, 1988.)*

THE AIMS AND LIMITATIONS OF SUBSEQUENT P300-BASED BCI STUDIES

The central goal of almost all these subsequent studies has been to improve the speed, accuracy, capacity, and/or clinical practicality of P300-based BCIs so that they can provide important new communication and control options for people whose severe motor disabilities prevent them from using conventional (i.e., muscle-based) assistive communication technology.

In considering these efforts to improve the performance of P300-based BCIs, it should be remembered that the core of the evaluation should be the improvement that the BCI can make to the quality of life of users with severe disabilities. In this regard, the fact that the BCI can restore a measure of independent communication may be more important than the BCI's exact accuracy or bitrate (i.e., speed). Furthermore, it is

not possible to conclude that a new design is superior to previous ones until it has been evaluated and validated in actual use by people with severe disabilities. These caveats must be emphasized as we proceed to discuss the extensive work exploring possible improvements in P300-based BCIs.

Most P300-based BCI studies have focused on offline analyses of data previously collected. Although offline analysis can enable very efficient comparison of different alternatives, it can only predict how the alternatives *may* perform in actual online usage. Even with leave-one-out cross-validation, offline analysis cannot reveal exactly how future performance may change when a method is actually used online. To the extent that the new method changes the classification, and thus the feedback provided to the BCI user, it may affect subsequent EEG and thereby affect subsequent performance in ways only assessable by online testing. The critical importance of online validation of new methods is discussed in greater detail in chapter 8 of this volume. In sum, while offline analysis is the workhorse of BCI research, online testing must be considered the gold standard. About 25% of the studies that have used offline analyses to evaluate alternative P300-based BCI methods have also included online validation of their results.

ALTERNATIVE ELECTRODE MONTAGES

As reviewed in Fabiani et al. (1987), P300 has traditionally been recorded from electrodes Fz, Cz, and Pz, according to the 10–20 electrode system (Jasper, 1958). Figure 12.2 shows examples of several electrode montages that have been used in P300-based BCI studies (Krusienski et al., 2008). The original Farwell and Donchin (1988) study used only the EEG recorded from electrode Pz. Studies since then have explored other recording montages: three or four midline electrodes, Fz, Cz, Pz, or Oz (Piccione et al., 2006; Sellers & Donchin, 2006; Serby et al., 2005); the International 10–20 system (Citi et al., 2008); a set of 10 midline and parietal/occipital electrodes (Kaper et al., 2004; Lenhardt et al., 2008); a set of 11 electrodes (Neshige et al., 2007); and a set of 25 central and parietal electrodes (Thulasidas et al., 2006).

Krusienski et al. (2008) compared the performances of SWLDA classification algorithms based on the EEG from: locations Fz, Pz, and Cz; locations PO7, PO8, and Oz; or all six of these locations. These locations are shown in figure 12.2. The algorithms that used either set of three EEG electrode locations achieved accuracies of about 65% on the 6 × 6 matrix, whereas the algorithm that used all six locations achieved an accuracy of 90%. At the same time, they also found that SWLDA classification was not further improved by using a still larger set of 19 electrodes (fig. 12.2) that included the original 6 electrodes. The high performance of these 6 electrodes in offline analyses was also confirmed in online testing.

These results are supported by the results of Hoffmann et al. (2008), who investigated the 4 midline electrodes, a set containing four additional parietal electrodes, as well as sets that included 16 and 32 electrodes. In general, the set using the midline and parietal electrodes performed as well as the 16- and 32-electrode montages. Meinicke et al. (2002) also examined the effects of various numbers of electrodes on the resulting classification. They found that with one or three electrodes, 30 sec were needed to achieve 85% accuracy; in contrast, 7 or 10 electrodes reached accuracy above 95% after 15 sec.

ALTERNATIVE SIGNAL-PROCESSING METHODS

Numerous studies have evaluated and compared the performances of a variety of different classification algorithms, for example:

- Independent components analysis (chapter 7, this volume) (Beverina et al., 2003; Khan et al., 2009; Li et al., 2009; Serby, et al., 2005)

- Support vector machines (chapter 8, this volume) (Beverina, et al., 2003; Garrett et al., 2003; Guo et al., 2010; Hong, Guo, et al., 2009; Hong, Lou, et al., 2009; Kaper, et al., 2004; Krusienski et al., 2006; Lal et al., 2004; Lenhardt et al., 2008; Lima et al., 2010; Meinicke, et al., 2002; Olson et al., 2005; Qin et al., 2007; Salvaris & Sepulveda, 2009; Salvaris & Sepulveda, 2007; Serby et al., 2005; Thulasidas et al., 2006)

- Stepwise linear discriminant analysis (SWLDA) (see chapter 8, this volume) (Bianchi et al., 2010; Brouwer & van Erp, 2010; Dias et al., 2007; Garrett et al., 2003; Hoffmann et al., 2008; Krusienski et al., 2006; Nijboer et al., 2008; Sellers & Donchin, 2006; Sellers et al., 2006; Townsend et al., 2010)

- Fisher's linear discriminant (chapter 8, this volume) (Babiloni et al., 2001; Gutierrez & Escalona-Vargas, 2010; Hoffmann, et al., 2008; Nazarpour et al., 2009; Salvaris & Sepulveda, 2009, 2010)

In an extensive offline analysis, Krusienski et al. (2006) compared classification by SWLDA, linear support vector machines, Gaussian support vector machines, Pearson's correlation method, and Fisher's linear discriminant analysis. Although all five methods performed reasonably well, the SWLDA and Fisher's linear discriminant methods were significantly better than the other three (approximately 88% accuracy vs. 80–83% accuracy). Meinicke et al. (2002) also compared three different classification methods: area; peak picking; and SVMs. They used electrode Pz and showed that the SVM solution reached about 78% accuracy in 30 sec, whereas the area and peak-picking methods reached about 78% accuracy in 1 min.

In addition to the kinds of studies described above, several Internet-based BCI data competitions (e.g., Blankertz, 2005; Blankertz et al., 2004; Blankertz et al., 2006; Bradshaw et al., 2001; Rakotomamonjy & Guigue, 2008) have motivated many research groups from all over the world to try to develop better P300-based BCI algorithms. Although a number of the new algorithms may achieve small improvements in performance, the overall result of now fairly extensive studies is that various signal-processing methods, when properly employed, provide roughly similar performance in offline analyses. At the same time, some algorithms are likely to be easier than others to use in online applications. Taken as a whole, these studies suggest that individual differences among BCI users may be a more critical determinant of performance than the exact choice of classification algorithm, provided that the algorithm is properly parameterized (chapter 8, this volume). This overall result implies that major improvements in the current performance of P300-based BCIs are likely to come from other kinds of changes, as addressed later in this chapter.

ALTERNATIVE STIMULI AND STIMULUS PRESENTATION PARAMETERS

A number of studies have focused on the standard visual matrix with row/column presentation and explored the impact of variations in basic parameters such as item size and number, the rapidity of row/column flashing, flash duration, and the number of repetitions per selection (Salvaris & Sepulveda, 2009; Sellers et al., 2006).

For example, Sellers et al. (2006) compared two different values of stimulus onset asynchrony (i.e., the time from the beginning of one stimulus to the beginning of the next) (175 msec and 350 msec), as well as two different matrices (3×3 and 6×6). In contrast to the findings of Farwell and Donchin (1988), but consistent with the findings of Meinicke et al. (2002), they found that the higher stimulus rate yielded higher classification accuracy regardless of whether the conditions were matched for the number of stimulus presentations or the time per selection was held constant. In addition, P300 amplitude was larger with the 6×6 matrix than with the 3×3 matrix. This is consistent with the many studies showing that P300 amplitude is inversely related to target probability (e.g., Allison & Pineda, 2003, 2006; Duncan-Johnson & Donchin, 1977). On the other hand, Guger et al. (2009) compared the 6 $\times$ 6 matrix format to a single-item presentation format. Although P300 amplitude was higher with the single-item format, the matrix format yielded higher accuracy and higher bit rate (chapter 8, in this volume).

Using the Farwell and Donchin matrix format, other studies have explored other variations in the presentation. Takano et al. (2009) varied the contrast between the stimuli and the background. They compared a white/gray pattern (luminance condition); a green/blue isoluminance pattern (color condition); and a green/blue luminance pattern (luminance/color condition). In online testing the third condition (luminance/color) provided higher accuracy. Salvaris and Sepulveda (2009) varied the item/background colors, the item size, and the distance between items. Although a white background yielded the best performance, and small items yielded the lowest performance, no single option was best for all subjects.

Perhaps the most important practical implication of these and other studies of basic format parameters is that the optimal parameter settings vary across users, and thus they should be optimized for each new BCI user (Sellers & Donchin, 2006).

Other researchers have explored modifications in the nature of the visual stimulus. In an effort to reduce the impact of the overlapping analysis epochs associated with rapid stimulus presentation rates, Martens et al. (2009) tested an apparent-motion paradigm in which the matrix items were in rectangles and the stimulus was a sudden 90° rotation of the rectangle. The user's task was to count the number of times the rectangle containing the desired item rotated. This paradigm showed a statistical improvement in performance for two of six subjects. In a similar effort, Hong et al. (2009) explored a stimulus designed to elicit a motion-specific ERP component (i.e., N200) that is most prominent at parietal electrodes P3 and P7. Although offline analyses found performance similar to that of the standard P300-based BCI format, the results suggested that the new design might reduce the number of scalp electrodes needed.

Several studies have addressed two problems associated with the row/column stimulation format. First, the desired item (i.e., the target stimulus) sometimes flashes twice in succession (once as part of a column and once as part of a row). As a result, the P300 ERP evoked by the second flash is likely to be attenuated (Squires et al., 1976); and, because their analysis epochs overlap, the two ERPs may distort each other (Martens et al., 2009; Woldorff, 1993). Furthermore, depending on the subject and particularly with higher stimulus-presentation rates, the subject may not even notice the second flash of the target. Another problem is that, with the row-column format, it is the target's row or column, not the target alone, that evokes the P300 ERP. As a result, although items not in the target's row or column are seldom selected by mistake, items that are in the target's row or column are selected by mistake much more often (Donchin et al., 2000; Fazel-Rezai, 2007).

To address these two problems, Townsend et al. (2010) developed a format in which groups of items (e.g., six items from an 8×9 matrix of alphanumeric symbols and commands) were presented simultaneously. The groups were selected to satisfy two constraints. First, no item could be presented a second time until at least six intervening groups of flashes had occurred. Second, two adjacent items were never presented at the same time. This *checkerboard* presentation format eliminated the two problems of successive target presentations and adjacent item presentations. In an online comparison in 18 subjects that took into account the need to correct for any errors that occurred, the checkerboard format performed significantly better than the standard row/column format. In addition, most users, including several people with ALS, reported that they liked the checkerboard format better. Further explorations of alternative presentation formats are likely to produce further improvements.

THE POSSIBLE ROLE OF GAZE DIRECTION IN P300-BASED BCI PERFORMANCE

As described above, the P300 is evoked by stimuli of special significance. In the case of P300-based BCIs, the special significance is that the stimulus represents the BCI output desired by the user. Thus, P300 elicitation does not require that the user look directly at (i.e., fixate) the stimulus, and P300-based BCIs should be usable by people with limited or even absent eye movements, such as many of those with late-stage ALS. At the same time, some recent evidence suggests that the performance of P300-based BCIs that use a matrix format may depend to some extent on the user's ability to fixate the desired item.

Brunner et al. (2010) and Treder and Blankertz (2010) compared P300-based BCI performance when the user fixated a central point to that when the user fixated the target. In both studies, performance was better when the user fixated the target. However, as noted previously, it is well known that P300 amplitude is decreased when the subject is assigned a second task (Donchin, 1987b; Fowler, 1994; Gopher, 1986; Kramer et al., 1986; Kramer et al., 1983; Kramer et al., 1985; Sirevaag et al., 1989; Wickens et al., 1983; Wickens et al.,1984). By asking that the subject fixate a point other than the target during BCI use, Brunner et al (2010) and Treder and Blankertz (2010) essentially imposed a second task. Thus, although accuracy was significantly higher when the target was fixated, it is not surprising that the gaze requirement yielded lower P300 amplitude and reduced accuracy. Although Brunner et al. (2010) concluded that the higher classification accuracy in the fixate-target condition indicates that P300-based BCI performance depends on the subject's ability to fixate the target character, it is evident from their results that classification does not require fixation. Moreover, using a paradigm similar to that of Treder and Blankertz (2010), Liu et al. (2010) reported mean accuracy higher than 96% for a covert attention task. These results demonstrate that optimizing the presentation paradigm can yield highly accurate results even when the subject does not fixate the target.

Nearly all P300-based BCI studies since 2004 have incorporated relatively short-latency (e.g., 150–250 msec) features recorded from occipital scalp locations (i.e., over visual cortex). The clear value of such early-latency posterior scalp features suggests that the responses elicited by the matrix P300-based BCI, and the accuracy of the classification they achieve, may depend to some degree on occipital visual evoked potentials (e.g., P100 and N200 see The Oddball Paradigm above), in addition to the P300. On the other hand, it should be noted that occipital VEP components are affected by attention (Eason, 1981; Harter et al., 1982; Hillyard & Munte, 1984; Mangun et al., 1993). It has also been noted that P300-related activity occurring in the temporal-parietal cortical junction may contribute to the EEG recorded from occipital electrodes (Dien et al., 2003; Polich, 2007).

The practical implications of these results for the clinical usefulness of P300-based BCIs are not clear. Whereas P300-based BCI performance may depend to some degree on the user's ability to look directly at the desired item, the importance of this factor in determining the usefulness of these BCIs for people with eye-movement impairments remains to be determined. In this regard it is relevant to note that one person with ALS who could no longer use his eye-tracker communication device was able to use a P300-based BCI very effectively (Sellers et al., 2010). In a more general sense, it is important to appreciate that the performance of any BCI that depends on the user's vision is likely to be affected by loss of eye-movement control. For example, a sensorimotor-rhythm-based BCI (chapter 13, this volume) that controls cursor movement may not perform as well when the user's gaze is not able to follow the moving cursor. This practical reality brings us to the next section.

P300-BASED BCIs THAT USE AUDITORY STIMULI

Some of the people who need the basic communication capacity that a P300-based BCI could provide may find it impractical or impossible to use a system that requires vision. For example, in addition to weak eye-movement control, people with advanced ALS may have visual difficulties due to diplopia (double vision), ptosis (drooping eyelids), or dry eyes. In response to this problem, several research groups have begun developing P300-based BCIs that use auditory stimuli instead of, or in addition to, visual stimuli (Hill, 2005; Nijboer et al., 2008; Pham et al., 2005). The major limitation of these paradigms is the low number of possible selections (e.g., two or four) compared to the much higher number available with standard visual P300-based BCIs (e.g., 6 × 6 = 36). Thus, the rate of communication is necessarily slow. Nevertheless it might still be extremely valuable for people who lack other effective options.

In an effort to improve the bitrate, several studies have presented auditory stimuli that map onto a visual matrix. Furdea et al. (2009) used a 5 × 5 visual matrix in one condition, and a 5 × 5 auditory (i.e., the spoken words "one" to "ten") and visual matrix in another condition. The auditory stimuli mapped to the five rows and five columns of the matrix, which were labeled 1–10. Nine of 13 subjects were able to use the auditory and visual matrix with accuracy of 70% or higher. In contrast, all 13 subjects achieved accuracy of 75% or higher in the visual condition, and 11 of the 13 were above 95%. In a similar design, Klobassa et al. (2009) used a 6 × 6 matrix and presented environmental sounds that correspond to the rows and columns. This study showed that subjects were eventually able to use the system with the auditory stimuli alone. However, the communication rates were still relatively low next to those of visual P300-based BCIs.

These early studies have established the feasibility of auditory P300-based BCIs. This achievement, combined with the clinical need for such systems, should encourage their further development.

PROSPECTS FOR IMPROVING P300-BASED BCIs

Current P300-based BCI designs provide relatively modest rates of communication. Many research groups are working to improve P300-based BCIs by exploring new electrode selection methods, presentation paradigms, and applications.

Cecotti et al. (2011) introduced a new electrode-selection algorithm to reduce the number of electrodes necessary for a given person to use a P300-based BCI. Electrode selection, more specifically reduction, will be a valuable asset in terms of cost, convenience, and portability as more people begin to use BCIs. In theory, a small number of electrodes should be sufficient for P300-based control; however, due to individual differences, it may be advantageous to start with a somewhat larger array and then prune it to as few electrodes as possible.

Other studies have explored variations in contrast and color (Salvaris & Sepulveda, 2009; Takano et al., 2009), overlapping stimuli and apparent (Martens et al., 2009) or actual (Hong et al., 2009) motion, stimulus presentation modifications (Jin et al., 2011; Townsend et al., 2010), suppressing characters that surround the target during calibration (Frye et al., in press), and using mindfulness induction to increase attentional resources (Lakey et al., 2011). Schreuder et al. (2010) designed a five-choice auditory BCI by giving each stimulus a unique tone and a unique spatial location. The study showed that the system produced speed and accuracy comparable to some visual P300-based BCIs. Brouwer and van Erp (2010) showed that a tactile P300-based BCI using stimulating electrodes placed around the waist can achieve speed and accuracy similar to that of most auditory BCIs.

New applications are also emerging. For example, Münssinger et al. (2010) showed that a P300-based BCI can be used as a creative tool as well as a communication device. Subjects performed copy-spelling, copy-painting, and free-painting tasks. We have seen advances toward a P300-based Internet browser (Bensch et al., 2007; Mugler et al., 2008; Mugler et al., 2010) and also how a predictive spelling program can increase throughput (Ryan et al., 2011).

INDEPENDENT HOME USE OF P300-BASED BCIs

Because P300-based BCI systems are noninvasive, relatively portable and inexpensive, and perform reliably, they are the first BCIs being taken out of the laboratory and used independently by severely disabled people in their daily lives for basic communication and environmental control. Although the first report of in-home testing is provided in Farwell and Donchin (1988), the concept was first described earlier by Donchin in a 1985 lecture (see Donchin, 1987a, for a transcript of the lecture). Birbaumer et al. (1999) reported the first long-term home usage of a BCI system by a man with ALS. However, it is only recently that a larger-scale effort to implement home use independent of close oversight by a research team has begun (Sellers et al., 2010; Vaughan et al., 2006). Even though the system is slow compared to conventional means of communication, it should be noted that, for severally disabled users, communication speed is often less important than accuracy and reliability and the fact that the BCI restores a measure of independence (Kübler & Neumann, 2005; Nijboer et al., 2008; Sellers & Donchin, 2006) (although most BCI users would presumably opt for faster communication if it were available).

These first efforts have encountered, defined, and begun to address the myriad difficult issues that arise when a new technology is taken out of the simple, highly controlled laboratory environment and placed into the complex, changing, and unpredictable environments in which people, including those with severe disabilities, actually live. These issues include (but are certainly not limited to): the capacities, expectations, and desires of the prospective users and their caregivers; the need for extremely simple and robust hardware and software and for simple and convenient usage procedures; the difficulty of evaluating prospective users who currently can communicate very little if at all; the impact of the user's disease process on P300 generation; the selection of the proper point in the disease process to introduce BCI usage; the physical and mental state of the user; the physical and social features and stability of the home environment; the presence of electromagnetic noise or instability; the need for prompt and effective technical support; the impact of other illnesses; and the practical and ethical issues that arise if and when disease progression degrades BCI performance. These many issues are addressed more fully in chapters 20 and 24 of this volume. Indeed, although the subject of chapter 20 is the clinical usage of BCIs in general, its substance is of necessity drawn almost entirely from experience with P300-based BCIs.

One issue important for home use is addressed here because it applies to P300-based systems specifically. That issue is the extent to which long-term intensive home use (i.e., many hours per day over months and years) will degrade performance. The amplitude, form, or stability of the P300 might conceivably degrade over the hours of use within a day and/or over many days and weeks of use. For example, habituation, or decreased amplitude with repeated stimulus presentation, occurs with many ERP phenomena (Kinoshita et al., 1996; Ravden & Polich, 1998, 1999). The initial results for P300-based BCI use are encouraging. Sellers and Donchin (2006) showed reliable use of the P300-based BCI by six people, three with ALS, over a period of 10 weeks. Most notably, despite frequent lengthy daily use over 3 years, P300-based BCI performance by a person with ALS did not deteriorate (Sellers et al., 2010). The amplitude and form of the target and nontarget ERPs remained stable. Furthermore, even though the SWLDA algorithm was reparameterized periodically, the optimal parameters changed very little over time.

One important finding from efforts to provide the P300-based BCI to people who are very severely disabled is that it is useful to conduct an initial test of the extent to which the person can generate a P300 in the simplest and most straightforward form of the oddball paradigm, such as a protocol in which a succession of two pictures (e.g., a zebra or an elephant) are presented, with one appearing 80% of the time and the other 20%. If the rare event fails to elicit a P300, it is very unlikely that the person will be able to use a visual P300-based BCI. A recent innovation is the development of a screening method to evaluate more thoroughly within a few sessions whether a severely disabled person has the ability to use the P300-based BCI (McCane et al., 2009).

SUMMARY

An *event-related potential* (ERP) is a distinctive pattern of voltage changes that is time-locked to a specific event. The most prominent ERP BCI is the P300-based BCI. The P300 is a positive potential that occurs over central-parietal scalp 250–700 msec after a rare event occurs in the context of the *oddball* paradigm. This paradigm has three essential attributes:

- A subject is presented with a series of events (i.e., stimuli), each of which falls into one of two classes.

- The events that fall into one of the classes are less frequent than those that fall into the other class.

- The subject performs a task that requires classifying each event into one of the two classes.

In 1988, Farwell and Donchin described a BCI based on the oddball paradigm. The rows and columns of a 6 × 6 matrix of letters and commands flashed rapidly, and the rare events were the flashes of the row and column that contained the item the subject wanted to select. This P300-based BCI provided relatively slow but effective communication.

Over the past two decades, the original P300-based BCI design has provided a robust basis for continued development by many groups. It has been further refined through studies of alternative recording sites, signal-processing methods, and stimulus presentation parameters and formats; and P300-based BCIs that use auditory rather than visual stimuli have been described.

Because P300-based BCIs are noninvasive, relatively simple and inexpensive, and provide stable performance, they are the first BCIs being taken out of the laboratory and used independently by severely disabled people for basic communication and control in their daily lives. This clinical translation effort is revealing, and spurring solutions to, the many problems associated with moving BCI systems from the laboratory to the home.

The relatively slow communication rates of current clinically practical BCIs mean that they are likely to be useful mainly for people whose severe disabilities largely preclude their use of other assistive communication technologies. Further exploration of promising new options may substantially increase the speed of P300-based BCIs and thereby expand their communication and control applications and their user populations.

REFERENCES

Adrover-Roig, D., & Barcelo, F. (2010). Individual differences in aging and cognitive control modulate the neural indexes of context updating and maintenance during task switching. *Cortex, 46*(4), 434–450.

Allison, B. Z., & Pineda, J. A. (2003). ERPs evoked by different matrix sizes: implications for a brain computer interface (BCI) system. *IEEE Trans Neural Syst Rehabil Eng, 11*(2), 110–113.

Allison, B. Z., & Pineda, J. A. (2006). Effects of SOA and flash pattern manipulations on ERPs, performance, and preference: implications for a BCI system. *Int J Psychophysiol, 59*(2), 127–140.

Babiloni, F., Cincotti, F., Bianchi, L., Pirri, G., del, R. M. J., Mourino, J., et al. (2001). Recognition of imagined hand movements with low resolution surface Laplacian and linear classifiers. *Med Eng Phys, 23*(5), 323–328.

Barcelo, F., & Knight, R. T. (2007). An information-theoretical approach to contextual processing in the human brain: evidence from prefrontal lesions. *Cereb Cortex, 17 Suppl 1*, i51–60.

Barcelo, F., Perianez, J. A., & Nyhus, E. (2007). An information theoretical approach to task-switching: evidence from cognitive brain potentials in humans. *Front Hum Neurosci, 1*, 13.

Bashore, T. R., & Van der Molen, M. W. (1991). Discovery of the P300: a tribute. *Biol Psychol, 32*, 155–171.

Bensch, M., Karim, A. A., Mellinger, J., Hinterberger, T., Tangermann, M., Bogdan, M., et al. (2007). Nessi: an EEG-controlled Web browser for severely paralyzed patients. *Comput Intell Neurosci, 71863.* Published online 2007 September 10. doi: 10.1155/2007/71863.

Beverina, F., Palmas, G., Silvoni, S., & Piccione, F. (2003). User adaptive BCIs: SSVEP and P300 based interfaces. *Psychol J, 1*(4), 23.

Bianchi, L., Sami, S., Hillebrand, A., Fawcett, I. P., Quitadamo, L. R., & Seri, S. (2010). Which physiological components are more suitable for visual ERP based brain-computer interface? A preliminary MEG/EEG study. *Brain Topogr, 23*(2), 180–185.

Blankertz, B. (2005). BCI competition III: data set II; Results. From http://ida.first.fraunhofer.de/projects/bci/competition_iii/results/

Blankertz, B., Müller, K. R., Curio, G., Vaughan, T. M., Schalk, G., Wolpaw, J. R., et al. (2004). The BCI Competition 2003: progress and perspectives in detection and discrimination of EEG single trials. *IEEE Trans Biomed Eng, 51*(6), 1044–1051.

Blankertz, B., Müller, K. R., Krusienski, D. J., Schalk, G., Wolpaw, J. R., Schlogl, A., et al. (2006). The BCI competition. III: Validating alternative approaches to actual BCI problems. *IEEE Trans Neural Syst Rehabil Eng, 14*(2), 153–159.

Bledowski, C., Prvulovic, D., Hoechstetter, K., Scherg, M., Wibral, M., Goebel, R., et al. (2004). Localizing P300 generators in visual target and distractor processing: a combined event-related potential and functional magnetic resonance imaging study. *J Neurosci, 24*(42), 9353–9360.

Bradshaw, L. A., Wijesinghe, R. S., & Wikswo, J. P., Jr. (2001). Spatial filter approach for comparison of the forward and inverse problems of electroencephalography and magnetoencephalography. *Ann Biomed Eng, 29*(3), 214–226.

Brouwer, A. M., & van Erp, J. B. (2010). A tactile p300 brain-computer interface. *Front Neurosci, 4*, 19.

Brunner, P., Joshi, S., Briskin, S., Wolpaw, J. R., Bischof, H., & Schalk, G. (2010). Does the "P300" speller depend on eye gaze? *J Neural Eng, 7*(5), 056013.

Cecotti, H., Rivet, B., Congedo, M., Jutten, C., Bertrand, O., Maby, E., et al. (2011). A robust sensor-selection method for P300 brain-computer interfaces. *J Neural Eng, 8*(1), 016001.

Citi, L., Poli, R., Cinel, C., & Sepulveda, F. (2008). P300-based BCI mouse with genetically-optimized analogue control. *IEEE Trans Neural Syst Rehabil Eng, 16*(1), 51–61.

Comerchero, M. D., & Polich, J. (1999). P3a and P3b from typical auditory and visual stimuli. *Clin Neurophysiol, 110*(1), 24–30.

Dias, N. S., Kamrunnahar, M., Mendes, P. M., Schiff, S. J., & Correia, J. H. (2007). Comparison of EEG pattern classification methods for brain-computer interfaces. *Conf Proc IEEE Eng Med Biol Soc, 2007*, 2540–2543.

Dien, J., Spencer, K. M., & Donchin, E. (2003). Localization of the event-related potential novelty response as defined by principal components analysis. *Brain Res Cogn Brain Res, 17*(3), 637–650.

Donchin, E. (1969). Discriminant analysis in average evoked response studies: the study of single trial data. *Electroencephalogr Clin Neurophysiol, 27*(3), 311–314.

Donchin, E. (1981). Presidential address, 1980. Surprise! . . .Surprise? *Psychophysiology, 18*(5), 493–513.

Donchin, E. (1987a). Can the mind be read in the brain waves? In F. Farley & C. H. Null (Eds.), *Using Psychological Science: Making the Public Case* (pp. 25–47). Washington, DC: Federation of Behavioral, Psychological, and Cognitive Sciences.

Donchin, E. (1987b). The P300 as a metric for mental workload. *Electroencephalogr Clin Neurophysiol Suppl, 39*, 338–343.

Donchin, E., Callaway, E., 3rd, & Jones, R. T. (1970). Auditory evoked potential variability in schizophrenia. II. The application of discriminant analysis. *Electroencephalogr Clin Neurophysiol, 29*(5), 429–440.

Donchin, E., & Coles, M. G. H. (1988). Is the P300 component a manifestation of context updating? *Behav Brain Sci, 11*, 357–374.

Donchin, E., & Herning, R. I. (1975). A simulation study of the efficacy of stepwise discriminant analysis in the detection and comparison of event related potentials. *Electroencephalogr Clin Neurophysiol, 38*(1), 51–68.

Donchin, E., & Isreal, J. B. (1980). Event-related potentials and psychological theory. *Prog Brain Res, 54*, 697–715.

Donchin, E., Spencer, K. M., & Wijesinghe, R. (2000). The mental prosthesis: assessing the speed of a P300-based brain-computer interface. *IEEE Trans Rehabil Eng, 8*(2), 174–179.

Duncan-Johnson, C. C., & Donchin, E. (1977). On quantifying surprise: the variation of event-related potentials with subjective probability. *Psychophysiology, 14*(5), 456–467.

Duncan, C. C., Barry, R. J., Connolly, J. F., Fischer, C., Michie, P. T., Naatanen, R., et al. (2009). Event-related potentials in clinical research: guidelines for eliciting, recording, and quantifying mismatch negativity, P300, and N400. *Clin Neurophysiol, 120*(11), 1883–1908.

Eason, R. G. (1981). Visual evoked potential correlates of early neural filtering during selective attention. *Bulletin of the Psychonomic Society, 18*, 203–206.

Fabiani, M., Gratton, G., Karis, D., & Donchin, E. (1987). Definition, identification, and reliability of measurement of the P300 component of the event related potential. *Adv Psychophysiol, 2*, 1–78.

Farwell, L. A., & Donchin, E. (1988). Talking off the top of your head: toward a mental prosthesis utilizing event-related brain potentials. *Electroencephalogr Clin Neurophysiol, 70*(6), 510–523.

Fazel-Rezai, R. (2007). Human error in P300 speller paradigm for brain-computer interface. *Conf Proc IEEE Eng Med Biol Soc, 2007*, 2516–2519.

Fowler, B. (1994). P300 as a measure of workload during a simulated aircraft landing task. *Hum Factors, 36*(4), 670–683.

Frye, G. E., Hauser, C. K., Townsend, G., & Sellers, E. W. (2011). Suppressing flashes of items surrounding targets during calibration of a P300-based brain-computer interface improves performance. *J Neural Eng. 8*(2) 025024 (5pp). doi:10.1088/1741-2560/8/2/025024

Furdea, A., Halder, S., Krusienski, D. J., Bross, D., Nijboer, F., Birbaumer, N., et al. (2009). An auditory oddball (P300) spelling system for brain-computer interfaces. *Psychophysiology, 46*(3), 617–625.

Garrett, D., Peterson, D. A., Anderson, C. W., & Thaut, M. H. (2003). Comparison of linear, nonlinear, and feature selection methods for EEG signal classification. *IEEE Trans Neural Syst Rehabil Eng, 11*(2), 141–144.

Gopher, D., & Donchin, E. (1986). Workload: an examination of the concept. In K. R. Boff, L. Kaufman, & J. P. Thomas. (Eds.), *Handbook of Perception* and Human Performance, Vol. 2: Cognitive Processes and Performance (pp. 1–49). Oxford: John Wiley & Sons.

Guo, J., Gao, S., & Hong, B. (2010). An auditory brain-computer interface using active mental response. *IEEE Trans Neural Syst Rehabil Eng, 18*(3), 230–235.

Gutierrez, D., & Escalona-Vargas, D. I. (2010). EEG data classification through signal spatial redistribution and optimized linear discriminants. *Comput Methods Programs Biomed, 97*(1), 39–47.

Harter, M. R., Aine, C., & Schroeder, C. (1982). Hemispheric differences in the neural processing of stimulus location and type: effects of selective attention on visual evoked potentials. *Neuropsychologia, 20*(4), 421–438.

Heinze, H. J., Mangun, G. R., Burchert, W., Hinrichs, H., Scholz, M., Munte, T. F., et al. (1994). Combined spatial and temporal imaging of brain activity during visual selective attention in humans. *Nature, 372*(6506), 543–546.

Hill, N. J., Lal, T. N., Bierig, K., Birbaumer, N., & Schölkopf, B. (2005). An auditory paradigm for brain-computer interfaces. *Advances in Neural Information Processing Systems, 17*, 569–576.

Hillyard, S. A., & Munte, T. F. (1984). Selective attention to color and location: an analysis with event-related brain potentials. *Percept Psychophys, 36*(2), 185–198.

Hoffmann, U., Vesin, J. M., Ebrahimi, T., & Diserens, K. (2008). An efficient P300-based brain-computer interface for disabled subjects. *J Neurosci Methods, 167*(1), 115–125.

Hong, B., Guo, F., Liu, T., Gao, X., & Gao, S. (2009). N200-speller using motion-onset visual response. *Clin Neurophysiol, 120*(9), 1658–1666.

Hong, B., Lou, B., Guo, J., & Gao, S. (2009). Adaptive active auditory brain computer interface. *Conf Proc IEEE Eng Med Biol Soc, 2009*, 4531–4534.

Horst, R. L., & Donchin, E. (1980). Beyond averaging. II. Single-trial classification of exogenous event-related potentials using stepwise discriminant analysis. *Electroencephalogr Clin Neurophysiol, 48*(2), 112–126.

Horst, R. L., Johnson, R., Jr., & Donchin, E. (1980). Event-related brain potentials and subjective probability in a learning task. *Mem Cognit, 8*(5), 476–488.

Isreal, J. B., Chesney, G. L., Wickens, C. D., & Donchin, E. (1980). P300 and tracking difficulty: evidence for multiple resources in dual-task performance. *Psychophysiology, 17*(3), 259–273.

Isreal, J. B., Wickens, C. D., & Donchin, E. (1980). The dynamics of P300 during dual-task performance. *Prog Brain Res, 54*, 416–421.

Jasper, H. (1958). The ten-twenty electrode system of the international Federation. *Electroencephalogr Clin Neurophysiol, 10*, 371–375.

Jin, J., Allison, B. Z., Sellers, E. W., Brunner, C., Horki, P., Wang, X., et al. (2011). Optimized stimulus presentation patterns for an event-related potential EEG-based brain-computer interface. *Med Biol Eng Comput, 49*(2), 181–191.

Kaper, M., Meinicke, P., Grossekathoefer, U., Lingner, T., & Ritter, H. (2004). BCI Competition 2003—Data set IIb: support vector machines for the P300 speller paradigm. *IEEE Trans Biomed Eng, 51*(6), 1073–1076.

Khan, O. I., Kim, S. H., Rasheed, T., Khan, A., & Kim, T. S. (2009). Extraction of P300 using constrained independent component analysis. *Conf Proc IEEE Eng Med Biol Soc, 1*, 4031–4034.

Kinoshita, S., Inoue, M., Maeda, H., Nakamura, J., & Morita, K. (1996). Long-term patterns of change in ERPs across repeated measurements. *Physiol Behav, 60*(4), 1087–1092.

Klobassa, D. S., Vaughan, T. M., Brunner, P., Schwartz, N. E., Wolpaw, J. R., Neuper, C., et al. (2009). Toward a high-throughput auditory P300-based brain-computer interface. *Clin Neurophysiol, 120*(7), 1252–1261.

Knight, R. T., & Scabini, D. (1998). Anatomic bases of event-related potentials and their relationship to novelty detection in humans. *J Clin Neurophysiol, 15*(1), 3–13.

Knight, R. T., Scabini, D., Woods, D. L., & Clayworth, C. C. (1989). Contributions of temporal-parietal junction to the human auditory P3. *Brain Res, 502*(1), 109–116.

Kramer, A., Schneider, W., Fisk, A., & Donchin, E. (1986). The effects of practice and task structure on components of the event-related brain potential. *Psychophysiology, 23*(1), 33–47.

Kramer, A. F., Wickens, C. D., & Donchin, E. (1983). An analysis of the processing requirements of a complex perceptual-motor task. *Hum Factors, 25*(6), 597–621.

Kramer, A. F., Wickens, C. D., & Donchin, E. (1985). Processing of stimulus properties: evidence for dual-task integrality. *J Exp Psychol Hum Percept Perform, 11*(4), 393–408.

Krusienski, D. J., Sellers, E. W., Cabestaing, F., Bayoudh, S., McFarland, D. J., Vaughan, T. M., et al. (2006). A comparison of classification techniques for the P300 Speller. *J Neural Eng, 3*(4), 299–305.

Krusienski, D. J., Sellers, E. W., McFarland, D. J., Vaughan, T. M., & Wolpaw, J. R. (2008). Toward enhanced P300 speller performance. *J Neurosci Methods, 167*(1), 15–21.

Kübler, A., & Neumann, N. (2005). Brain-computer interfaces—the key for the conscious brain locked into a paralyzed body. *Prog Brain Res, 150*, 512–525.

Kutas, M., McCarthy, G., & Donchin, E. (1977). Augmenting mental chronometry: the P300 as a measure of stimulus evaluation time. *Science, 197*(4305), 792–795.

Lakey, C. E., Berry, D. R., & Sellers, E. W. (2011). Manipulating attention via mindfulness induction improves P300-based brain-computer interface performance. *J Neural Eng. 8*(2) 025019 (7pp) doi:10.1088/1741-2560 /8/2/025019

Lal, T. N., Schroder, M., Hinterberger, T., Weston, J., Bogdan, M., Birbaumer, N., et al. (2004). Support vector channel selection in BCI. *IEEE Trans Biomed Eng, 51*(6), 1003–1010.

Lenhardt, A., Kaper, M., & Ritter, H. J. (2008). An adaptive P300-based online brain-computer interface. *IEEE Trans Neural Syst Rehabil Eng, 16*(2), 121–130.

Li, K., Sankar, R., Arbel, Y., & Donchin, E. (2009). Single trial independent component analysis for P300 BCI system. *Conf Proc IEEE Eng Med Biol Soc, 1*, 4035–4038.

Lima, C. A., Coelho, A. L., & Eisencraft, M. (2010). Tackling EEG signal classification with least squares support vector machines: a sensitivity analysis study. *Comput Biol Med, 40*(8), 705–714.

Lin, E., & Polich, J. (1999). P300 habituation patterns: individual differences from ultradian rhythms. *Percept Mot Skills, 88*(3 Pt 2), 1111–1125.

Linden, D. E. (2005). The p300: where in the brain is it produced and what does it tell us? *Neuroscientist, 11*(6), 563–576.

Liu, Y., Zhou, Z., & Hu, D. (2010). Gaze independent brain-computer speller with covert visual search tasks. *Clin Neurophysiol. 122*(6), 1127–1136.

Luu, P., Tucker, D. M., & Stripling, R. (2007). Neural mechanisms for learning actions in context. *Brain Res, 1179*, 89–105.

Magliero, A., Bashore, T. R., Coles, M. G., & Donchin, E. (1984). On the dependence of P300 latency on stimulus evaluation processes. *Psychophysiology, 21*(2), 171–186.

Mangun, G. R. (1995). Neural mechanisms of visual selective attention. *Psychophysiology, 32*(1), 4–18.

Mangun, G. R., Hillyard, S. A., & Luck, S. J. (1993). Electrocortical substrates of visual selective attention. In D. Meyer & S. Kornblum (Eds.), *Attention and Performance XIV* (pp. 219–243). Cambridge, MA: MIT Press.

Martens, S. M., Hill, N. J., Farquhar, J., & Scholkopf, B. (2009). Overlap and refractory effects in a brain-computer interface speller based on the visual P300 event-related potential. *J Neural Eng, 6*(2), 026003.

McCane, L., Vaughan, T. M., McFarland, D. J., Zeitlin, D., Tenteromano, L., Mak, J., et al. (2009). Evaluation of individuals with ALS for in home use of a P300 brain computer. Program No. 664.7 *Society of Neuroscience Annual Meeting (Chicago, IL).*

McCarthy, G., & Donchin, E. (1981). A metric for thought: a comparison of P300 latency and reaction time. *Science, 211*(4477), 77–80.

Meinicke, P., Kaper, M., Hoppe, F., Huemann, M., & Ritter, H. (2002). Improving transfer rates in brain computer interface: A case study. *Adv Neural Info Proc Syst.*, pp. 1107–1114.

Mugler, E., Bensch, M., Hadler, S., Rosenstiel, W., Bogdan, M., Birnauner, N., et al. (2008). Control of an Internet browser using the P300 event-related potential. *International Journal of Bioelectromagnetism, 10*(1), 7.

Mugler, E. M., Ruf, C. A., Halder, S., Bensch, M., & Kübler, A. (2010). Design and implementation of a P300-based brain-computer interface for controlling an internet browser. *IEEE Trans Neural Syst Rehabil Eng, 18*(6), 599–609.

Mulert, C., Jager, L., Schmitt, R., Bussfeld, P., Pogarell, O., Moller, H. J., et al. (2004). Integration of fMRI and simultaneous EEG: towards a comprehensive understanding of localization and time-course of brain activity in target detection. *Neuroimage, 22*(1), 83–94.

Münssinger, J. I., Halder, S., Kleih, S. C., Furdea, A., Raco, V., Hosle, A., et al. (2010). Brain painting: first evaluation of a new brain-computer interface application with ALS-patients and healthy volunteers. *Front Neurosci, 4*, 182.

Nazarpour, K., Praamstra, P., Miall, R. C., & Sanei, S. (2009). Steady-state movement related potentials for brain-computer interfacing. *IEEE Trans Biomed Eng, 56*(8), 2104–2113.

Neshige, R., Murayama, N., Igasaki, T., Tanoue, K., Kurokawa, H., & Asayama, S. (2007). Communication aid device utilizing event-related potentials for patients with severe motor impairment. *Brain Res, 1141*, 218–227.

Nijboer, F., Furdea, A., Gunst, I., Mellinger, J., McFarland, D. J., Birbaumer, N., et al. (2008). An auditory brain-computer interface (BCI). *J Neurosci Methods, 167*(1), 43–50.

Nijboer, F., Sellers, E. W., Mellinger, J., Jordan, M. A., Matuz, T., Furdea, A., et al. (2008). A P300-based brain-computer interface for people with amyotrophic lateral sclerosis. *Clin Neurophysiol, 119*(8), 1909–1916.

Olson, B. P., Si, J., Hu, J., & He, J. (2005). Closed-loop cortical control of direction using support vector machines. *IEEE Trans Neural Syst Rehabil Eng, 13*(1), 72–80.

Pan, J., Takeshita, T., & Morimoto, K. (2000). P300 habituation from auditory single-stimulus and oddball paradigms. *Int J Psychophysiol, 37*(2), 149–153.

Pham, M., Hinterberger, T., Neumann, N., Kübler, A., Hofmayer, N., Grether, A., et al. (2005). An auditory brain-computer interface based on the self-regulation of slow cortical potentials. *Neurorehabil Neural Repair, 19*(3), 206–218.

Piccione, F., Giorgi, F., Tonin, P., Priftis, K., Giove, S., Silvoni, S., et al. (2006). P300-based brain computer interface: reliability and performance in healthy and paralysed participants. *Clin Neurophysiol, 117*(3), 531–537.

Polich, J. (1986). Normal variation of P300 from auditory stimuli. *Electroencephalogr Clin Neurophysiol, 65*(3), 236–240.

Polich, J. (1990). Probability and inter-stimulus interval effects on the P300 from auditory stimuli. *Int J Psychophysiol, 10*(2), 163–170.

Polich, J. (2007). Updating P300: an integrative theory of P3a and P3b. *Clin Neurophysiol, 118*(10), 2128–2148.

Polich, J., & Bondurant, T. (1997). P300 sequence effects, probability, and interstimulus interval. *Physiol Behav, 61*(6), 843–849.

Posner, M. I. (1980). The orienting of attention. *Q J Exp Psychol, 32*, 3–25.

Pritchard, W. S. (1981). Psychophysiology of P300. *Psychol Bull, 89*(3), 506–540.

Qin, J., Li, Y., & Sun, W. (2007). A semisupervised support vector machines algorithm for BCI systems. *Comput Intell Neurosci*, 94397.

Rakotomamonjy, A., & Guigue, V. (2008). BCI competition III: dataset II—ensemble of SVMs for BCI P300 speller. *IEEE Trans Biomed Eng, 55*(3), 1147–1154.

Ravden, D., & Polich, J. (1998). Habituation of P300 from visual stimuli. *Int J Psychophysiol, 30*(3), 359–365.

Ravden, D., & Polich, J. (1999). On P300 measurement stability: habituation, intra-trial block variation, and ultradian rhythms. *Biol Psychol, 51*(1), 59–76.

Ryan, D. B., Frye, G. E., Townsend, G., Berry, D. R., Mesa, G. S., Gates, N. A., et al. (2011). Predictive spelling with a P300-based brain-computer interface: increasing the rate of communication. *Int J Hum Comput Interact, 27*(1), 69–84.

Salvaris, M. S., & Sepulveda, F. (2007). Robustness of the Farwell & Donchin BCI protocol to visual stimulus parameter changes. *Conf Proc IEEE Eng Med Biol Soc, 2007*, 2528–2531.

Salvaris, M., & Sepulveda, F. (2009). Visual modifications on the P300 speller BCI paradigm. *J Neural Eng, 6*(4), 046011.

Salvaris, M., & Sepulveda, F. (2010). Classification effects of real and imaginary movement selective attention tasks on a P300-based brain-computer interface. *J Neural Eng, 7*(5), 056004.

Schreuder, M., Blankertz, B, & Tangermann, M. (2010). A new auditory multi-class brain-computer interface paradigm: spatial hearing as an informative cue. *PLoS One, 5*(4), e9813.

Sellers, E. W., & Donchin, E. (2006). A P300-based brain-computer interface: initial tests by ALS patients. *Clin Neurophysiol, 117*(3), 538–548.

Sellers, E. W., Krusienski, D. J., McFarland, D. J., Vaughan, T. M., & Wolpaw, J. R. (2006). A P300 event-related potential brain-computer interface (BCI): the effects of matrix size and inter stimulus interval on performance. *Biol Psychol, 73*(3), 242–252.

Sellers, E. W., Vaughan, T. M., & Wolpaw, J. R. (2010). A brain-computer interface for long-term independent home use. *Amyotroph Lateral Scler, 11*(5), 449–455.

Serby, H., Yom-Tov, E., & Inbar, G. F. (2005). An improved P300-based brain-computer interface. *IEEE Trans Neural Syst Rehabil Eng, 13*(1), 89–98.

Sirevaag, E. J., Kramer, A. F., Coles, M. G., & Donchin, E. (1989). Resource reciprocity: an event-related brain potentials analysis. *Acta Psychol (Amst), 70*(1), 77–97.

Soltani, M., & Knight, R. T. (2000). Neural origins of the P300. *Crit Rev Neurobiol, 14*(3–4), 199–224.

Squires, K. C., & Donchin, E. (1976). Beyond averaging: the use of discriminant functions to recognize event related potentials elicited by single auditory stimuli. *Electroencephalogr Clin Neurophysiol, 41*(5), 449–459.

Squires, K. C., Donchin, E., Herning, R. I., & McCarthy, G. (1977). On the influence of task relevance and stimulus probability on event-related-potential components. *Electroencephalogr Clin Neurophysiol, 42*(1), 1–14.

Squires, K. C., Wickens, C., Squires, N. K., & Donchin, E. (1976). The effect of stimulus sequence on the waveform of the cortical event-related potential. *Science, 193*(4258), 1142–1146.

Sutton, S., Braren, M., Zubin, J., & John, E. R. (1965). Evoked-potential correlates of stimulus uncertainty. *Science, 150*(700), 1187–1188.

Sutton, S., Tueting, P., Zubin, J., & John, E. R. (1967). Information delivery and the sensory evoked potential. *Science, 155*(768), 1436–1439.

Takano, K., Komatsu, T., Hata, N., Nakajima, Y., & Kansaku, K. (2009). Visual stimuli for the P300 brain-computer interface: a comparison of white/gray and green/blue flicker matrices. *Clin Neurophysiol, 120*(8):1562–1566.

Thulasidas, M., Guan, C., & Wu, J. (2006). Robust classification of EEG signal for brain-computer interface. *IEEE Trans Neural Syst Rehabil Eng, 14*(1), 24–29.

Townsend, G., LaPallo, B. K., Boulay, C. B., Krusienski, D. J., Frye, G. E., Hauser, C. K., et al. (2010). A novel P300-based brain-computer interface stimulus presentation paradigm: moving beyond rows and columns. *Clin Neurophysiol, 121*(7), 1109–1120.

Treder, M. S., & Blankertz, B. (2010). (C)overt attention and visual speller design in an ERP-based brain-computer interface. *Behav Brain Funct, 6*, 28.

Vaughan, T. M., McFarland, D. J., Schalk, G., Sarnacki, W. A., Krusienski, D. J., Sellers, E. W., et al. (2006). The Wadsworth BCI Research and Development Program: at home with BCI. *IEEE Trans Neural Syst Rehabil Eng, 14*(2), 229–233.

Vidal, J. J. (1977). Real-time detection of brain events in EEG. *Proc IEEE, 5*, 633–641.

Wickens, C. D., Kramer, A. F., & Donchin, E. (1984). The event-related potential as an index of the processing demands of a complex target acquisition task. *Ann N Y Acad Sci, 425*, 295–299.

Wickens, C., Kramer, A., Vanasse, L., & Donchin, E. (1983). Performance of concurrent tasks: a psychophysiological analysis of the reciprocity of information-processing resources. *Science, 221*(4615), 1080–1082.

Woldorff, M. G. (1993). Distortion of ERP averages due to overlap from temporally adjacent ERPs: analysis and correction. *Psychophysiology, 30*(1), 98–119.

13 | BCIs THAT USE SENSORIMOTOR RHYTHMS

GERT PFURTSCHELLER AND DENNIS J. McFARLAND

Brain-computer interfaces (BCIs) based on sensorimotor rhythms (SMRs) have been the focus of research and development for many years because of the long history of evidence that the execution or imagination of limb movement induces changes in rhythmic activity recorded over sensorimotor cortex (Pfurtscheller and Aranibar, 1979; Neuper and Pfurtscheller, 1999). These changes in SMRs can be detected on the scalp by electroencephalography (EEG) or magnetoencephalography (MEG) or on the surface of the brain by electrocorticography (ECoG) (McFarland et al., 2000; Jurkiewicz et al., 2006; Graimann et al., 2002). SMRs are recorded and their useful features are extracted and translated as described in chapters 6, 7, and 8 of this volume, and the resulting outputs are then used to control one or more of a variety of potentially useful BCI applications (e.g., movement control in one, two, or three dimensions).

This chapter discusses BCI usage of SMRs. It begins by reviewing their nature and basic characteristics, goes on to address the issues critical for recording and analyzing them, and then reviews their existing and possible future BCI applications.

SENSORIMOTOR RHYTHMS

SMRs are oscillations in the electric or magnetic fields recorded over sensorimotor cortices (i.e., posterior frontal and anterior parietal areas) (see chapter 3 of this volume and Pfurtscheller and Lopes da Silva, 1999). SMRs typically fall into three major frequency bands: mu (8–12 Hz), beta (18–30 Hz), and gamma (30–200+ Hz). EEG recording is largely limited to mu, beta, and lower-frequency gamma activity, but ECoG and MEG can detect higher-frequency activity. Most SMR studies to date have used EEG, and this is reflected in this chapter's focus on mu and beta SMRs. Gamma activity in ECoG recording is discussed extensively in chapter 15.

Beginning with the early studies of Berger (1930), Jasper and Andrew (1938), and Jasper and Penfield (1949), it has been shown repeatedly that SMRs change with motor behavior. Chatrian et al. (1959) described the decrease, or *desynchronization*, of the Rolandic *wicket rhythm* (i.e., the mu rhythm) during movement. Subsequent studies confirmed that SMRs decrease during motor behaviors. This decrease, known as *event-related desynchronization* (ERD) (Pfurtscheller and Aranibar, 1979), consists of a reduction in rhythmic activity related to an internally or externally paced event such as a voluntary movement. ERD is also referred to as *blocking* of a rhythm. SMR ERDs can be seen as correlates of activated cortical networks.

SMRs can also be *increased* in association with sensorimotor events (e.g., immediately after movement). This is called *event-related synchronization* (ERS) (Pfurtscheller, 1992). ERS may be, at least under certain circumstances, a correlate of a deactivated or inhibited cortical network. Figure 13.1 illustrates the ERD and ERS patterns associated with actual or imagined movements of foot or hand. Note the similarities between the patterns for actual and imagined movements. As also illustrated in figure 13.1, SMR ERDs and ERSs are both characterized by localized cortical (or scalp) topographies and specificities in frequency. These phenomena can be studied with time courses, time-frequency representations, and topographic maps (e.g., Pfurtscheller and Lopes da Silva, 1999).

The extensive networks responsible for the SMRs recorded over the cortex include both cortical and subcortical structures. Thus, recordings from depth electrodes reveal mu- and beta-range activity in the thalamus, subthalamic nucleus, and pedunculopontine area (Androulidakis et al., 2008; Klostermann et al., 2007; Williams et al., 2002). The relationships among these areas are complex. For example, with movement, mu ERD occurs in motor cortex and mu ERS occurs in the subthalamic nucleus, whereas beta ERD occurs uniformly in motor cortex, thalamus, and the subthalamic nucleus (Klostermann et al., 2007).

SMRs DURING SENSORIMOTOR BEHAVIORS

Over the past several decades, many studies have described in detail how voluntary movements are associated with mu and beta ERD localized over sensorimotor cortical areas (Pfurtscheller and Aranibar, 1979; Pfurtscheller and Berghold, 1989; Derambure et al., 1993; Toro et al., 1994; Stancák and Pfurtscheller, 1996b; Neuper and Pfurtscheller, 2001a; Pfurtscheller, Graimann, Huggins et al., 2003; Cassim et al., 2001; Alegre et al., 2002). For example, more than two seconds prior to a finger flexion, mu ERD appears over the contralateral Rolandic region (i.e., over the central sulcus) and becomes bilaterally symmetrical during actual execution of movement (Stancák and Pfurtscheller, 1996a). These effects are illustrated in figure 13.2.

Mu rhythms display two distinct ERD patterns. Lower-frequency (8–10 Hz) mu-rhythm ERD occurs during almost any kind of motor behavior, is widespread over the entire sensorimotor cortex, and probably reflects general motor preparation and attentional processes. In contrast, higher-frequency

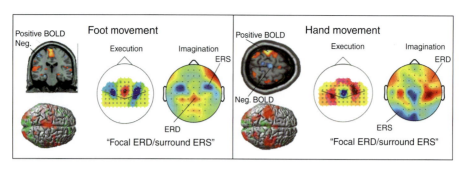

Figure 13.1 Examples of ERD and ERS patterns (obtained from EEG and fMRI data) during actual and imagined movements of the foot (left) or hand (right). Clearly visible are the antagonistic pattern of activation (ERD, positive BOLD signal [see chapter 4]) and deactivation (ERS, negative BOLD signal). Note also the similarity of the ERD maps for actual and imagined movements. (From Pfurtscheller and Lopes da Silva, 2011.)

(10–13 Hz) mu-rhythm ERD is topographically restricted and is related to task-specific aspects of performance. In sum, lower-frequency mu ERD appears to be nonspecific, whereas higher-frequency mu ERD is topographically and functionally specific (Pfurtscheller, Neuper & Kraus, 2000).

Like the mu rhythm, the beta rhythm exhibits desynchronization (ERD) in association with somatosensory stimulation and motor behaviors. In addition to this ERD, beta rhythms also display a brief ERS following movement, which is called *beta rebound* (Pfurtscheller, 1981; Pfurtscheller et al. 1996a). Figure 13.3 illustrates this phenomenon. It shares with other event-related responses characteristics such as: strict somatotopic organization (Salmelin et al., 1995; Pfurtscheller and Lopes da Silva, 1999; Jurkiewicz, 2006); somatotopically specific frequencies (e.g., slightly lower frequencies over hand area than over foot area [Neuper and Pfurtscheller, 2001b]); similar patterns after active and passive movements (Cassim et al., 2001; Alegre et al., 2002), electrical nerve stimulation (Neuper and Pfurtscheller, 2001b), or motor imagery (Pfurtscheller et al., 2005); and coincidence with reduced excitability of neurons in motor cortex, as measured with transcranial magnetic stimulation (Chen et al., 1998).

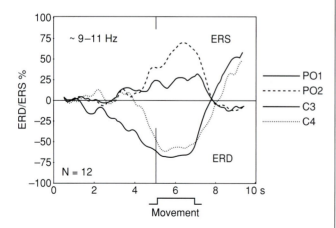

Figure 13.2 Grand average ERD and ERS time courses during slow voluntary movements of the right index finger. The movement period is indicated below the x-axis. Note that the ERD starts over the left motor area several seconds prior to movement. Also note the ERS over posterior areas. (From Neuper and Pfurtscheller, 2001a.)

Localized mu ERD related to a specific sensorimotor event does not usually occur in isolation. It is typically accompanied by simultaneous ERS in neighboring cortical areas. To describe this phenomenon, Suffczynski et al. (1999) introduced the term *focal-ERD/surround-ERS* (also referred to as *center/surround*). There are numerous examples of this phenomenon. Figure 13.1A shows hand-area ERD and foot-area ERS during hand movement, whereas figure 13.1B shows hand-area ERS and foot-area ERD during foot movement. The phenomenon may also involve cortical areas representing different sensory modalities. For example, Gerloff et al. (1998) reported that the mu ERD occurring during repetitive finger movement was accompanied by ERS of the 8–12 Hz visual alpha rhythm rhythm recorded over parieto-occipital (i.e., visual) cortex. Conversely, Koshino and Niedermeyer (1975) and Kreitmann and Shaw (1965) reported that the alpha ERD over occipital cortex during visual stimulation was accompanied by mu ERS over sensorimotor cortex. Metabolic imaging studies provide additional evidence of focal ERD/surround ERS. For example, Ehrsson et al. (2003) showed that actual or imagined toe movements increased the BOLD signal (see chapter 4) in a foot representation area and decreased it in a hand area.

The focal ERD/surround ERS phenomenon may reflect a mechanism that accentuates attention to a specific sensorimotor subsystem by inhibiting other cortical areas that are not directly involved in the specific behavior (Pfurtscheller et al.,1996b). In this process the interplay between thalamocortical modules and the inhibitory reticular thalamic nucleus neurons may play an important role (Lopes da Silva, 1991, 2006).

SMRs DURING MOTOR IMAGERY

Early clinical studies by Jasper and Penfield (1949) show that SMR ERD is associated with motor imagery as well as with actual movement. Gastaut et al. (1965) observed mu ERD when subjects with amputated limbs imagined moving their missing limbs.

More recent studies have further documented the ERDs associated with movement imagery and have demonstrated their similarity to the ERDs associated with actual movements.

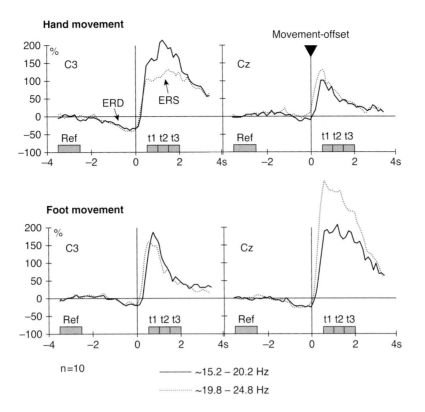

Figure 13.3 *Grand average ERD and ERS patterns over hand and foot areas. The time courses for electrodes C3 and Cz are shown separately for finger and foot movement. The vertical lines indicate the movement offset. Band-power increase is indicated by upward deflections. Note the ERD prior to movement and the ERS following movement. Also note that the effects of finger movement are greater over C3 and the effects of foot movement are greater over Cz. (From Neuper and Pfurtscheller, 2001b.)*

Figure 13.1 illustrates this similarity. For example, imagery of right- and left-hand movements is associated with ERD of mu and beta rhythms over the contralateral hand area that is comparable to the premovement ERD seen during execution of self-paced movements (Pfurtscheller and Neuper 1997, 2006, 2010). Further support for somatotopically localized ERD with imagery comes from studies in patients with impaired motor function (Neuper and Pfurtscheller, 1999; Neuper et al., 2006). Furthermore, foot motor imagery, like actual foot movement, is followed by beta ERS (Pfurtscheller and Solis-Escalante, 2009).

Many other studies using a variety of recording techniques provide further evidence for the participation of sensorimotor cortex in motor imagery and for the similarities of the activity associated with imagery to that associated with actual movement. These include studies using EEG (McFarland et al., 2000; Caldara et al., 2004; Neuper et al., 2005; Pfurtscheller, Brunner, Schlögl et al., 2006; Neuper et al., 2009), ECoG (Leuthardt et al., 2004), MEG (Mellinger et al., 2007), functional magnetic resonance imagery (fMRI) (Porro et al., 1996; Lotze et al., 1999; Dechent et al., 2004; Ehrsson et al., 2003), and near-infrared spectroscopy (fNIRS) (Wriessnegger et al., 2008).

The strong similarities between actual movement and movement imagery in the activity patterns found in sensorimotor cortical areas are consistent with the concept that motor imagery is realized via the same brain structures involved in movement preparation and performance (Jeannerod, 2001; Decety, 1994).

ANALYZING SENSORIMOTOR CORTEX ACTIVITY

FREQUENCY ANALYSIS

Since SMRs consist of rhythmic oscillations, their quantification begins with frequency analysis. For EEG, the relevant range is 5–40 Hz, whereas for ECoG and MEG the relevant range extends considerably higher, to at least 200 Hz (Graimann and Pfurtscheller, 2006). The classical approach to quantifying SMRs and tracking their ERD and ERS is simple bandpass filtering (see chapter 7 of this volume) in one or more specific frequency bands. The standard ERD/ERS calculation as defined by Pfurtscheller and Aranibar (1979) is accomplished by bandpass filtering each trial, squaring the samples, and then averaging over multiple trials. The results are used to define the proportional power decrease (ERD) or power increase (ERS) relative to a specific reference interval that is usually a period of several seconds shortly before the onset of the event (e.g., movement or movement imagery; fig. 13.3). Since time-domain evoked potentials can mask SMR ERD or ERS, the mean value of the samples to be averaged is typically subtracted from each sample before squaring them. The results can be used to produce time-frequency maps (Graimann et al., 2002).

A variety of other frequency-analysis methods have been applied to SMRs. These include the Fourier transform (Makeig, 1993), the continuous wavelet transform (Tallon-Baundry and Bertrand, 1999), matching pursuit (Durka et al., 2001), and autoregressive models (Marple, 1987). Further information on these techniques, their unique features, and their particular advantages and disadvantages is provided in chapters 7 and 8 of this volume. In general, the choice of a particular method for a given application is frequently determined by the trade-off that the method provides between frequency resolution and time resolution.

SPATIAL ANALYSIS

SMRs and their associated time-domain evoked potentials are usually localized over specific cortical regions. Thus, spatial-filtering methods that emphasize localized signal features (i.e., features with high spatial frequency) and de-emphasize widespread features (i.e., features with low spatial frequency), can substantially improve the recognition and measurement of SMRs (McFarland, McCane et al., 1997). The conventional monopolar (i.e., referential) EEG method has minimal spatial resolution and is thus not well suited for revealing localized ERD/ERS patterns over sensorimotor areas. Other spatial-filtering techniques such as the common average reference (CAR or AVE) and Laplacian derivations or simple bipolar derivations are more suitable. Spatial filtering principles and alternatives are discussed fully in chapter 7 of this volume. Figure 13.4 illustrates the importance of appropriate spatial filtering for recording SMRs. It shows the SMR localization achieved by analyzing the same EEG data with three different spatial filters. The superior signal quality provided by the CAR and large Laplacian methods is clear. Independent component analysis (ICA) is another technique that can be used for spatial filtering aimed at improving SMR recognition and quantification. It is a statistical signal-processing method that decomposes a multivariate input signal into statistically independent components (Naeem et al., 2006). ICA is addressed more fully in chapter 7.

ANALYSES OF RELATIONSHIPS BETWEEN DIFFERENT CHANNELS

Currently, almost all BCIs use signal features obtained from single recording sites (e.g., power in a specific frequency band, voltage at a specific time point). Nevertheless, a number of studies suggest that features consisting of the relationships between the signals from different recording sites may be valuable for BCI applications that use SMRs (e.g., Lachaux et al., 1999; Gysel and Celka, 2004; Brunner et al., 2006). Brunner et al. (2006) found that phase locking value (PLV), which reflects the level of phase synchronization between signals from different locations, can be useful in distinguishing among different mental states. Pairs of electrodes within one hemisphere (e.g., electrodes over premotor and primary motor cortices) appeared to be more useful than interhemispheric electrode pairs. PLV methods are described in chapter 7.

TRANSLATING SMR ACTIVITY INTO DEVICE CONTROL

Early SMR-based BCI applications often used linear regression algorithms to translate SMR amplitudes into cursor movements (e.g., Wolpaw et al., 1994). Further developments of this approach have yielded the most complex SMR-based BCI control realized to date (Wolpaw and McFarland, 2004; McFarland et al., 2008, 2010). Regression algorithms have the advantage of

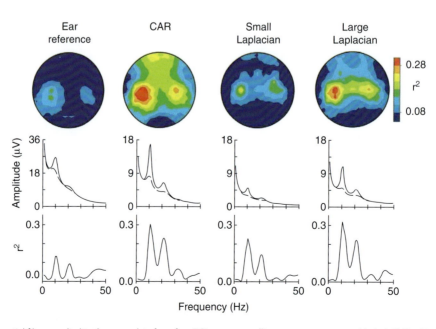

Figure 13.4 Three different spatial filters applied to the same data from four BCI users controlling cursor movement with their SMRs. (Top) Average topographies of r^2 for top/bottom target differences. (Bottom) Average spectra of r^2 for the channel used for cursor control. (From McFarland et al., 1997.)

being able to support acquisition of many different targets with a single function; and thus they can readily generalize across different numbers of targets (McFarland and Wolpaw, 2005). Consider, for example, the icons on modern video desktop displays and graphical user interfaces, which often change with context. Any number of icons (i.e., targets) can be mapped by two regression functions. In contrast, many SMR-based BCI applications to date have used classification algorithms, for which each change in the number of possible selections necessitates deriving new classification parameters (e.g., Pfurtscheller, Neuper, Flotzinger et al., 1997; see Lotte et al., 2007 for review).

Adaptation of the translation algorithm to the changing characteristics of individual users is a desirable attribute for BCI systems (McFarland, Lefkowitz et al., 1997). Vidaurre et al. (2006) and Shenoy et al. (2006) have characterized the changing statistics of the signal features of individual users. McFarland et al. (2006) discussed the multiple parameters that can be adaptively controlled in a sensorimotor BCI system. The method by which this is done may vary with the parameter in question. For example, an adaptive estimate of the slope and intercept of the equation that translates EEG into cursor movement considers only simple statistics of the signal (e.g., Ramoser et al., 1997). In contrast, feature-selection algorithms often consider the covariances between signal features (e.g., McFarland and Wolpaw, 2005; Shenoy et al., 2006; Vidaurre et al., 2006). Several recent studies have further demonstrated the impressive performance of SMR-based BCIs that use adaptive algorithms (McFarland et al., 2011; Thomas et al., 2011; Vidaurre et al., 2011).

ONLINE AND OFFLINE ANALYSES

Communication is an interactive process that requires the user to track the process continually and correct mistakes. Control applications require the user to navigate on the basis of their current state (e.g., cursor position) and make necessary corrections during the course of performance. Thus a BCI device that is used for communication or control applications runs in real time and provides feedback to the user. Whereas early SMR-based BCI studies described results for real-time operation (e.g., Wolpaw et al., 1991; Pfurtscheller et al., 1993), much subsequent BCI research has focused on offline analyses of prerecorded data (e.g., Blankertz et al., 2006). Indeed, in the Lotte et al. (2007) review of BCI classification algorithms, most of the studies considered used offline analyses.

Although offline studies are convenient and efficient, and can often guide subsequent online studies, offline results may not generalize to online performance. BCI operation depends on ongoing real-time interaction between the brain signals the user produces and the outputs into which the BCI translates these signals. Thus, the outputs that a particular translation algorithm produces are likely to affect subsequent brain signals, and these will in turn affect subsequent BCI outputs. These interactive effects are not accessible to offline analyses in which data obtained with a particular algorithm are reanalyzed with promising new algorithms. As a result, the value of a particular algorithm can only be fully assessed through actual online testing. This crucial issue is considered in more detail in chapter 8 of this volume.

ARTIFACTS

Artifacts produced by nonbrain signals, whether originating from power lines, muscle activity, or other sources, are a major source of concern in BCI research and development (see Fatourechi et al., 2007 for review). Chapter 7 addresses artifact issues more completely. Here we discuss those aspects that are of particular concern for BCIs that use SMRs.

Electromagnetic signals recorded from the scalp may be produced by brain or nonbrain activity. Electromyographic activity (EMG) from cranial, facial, and neck muscles and electrooculographic activity (EOG) from eye movements and eye blinks are the most prominent and important nonbrain artifacts. Furthermore, mental efforts, such as those often associated with BCI usage, often produce changes in these nonbrain signals (e.g., Ichikawa and Ohira, 2004; Silvestrini and Gendolla, 2007; Whitham et al., 2008).

EMG presents a particularly difficult problem as it produces broadband signals that may extend over widespread areas of scalp, including the vertex (Goncharova et al., 2003). Because EMG activity can overlap with SMRs in both frequency and location (and may greatly exceed them in amplitude), simple low-pass filtering (see chapter 7) is generally not an adequate remedy. Consequently, without sufficient topographic and spectral analysis, EMG signals may obscure, or may masquerade as, actual SMRs.

For example, McFarland et al. (2005) describe how cranial EMG can interfere during the initial training of users operating an SMR-based BCI application. As illustrated in that study, EMG contamination can be readily identified and differentiated from actual brain signals by appropriately comprehensive topographical and spectral analysis. In the absence of such analysis (e.g., if the data are limited to one or two locations or to a limited frequency range), it is often not possible to determine whether the signals used by the BCI are actual brain signals or EMG. Topographic and spectral characteristics of SMRs and EMG are illustrated in figure 13.5. This issue has recently become even more important as studies have begun to focus on gamma-range (i.e., >30 Hz) brain activity (e.g., Palaniappan, 2006), which is very weak in the scalp-recorded EEG (Pfurtscheller and Cooper, 1975). (Whitman et al. [2008] have even suggested that all scalp-recorded gamma-range signals may be due to EMG activity.) In sum, essentially all SMR-based BCI research and development efforts that use scalp recording should incorporate the comprehensive topographical and spectral analyses needed to recognize artifacts produced by cranial and facial EMG. Scherer et al. (2007) have suggested an interesting additional measure in which EMG detection is based on the residual variance in the signal not explained by an autoregressive model. Recently, Halder et al (2011) supported the brain origin of the signals used by a SMR-based BCI by showing concurrent fMRI activation of the appropriate brain regions.

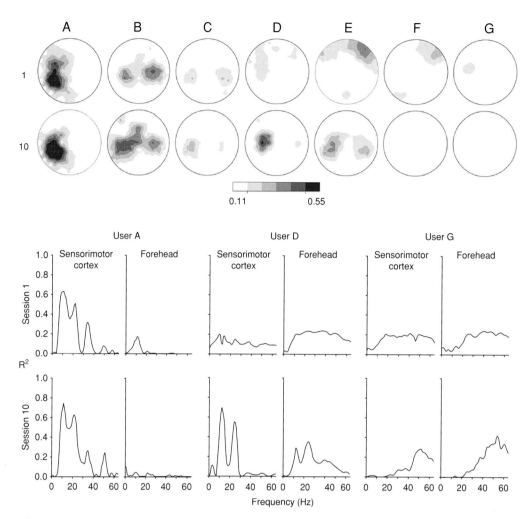

Figure 13.5 *(Top) Average topographies of r^2 (in the frequency band used for control) for top/bottom target differences from seven BCI users (A–G) during their first and 10th sessions of SMR training. Note the localized control over sensorimotor areas in users A–E by the 10th session. In contrast, Users F and G did not develop such SMR control. Note also the probable EMG activity over frontal areas in users D–F early in training. This activity disappeared with training. (Bottom) Spectra over sensorimotor cortex and forehead of BCI users A, D, and G. Note the broadband probable EMG activity over forehead areas early in training in users D and G. In User D, this decreased markedly with training, whereas in User G it did not. True SMR control is spatially and spectrally focused (e.g., user A throughout and user D later in training). (From McFarland et al., 2005.)*

Unlike EMG artifacts, which may occur over a very broad spectral range, EOG artifacts are mainly at lower frequencies (i.e., 1–4 Hz), except at frontal polar sites (Hagemann and Naumann, 2001). As a result, EOG is generally not a major concern for BCIs that use SMRs. A number of methods for removing EOG artifacts have been described (e.g., Croft et al., 2005; Fatourechi et al., 2007).

Although cranial and facial EMG is a major potential source of artifacts, muscle activity is a concern for another reason as well. Because SMRs are often affected by motor actions, muscle activity in the limbs or elsewhere in the body can affect these rhythms. The possibility of peripheral mediation of SMR changes has been a concern in the development of SMR-based BCI applications, particularly in regard to their potential usefulness for people who lack voluntary motor function. Thus, a number of studies have included careful ancillary experiments to demonstrate that the SMR control they report does not depend on muscle activity elsewhere in the body

(e.g., Vaughan et al., 1998; Wolpaw and McFarland, 2004; McFarland et al., 2010).

BCI USES OF SMRs

Over the past 20 years, SMRs have been applied to BCI applications in a variety of different ways. Essentially all of these efforts have started from the observation that SMRs change with motor imagery as well as with actual movements. Thus, the prospective BCI user is asked to imagine particular actions and the resultant changes in SMR amplitudes are translated into outputs such as cursor movement.

Although SMR-based BCIs generally use imagery in some way, they differ substantially in how they do this. At one end of the spectrum are BCIs that simply use imagery as a starting point that enables the user to gain initial control of the BCI's output. Then, from this point on, these BCIs rely on progressive adaptive interactions between the user (who gradually improves SMR control) and the BCI (which gradually improves its translation of that control into outputs such as cursor movement). In this approach, successful BCI operation is based on the continued mutual adaptation of user to system and system to user. As this process proceeds, imagery typically begins to be less important and often disappears entirely, so that BCI use appears to become automatized like a well-learned muscle-based action (e.g., Wolpaw and McFarland, 2004; McFarland et al., 2010).

At the other end of the spectrum are BCIs that rely on specific imagery or other mental tasks initially (e.g., foot movement vs. hand movement, calculation vs. mental visualization of object rotation), define the SMR changes associated with each task, and continue to rely on these relationships throughout subsequent BCI operation (e.g., Curran and Stokes, 2003; Curran et al., 2004; Krauledat et al., 2008). This approach assumes that the SMR patterns associated with the chosen tasks do not change with repeated BCI usage, and/or that any changes can readily be accommodated by recalibrations. It does not try to actively engage the adaptive properties of the user's brain in order to improve BCI operation. These two different approaches are illustrated in this chapter's next subsections, which describe the different kinds of SMR-based BCI applications that have been implemented.

It should be noted that efforts to develop SMR-based BCIs were also encouraged by evidence that people could learn to change SMR amplitudes in one direction (i.e., increase or decrease) (e.g., Kulman, 1978; Elder et al., 1986). Since these early studies had therapeutic goals (e.g., decreased seizure frequency in epileptic patients), they did not attempt to show that people can learn to change SMR amplitudes rapidly and accurately in either direction, up or down. Such rapid bidirectional control is essential for BCI communication and control applications. The initial demonstration and subsequent refinements of rapid bidirectional SMR control have been the central achievement of SMR-based BCI research over the past 20 years.

CURSOR MOVEMENT IN ONE OR MORE DIMENSIONS

In 1991, Wolpaw et al. (1991) described an SMR-based BCI in which users moved a cursor to hit a target located on the top or bottom edge of a video screen. Cursor movement was controlled by the amplitude of mu-rhythm (8–12 Hz) activity recorded over sensorimotor areas. After an initial screening session to identify the locations and frequencies of SMR changes associated with actual limb movements and/or movement imagery, cursor movement direction (i.e., up or down) was made dependent on these changes, and users were encouraged to find motor imagery that would move the cursor toward the target. Subjects reported using a variety of kinds of imagery for moving in one direction or the other (e.g., imagining running, floating, shooting baskets, etc.) As their control improved, and as the translation algorithm was adapted to use the growing control as effectively as possible, users typically reported that the imagery became less important, and their control over cursor movement became more like a normal muscle-based action. This observation is consistent with the learning of many conventional (i.e., muscle-based) tasks in which, with continued practice, performance becomes automatized (e.g., Bebko et al., 2003; Poldrack et al., 2005). Furthermore, it bodes well for the eventual practical success of SMR-based BCIs, since automatized performance is less likely to interfere with concurrent mental operations. For example, in composing a manuscript an experienced typist does not need to think about each individual keystroke.

Subsequent to this first demonstration, one-dimensional SMR-based cursor control was extended to allow selection among more than two targets (e.g., McFarland et al., 1993; McFarland et al., 2003; Pfurtscheller, Müller-Putz, Schlögl et al., 2006). In addition, SMRs detected by MEG were applied to cursor control (Mellinger et al., 2007). More complex training protocols have enabled people to learn to control two SMR signals simultaneously and to use this control to move a cursor in two dimensions (Wolpaw and McFarland, 1994, 2004; Kostov and Polak, 2000; Cincotti et al., 2008). In Wolpaw and McFarland (1994, 2004), movement in each dimension was controlled by a linear equation that translated SMR features (i.e., the independent variables) into cursor movement (i.e., the dependent variable). The SMR features used (i.e., amplitudes in specific frequency bands at specific locations) and the weights assigned to them were the result of continued adaptive interaction between the user and the BCI over the course of training sessions. As discussed in Wolpaw (2010), this SMR-based two-dimensional cursor control is comparable in speed and accuracy to that achieved in humans with intracortical microelectrode implants (Hochberg et al., 2006). It has been supplemented by an SMR-based "select" function to provide mouse-like operation that enables a BCI user to move a cursor to a target and to then decide whether to select it (McFarland et al., 2008). Most recently, SMR-based cursor control has been extended to three dimensions (McFarland et al., 2010), and two-dimensional control has been combined with a constant progression in a third dimension to enable movement in three dimensions (Royer et al., 2010). Figure 13.6 illustrates simultaneous independent control of three movement dimensions. These and related studies show that SMRs can provide rapid and accurate control of one output or parallel control of several independent simultaneous outputs.

COMMUNICATION APPLICATIONS

Spelling systems are communication aids that allow users to express themselves by selecting letters or other items, thus forming words and sentences. People with ALS have learned to use SMRs to operate a spelling device (Neuper et al., 2003; Kübler et al., 2005). One SMR-based BCI spelling application divided the alphabet into four parts, and users reached a single letter through a series of three successive selections (Wolpaw et al., 2003). Millán et al. (2003) reported an average spelling rate of ~3.0 letters/min for a BCI that differentiated among the EEG patterns associated with imagination of left hand

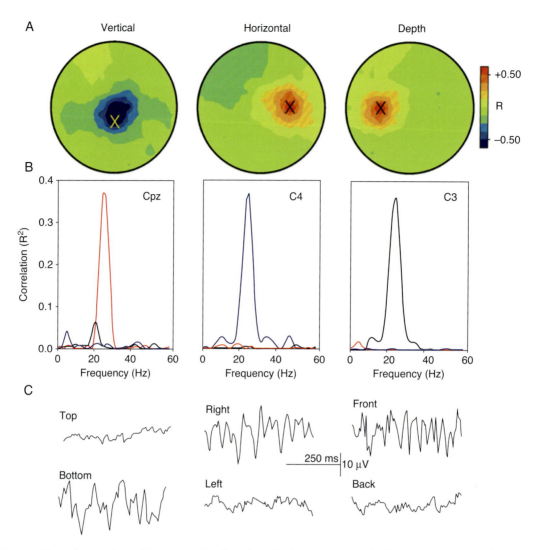

Figure 13.6 *SMR topographies and spectra from a BCI user controlling three-dimensional cursor movement. In this case, movement in each dimension was controlled by 26-Hz EEG activity at one or two specific electrodes. (A) Scalp topographies (nose at top) of the correlations of the 26-Hz frequency band with the vertical, horizontal, and depth target locations, respectively. (The correlations are shown as R in order to distinguish negative and positive correlations.) The electrodes that controlled each dimension of movement are marked with an X. (B) Spectra corresponding to the correlations (r^2) of the activities at the scalp electrode that made the largest contributions to the control signal are shown. The correlations with the vertical, horizontal, and depth dimensions are presented as red, blue, and black lines, respectively. The activity at the electrode that provided a given control signal correlated strongly with the corresponding dimension of the target location and did not correlate with the other dimensions. (C) Samples of EEG activity at the marked electrodes from single trials; these illustrate the control in each dimension that the user employed to move the cursor to the target. (From McFarland et al., 2010.)*

movement, right hand movement, and cube rotation. Müller and Blankertz (2006) described an intriguing BCI application ("Hex-O-Spell") in which the BCI differentiated among six possible choices, and two successive selections were used to arrive at the desired letter (as illustrated in fig. 13.7). More recently, Friedrich et al. (2009) described an application in which an automatic scanning protocol proceeded through a set of choices and the user produced a specific SMR change when the desired selection was reached.

CONTROL APPLICATIONS

In an early application, an SMR-based BCI was used to restore hand grasp in a person paralyzed by spinal cord injury (Pfurtscheller, Guger, Müller, et al., 2000). The BCI controlled an orthosis that opened and closed the user's paralyzed hand. This BCI was subsequently combined with the Freehand (Keith et al., 1989), an implanted neuroprosthesis that uses functional electrical stimulation (FES) of hand muscles to restore grasp. Using this BCI/FES system, a paralyzed person was able to use foot motor imagery to modulate SMRs in order to perform hand grasp (Pfurtscheller et al., 2003b; Müller-Putz et al., 2005).

Virtual reality (VR) provides an excellent training and testing environment for simulating BCI control applications that would be very costly, potentially dangerous, or even impossible to realize at present. In a simulation of wheelchair control, the BCI controls not an actual wheelchair but rather the movement of a virtual wheelchair through an immersive virtual environment that simulates the real wheelchair movement as realistically as possible. Recently, Leeb et al. (2007) reported an

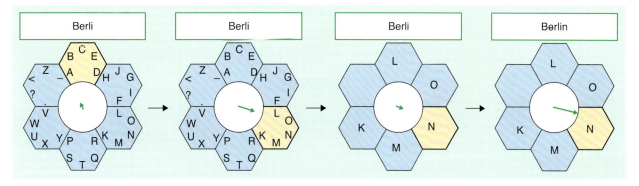

Figure 13.7 *The Hex-o-Spell. The two states classified by the BCI system control the turning and lengthening, respectively, of the green arrow. Letters could be chosen in a two-step procedure. First a subgroup is selected, and then the hexagon that contains the desired letter is selected. (From Müller and Blankertz, 2006.)*

experiment in which a person paralyzed by spinal cord injury was placed with his wheelchair in the middle of a multiprojection-based stereo and head-tracked VR system that simulated a street with shops populated by 15 people (i.e., avatars). By using foot vs. hand motor imagery to modulate power in a 15–19 Hz frequency band recorded over sensorimotor cortex, the BCI user was able to move forward from avatar to avatar in the virtual environment. This paradigm is illustrated in figure 13.8. Figure 13.9 shows examples of time-frequency maps during hand and foot motor imagery in this BCI VR application.

ASYNCHRONOUS BCIs

BCIs may be *synchronous* or *asynchronous*. In a *synchronous* BCI, the system specifies the timing of operation. In an *asynchronous* BCI, the user determines timing. Chapter 10 in this volume discusses these two alternative designs more fully. Although the asynchronous design may be preferable for some applications (especially those most likely to be useful for people who are severely paralyzed), it is much more difficult to realize. Thus, almost all BCIs described to date are synchronous.

Several studies have explored the use of SMRs and related activity to realize asynchronous BCI applications. Mason and

Birch (2000) described an asynchronous BCI that uses time-domain motor-related potentials, and subsequently applied it to the real-time control of a video game (Mason et al., 2004). Scherer et al. (2004) described an asynchronous protocol based on left hand, right hand, and foot motor imagery that they applied to a spelling application. In a later study, Scherer et al. (2007) developed an asynchronous SMR-based BCI by training two independent classifiers. One classifier detected the onset of a motor-imagery task and the second determined which movement imagery task (among several possibilities) the subject was performing. With the resultant outputs, the BCI user could navigate in a virtual environment or use the Google Earth website. Most recently, Solis-Escalante (2009) and Pfurtscheller et al. (2010) provided evidence that the beta-range SMR ERS that occurs immediately after foot motor imagery might support effective asynchronous BCI operation and Hema et al (2011) used an asynchronous SMR-based BCI to control a wheelchair.

POTENTIAL USERS OF SMR-BASED BCIs

An important practical issue for SMR-based BCIs is whether their most likely prospective users will be able to operate them. Although early observations suggested that SMRs occurred in

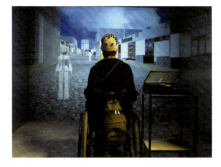 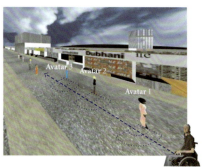

Figure 13.8 *(Left) A virtual street populated with 15 avatars and a user with tetraplegia in his wheelchair in the middle of a multiprojection wall virtual reality system. The BCI user wore the electrode cap with one bipolar channel connected to the BCI system (amplifier and laptop on the right side). (Right) The task of the participant was to go from avatar to avatar in the direction of the end of the street (outlined with a dashed line). The avatars were lined up, and each avatar had an invisible communication sphere (drawn as dotted lines here). The BCI user had to stop within this sphere, not too close and not too far away from the avatar. (From Leeb et al., 2007.)*

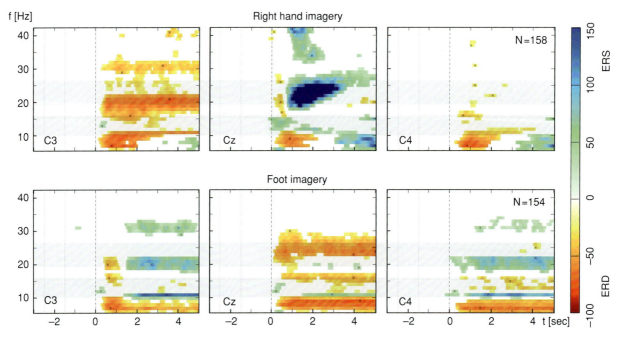

Figure 13.9 *Examples of time-frequency maps from an online BCI experiment with right hand (upper panel) versus foot (lower panel) motor imagery in a trained subject. The task was to use only motor imagery to walk along a virtual street (Pfurtscheller, Leeb, Keinrath, et al.,2006). The cue was presented at t = 0, and the motor imagery process lasted several seconds. Only trials without artifact (N = 158 and N = 154) were used for the calculation of the time-frequency maps. Different reactivity patterns occurred during right hand versus foot motor imagery. Hand motor imagery showed a broadband contralateral (C3) 10-Hz and 20-Hz ERD and a midcentral (Cz) beta ERS, while foot motor imagery displayed narrowband 11-Hz, 22-Hz, and 33-Hz ERS at electrode positions C3 and C4 and a broadband midcentral beta ERD. (For details see Leeb, 2008.)*

only a minority of people (Chatrian, 1976), subsequent computer-based analyses demonstrated that SMRs occur in most adults (Pfurtscheller, 1989). Furthermore, Guger et al. (2003) tested the ability of 99 healthy adults to use SMR activity from one bipolar EEG channel over sensorimotor cortex to perform a two-choice task. After brief training, 93% achieved accuracies of >60%. Thus, it appears likely that most people without disabilities are able to use SMR-based BCIs.

At the same time, the most critical issue is whether people with severe disabilities, who are the primary users of assistive BCI devices, can use SMR-based systems. It is possible that a pathological process that causes severe motor disabilities may also impair SMR control. For example, although ALS is traditionally considered a disease that mainly affects spinal cord motoneurons, it can also affect motor cortex and related areas of frontal cortex, and may also be associated with dementia (Witgert et al., 2010; Yoshida, 2004). Nevertheless, the available data, although limited, suggest that most of the major target user groups retain the capacity for SMR control. Kübler et al. (2005) showed that four people severely disabled by ALS could operate an SMR-based BCI, although their training rates and eventual performance tended to be at the low end of the range for people without disabilities. Cincotti et al. (2008) reported that four people with muscular dystrophy or spinal muscular atrophy could use an SMR-based BCI.

EEG changes have been described in people with spinal cord injuries (Cramer et al., 2005) or cerebral palsy (e.g., Jaseja, 2007). Nevertheless, several people with spinal cord injuries

were as successful as people without disabilities in mastering SMR-based control of two- and three-dimensional cursor movements, and at least one individual with severe cerebral palsy was able to use a simple SMR-based BCI application (Wolpaw and McFarland, 2004; McFarland, Krusienski, et al., 2003; McFarland et al., 2008, 2010). Enzinger et al. (2008) suggest that BCI use might actually serve to restore more normal EEG following spinal cord injury.

BCI use by individuals with severe disabilities may be constrained by other factors related to their disease or disability. For example, people with ALS may have visual difficulties (e.g., diplopia, ptosis, dry eyes, gaze instability) that interfere with their use of BCIs that require effective vision. Spurred by this problem, Nijboer et al. (2008) described an interesting auditory BCI design in which users learned to control SMRs in order to select from among a set of different sounds. Such auditory BCIs might be particularly useful for people whose disabilities interfere with their vision or their ability to maintain gaze.

Birbaumer and Cohen (2007) have suggested that an additional problem may arise in people whose severe disabilities have left them with no remaining useful muscle control. The continued existence of this totally locked-in state (see chapters 11 and 19 of this volume), in which no intentional behaviors can occur, might conceivably produce a state of learned helplessness (Seligman, 1972) that precludes effective BCI operation. If this is the case, BCI usage might be possible only if it begins before the individual becomes totally locked-in (i.e., so that the person never becomes helpless).

FUTURE DIRECTIONS

As the preceding subsection of this chapter illustrates, SMRs are promising features for BCI use. They might provide the multichannel outputs needed to control devices such as wheelchairs, robotic arms, or neuroprostheses. Their ultimate value for these and other purposes will depend primarily on the reliability, accuracy, and speed of the control they provide. Clearly, much work remains to be done in these areas.

Improvements in feature selection and extraction, and in the translation algorithms applied to the EEG features are certainly important. The incorporation of features derived from relationships between individual channels (e.g., coherences) is a particularly promising area for study. Perhaps the most complex aspect of feature extraction and translation is the appropriate management of the initial and ongoing adaptations of the BCI system to the user and of the user to the BCI system. Appropriate management of these interactions can augment the control achieved, and is likely to be essential for ensuring reliable BCI performance.

One intriguing area that needs further exploration is based on the observation that SMRs can display either long-lasting (several sec) or brief (<one sec) ERD and/or ERS changes. Long-lasting changes are associated with focused attention or with voluntary actions such as actual or imagined slow finger extension and flexion. Brief changes are automatic responses to specific external stimuli (e.g., the brief ERD/ERS pattern triggered by visually cued motor imagery (Pfurtscheller et al., 2008) or the brief beta rebound (ERS) that follows a motor task (Pfurtscheller and Lopes da Silva, 1999). Both long-lasting and brief SMR changes typically display clear somatotopical organization. Blankertz et al. (2008) and Scherer (2008) used the brief ERD after visually cued motor imagery to discriminate among different motor imagery tasks. By focusing on these two different classes of SMR changes (i.e., brief vs. long-lasting), future studies may improve BCI designs.

SUMMARY

Movement and motor imagery are accompanied by changes in rhythmic activity recorded over sensorimotor cortex. Decreases and increases in these *sensorimotor rhythms* (SMRs) are referred as *event-related desynchronization* (ERD) and *event-related synchronization* (ERS), respectively. These changes are typically somatotopically localized.

Over the past 20 years, many studies have shown that SMR changes associated with motor imagery can serve as useful control signals for BCIs. SMR-based BCIs have controlled cursor movements in one, two, or three dimensions and have supported a variety of other communication and control applications.

Successful development and implementation of SMR-based BCI applications require appropriate frequency analysis and spatial filtering, effective translation algorithms, and adequate attention to online testing. Recognition and elimination of artifacts, particularly EMG activity from cranial muscles, is extremely important, and usually requires comprehensive frequency and topographical analyses.

Data to date suggest that many people with severe motor disabilities, such as those due to ALS or spinal cord injury, are able to use SMR-based BCIs.

The eventual value of SMR-based BCIs will hinge on improvements in speed, accuracy, and reliability. Better encouragement and guidance of the mutual adaptation of the user to the BCI and the BCI to the user are likely to be particularly important. The development of asynchronous BCI designs, use of relationships between channels as signal features, and attention to the distinctive characteristics of specific SMRs should also prove productive.

REFERENCES

Alegre, M., Labarga, A., Gurtubay, I.G., Iriarte, J., Malanda, A., and Artieda, J. (2002). Beta electroencephalograph changes during passive movements: sensory afferences contribute to beta event-related desynchronization in humans. *Neurosci Lett, 331*(1), 29–32.

Androulidakis, A.G., Mazzone, P., Litvak, V., Penny, W., Dileone, M., Gaynor, L.M., Tisch, S., Di Lazzaro, V., and Brown, P. (2008). Oscillatory activity in the pedunculopontine area of patients with Parkinson's disease. *Exp Neurol, 211*, 59–66.

Bebko, J.M., Demark, J.L., Osborn, P.A., Majumder, S., Ricciuti, C.J., and Rhee, T. (2003). Acquisition and automatization of a complex task: an examination of three-ball cascade juggling. *J Mot Behav, 35*, 109–118.

Berger, H. (1930). Uber das Elektrenkephalogramm des Menschen II. *J Psychol Neurol, 40*, 160–179.

Birbaumer, N. and Cohen, L.G. (2007). Brain-computer interfaces: communication and restoration of movement in paralysis. *J. Physiol, 579*, 621–636.

Blankertz, B., Losch, F., Krauledat, M., Dornhege, G., Curio, G., and Müller, K.R. (2008). The Berlin brain-computer interface: accurate performance from first-session in BCI-naive subjects. *IEEE Trans Biomed Eng, 55*, 2452–2462.

Blankertz, B. Müller, K.R., Krusienski, D.J., Schalk, G., Wolpaw, J.R., Schlogl, A., Pfurtscheller, G., Millán, J. del R., Schroder, M., and Birbaumer, N. (2006). The BCI competition III: validating alternative approaches to actual BCI problems. *IEEE Trans Neural Syst Rehabil Eng, 14*, 153–159.

Brunner, C., Graimann, B., Huggins, J.E., Levine, S.P., and Pfurtscheller, G. (2005). Phase relationships between different subdural electrode recordings in man. *Neurosci Lett, 375*, 69–74.

Brunner,C. Scherer,R.,Graimann, B., Supp, G., and Pfurtscheller, G. (2006). Online control of a brain computer interface using phase information. *IEEE Trans Biomed Eng, 53*, 2501–2406.

Caldara, R., Deiber, M.P., Andrey, C., Michel, C.M., Thut, G., and Hauert, C.A. (2004). Actual and mental motor preparation and execution: a spatiotemporal ERP study. *Exp Brain Res, 159*, 389–399.

Cassim, F., Monaca, C., Szurhaj, W., Bourriez, J.L., Defebvre, L., Derambure, P., and Guieu, J.D. (2001). Does post-movement beta synchronization reflect an idling motor cortex? *Neuroreport, 12*(17), 3859–3863.

Chatrian, G.E., Petersen, M.C., and Lazarte, J.A. (1959). The blocking of the rolandic wicket rhythm and some central changes related to movement. *Electroencephalogr Clin Neurophysiol, 11*, 497–510.

Chatrian, G.E. (1976). The mu rhythm. In: A. Remond (Ed.). *Handbook of electroencephalography and clinical neurophysiology: the EEG of the waking adult.* Amsterdam: Elsevier, pp. 46–69.

Chen, R., Yaseen, Z., Cohen, L.G., and Hallett, M. Time course of corticospinal excitability in reaction time and self-paced movements. *Ann Neurol 44*, 317–325, 1998.

Cincotti, F., Mattia, D., Aloise, F., Bufalari, S., Schalk, G., Oriolo, G., Cherubini, A., Marciani, M.G., and Babiloni, F. (2008). Non-invasive brain-computer interface system: towards its application as assistive technology. *Brain Res Bull, 75*, 796–803.

Cramer, S.C., Lastra, L., Lacourse, M.G., and Cohen, M.J. (2005). Brain motor system function after chronic, complete spinal cord injury. *Brain, 128*, 2941–2950.

Croft, R.J., Chandler, J.S., Barry, R.J., Cooper, N.R., and Clarke, A.R. (2005). EOG correction: a comparison of four methods. *Psychophysiology, 42*, 16–24.

Curran, E.A. and Stokes, M.J. (2003). Learning to control brain activity: a review of the production and control of EEG components for driving brain-computer interface (BCI) systems. *Brain Cogn, 51*, 326–336.

Curran, E., Sykacek, P., Stokes, M., Roberts, S.J., Penny, W., Johnsrude, I., and Owen, A.M. (2004). Cognitive tasks for driving a brain-computer interfacing system: a pilot study. *IEEE Trans Neural Syst Rehabil Eng, 12,* 48–54.

Decety, J. (1996). Do imagined and executed actions share the same neural substrate? *Brain Research: Cognitive Brain Research, 3(2),* 87–93.

Dechent, P., Merboldt, K.D., and Frahm, J. (2004). Is the human primary motor cortex involved in motor imagery? *Cogn Brain Res, 19,* 138–144.

Derambure, P., Defebvre, L., Dujardin, K., Bourriez, J.L., Jacquesson, J.M., Destee, A. and Guieu, J.D. (1993). Effect of aging on the spatio–temporal pattern of event–related desynchronization during a voluntary movement. *Electroencephalogr Clin Neurophysiol, 89,* 197–203.

Dewan, E.M. (1967). Occipital alpha rhythm eye position and lens accommodation. *Nature, 214,* 975–977.

Durka, P.J., Ircha, D., Neuper, C., Pfurtscheller, G. (2001). Time-frequency microstructure of electroencephalogram desynchronization and synchronization. *Med Biol Eng Comput, 39(3),* 315–321.

Ehrsson, H.H., Geyer, S., and Naito, E. (2003). Imagery of voluntary movement of fingers, toes, and tongue activates corresponding body-part-specific motor representations. *J Neurophysiol, 90,* 3304–3316.

Elder, S.T., Lashley, J.K., Kedouri, N., Regenbogen, D., Martyn, S., Roundtree, G., and Grenier, C. (1986). Can subjects be trained to communicate through the use of EEG biofeedback? *Clin Biofeedback Health, 9,* 42–47.

Enzinger C.,Ropele S. Fazekas F., Loitfelder M., Gorani F., Seifert T., Reiter G., Neuper C., Pfurtscheller G. and Müller-Putz G. (2008) Brain motor system function in a patient with complete spinal cord injury following extensive brain-computer interface training. Exp Brain Res *190*(2), 215–223.

Fatourechi, M., Bashashati, A., Ward, R.K., and Birch, G.E. (2007). EMG and EOG artifacts in brain computer interface systems: a survey. *Clin Neurophysiol, 118,* 480–494.

Friedrich, E.V., McFarland, D.J., Neuper, C., Vaughan, T.M., Brunner, P., and Wolpaw, J.R. (2009). A scanning protocol for a sensorimotor rhythm-based brain-computer interface. *Biol Psychol, 80,* 169–175.

Gastaut, H., Naquet, R., Gastaut, Y. (1965). A study of the mu rhythm in subjects lacking one or more limbs. *Electroencephalogr. Clin. Neurophysiol, 18,* 720–721.

Gerloff, C., Hadley, J., Richard, J., Uenishi, N., Honda, M., and Hallett, M., (1998). Functional coupling and regional activation of human cortical motor areas during simple, internally paced and externally paced finger movements. *Brain, 121,* 1513–1531.

Goncharova, I. I., McFarland, D. J., Vaughan, T. M., and Wolpaw, J. R. (2003). EMG Contamination of EEG: Spectral and Topographical Characteristics. *Clin Neurophysiol, 114,* 1580–1593.

Graimann, B., Huggins, J. E., Levine S. P., and Pfurtscheller G. (2002). Visualization of significant ERD/ERS patterns in multichannel EEG and ECoG data. *Clin Neurophysiol, 113*(1), 43–47.

Graimann, B., and Pfurtscheller, G. (2006). Quantification and visualization of event-related changes in oscillatory brain activity in the time-frequency domain. *Prog Brain Res, 159,* 79–97.

Guger, C., Edlinger, G., Harkam, W., Niedermayer, I., and Pfurtscheller, G. (2003). How many people are able to operate an EEG-based brain-computer interface. *IEEE Trans Neural Sys Rehab Eng, 11,* 145–147.

Gysels, E., and Celka, P. (2004). Phase synchronization for the recognition of mental tasks in a brain computer interface. *IEEE Trans Neural Syst Rehab Eng, 12,* 406–415.

Hagemann, D., and Naumann, E. (2001). The effects of ocular artifacts on (lateralized) broadband power in the EEG. *Clin Neurophysiol, 112,* 215–231.

Halder, S., Agorastos, D., Veit, R., Hammer, E.M., Lee, S., Varkuit, B., Bogdan, M., Rosenstiel, W., Birbaumer, N., and Kübler, A. (2011). Neural mechanisms of brain-computer interface control. *Neuroimage, 55,* 1779–1790.

Hema, C.R., Paulraj, M.P., Yaacob, S., Adom, A.H., and Nagarajan, R. (2011). Asynchronous brain machine interface-based control of a wheelchair. *Adv Exp Med Biol, 696,* 565–572.

Hochberg, L.R., Serruya, M.D., Friehs, G.M., Mukand, J.A., Saleh, M., Caplan, A.H., Branner, A., Penn, R.D., and Donoghue, J.P. (2006). Neuronal ensemble control of prosthetic devices by a human with tetraplegia. *Nature, 442,* 164–171.

Ichikawa, N., and Ohira, H. (2004). Eyeblink activity as an index of cognitive processing: temporal distribution of eyeblinks as an indicator of expectancy in semantic priming. *Percept Mot Skills, 98,* 131–140.

Jaseja, H. (2007). Cerebral palsy: Interictal epileptiform discharges and cognitive impairment. *Clin Neurol Neurosurg, 109,* 549–552.

Jasper, H.H., and Andrew, H.L. (1938). Electro–encephalography III. normal differentiation of occipital and precentral regions in man. *Arch Neurol Psychiat, 39,* 96–115.

Jasper, H.H. and Penfield, W. (1949). Electrocorticograms in man: effect of the voluntary movement upon the electrical activity of the precentral gyrus. *Arch Psychiat Z Neurol, 183,* 163–174.

Jeannerod, M. (2001). Neural simulation of action: a unifying mechanism for motor cognition. *Neuroimage, 14,* 103–109.

Jurkiewicz, M.T., Gaetz, W.C., Bostan, A.C., and Cjeyme. D. (2006). Post-movement beta rebound is generated in motor cortex: Evidence from neuromagnetic recordings. *Neuroimage, 32,*1281–1289.

Keith, M.W., Peckham, P.H., Thrope, G.B., Stroh, K.C., Smith, B., Buckett, J.R., Kilgore, K.L., and Jatich, J.W. (1989). *J Hand Surg, 14,* 524–530.

Klostermann, F., Nikulin, VV, Kuhn, AA, Marzinzik, F, Wahl, M, Pogosyan, A, Kupsch, A, Schneider, GH, Brown, P, and Curio, G, (2007). Task-related differential dynamics of EEG alpha- and beta-band synchronization in cortico-basal motor structures. *Eur J Neurosci, 25,* 1604–1615.

Koshino, Y. and Niedermeyer, E. (1975). Enhancement of rolandic mu–rhythm by pattern vision, *Electroenceph. Clin. Neurophysiol, 38,* 535–538.

Kostov, A. and Polak, M. (2000). Parallel man-machine training in development of EEG-based cursor control. *IEEE Trans Rehabil Eng, 8,* 203–205.

Krauledat, M., Tangermann, M., Blankertz, B., and Müller, K.R. (2008). Towards zero training for brain-computer interfacing. *PLoS ONE, 13,* e2967.

Kreitmann, N. and Shaw, J.C. (1965). Experimental enhancement of alpha activity. *EEG Clin Neurophysiol, 18,* 147–155.

Kübler, A., Nijboer, F., Mellinger, J., Vaughan, T.M., Pawelzik, H., Schalk, G. McFarland, D.J., Birbaumer, N., and Wolpaw, J.R. (2005). Patients with ALS can use sensorimotor rhythms to operate a brain-computer interface. *Neurol, 64,*1775–1777.

Kuhlman, W.N. (1978). EEG feedback training: enhancement of somatosensory cortical activity. *Electroenceph Clin Neurophysiol, 45,* 290–294.

Lachaux, JP., Rodriguez, E., Martinerie, J., and Varela, FJ. (1999). Measuring phase synchrony in brain signals. *Hum Brain Mapp, 8,* 194–208.

Leeb, R.; Friedman, D.; Müller-Putz, G. R.; Scherer, R.; Slater, M. and Pfurtscheller, G. (2007). Self-paced (asynchronous) BCI control of a wheelchair in virtual environments: a case study with a tetraplegics. *Comput Intell Neurosci,* 2007, Article ID 79642.

Leeb, R.(2008). Brain-Computer Communication: Motivation, Aim and Impact of Virtual Feedback. PhD Thesis, Graz University of Technology.

Leuthardt, E.C., Schalk, G., Wolpaw, J.R., Ojemann, J.G., and Moran, D.W. (2006). A brain-computer interface using electrocorticographic signals in humans. *J Neural Eng, 1,* 63–71.

Lopes da Silva, F.H. (1991). Neural mechanisms underlying brain waves: from neural membranes to networks, *Electroenceph Clin Neurophysiol, 79,* 81–93.

Lopes da Silva, F.H. (2006). Event-related neural activities: what about phase? *Prog Brain Res, 159,* 3–17.

Lotte, F., Congedo, M., Lecuyer, A., Lamarche, F., and Arnaldi, B. (2007). A review of classification algorithms for EEG-based brain-computer interfaces. *J Neural Eng, 4,* 1–14.

Lotze, M., Montoya, P., Erb, M., et al. (1999). Activation of cortical and cerebellar motor areas during executed and imagined hand movements: an fMRI study. *J Cogn Neurosci 11,* 491–501.

Makeig, S. (1993). Auditory event-related dynamics of the EEG spectrum and effects of exposure to tones. *Electroenceph Clin Neurophysiol, 86,* 283–293.

Marple, S.L. *Digital spectral analysis with applications.* Englewood Cliffs, NJ: Prentice-Hall, 1987.

Mason, S.G. and Birch, G.E. (2000). A brain-controlled switch for asynchronous control applications. *IEEE Trans Biomed Eng, 47,* 1297–1307.

Mason, S.G., Bohringer, R., Borisoff, J.F., and Birch, G.E. (2004). Real-time control of a video game with a direct brain-computer interface. *J Clin Neurophysiol, 21,* 404–408.

McFarland, D.J., Krusienski, D.J., Sarnacki, W.A., and Wolpaw, J.R. (2008). Emulation of computer mouse control with a noninvasive brain-computer interface. *J Neural Eng, 5,* 101–110.

McFarland, D.J., Krusienski, D.J., and Wolpaw, J.R. (2006). Brain-computer interface signal processing at the Wadsworth Center: mu and sensorimotor beta rhythms. In: Neuper, K. and Klimesch, W. (Eds). *Prog Brain Res, 159,* 411–419.

McFarland, D.J., Lefkowitz, A.T., and Wolpaw, J.R. (1997). Design and operation of an EEG-based brain-computer interface with digital signal processing technology. *Behav Res Meth Inst Comput, 27,* 337–345.

McFarland, D.J., McCane, L.M., David, S.V., and Wolpaw, J.R. (1997). Spatial filter selection for EEG-based communication. *Electroenceph Clin Neurophysiol, 103,* 386–394.

McFarland D.J., Miner L.A., Vaughan T.M., and Wolpaw J.R. (2000). Mu and Beta Rhythm Topographies During Motor Imagery and Actual Movements. *Brain Topogr, 12,* 177–186.

McFarland, D.J., Neat, G.W., Read, R.F., and Wolpaw, J.R. (1993). An EEG-based method for graded cursor control. *Psychobiol, 21,* 77–81.

McFarland, D.J., Sarnacki, W.W., Vaughan, T.M., and Wolpaw, J.R. (2005). Brain-computer interface (BCI) operation: Signal and noise during early training sessions. *Clin Neurophysio, 116,* 56–62.

McFarland, D.J., Sarnacki, W.A., and Wolpaw, J.R. (2003). Brain-computer interface (BCI) operation: optimizing information transfer rates. *Biol Psychol, 63,* 237–251.

McFarland, D.J., Sarnacki, W.A., and Wolpaw, J.R. (2010). Electroencephalographic (EEG) control of three-dimensional movement. *J Neural Eng, 7,* 036007.

McFarland, D.J., Sarnacki, W.A., and Wolpaw, J.R. (2011). Should the parameters of a BCI translation algorithm be continually adapted? *J Neurosci Meth, 199,* 103–107.

McFarland, D.J., and Wolpaw, J.R., (2005). Sensorimotor rhythm-based brain-computer interface (BCI): Feature selection by regression improves performance. *IEEE Trans Neural Syst Rehabil Eng, 13,* 372–379.

Mellinger, J., Schalk, G., Braun, C., Preissl, H., Rosenstiel, W., Birbaumer, N., and Kübler, A. (2007). An MEG-based brain–computer interface (BCI). *NeuroImage, 36,* 581–593.

Millán, J. and Mouriño, J. (2003). Asynchronous BCI and local neural classifiers: an overview of the Adaptive Brain Interface project *IEEE Trans Neural Syst Rehabil Eng, 11,* 159–161.

Müller, K.-R. and Blankertz, B. (2006). Toward noninvasive brain computer interfaces. *IEEE Signal Proc Mag, 23,* 125–128.

Müller-Putz, G. R., Scherer, R, Pfurtscheller, G., and Rupp, R. (2005). EEG-based neuroprosthesis control: a step into clinical practice. *Neurosci Lett, 382,* 169–174.

Naeem, M., Brunner, C., Leeb, R., Graimann, B., and Pfurtscheller, G. (2006). Seperability of four-class motor imagery data using independent components analysis. *J Neural Eng, 3,* 208–216.

Neuper, C., Scherer, R., Reiner, M., and Pfurtscheller, G. (2005). Imagery of motor actions: differential effects of kinesthetic and visual-motor mode of imagery in single-trial EEG. *Cogn Brain Res, 25,* 668–677

Neuper, C., Müller, G.R., Kübler, A., Birbaumer, N., and Pfurtscheller, G. (2003). Clinical application of an EEG-based brain-computer interface: a case study in a patient with severe motor impairment. *Clin Neurophysiol, 114,* 399–409.

Neuper, C. and Pfurtscheller, G. (1999). Motor imagery and ERD, In: G. Pfurtscheller and F.H. Lopes da Silva (ed.), *Event-Related Desynchronization. Handbook of Electroencephalography and Clinical Neurophysiology.* Revised Edition *Vol. 6.* pp. 303–325 (Amsterdam: Elsevier).

Neuper, C. and Pfurtscheller, G. (2001a). Event-related dynamics of cortical rhythms: frequency-specific features and functional correlates. *Int J Psychophysiol, 43,* 41–58.

Neuper, C. and Pfurtscheller, G. (2001b). Evidence for distinct beta resonance frequencies related to specific sensorimotor cortical areas. *Clin Neurophysiol 112(11),* 2084–2097.

Neuper, C., Mueller-Putz, G.R., Scherer, R., and Pfurtscheller G. (2006). Motor imagery and EEG-based control of spelling devices and neuroprostheses. *Prog Brain Res, 159,* 393–409.

Neuper, C., Scherer, R., Wriessnegger, S., and Pfurtscheller, G. (2009). Motor imagery and action observation: Modulation of sensorimotor brain rhythms during mental control of a brain-computer interface. *Clin Neurophysiol, 120,* 239–247.

Nijboer, F., Furdea, A., Gunst, I., Mellinger, J., McFarland, D.J., Birbaumer, N., and Kübler, A. (2008). An auditory brain-computer interface (BCI). *J Neurosci Meth, 167,* 43–50.

Palaniappan, R. (2006). Utilizing gamma band to improve mental task based brain-computer interface design. *IEEE Trans Neural Syst Rehabil Eng, 14,* 299–303.

Pfurtscheller, G. (1981). Central beta rhyhm during sensorimotor activitiesin man. *Electroencephalogr Clin Neurophysiol 51,* 253–264.

Pfurtscheller, G. (1989). Functional topography during sensorimotor activation studied with event-related desynchronization mapping. *J Clin Neurophysiol, 6,* 75–84.

Pfurtscheller, G. (1992). Event–related synchronization (ERS): an electrophysiological correlate of cortical areas at rest. *Electroenceph Clin Neurophysiol, 83,* 62–69.

Pfurtscheller, G. and Aranibar, A. (1979). Evaluation of event–related desynchronization (ERD) preceding and following voluntary self–paced movements. *Electroenceph Clin Neurophysiol, 46,* 138–146.

Pfurtscheller, G. and Berghold, A. (1989). Patterns of cortical activation during planning of voluntary movement. *Electroenceph Clin Neurophysiol, 72,* 250–258.

Pfurtscheller, G., Brunner, C., Schlögl, A., and Lopes da Silva, F.H. (2006a). Mu rhythm (de)synchronization and EEG single-trial classification of different motor imagery tasks. *NeuroImage, 31,* 153–159.

Pfurtscheller, G., Flotzinger, D., and Kalcher, J. (1993). Brain-computer interface- a new communication device for handicapped persons. *J Microcomp Appl, 16,* 293–299.

Pfurtscheller, G., Graimann, B., Huggins, J.E., Levine, S.P., and Schuh, L.A. (2003). Spatiotemporal patterns of beta desynchronization and gamma synchronization in corticographic data during self-paced movement. *Clin Neurophysiol, 114,* 1226–1236.

Pfurtscheller, G., Guger, C., Müller, G., Krausz, G., and Neuper, C. (2000). Brain oscillations control hand orthosis in a tetraplegic. *Neurosci Lett, 292,* 211–214.

Pfurtscheller, G., Leeb, R., Keinrath, C., et al. (2006). Walking from thought. *Brain Res, 1071,* 145–152.

Pfurtscheller, G. and Lopes da Silva, F.H. (1999). Event-related EEG/MEG synchronization and desynchronization: basic principles. *Clin Neurophysiol, 110,* 1842–1857.

Pfurtscheller, G. and Lopes da Silva, F.H. (2011). EEG event-related desynchronization (ERD) and event-related synchronization ERS). In: *Niedermeyer`s Electroencephalography* 6th edition (Eds. D. Schoner and F. Lopes a Silva), Wolters Kluver, pp. 935–948.

Pfurtschelle r, G., Müller, G. R., Rupp, R., and Gerner, H. J. (2003b). "Thought"-control of functional electrical stimulation to restore hand grasp in a tetraplegic. *Neurosci Lett, 351(1),* 33–36.

Pfurtscheller, G., Müller-Putz, G.R., Schlögl, A., et al. (2006). 15 years of BCI research at Graz University of Technology: current projects. *IEEE Trans Neural Sys Rehabil Eng, 14,* 205–210.

Pfurtscheller, G. and Neuper, C. (1997). Motor imagery activates primary sensorimotor area in humans. *Neurosci Lett, 239,* 65–68.

Pfurtscheller, G. and Neuper, C. (2006). Future prospects of ERD/ERS in the context of brain-computer (BCI) developments. *Prog Brain Res, 159,* 433–437.

Pfurtscheller, G., Neuper, C., Brunner, C., and Lopes da Silva, F.H. (2005). Beta rebound after different types of motor imagery in man. *Neurosci Lett, 378,* 156–159.

Pfurtscheller, G., Neuper, C., Flotzinger, D., and Pregenzer, M. (1997). EEG-based discrimination between imagination of right and left hand movement. *Electroencephalogr Clin Neurophysiol, 103,* 642–651.

Pfurtscheller, G., Neuper, C., and Krausz, G. (2000). Functional dissociation of lower and upper frequency mu rhythms in relation to voluntary limb movement. *Clin Neurophysiol., 111,* 1873–1879.

Pfurtscheller, G., Scherer, R., Müller-Putz, G., and Lopes da Silva, F.H. (2008). Short-lived brain state after cued motor imagery in naïve subjects. *Eur J Neurosci 28,*1419–1426.

Pfurtscheller, G., and Solils-Escalante, T. (2009). Could the beta rebound in the EEG be suitable to realize a "brain switch"? *Clin Neurophysiol, 120,* 24–29

Pfurtscheller, G., Stancák Jr., A., and Neuper, C. (1996a). Post–movement beta synchronization. A correlate of an idling motor area? *Electroenceph Clin Neurophysiol, 98,* 281–293.

Pfurtscheller, G., Stancák, A., and Neuper, C. (1996). Event-related synchronization (ERS) in the alpha band–an electrophysiological correlate of cortical idling: A review. *Int J Psychophysiol., 24,* 39–46.

Pfurtscheller, G., and Neuper, C. (2010). Dynamics of sensorimotor oscillations in a motor task. In: B. Graimann, B. Allison, and G. Pfurtscheller (Eds.), *Brain-Computer Interfaces—Non-Invasive and Invasive Technologies.* Berlin, Springer, 47–64.

Pfurtscheller G., Solis-Escalante T., Ortner R. Lintortner P. and Müller-Putz G. (2010). Self-paced operation of an SSVEP-based orthosis with and without an imagery-based brain switch: "A feasibility study towards a hybrid BCI. *IEEE Trans Neural Systems Rehab Engng, 18/4,* 409–414.

Poldrack, R.A., Sabb, F.W., Foerde, K., Tom, S.M., Asarnow, R.F., Bookheimer, S.Y., and Knowlton, B.J. (2005). The neural correlates of motor skill automaticity. *J Neurosci, 25,* 5356–5364.

Porro, C.A., Francescato, M.P., Cettolo, V., Diamond, M.E., Baraldi, P., Zuiani, C., Bazzocchi, M., and di Prampero, P.E. (1996). Primary motor and sensory cortex activation during motor performance and motor imagery: a functional magnetic resonance imaging study. *J Neurosci 16,* 7688–7698.

Ramoser, H., Wolpaw, J.R., and Pfurtscheller, G. (1997). EEG-based communication: evaluation of alternative signal prediction methods. *Biomed Tech, 42,* 226–233.

Royer, A.S., Doud, A.J., Rose, M.L., and He, B. (2010). EEG control of a virtual helicopter in 3-dimensional space using intelligent control strategies. *IEEE Trans Neural Syst Rehab Eng, 18,* 581–589, 2010.

Salmelin, R., Hämäläinen, M., Kajola, M., and Hari, R. (1995). Functional segregation of movement related rhythmic activity in the human brain. *Neuroimage, 2,* 237–243.

Scherer, R., Müller, G.R., Neuper, C., Graimann, B., and Pfurtscheller, G. (2004). An asynchronously controlled EEG-based virtual keyboard: improvement of the spelling rate. *IEEE Trans Biomed Eng, 51,* 979–984

Scherer, R., Schlogl, A., Lee, F., Bischof, H., Jansa, J., and Pfurtscheller, G. (2007). The self-paced Graz brain-computer interface: methods and applications. *Comput Intell Neurosci,* 79826.

Scherer R. (2008). Towards practical Brain-Computer Interfaces: Self-paced operation and reduction of the number of EEG sensors. PhD Thesis, Graz University of Technology.

Seligman, M.E. (1972). Learned helplessness. *Annual Review of Medicine, 23,* 407–412.

Shenoy, P., Krauledat, M., Blankertz, B., Rao, R.P., and Müller, K.R. (2006). Towards adaptive classification for BCI. *J Neural Eng, 3,* 13–23.

Silvestrini, N., and Gendolla, G.H.E. (2007). Mood effects on autonomic activity in mood regulation. *Psychophysiol, 44,* 650–659.

Stancák Jr., A. and Pfurtscheller, G. (1996). Mu–rhythm changes in brisk and slow self–paced finger movements. *Neuroreport, 7,* 1161–1164.

Stancák Jr., A. and Pfurtscheller, G. (1996b). The effects of handedness and type of movement on the contralateral preponderance of mu–rhythm desynchronization. *Electroenceph Clin Neurophysiol, 99,* 174–182.

Suffczynski, P., Pjin, J., Pfurtscheller, G., and Lopes da Silva, F. (1999). Event-related dynamics of alpha band rhythms: a neuronal network model of focal ERD/surround ERS. In: G. Pfurtscheller and F. Lopes da Silva (Eds.), *Event-Related Desynchronization. Handbook of Electroencephalography and Clinical Neurophysiology,* Vol. 6 (pp. 67–85). Amsterdam: Elsevier.

Tallon-Baudry, C. and Bertrand, O. (1999). Oscillatory gamma activity in humans and its role in object representations. *Trends Cogn Sci 3*(4), 151–162.

Thomas, K.P., Guan, C., Lau, C.T., Vinod, A.P., and Ang, K.K. (2011). Adaptive tracking of discriminative frequency components in electroencephalograms for a robust brain-computer interface. *J Neur Eng, 8,* 036007.

Toro, C., Deuschl, G., Thatcher, R., Sato, S., Kufta, C., and Hallett, M. (1994). Event–related desynchronization and movement–related cortical potentials on the ECoG and EEG. *Electroenceph Clin Neurophysiol, 93,* 380–389.

Vaughan, T.M., Miner, L. A., McFarland, D. J. and Wolpaw, J. R. (1998). EEG-based communication: analysis of concurrent EMG activity. *Electroenceph Clin Neurophysiol, 107,*428–433.

Vidaurre, C., Sannelli, C., Miller, K.R., and Blankertz, B. (2011). Co-adaptive calibration to improve BCI efficiency. *J Neur Eng, 8,* 025009.

Vidaurre, C., Schlogl, A., Cabeza, R., Scherer, R., and Pfurtscheller, G. (2006). A fully on-line adaptive BCI. *IEEE Trans Biomed Eng, 53,* 1214–1219.

Whitham, E.M., Lewis, T., Pope, K.J., Fitzgibbon, S.P., Clark, C.R., Loveless, S., DeLosAngeles, D., Wallace, A.K., Broberg, M., and Willoughby, J.O. (2008). Thinking activates EMG in scalp electrical recordings. *Clin Neurophysiol, 119,* 1166–1175.

Williams, D., Tijssen, M., van Bruggen, G., Bosch, A., Insola, A., Lazzaro, V., Mazzone, P., Oliviero, A., Quartarone, A., Speelman, H., and Brown, P.,(2002). Dopamine-dependent changes in the functional connectivity between basal ganglia and cerebral cortex in humans. *Brain, 125,* 1558–1569.

Witgert, M., Salamone, A.R., Strutt, A.M., Jawaid, A., Massman, P.J., Bradshaw, M., Mosnik, D., Appel, S.H., and Schulz, P.E. (2010). Frontal-lobe mediated behavioral dysfunction in amyotrophic lateral sclerosis. *Eur J Neurosci, 17,* 103–110.

Wolpaw, J.R. (2010). Brain-computer interface research comes of age: traditional assumptions meet emerging realities. *J Motor Behav, 42,* 351–353.

Wolpaw, J. R., Birbaumer, N., McFarland, D. J., Pfurtscheller, G., and Vaughan, T. M. (2002). Brain-computer interfaces for communication and control. *Clin Neurophysiol, 113,* 767–791.

Wolpaw, J. R. and McFarland, D. J. (1994). Multichannel EEG-based brain-computer communication. *Electroencephal Clin Neurophysiol, 90,* 444–449.

Wolpaw, J.R and McFarland, D.J. (2004). Control of a two-dimensional movement signal by a non-invasive brain-computer interface in humans. *Proc Nat Acad Sci, 101,*17849–17854.

Wolpaw, J.R., McFarland, D.J., Neat, G.W., and Forneris, C.A. (1991). An EEG-based brain-computer interface for cursor control. *Electroencephal Clin Neurophysiol, 78,* 252–259

Wolpaw, J.R., McFarland, D.J., Vaughan, T.M., and Schalk, G. (2003). The Wadsworth Center brain-computer interface (BCI) research and development program. *IEEE Trans Neural Sys Rehabil Eng, 11,* 204–207

Wriessnegger, S.C, Kurzmann, J., and Neuper, C. (2008). Spatio-temporal differences in brain oxygenation between movement execution and imagery: a multichannel near-infrared spectroscopy study. *Int J Psychophysiol. 67*(1), 54–63

Yoshida, M. (2004). Amyotropic lateral sclerosis with dementia: the clinico-pathological spectrum. *Neuropathol, 24,* 87–102.

14 | BCIs THAT USE STEADY-STATE VISUAL EVOKED POTENTIALS OR SLOW CORTICAL POTENTIALS

BRENDAN Z. ALLISON, JOSEF FALLER, AND CHRISTA NEUPER

Although P300 evoked responses and sensorimotor rhythms (see chapters 12 and 13 in this volume) have received the most attention as EEG features for BCIs, they are not the only EEG features that have been or are being used for BCI development. Indeed, several of the earliest BCIs used two other kinds of features, steady-state visual evoked potentials (SSVEPs) and slow cortical potentials (SCPs), and these features, particularly SSVEPs, continue to be relevant to BCI development. They are addressed in this chapter.

STEADY-STATE VISUAL EVOKED POTENTIALS AND SSVEP-BASED BCIs

An EEG *evoked potential* (EP) is a distinctive pattern of positive and negative voltage deflections that is time-locked to a specific sensory stimulus or event (see chapter 3 in this volume). Visual evoked potentials (VEPs) are those evoked by sudden visual stimuli, such as a light flash, the appearance of an image, or an abrupt change in color or pattern. The most prominent VEP deflections, or *components*, include N70 and P100, which tend to occur about 70 and 100 ms after the eliciting visual stimulus, respectively (Celesia and Peachey, 2005). They are generated in or near the primary visual cortex and thus are most prominent over occipital scalp areas.

Steady-state VEPs (SSVEPs) are stable oscillations in voltage that are elicited by rapid repetitive stimulation such as a strobe light, a light-emitting diode (LED), or a pattern-reversing checkerbox presented on a monitor. The successive stimulus presentations evoke similar responses, and the overlap of these responses produces a steady-state oscillation. SSVEPs may be analyzed by conventional averaging methods or by frequency analysis. Frequency analysis normally reveals a peak at the frequency of stimulation, as well as peaks at higher harmonic frequencies.

SSVEP AND RELATED PARADIGMS

In a standard SSVEP-based BCI, the user is presented with a display of concurrent repetitive stimuli (e.g., several LEDs) that are located at different places in the visual field. Each stimulus is presented at a fixed frequency that differs from the other stimuli. Each stimulus represents a specific BCI output (e.g., type a specific letter, move the wheelchair in a specific direction, etc.). The user typically makes a selection by fixating on (i.e., gazing at) the stimulus that represents the desired BCI output. The BCI computes the frequency spectrum of the occipital EEG. The frequency spectrum usually shows a peak that matches the rate of the stimulus on which the user is fixating, and the BCI then produces the output represented by that stimulus. Figure 14.1 depicts a user who fixates on the box that flickers at 8 Hz, shows the frequency spectrum of the EEG recorded from occipital location O2, the development over time of the power in each frequency band, and the topographical distribution of power in the band at 8 Hz (i.e., the frequency of the stimulus the user is gazing at). EEG power is concentrated at that frequency and its harmonic frequencies, and the 8-Hz activity is focused over occipital cortex.

The standard SSVEP BCI paradigm, in which each of the repetitive stimuli occurs at a specific frequency, is called the *frequency-modulated visual evoked potential* (f-VEP) BCI paradigm (Bin et al., 2009). It is shown in figure 14.2, which also shows two arrhythmic repetitive stimulation paradigms that have been used in BCIs. In a *t-VEP paradigm*, the different stimuli are mutually independent and nonoverlapping. The BCI computes the average VEP for each stimulus and produces the output represented by the stimulus that elicits the largest VEP. In a *c- (or m-sequence) VEP paradigm*, each stimulus occurs in a pseudorandom pattern that is nearly orthogonal to the patterns of all the other stimuli. The BCI computes the correlation between the EEG and a template computed for each stimulus. Typically, the stimulus on which the user is fixating produces the highest correlation.

Bin et al. (2009) compared the accuracy and speed of BCIs that used f-, c-, and t-VEP paradigms. They found that the c-VEP paradigm performed best, with the f-VEP paradigm yielding intermediate performance, and the t-VEP BCI much worse. One major advantage of the f-VEP paradigm is that it does not require stimulus time- or phase-locked recording of the EEG, and hence it is well suited to user-paced, asynchronous operation, which is a very natural way of interacting with a computer system. Future SSVEP BCI development will probably further explore c-(m-sequence) paradigms and other stimulus presentation variants. Although these alternatives are technically not SSVEP paradigms (i.e., their stimuli are not rhythmic), they are typically grouped with SSVEP BCIs for convenience.

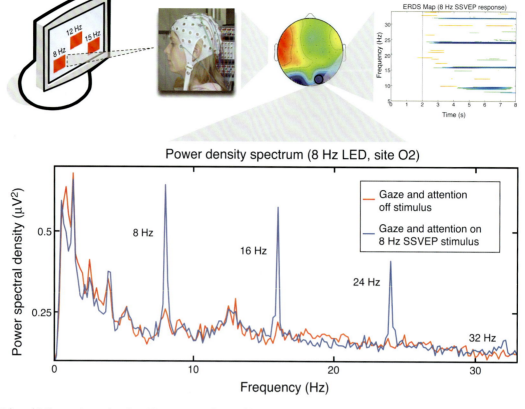

Figure 14.1 *SSVEP-based BCI operation and analysis. The user views three red boxes each of which flickers at a different frequency. By choosing to focus on the 8-Hz box, she elicits EEG activity at 8 Hz and its harmonic frequencies (as shown in the frequency spectrum of EEG activity at occipital location O2; blue trace in bottom panel). Also shown for comparison is the spectrum produced when the user is not looking at one of the boxes (red trace). It lacks the 8-Hz and harmonic peaks but is otherwise similar. The 8-Hz activity is focused over occipital areas (as shown in the topographical plot [top middle] of power at 8 Hz [with blue indicating higher power]). The top right panel shows that this increased activity does not occur immediately. The vertical line indicates the time at which the user decides to look at the 8-Hz box. Power at 8 Hz and its harmonic frequencies increase significantly (p < 0.01 indicated by blue-green) over the next 2 sec. (Yellow indicates significant power decrease.)*

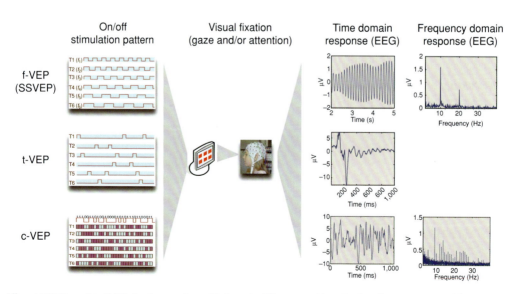

Figure 14.2 *Three different SSVEP or related VEP stimulus paradigms. T1–6 are six different repetitive stimuli each representing a different BCI output. The left panels indicate when the stimuli turn on (trace high) or off (trace low). Note that only the f-VEP (i.e., SSVEP) paradigm uses rhythmic stimuli (as indicated by the evenly spaced square pulses). The right panels show the resulting EEG measures. Note that the frequency-domain response is not shown in the t-VEP case since t-VEPs are typically analyzed only in the time domain. See text for explication. (Adapted from Bin et al., 2009.)*

EARLY SSVEP-LIKE BCIs

Early BCI studies used VEPs as an input for BCI systems. In the first BCI described in the published literature (Vidal 1973, 1977), the user viewed a maze and a checkerbox stimulus. By directing gaze at one of four fixation points surrounding the checkerbox stimulus (and thus producing a VEP that reflected which quadrant of the visual field the stimulus was in), the user could move a cursor in one of four directions and thereby move through the maze. The system recorded bipolar EEG from four occipital electrode pairs and could identify the correct fixation point (and thus the correct direction) with >90% accuracy.

Sutter (1992) developed a BCI that used an m-sequence (c-VEP) stimulation paradigm. As shown in figure 14.3 (lower right), the user viewed a display with 64 selections (i.e., 64 different stimuli). The system was programmable such that each of these 64 selections could lead to another menu of new selections. For example, selecting a letter could bring up a second menu with words beginning with that letter. This early, very thorough BCI research effort explored epidural recording electrodes and wireless signal transmission, evaluated use by people who were severely disabled, and achieved performance that remains impressive.

RECENT SSVEP-BASED BCI DESIGNS

Over the last 12 years, a wide variety of studies have applied standard (f-VEP) SSVEP-based BCIs to a range of different applications and further defined their main characteristics. Middendorf et al. (2000) developed an SSVEP-based BCI that could control a functional electrical stimulator (FES) to initiate knee flexion. The same article also described an SSVEP BCI that could control the roll position of a flight simulator, and explored the effects of discrete (intermittent) versus proportional (continuous) feedback during training. Although the type of feedback did not matter, performance did improve with training, an important observation that was subsequently confirmed (Allison et al., 2006).

Many other SSVEP-based BCI studies have explored aeronautical or other navigation applications. For example, Lalor et al. (2005) introduced a game in which players could use an SSVEP BCI to help an avatar called a "Mawg" to walk a tightrope. As the Mawg crossed the tightrope, it sometimes leaned to its left or right. Players were instructed to help stabilize the Mawg by focusing on one of two oscillating (i.e., pattern reversing) checkerboxes. (The authors commented that some players purposely focused on the wrong checkerbox, causing the Mawg to fall more quickly. This anecdote underscores a concern in BCI research, which is the difficulty of knowing whether users are actually complying with instructions.)

Müller-Putz et al. (2005) found that basing selection on three rather than two of the harmonic peaks in the frequency spectrum significantly improved accuracy for a four-choice SSVEP-based BCI. Subsequent studies confirmed the value of using harmonic peaks and also showed that some subjects had strong third-harmonic peaks (Allison et al., 2008; Müller-Putz et al., 2008; Brunner et al., 2010a).

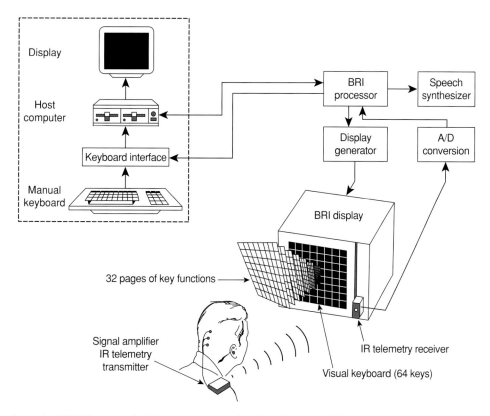

Figure 14.3 Overview of an early c-VEP BCI system called a brain-response interface (BRI). The user could select one of 64 choices in an 8 × 8 matrix by focusing on the corresponding cell. Each cell blinked in a different phase of a pseudorandom binary sequence (more specifically, a maximum length sequence pattern). As indicated, this BCI supports an elaborate menu structure and uses wireless signal transmission. (From Sutter, 1992.)

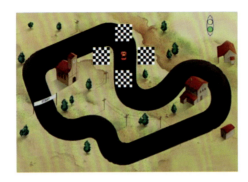

Figure 14.4 *Screenshot of an SSVEP BCI to navigate a virtual car around a racetrack. The subject focuses on one of the four checkerboard patterns. Each of the 36 subfields switches between black and white at a different stimulus frequency. The four checkerboxes move with the car. (From Martinez et al., 2007.)*

Trejo et al. (2006) and Martinez et al. (2007) (see fig. 14.4) described SSVEP-based BCIs that allowed the user to move a map and a car, respectively, in one of four directions by focusing on one of four oscillating checkerboxes. Such BCIs might provide hands-free functioning for people such as astronauts. With such designs, performance might be improved by simultaneously focusing on two different stimuli to produce diagonal movements (Müller et al., 2003; Allison et al., 2007a).

Faller et al. (2010) described two SSVEP-based BCIs that allowed users to navigate an avatar through immersive virtual-reality or augmented-reality environments by focusing on one of four oscillating stimuli each of which corresponded to a movement command. For example, users could move through a virtual-reality slalom course. The slalom course included a rest area in which the user did not move. This element tested the performance of a "no-control state", which is especially important for BCIs (including SSVEP-based BCIs) that use asynchronous operating protocols (see discussion in chapter 10), since unintended (i.e., false-positive) outputs may be a major problem for asynchronous BCI systems (e.g., Pfurtscheller et al., 2010b).

IMPORTANT ISSUES FOR SSVEP-BASED BCIs

The traditional understanding is that SSVEP-based BCIs operate by determining which stimulus the user is fixating on. For this reason, SSVEP-based BCIs have been described as *dependent BCIs* (see chapter 1 in this volume), that is, they depend on the user's muscle-based control of gaze direction and they might thus be of limited value to users who lack reliable gaze control (Wolpaw et al., 2002; Gao et al., 2003).

However, it has become clear that SSVEPs are not entirely dependent on muscle-based gaze. Recent work shows that SSVEP BCIs can function without gaze fixation (although fixation gaze can considerably improve performance) (Kelly et al., 2005; Allison et al., 2008). SSVEP-based BCIs can detect which stimulus the user is attending to, even if the user is not gazing directly at it. Attending to the stimulus, even when not gazing at it, increases the amplitude in the fundamental and harmonic spectral peaks associated with that stimulus. This effect can be detected in a number of ways, including spectral analysis,

bandpower, or correlation analysis (Kelly et al., 2005; Brunner et al., 2010a). Hence, the BCI can determine which stimulus the user is attending to by detecting frequencies in occipital EEG that correspond to one of the oscillating stimuli (see fig. 14.1).

In practice, people typically do look at the stimulus that represents the desired BCI output, unless disability prevents them from doing so or the experimenter asks them not to do so. Thus, in many situations and applications, SSVEP BCIs operate essentially as eye-tracking systems.

Although the rapid visual stimuli used by SSVEP-based BCIs do not appear to be annoying or fatiguing to most people, they may annoy elderly users (Allison et al., 2010c). With higher stimulus rates (above about 35 Hz), the stimuli do not appear to flicker and they produce less annoyance or fatigue. However, the SSVEPs resulting from these high-frequency stimuli are harder to detect. One method of dealing with this is the phase-rectified signal averaging (PRSA) technique, which effectively enhances quasiperiodic oscillations in nonstationary signals (like the EEG). The method aligns (i.e., phase-rectifies) and averages equal-length signal segments relative to automatically selected anchor points. The power density spectrum of the resulting EEG shows pronounced peaks at the frequencies of quasiperiodic oscillations (i.e., the stimulus the user is fixating on) while other spectral components are attenuated (Bauer et al., 2006). Garcia-Molina and Mihajlovic (2010) showed that PRSA improved performance for high-frequency SSVEP stimuli—but not to the level achieved with standard lower-frequency stimuli.

FUTURE DIRECTIONS FOR SSVEP-BASED BCIs

SSVEP BCIs are likely to have a bright future. They involve a straightforward user task (i.e., to focus on the stimulus that represents the desired BCI output), do not require significant training, and work in most prospective users (Allison et al., 2010a, 2010b, 2010c; Brunner et al., 2011). They have long been appreciated for their high information-transfer rate (ITR) (e.g., Sutter 1992), which continues to improve (e.g., Wang et al., 2010) and will probably increase further in the near future.

Gaze dependence remains an issue. Efforts continue to explore this question for SSVEP-based BCIs as well as for P300-based BCIs (e.g., Brunner et al., 2010b; Treder and Blankertz, 2010) (see chapter 12). Integrating the stimuli within monitor-based applications and placing them near the center of the visual field could reduce the need to shift gaze. Indeed, embedding oscillating stimuli within graphically immersive environments is a major challenge for future SSVEP BCIs (Faller et al., 2010).

At the same time, SSVEP-based BCIs may not be useful to people with severely compromised vision. For this reason, BCIs that use steady-state tactile or auditory stimuli are being explored. Müller-Putz et al. (2006) described a BCI that used attention-driven amplitude modulation of steady-state somatosensory evoked potentials (SSSEPs) to discriminate between two different repetitive tactile stimuli. The system stimulated each of the user's index fingers at a different frequency. As with

SSVEPs, frequency analysis of the SSSEPs showed fundamental and harmonic spectral peaks that corresponded to the frequency of the attended stimulus. By concentrating on the left or right finger, users could increase the spectral peaks associated with the left or right stimulus, respectively. The change was detected by linear discriminant analysis (LDA) (see chapter 8).

Kim et al. (2011) tested a BCI based on auditory steady-state evoked potentials (ASSEP). Subjects heard pure tones from two different sources. One source switched on and off at 37 Hz, and the other one at 43 Hz. The frequency spectrum of the ASSEP depended on which stimulus the user was attending to. Although the accuracy and speed of these two nonvisual steady-state evoked potential-based BCIs were low relative to most other BCIs, they represent initial research efforts and there are many possible options for improving their performance. These nonvisual BCIs could provide communication and control to users with severely impaired vision and, perhaps, also to healthy users whose vision is engaged in other tasks (e.g., driving, watching a movie, or using another kind of BCI).

In recent years *hybrid BCIs* have drawn considerable attention (for review, see Pfurtscheller et al., 2010a; Millán et al., 2010). As defined in chapter 1, a hybrid BCI combines two different kinds of BCIs or combines a BCI with a conventional muscle-based control device (e.g., a keyboard, a mouse, a joystick). Many hybrid BCIs include an SSVEP-based BCI output.

In one hybrid design, the user could turn an SSVEP-based BCI on or off by using a sensorimotor-rhythm (SMR)-based switch operated by imagining foot movements (Pfurtscheller et al., 2010b). Horki et al. (2011) described a hybrid BCI in which motor imagery controlled grasp function and an SSVEP-based BCI controlled elbow function. Panicker et al. (2011) used SSVEP activity to ascertain whether the user was paying attention to a P300-based BCI. If no SSVEP activity was detected, the P300-based BCI did not output any target character but simply indicated a "no-control" state by providing an "=" symbol as feedback. Hence, the SSVEP signal effectively turned the P300 BCI into an asynchronous BCI. Finally, a series of recent studies explored hybrid BCIs that use SSVEP and SMR activity simultaneously (Allison et al., 2010a and 2010b; Brunner et al., 2010a and 2011). They showed that the combination could improve accuracy and that it could enable the user to simultaneously move a cursor in one dimension with SMR activity and in a second dimension with SSVEP activity.

SLOW CORTICAL POTENTIALS AND SCP-BASED BCIs

SLOW CORTICAL POTENTIALS

Chapter 13 in this volume discussed BCIs that use SMRs, which are recorded over sensorimotor cortex and are affected by actual or imagined movement. SMRs are EEG features that are analyzed in the frequency domain (e.g., frequency on the x-axis) and thus are often referred to as frequency-domain activity. Additional EEG features associated with motor

function are measured in the time domain and thus are referred to as time-domain activity. Movement or movement imagery is typically associated with relatively slow changes in the voltages recorded over sensorimotor cortex. These are called *slow cortical potentials* (SCPs). SCPs are event-related potentials that are time-locked and phase-locked to specific sensorimotor events (i.e., they occur at predictable times before, during, or after specific events). SCPs typically consist of negative potential shifts that precede actual or imagined movement or cognitive tasks (e.g., mental arithmetic). They are thought to represent cortical activation in preparation for action (Birbaumer et al., 1990; Shibasaki and Hallett, 2006). An SCP is typically followed by a biphasic wave referred to as the *movement-related potential* (Colebatch, 2007).

The *Bereitschaftspotential* (or *readiness potential*) is a negative SCP that usually begins 500–1000 ms before a self-initiated movement (Kornhuber and Deecke, 1965; Altenmüller et al. 2005; Shibasaki and Hallett, 2006). It has several components that differ in onset time and topographical distribution and probably reflect activity in the supplementary motor area and in primary motor and sensory cortices. Its amplitude and topography are affected by movement type and the muscles involved, as well as by psychological variables.

The *contingent negative variation (CNV)* is a negative SCP that begins 200–500 ms after a stimulus (*S1*) that warns that an imperative stimulus (*S2*) (i.e., a stimulus that requires a particular action) will occur one to several seconds later (Walter et al. 1964). The action may be motor or cognitive. The CNV is distributed over frontal areas and over the regions directly involved in the action, and it is affected by motivational and task-specific factors (Altenmüller et al., 2005).

Like SMRs, SCPs and related potentials over sensorimotor areas are associated with motor imagery as well as with actual movements (Beisteiner et al., 1995; Cunnington et al., 1996). The involvement of primary motor areas in movement imagery is supported by dipole-source analysis of electric and magnetic fields (Lang et al., 1996). Thus, these time-domain phenomena provide further evidence that sensorimotor cortical areas are involved not only in actual limb movements, but also in imagination of the same movements.

Although SCPs are typically recorded from the scalp and are thought to reflect the activity of cortical sensorimotor areas (Colebatch, 2007), recent studies in patients with electrodes implanted for therapeutic deep-brain stimulation find similar activity in subcortical brain structures. For example, SCPs comparable to those recorded over the cortex can be recorded from the subthalamic nucleus (Paradiso et al., 2003).

SCP-BASED BCIs

As noted, SCP activity may be modulated by many cognitive activities, such as moving or performing arithmetic. SCP BCI users learn to perform mental tasks to produce SCP changes that can be detected by a BCI and used for control. This training, which is essentially operant conditioning (Kübler et al., 2001; Allison et al., 2007b; Neuper and Pfurtscheller, 2010), requires repeated sessions over weeks or months and is not effective in some prospective users.

In early studies, subjects used their SCP control to move a rocket ship icon up or down on a computer screen in response to a tone cue indicating the correct direction (e.g., Lutzenberger et al., 1979; Elbert et al., 1980). These studies used this paradigm to explore the impact of SCP training on a variety of disorders, including epilepsy, alcohol dependency, schizophrenia, and different types of depression (Schneider et al., 1992a, 1992b, 1993; Kotchoubey et al., 1996; Leins et al., 2007). They generally had clinical or basic-science (rather than communication and control) goals, and although the publications reporting these studies did not mention the term "BCI" in the title or abstract, their paradigm clearly qualifies as a BCI paradigm.

In a typical SCP-based BCI, the user communicates through a series of trials. In each trial a possible selection is offered. Each trial has two time intervals: a baseline interval followed by an active-control interval (Lutzenberger et al., 1979; Kübler et al., 1999). During the baseline interval, the user rests. During the active control interval, the user either generates an SCP (e.g., by performing a specific mental task) in order to make the selection or does not generate one (i.e., continues to rest) in order to ignore the selection. For example, a user spelling a letter selects the first half of the alphabet (if it contains the desired letter) or ignores it and waits for the second half to be offered in the next trial. In subsequent trials the chosen half of the alphabet is progressively subdivided until a single letter is selected.

These early SCP BCIs were especially slow because users could make only one selection every 10 sec (at best). Subsequently Kübler et al. (1999) described an SCP-based BCI that allowed a selection every 4 sec. The baseline interval and active control interval were each 2 sec. Since only the last 500 msec of the baseline interval were used in data analysis, the first 1.5 sec gave the user time to return to a resting state. Three users with ALS were trained on a task in which they directed a ball from the center of the screen toward a rectangular box located at one of the edges of the screen. All subjects were able to control the ball's vertical position through SCP activity recorded from site Cz, referenced against both mastoids (in two subjects) or the nasion (in the other subject). Depending on training, some subjects were also able to control the horizontal axis via SCP differences between channels C3 and C4.

Subjects were trained until they reached 70% accuracy on a three-trial sequence, such as "keep the ball in the center" twice and then "hit the rectangle at the bottom." This required months of training. They were then switched to a language support program (LSP) that allowed spelling. The LSP presented letters or groups of letters on the bottom half of the monitor. Whenever a letter or group of letters appeared on the bottom, subjects could move the ball toward it with SCP activity or they could ignore it. If subjects chose to ignore it, another choice was presented. This process continued until subjects made a selection that contained the target letter. Then, this group of letters was split into two halves presented sequentially on the bottom of the monitor, and the process continued until the target letter was selected. This study and the concurrently published study by Birbaumer et al. (1999) were among the first to validate BCIs as assistive technologies for severely disabled users in real-world settings. This article also suggested that such users might require more training than healthy users, since 13 healthy users who were also assessed showed more promising results with less training.

Birbaumer et al. (1999) described a SCP-based BCI spelling system. Two users with severe ALS learned to use SCPs to control an LSP system similar to that used by Kübler et al., (1999). The report included the first full message written by one user, named in the article as Hans Peter Salzmann. Mr. Salzmann produced about two characters per min, and his message clearly reflects that he was both mentally active and very grateful for his BCI communication system. He continued to use this BCI until his death in 2007.

Later work expanded the range of applications available to an SCP-based BCI. These included an alternate spelling system, a web browser that was later upgraded in numerous ways, and a three-layer selection system (Kaiser et al., 2002; Hinterberger et al., 2004a; Bensch et al., 2007). Additional SCP studies explored basic-science issues and investigated SCPs in conjunction with functional magnetic resonance imaging (fMRI) and transcranial magnetic stimulation (TMS) (Kübler et al., 2002; Hinterberger et al., 2004b, 2005).

POSSIBLE FUTURE USES OF SCP-BASED BCIs

For about 25 years, SCP BCIs were among the dominant BCI research approaches (e.g., Lutzenberger et al., 1979; Birbaumer et al., 1999; Kübler et al., 2001; Wolpaw et al., 2002; Hinterberger et al., 2004a; Birbaumer and Cohen, 2007). SCP-based BCIs were grounded in extensive basic and clinical research and have been validated in people with severe disabilities and in home settings. However, over the past decade several fundamental problems with SCP-based BCIs have greatly limited interest in their further development. First, as is clearly evident from the studies described here, they are quite slow. Although Kübler et al. (1999) did succeed in shortening the time per selection from 10 sec to 4 sec, they reported that efforts to further reduce the time per selection were not successful because the users said that shorter trials were exhausting. Second, SCP BCIs do not allow good multidimensional control. Although efforts to attain multidimensional control with SMR BCIs have been successful (e.g., Wolpaw and McFarland, 1994, 2004; Scherer et al., 2004; McFarland et al., 2010; Royer et al., 2010), SCP BCIs that allow successful simultaneous control of more than one dimension have been less successful (Kübler et al., 1999). Third, SCP BCIs are very prone to error, and fourth, extensive training is necessary. Moreover, when subjects who used SCP BCIs were also given an opportunity to try an SMR or P300 BCI, they preferred one of the two latter approaches (Birbaumer and Cohen, 2007; Allison et al., 2010b). Taken together, these factors explain why interest in SCP-based BCIs has diminished.

However, new SCP-based BCI designs might serve to enhance (see chapter 1 of this volume) other kinds of BCI control or muscle-based control. In an offline study Garipelli et al. (2009) showed changes in the CNV associated with anticipation. Such technology could be very useful in various ways. For example, the authors suggested that a BCI wheelchair-control system could use such a CNV-based anticipation measure to determine whether the user wanted to enter the next room or to continue down the corridor. By recognizing anticipation, SCP analysis might improve the performance of the SMR-based system described by Friedrich et al. (2009). Similar BCI designs might also be valuable for marketing studies, usability testing, basic research, and other applications. In recent work Bai et al. (2011) explored SCPs and SMR changes that precede voluntary movement (Kornhuber and Deecke, 1965; Pfurtscheller and Aranibar, 1979) (see chapter 13). The system detected movement onset an average of 0.62 sec before it occurred with a low false positive rate. Neurofeedback paradigms that train SCP activity might also prove useful in a variety of disorders (e.g., Leins et al., 2007).

SUMMARY

This chapter describes steady-state visual evoked potentials (SSVEPs), slow cortical potentials (SCPs), and BCIs based on these signals. SSVEPs are produced by repetitive stimuli (e.g., a flashing light or a pattern-reversing checkerboard) and are focused over occipital cortex. With a rhythmic stimulus, they typically display a peak at the frequency of the stimulus and at several harmonic frequencies.

In the standard SSVEP-based BCI, the user views a set of stimuli that are placed at different locations in the visual field and that flash at different rates. The user looks at the stimulus that represents the desired BCI output, and the frequency spectrum shows peaks corresponding to that stimulus. Although gaze fixation is extremely important in producing SSVEPs, SSVEPs can also reveal the stimulus that a user is simply attending to, even without gaze fixation.

BCIs based on SSVEPs and similar signals can provide relatively robust and rapid communication and have been applied to a variety of applications including word-processing, navigation tasks, and computer games. Steady-state evoked potentials evoked by somatosensory or auditory stimuli might also be used for BCIs, particularly for people with impaired vision.

Slow cortical potentials (SCPs) are slow, mainly negative, voltage shifts recorded over sensorimotor or frontal cortical areas. They precede and coincide with imagined or actual motor actions or cognitive tasks. With extensive training, people can learn to control SCPs and use them to operate spelling programs and other applications. Although SCP-based BCIs were used successfully in the past by people with severe disabilities (e.g., ALS), this BCI modality receives little attention at present because it is inherently slow, allows only one dimension of control, requires extensive training, and is prone to error. In the future, SCP-based BCI paradigms may prove useful as therapeutic neurofeedback tools or as adjuncts to other BCI or conventional control modalities (e.g., by allowing recognition of anticipation in the user).

REFERENCES

Allison, B. Z., Boccanfuso, J. B., Agocs, C., McCampbell, L. A., Leland, D. S., Gosch, C., et al. (2006). Sustained use of an SSVEP BCI under adverse conditions. *Proceedings of the 13th Annual Cognitive Neuroscience Society Meeting*, 129.

Allison, B. Z., Brunner, C., Grissmann, S., & Neuper, C. (2010a). Toward a multidimensional "hybrid" BCI based on simultaneous SSVEP and ERD activity. Program No. 227.4. *Society for Neuroscience Conference*. San Diego, CA.

Allison, B. Z., Brunner, C., Kaiser, V., Müller-Putz, G. R., Neuper, C., & Pfurtscheller, G. (2010b). Toward a hybrid brain-computer interface based on imagined movement and visual attention. *Journal of Neural Engineering, 7*, 026007.

Allison, B. Z., Graimann, B., Lüth, T., & Gräser, A. (2007a). An SSVEP brain-computer interface (BCI) with simultaneous attention to two targets. Program No. 770.9. *Society for Neuroscience Conference*. San Diego, CA.

Allison, B., Lüth, T., Valbuena, D., Teymourian, A., Volosyak, I., & Gräser, A. (2010c). BCI demographics: how many (and what kinds of) people can use an SSVEP BCI? *IEEE Transactions on Neural Systems Rehabilitation Engineering, 18*, 107–113.

Allison, B. Z., McFarland, D. J., Schalk, G., Zheng, S. D., Jackson, M. M., & Wolpaw, J. R. (2008). Towards an independent brain-computer interface using steady state visual evoked potentials. *Clinical Neurophysiology, 119*, 399–408.

Allison, B. Z., Wolpaw, E. W., & Wolpaw, J. R. (2007b). Brain-computer interface systems: progress and prospects. *Expert Review of Medical Devices, 4*, 463–474.

Altenmüller, E. O., Münte, T. F., & Gerloff, C. (2005). Neurocognitive functions and the EEG. In E. Niedermeyer & F. Lopes da Silva (Eds.), *Electroencephalography: basic principles, clinical applications and related fields*. Philadelphia: Lippincott Williams & Wilkins, 661–682.

Bai, O., Rathi, V., Lin, P., Huang, D., Battapady, H., Fei, D. Y., et al. (2011). Prediction of human voluntary movement before it occurs. *Clinical Neurophysiology, 122*, 364–372.

Bauer, A., Kantelhardt, J. W., Bunde, A., Barthel, P., Schneider, R., Malik, M., et al. (2006). Phase-rectified signal averaging detects quasi-periodicities in non-stationary data. *Physica A: Statistical Mechanics and its Applications, 364*, 423–434.

Beisteiner, R., Höllinger, P., Lindinger, G., Lang, W., & Berthoz, A. (1995). Mental representations of movements. Brain potentials associated with imagination of hand movements. *Electroencephalography and Clinical Neurophysiology, 96*, 83–193.

Bensch, M., Karim, A. A., Mellinger, J., Hinterberger, T., Tangermann, M., Bogda, M., et al. (2007). Nessi: an EEG-controlled web browser for severely paralyzed patients. *Computational Intelligence and Neuroscience, 2007*, 71863.

Bin, G., Gao, X., Wang, Y., Hong, B., & Gao, S. (2009). VEP-based brain-computer interfaces: time, frequency, and code modulations. *Computational Intelligence Magazine, IEEE, 4*, 22–26.

Birbaumer, N., & Cohen, L. G. (2007). Brain-computer interfaces: communication and restoration of movement in paralysis. *The Journal of Physiology, 579*, 621–636.

Birbaumer, N., Ghanayim, N., Hinterberger, T., Iversen, I., Kotchoubey, B., Kübler, A., et al. (1999). A spelling device for the paralysed. *Nature, 398*, 297–298.

Brunner, C., Allison, B. Z., Altstätter, C., & Neuper, C. (2011). A comparison of three brain-computer interfaces based on event-related desynchronization, steady state visual evoked potentials, or a hybrid approach using both signals. *Journal of Neural Engineering, 8*, 7–13.

Brunner, C., Allison, B. Z., Krusienski, D. J., Kaiser, V., Müller-Putz, G. R., Pfurtscheller, G., et al. (2010a). Improved signal processing approaches in an offline simulation of a hybrid brain-computer interface. *Journal of Neuroscience Methods, 188*, 165–173.

Brunner, P., Joshi, S., Briskin, S., Wolpaw, J. R., Bischof, H., & Schalk, G. (2010b). Does the P300 speller depend on eye gaze? *Journal of Neural Engineering, 7*(5), 056013.

Celesia, G. G., & Peachey, N. S. (2005). Visual evoked potentials and electroretinograms. In E. Niedermeyer, & F. Lopes da Silva (Eds.), *Electroencephalography—Basic principles, clinical applications and related fields*. Philadelphia: Lippincott Williams & Wilkins, 1017–1043.

Colebatch, J. G. (2007). Bereitschaftspotential and movement-related potentials: Origin, significance, and application in disorders of human movement. *Movement Disorders, 22*, 601–610.

Cunnington, R., Iansek, R., Bradshaw, J. L., & Phillips, J. G. (1996). Movement-related potentials associated with movement preparation and motor imagery. *Experimental Brain Research, 111*(3), 429–436.

Elbert, T., Rockstroh, B., Lutzenberger, W., & Birbaumer, N. (1980). Biofeedback of slow cortical potentials. I. *Electroencephalography and Clinical Neurophysiology, 48*, 293–301.

Faller, J., Leeb, R., Pfurtscheller, G., & Scherer, R. (2010). Avatar navigation in virtual and augmented reality environments using an SSVEP BCI.

International Conference on Applied Bionics and Biomechanics (ICABB) 2010, Venice, Italy.

Friedrich, E. V., McFarland, D. J., Neuper, C., Vaughan, T. M., Brunner, P., & Wolpaw, J. R. (2009). A scanning protocol for sensorimotor rhythm-based brain-computer interfaces. *Biological Psychology, 80,* 169–175.

Gao, X., Xu, D., Cheng, M., & Gao, S. (2003). A BCI-based environmental controller for the motion-disabled. *IEEE Transactions on Neural Systems and Rehabilitation Engineering,* 11, 137–140.

Garcia-Molina, G., & Mihajlovic, V. (2010). Spatial filters to detect steady state visual evoked potentials elicited by high frequency stimulation: BCI application. *Journal of Biomedizinische Technik/Biomedical Engineering, 3,* 173–182.

Garipelli, G., & Chavarriaga, R. (2009). Fast recognition of anticipation related potentials. *IEEE Transactions on Biomedical Engineering, 56,* 1257–1260.

Hinterberger, T., Schmidt, S., Neumann, N., Mellinger, J., Blankertz, B., Curio, G., et al. (2004a). Brain-computer communication and slow cortical potentials. *IEEE Transactions on Biomedical Engineering, 51,* 1011–1018.

Hinterberger, T., Weiskopf, N., Veit, R., Wilhelm, B., Betta, E., & Birbaumer, N. (2004b). An EEG-driven brain-computer interface combined with functional magnetic resonance imaging (fMRI). *IEEE Transactions on Biomedical Engineering, 51,* 971–974.

Hinterberger, T., Wilhelm, B., Mellinger, J., Kotchoubey, B., & Birbaumer, N. (2005). A device for the detection of cognitive brain functions in completely paralyzed or unresponsive patients. *IEEE Transactions on Neural Systems and Rehabilitation Engineering, 52,* 211–220.

Horki, P., Solis-Escalante, T., Neuper, C., & Müller-Putz, G. (2011). Combined motor imagery and SSVEP based BCI control of a 2 DoF artificial upper limb. *Medical and Biological Engineering and Computing,* 49, 1–11.

Kaiser, J., Kübler, A., Hinterberger, T., Neumann, N., & Birbaumer, N. (2002). A non-invasive communication device for the paralyzed. *Minimally Invasive Neurosurgery 45,* 19–23.

Kelly, S. P., Lalor, E. C., Reilly, R. B., & Foxe, J. J. (2005). Visual spatial attention tracking using high-density SSVEP data for independent brain-computer communication. *IEEE Transactions on Neural Systems and Rehabilitation Engineering, 13,* 172–178.

Kim, D.-W., Hwang, H.-J., Lim, J.-H., Lee, Y.-H., Jung, K.-Y., & Im, C.-H. (2011). Classification of selective attention to auditory stimuli: toward vision-free brain-computer interfacing. *Journal of Neuroscience Methods,* 197, 180–185.

Kornhuber, H. H., & Deecke, L. (1965). Changes in the brain potential in voluntary movements and passive movements in man: readiness potential and reafferent potentials. *Pflügers Archiv für die gesamte Physiologie des Menschen und der Tiere, 284,* 1–17.

Kotchoubey, B., Schneider, D., Schleichert, H., Strehl, U., Uhlmann, C., Blankenhorn, V., et al. (1996). Self regulation of slow cortical potentials in epilepsy: a retrial with analysis of influencing factors. *Epilepsy Research, 25,* 269–276.

Kübler, A., Kotchoubey, B., Hinterberger, T., Ghanayim, N., Perelmouter, J., Schauer, M., et al. (1999). The thought translation device: a neurophysiological approach to communication in total motor paralysis. *Experimental Brain Research, 124* (2), 223–232.

Kübler, A., Neumann, N., Kaiser, J., Kotchoubey, B., Hinterberger, T., & Birbaumer, N. (2001). Brain-computer communication: self-regulation of slow cortical potentials for verbal communication. *Archives of Physical Medicine and Rehabilitation, 82,* 1533–1539.

Kübler, A., Schmidt, K., Cohen, L. G., Lotze, M., Winter, S., Hinterberger, T., et al. (2002). Modulation of slow cortical potentials by transcranial magnetic stimulation in humans. *Neuroscience Letters, 324,* 205–208.

Lalor, E. C., Kelly, S. P., Finucane, C., Burke, R., Smith, R., Reilly, R. B., et al. (2005). Steady-state VEP-based brain-computer interface control in an immersive 3D gaming environment. *EURASIP Journal on Applied Signal Processing, 19,* 3156–3164.

Lang, W., Cheyne, D., Höllinger, P., Gerschlager, W., & Lindinger, G. (1996). Electric and magnetic fields of the brain accompanying internal simulation of movement. *Cognitive Brain Research, 3,* 125–129.

Leins, U., Goth, G., Hinterberger, T., Klinger, C., Rumpf, N., & Strehl, U. (2007). Neurofeedback for children with ADHD: a comparison of SCP and Theta/Beta protocols. *Applied Psychophysiology and Biofeedback, 32(2),* 73–88.

Lutzenberger, W., Elbert, T., Rockstroh, B., & Birbaumer, N. (1979). The effects of self-regulation of slow cortical potentials on performance in a signal detection task. *International Journal of Neuroscience, 9,* 175–183.

Martinez, P., Bakardjian, H., & Cichocki, A. (2007). Fully online multicommand brain-computer interface with visual neurofeedback using SSVEP paradigm. *Computational Intelligence and Neuroscience, 2007,* Vol. 2007, Article ID 94561.

McFarland, D. J., Sarnacki, W. A., & Wolpaw, J. R. (2010). Electroencephalographic (EEG) control of three-dimensional movement. *Journal of Neural Engineering, 7,* 036007.

Middendorf, M., McMillan, G., Calhoun, G., & Jones, K. S. (2000). Brain-computer interfaces based on the steady-state visual-evoked response. *IEEE Transactions on Rehabilitation Engineering, 8,* 211–214.

Millán, J. d., Rupp, R., Müller-Putz, G. R., Murray-Smith, R., Guigliemma, C., Tangermann, M., et al. (2010). Combining brain-computer interfaces and assistive technologies: state-of-the-art and challenges. *Frontiers of Neuroscience, 4,* 12.

Müller, M. M., Malinowski, P., Gruber, T., & Hillyard, S. A. (2003). Sustained division of the attentional spotlight. *Nature, 424,* 309–312.

Müller-Putz, G. R., Eder, E., Wriessnegger, S. C., & Pfurtscheller, G. (2008). Comparison of DFT and lock-in amplifier features and search for optimal electrode positions in SSVEP-based BCI. *Journal of Neuroscience Methods, 168,* 174–181.

Müller-Putz, G. R., Scherer, R., Brauneis, C., & Pfurtscheller, G. (2005). Steady-state visual evoked potential (SSVEP)-based communication: impact of harmonic frequency components. *Journal of Neural Engineering, 2,* 1–8.

Müller-Putz, G. R., Scherer, R., Neuper, C., & Pfurtscheller, G. (2006). Steady-state somatosensory evoked potentials: suitable brain signals for brain-computer interfaces? *IEEE Transactions on Neural Systems and Rehabilitation Engineering, 14,* 30–37.

Neuper, C., & Pfurtscheller, G. (2010). Brain-computer interfaces: non-invasive and invasive technologies. In B. Graimann, B. Z. Allison, & G. Pfurtscheller (Eds.), *Brain-Computer Interfaces: Non-invasive and Invasive Technologies.* Springer, Berlin Heidelberg, 65–78.

Panicker, R., Puthusserypady, S., & Sun, Y. (2011). An asynchronous P300 BCI with SSVEP-based control state detection. *IEEE Transactions on Biomedical Engineering, 58,* 1781–1788.

Paradiso, G., Saint-Cyr, J. A., Lozano, A. M., Lang, A. E., & Chen, R. (2003). Involvement of the human subthalamic nucleus in movement preparation. *Neurology, 61,* 1538–1545.

Pfurtscheller, G., Allison, B. Z., Brunner, C., Bauernfeind, G., Solis-Escalante, T., Scherer, R., et al. (2010a). The hybrid BCI. *Frontiers in Neuroscience, 4,* 30.

Pfurtscheller, G., & Aranibar, A. (1979). Evaluation of event-related desynchronization (ERD) preceding and following voluntary self-paced movements. *Electroencephalography and Clinical Neurophysiology, 46,* 138–146.

Pfurtscheller, G., Solis-Escalante, T., Ortner, R., Linortner, P., & Müller-Putz, G. R. (2010b). Self-paced operation of an SSVEP-based orthosis with and without an imagery-based brain switch: a feasibility study towards a hybrid BCI. *IEEE Transactions on Neural Systems and Rehabilitation Engineering, 18,* 409–414.

Royer, A. S., Doud, A. J., Rose, M. L., and He, B. (2010). EEG control of a virtual helicopter in 3-dimensional space using intelligent control strategies. *IEEE Transactions on Neural Systems and Rehabilitation Engineering, 18,* 581–589.

Scherer, R., Müller, G. R., Neuper, C., Graimann, B., & Pfurtscheller, G. (2004). An asynchronously controlled EEG-based virtual keyboard: improvement of the spelling rate. *IEEE Transactions on Neural Systems and Rehabilitation Engineering, 51,* 979–984.

Schneider, F., Elbert, T., Heimann, H., Welker, A., Stetter, F., Mattes, R., et al. (1993). Self-regulation of slow cortical potentials in psychiatric patients: alcohol dependency. *Applied Psychophysiology and Biofeedback, 18,* 23–32.

Schneider, F., Heimann, H., Mattes, R., Lutzenberger, W., & Birbaumer, N. (1992a). Self-regulation of slow cortical potentials in psychiatric patients: Depression. *Applied Psychophysiology and Biofeedback, 17,* 203–214.

Schneider, F., Rockstroh, B., Heimann, H., Lutzenberger, W., Mattes, R., Elbert, T., et al. (1992b). Self-regulation of slow cortical potentials in psychiatric patients: schizophrenia. *Applied Psychophysiology and Biofeedback, 17,* 4.

Shibasaki, H., & Hallett, M. (2006). What is the Bereitschaftspotential? *Clinical Neurophysiology, 117,* 2341–2356.

Sutter, E. E. (1992). The brain response interface: communication through visually-induced electrical brain responses. *Journal of Microcomputer Applications, 15,* 31–45.

Treder, M. S., & Blankertz, B. (2010). Covert attention and visual speller design in an ERP-based brain-computer interface. *Behavioral and Brain Functions, 6:28.*

Trejo, L. J., Rospial, R., & Matthews, B. (2006). Brain-computer interfaces for 1-D and 2-D cursor control: designs using volitional control of the EEG spectrum or steady-state visual evoked potentials. *IEEE Transactions on Neural Systems and Rehabilitation Engineering, 14,* 225–229.

Vidal, J. J. (1973). Toward direct brain-computer communication. *Annual Review of Biophysics and Bioengineering, 2,* 157–180.

Vidal, J. J. (1977). Real-time detection of brain events in EEG. *Proceedings of the IEEE, 65,* 633–641.

Walter, W. G., Cooper, R., Aldridge, V. J., McCallum, W. C., & Winter, A. L. (1964). Contingent negative variation: an electric sign of sensorimotor association and expectancy in the human brain. *Nature, 203*, 380–384.

Wang, Y., Wang, Y., & Jung, T. (2010). Visual stimulus design for high-rate SSVEP BCI. *Electronics Letters, 46*, 1057–1058.

Wolpaw, J. R., Birbaumer, N., McFarland, D. J., Pfurtscheller, G., & Vaughan, T. M. (2002). Brain-computer interfaces for communication and control. *Clinical Neurophysiology, 113*, 767–791.

Wolpaw, J. R., & McFarland, D. J. (1994). Multichannel EEG-based brain-computer communication. *Electroencephalography and Clinical Neurophysiology, 90*, 444–449

Wolpaw, J. R., & McFarland, D. J. (2004). Control of a two-dimensional movement signal by a noninvasive brain-computer interface in humans. *Proceedings of the National Academy of Science of the United States of America, 101*, 17849–17854.

15 | BCIs THAT USE ELECTROCORTICOGRAPHIC ACTIVITY

GERWIN SCHALK

Electrocorticography (ECoG), also sometimes called intracranial EEG or iEEG, is the technique of recording electrical signals from locations underneath the skull but not within the brain itself. On the continuum of invasiveness going from scalp-recorded EEG signals at one end to intracortically recorded single-unit action potentials and local field potentials (LFPs) at the other, ECoG represents a midway point: it involves surgery, but the electrodes do not penetrate into the brain (see fig. 15.1). ECoG can be recorded from the surface of the dura mater (i.e., *epidurally*) using electrodes placed on the dura or using screws that penetrate the skull and serve as electrodes. Alternatively, ECoG can be recorded from beneath the dura (i.e., *subdurally*) using electrodes placed directly on the surface of the brain. ECoG signals resemble EEG signals in that they are the result of field potentials from population activity rather than action potentials from individual neurons. ECoG is currently regarded as a highly promising modality for BCI development because it is greatly superior to EEG in amplitude, topographical resolution, frequency range, and resistance to artifacts, and may be superior to intracortical signals in long-term stability.

ECoG was first recorded from animals and humans in the late 19th century (Caton 1875). Interest has increased in recent decades, and a variety of animal studies (particularly in rats, rabbits, cats, and pigs) have appeared in the literature (e.g., Freeman 1978; Freeman and Schneider 1982; Freeman and van Dijk 1987; Hata et al. 1987; Peruche et al. 1995; Dési et al. 1996; Waters et al. 1996; Dias-dos Santos and Machado 1997; Shinozuka and Nathanielsz 1998; Fritz et al. 1999; Schürmann et al. 2000). Because placement of ECoG electrodes requires surgery, human studies are currently limited to people who are implanted with ECoG electrodes preparatory to brain surgery (usually to remove an epileptic focus or a tumor). There have been only a few exceptions to this general rule, most notably a 1992 study by Sutter (1992) in which visual evoked responses in ECoG recorded over occipital cortex allowed a person severely disabled by ALS to communicate at a rate of 10–12 words/min. Because the ECoG electrode arrays placed presurgically are implanted for clinical purposes, the configuration and location of the electrodes, as well as the duration of the implant, are determined solely by clinical requirements and without any regard for research needs. The electrodes are typically 4 mm (2.3 mm exposed) platinum electrodes and are configured in either a grid (e.g., 8 × 8 electrodes) or strip (e.g., four or six electrodes) configuration with an interelectrode distance of usually 10 mm (see fig. 15.2). They are typically implanted for periods of only several days to 1–2 weeks.

During these relatively short periods, research studies may be possible, when patients are interested in participating and when their baseline CNS function, current medical state, and current medications permit them to do so. Because these patients are under evaluation for brain surgery, many of the earlier human ECoG studies were conducted by research-oriented clinicians (Calvet and Bancaud 1976; Fried et al. 1981; Ojemann et al. 1989; Menon et al. 1996; Hirai et al. 1999; Aoki 1999). For this reason, and because in each case the ECoG array is placed in a location pertinent to the individual patient's clinical needs, these studies have most often focused on research topics relevant to the individual patient's clinical evaluation (e.g., topographical mapping of motor or language function). These early efforts culminated in the first comprehensive characterization of ECoG responses to visuomotor tasks (Crone, Miglioretti, Gordon, and Lesser 1998; Crone, Miglioretti, Gordon, Sieracki et al. 1998). As the growing interest in brain-computer interface (BCI) research began to draw multidisciplinary research teams, often including electrical and software engineers, applied mathematicians, and neuroscientists, evaluation of ECoG data began to extend to more comprehensive offline BCI studies (Huggins et al. 1999; Levine et al. 1999; Levine et al. 2000; Rohde et al. 2002; Graimann et al. 2003; Pfurtscheller et al. 2003). In 2004, an online study by Leuthardt et al. (2004) sparked substantial interest by showing that ECoG can support accurate BCI operation with little user training. This study also provided initial evidence that ECoG signals contain information about the direction of hand movements.

For BCI purposes, ECoG appears to avoid or reduce some of the shortcomings of the traditional noninvasive and invasive signal acquisition techniques. Although EEG is noninvasive and has been shown to support important BCI applications, including two- and three-dimensional movement control (Wolpaw and McFarland 1994, 2004; Farwell and Donchin 1988; Wolpaw et al. 1991; Sutter 1992; McFarland et al. 1993; Pfurtscheller et al. 1993; Birbaumer et al. 1999; Kübler et al. 1999; Pfurtscheller et al. 2000; Wolpaw et al. 2002; Millán et al. 2004; Kübler et al. 2005; Vaughan et al. 2006; Müller and Blankertz 2006; McFarland et al. 2008; Royer et al. 2010; McFarland et al. 2010), the highest-functioning EEG-based BCIs require substantial user training, and their performance is often not reliable. On the other end of the spectrum are BCIs that are based on intracortical recordings of action-potential firing rates or LFPs (Georgopoulos et al. 1986; Taylor et al. 2002; Serruya et al. 2002; Shenoy et al. 2003; Andersen et al. 2004; Lebedev et al. 2005; Santhanam et al. 2006; Hochberg et al. 2006; Donoghue et al. 2007; Velliste et al. 2008). Thus far, despite the dramatically better resolution of microelectrode

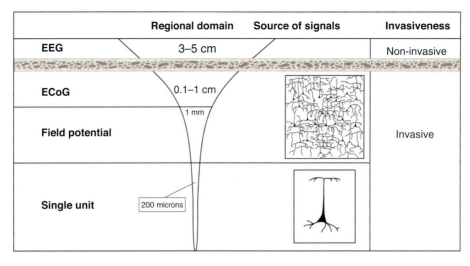

	Regional domain	Source of signals	Invasiveness
EEG	3–5 cm		Non-invasive
ECoG	0.1–1 cm		
Field potential	1 mm		Invasive
Single unit	200 microns		

Figure 15.1 *Recording domains for single-unit, LFP, ECoG, and EEG recording. (Modified from Leuthardt et al., 2006b.)*

recordings compared to EEG recordings, these BCIs have yet to greatly exceed the performance of EEG-based BCIs and still face significant and unresolved questions as to the long-term functional stability of intracortical electrodes, particularly for recording action potentials (Shain et al. 2003; Donoghue et al. 2004; Davids et al. 2005). Despite encouraging evidence that current noninvasive and invasive BCI technologies can actually be useful to severely disabled people (Kübler et al. 2005; Hochberg et al. 2006; Sellers et al. 2010), these shortcomings and uncertainties

remain substantial obstacles to their widespread clinical use in humans.

When compared to EEG, ECoG has several major advantages:

- higher spatial resolution (i.e., 1.25 mm for subdural recordings [Freeman et al. 2000] and 1.4 mm for epidural recordings [Slutzky et al. 2010] vs. several centimeters for EEG)

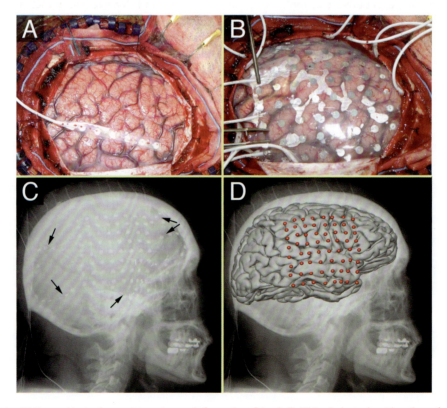

Figure 15.2 *ECoG array in situ. (A) Exposed brain after craniotomy (removal of a portion of the skull). (B) 8 × 8 electrode grid on the surface of the brain. (C) Lateral x-ray image; the electrode grid and several electrode strips (see arrows) are visible. (D) Average brain template and electrode locations co-registered to the x-ray image. (Modified from Schalk et al., 2008.)*

- higher signal amplitude (i.e., 50–100 μV maximum vs. 10–20 μV maximum for EEG)

- far less vulnerability to artifacts such as electromyographic (EMG) (Freeman et al. 2003) or electroocular (EOG) activity (Ball et al. 2009)

- broader bandwidth (i.e., 0–500 Hz [Staba et al. 2002; Gaona et al. 2011] vs. 0–40 Hz for EEG)

With respect to ECoG's larger bandwidth, it is important to note that this advantage may in part be directly related to the larger amplitude of ECoG. Although ECoG generally displays a 1/frequency drop-off in signal power (Miller et al. 2009a), task-related brain signals may still remain larger than the noise floor of the amplifier/digitizer, and thus they are detectable at higher frequencies than with EEG. In addition to these advantages of signal quality, ECoG electrodes (which do not penetrate cortex) may provide greater long-term functional stability (Loeb et al. 1977; Bullara et al. 1979; Yuen et al. 1987; Pilcher and Rusyniak 1993; Margalit et al. 2003) than intracortical electrodes (which induce complex local responses that may degrade or prevent neuronal recordings (see chapter 5 in this volume). A recent study by Chao and colleagues (2010) showed that the signal-to-noise ratio of ECoG signals, and the cortical representations of motor functions that can be identified with ECoG, are stable over several months (Schalk 2010). Thus, there is strong theoretical and empirical evidence that ECoG could enable BCIs that have high functional specificity and that are less susceptible to the problems of reliability and long-term stability that often affect other electrophysiological signal-acquisition methodologies.

ELECTROPHYSIOLOGICAL FEATURES DETECTED BY ECoG

With its detection of brain electrical activity over a wide frequency range, ECoG detects several electrophysiological features of potential use for BCIs. These include the mu and beta rhythms (Chatrian 1976) that are well described in the classical EEG literature, as well as in the numerous BCI studies in which they are used (see chapter 13). As discussed in chapter 13, mu and beta rhythms are oscillations in the 8–12 Hz (mu) and 18–26 Hz (beta) frequency bands. Changes in mu/beta amplitude typically occur in association with actual or imagined movements (see fig. 15.3) [Pfurtscheller and Cooper 1975; Crone et al. 1998]), and are relatively focused spectrally but relatively widespread spatially (see fig. 15.4). While mu/beta amplitude gives information about general aspects of movements (e.g., whether or not a hand is moved), it is thought to hold only modest information about the details of movements (e.g., kinematic parameters of hand movements) (Toro et al. 1994).

With a bandwidth that typically reaches as high as 30–40 Hz, EEG detects mu and beta activity very well. Although recent advances in recording hardware and analysis methods suggest that the frequency range of EEG may be extended (Jokeit and Makeig 1994; Darvas et al. 2010), EEG is largely insensitive to gamma activity, which begins at 30–40 Hz (Pfurtscheller and Neuper 1992) and extends as high as 400–500 Hz (Miller et al. 2009a). In contrast, ECoG can detect gamma activity very well. This is potentially a major advantage for BCI development because gamma activity, unlike mu and beta activity, displays high functional localization (e.g., see fig. 15.4). Many ECoG studies (Menon et al. 1996; Crone et al. 1998; Aoki et al. 1999; Freeman et al. 2000; Crone et al. 2001; Pfurtscheller et al. 2003; Leuthardt et al. 2004; Sinai et al. 2005; Schalk et al. 2007; Miller et al. 2007a; Leuthardt et al. 2007, Lachaux et al. 2007; Canolty et al. 2007; Sanchez et al. 2008; Kubánek et al. 2009; Miller, Schalk et al. 2010; Edwards et al. 2010; Pei et al. 2010; Chang et al. 2011) have reported that topographically focused gamma activity correlates closely with specific aspects of cortical function or with behavioral details such as the direction of limb movements (Leuthardt et al. 2004; Schalk et al. 2007; Pistohl et al. 2008; Kubánek et al. 2009; Miller et al. 2009b; Acharya et al. 2010) (see fig. 15.5).

In contrast to mu and beta activity, gamma activity usually has a broad spectral distribution. Although a somewhat arbitrary frequency-based division into "low" and "high" gamma activity has been proposed (Sinai et al. 2005), it has become increasingly apparent that gamma activity is a broadbanded noise-like phenomenon that declines in amplitude as frequency rises (Miller et al. 2009a; Miller et al. 2009b). However, the

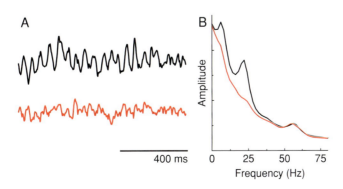

Figure 15.3 Example of ECoG signals during a task and rest. (A) Raw ECoG signals from one subject during rest (black trace) and while imagining saying the word "move" (red trace). The oscillations associated with rest decrease with imagery. (B) Frequency spectra for the corresponding conditions. Imagery is associated with decrease in the mu (8–12 Hz) and beta (18–26 Hz) frequency bands. (From Schalk, 2006.)

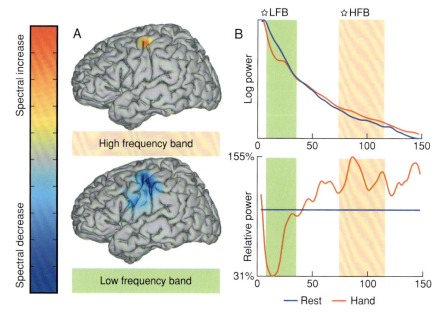

Figure 15.4 *Example of ECoG during the task of repetitively opening and closing of the hand and during rest. (A) Signals in the mu/beta band (5–30 Hz) decrease with the task and are spatially less specific (i.e., they are broadly distributed topographically), whereas signals in the gamma band (i.e., 70–116 Hz as measured here) increase with the task and are spatially more specific (i.e., they are sharply focused topographically). (B) The power spectrum on a logarithmic scale for the electrode marked with a star in the topographies illustrates the decrease in the mu/beta band (marked by the green bar) and increase in the gamma band (orange bar). (From Brunner et al., 2009.)*

most recent evidence suggests that this view may be an oversimplification (Gaona et al. 2011). Although gamma activity appears to be closely related to the firing rate of individual neurons (Kasanetz et al. 2006; Ray et al. 2008; Manning et al. 2009; Miller 2010), it remains unclear to what extent its amplitude depends on the respective contributions of neuronal firing rates and synaptic potentials, and of their relative phases. Gamma amplitude has also been closely linked to the blood oxygen level dependent (BOLD) signals detected by functional magnetic resonance imaging (fMRI) (Niessing et al. 2005; Lachaux et al. 2007, see chapter 4 in this volume). It is plausible, and even probable, that increased cortical activation is reflected directly in gamma activity and leads to the increased metabolic demand that is reflected in the BOLD signal detected

by fMRI (see chapter 4 in this volume). In summary, recent results suggest that gamma activity reflects local cortical-processing activity that occurs immediately beneath the ECoG electrodes. Thus, like LFPs detected within the brain, it reflects the activation of local neuronal and synaptic populations.

ECoG activity in the mu, beta, and gamma bands can be best displayed in the frequency domain (i.e., with frequency on the *x*-axis and amplitude on the *y*-axis). In the frequency domain, modulations in activity appear as amplitude changes in four major bands: theta (4–8 Hz), mu (8–12 Hz), beta (18–25 Hz), gamma (> 40 Hz) (Miller et al. 2009a; He et al. 2010).

ECoG also displays discrete (i.e., evoked) and continuous time-domain features (i.e., time on the *x*-axis and amplitude on the *y*-axis). Discrete time-domain ECoG features are

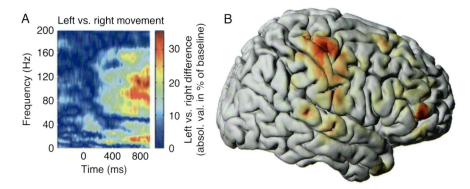

Figure 15.5 *ECoG recording reveals information about the direction of a hand movement. (A) ECoG signal in different frequency bands recorded at one location in the contralateral hand area of motor cortex from one subject differentiates left and right movement directions. (From Leuthardt et al., 2004.) (B) Color-coded shading of average data from five subjects illustrates the information about hand movement direction provided by ECoG recorded over different cortical areas. Most of the information is captured over the hand representations of motor cortex. (Modified from Schalk et al., 2007.)*

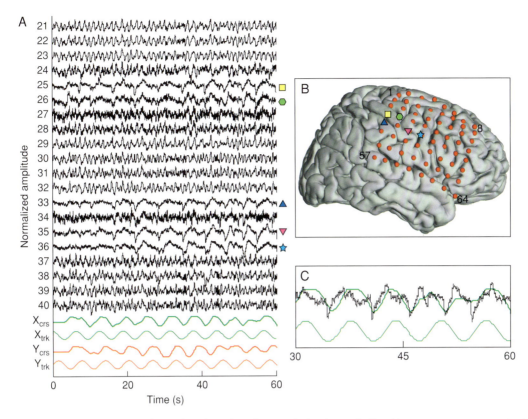

Figure 15.6 *Example ECoG time course during a tracking task. In this task, a subject used a hand-controlled joystick to move a cursor so as to track a target that moved on a computer screen. (A) Time courses for ECoG signals from 20 locations (see B) and (bottom four traces) for the horizontal and vertical positions of the cursor (X_{crs}, Y_{crs}) and the moving target (X_{trk}, Y_{trk}). Symbols along y-axis to the right of the plots indicate the five channels (i.e., 25, 26, 33, 35, and 36) in which the time course of ECoG activity (i.e., the local motor potential, LMP) correlates with the movement parameters X_{crs} or Y_{crs}. (B) Grid electrode locations with symbols at the channels that show the LMP as identified in the data of A. (C) Magnification of ECoG time course of channel 35 from 30 to 60 sec, as well as the horizontal positions of the cursor (dark green trace) and the moving target (light green trace). The (black) ECoG time course correlates better with the (dark green) cursor position than with the (light green) target position. (From Schalk et al., 2007.)*

usually evoked by a physical or cognitive stimulus, as in P300 evoked responses (e.g., [Farwell and Donchin 1988]) or in steady-state visual evoked potentials (SSVEPs) (e.g., Allison et al. 2008; see chapters 12 and 13 in this volume), or associated with the onset of a movement (e.g., Bereitschaftspotential [Kornhuber and Deecke 1965], contingent negative variation [Walter et al. 1964], or movement-related potentials [Levine et al. 2000]) (see chapter 13). Despite some early interest in the use of ECoG movement-related potentials for BCI purposes (Graimann et al. 2003) and a recent demonstration of rapid communication using ECoG-recorded evoked potentials (VEP and P300) (Brunner et al. 2011), discrete time-domain ECoG phenomena have to date received little attention from BCI researchers. On the other hand, a recent study (Schalk et al. 2007) describes a continuous time-domain ECoG feature, called the *local motor potential* (LMP), that encodes different aspects of movements (see fig. 15.6). Although this phenomenon has been confirmed by other studies (Kubánek et al. 2009; Acharya et al. 2010), its physiological origin and its potential BCI value remain to be defined.

As indicated above, increases in gamma activity appear to reflect highly localized cortical activation that correlates with different motor, sensory, and cognitive functions.

Recent studies have shown that gamma activity is also modulated by the phase of lower-frequency brain oscillations (e.g., in the theta, mu/alpha, and beta ranges) (Canolty et al. 2006; Canolty and Knight 2010; Miller, Hermes et al. 2010; He et al. 2010; i.e., by cross-frequency or phase-amplitude coupling). Although these relationships have many possible interpretations, they might provide a mechanism for coordinating fast processes (e.g., movements) with slower perceptual or cognitive processes (Canolty and Knight 2010). To what extent these coupling mechanisms could be useful in a BCI context remains unclear.

The picture of cortical function that emerges from established cortical research and from all of these studies is one in which: (1) local cortical processes can be detected in gamma activity (Miller, Schalk et al. 2010); (2) local cortical processes are synchronized with or modulated by signals from other areas and this is reflected in the interactions of rhythm phase with gamma amplitudes ([Canolty and Knight 2010], for review); (3) the function of a particular cortical system (e.g., hand area of motor cortex) is enabled or disabled by the thalamus through thalamocortical oscillations that express themselves in mu/beta rhythms (Niedermeyer and Lopes da Silva 1993). Figure 15.7 illustrates the current state of this evolving understanding of cortical function and the related ECoG signals.

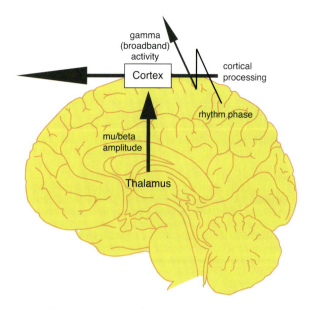

Figure 15.7 *Schematic of current and emerging understanding of the physiological origin of ECoG signals. The amplitude of mu/beta rhythm oscillations represents the level of thalamocortical interactions. Gamma activity represents the degree of local cortical processing. ECoG rhythm phase modulates local cortical processing.*

In summary, ECoG can detect brain electrical activity over a very wide frequency range. Although EEG-based studies have already shown that the lower frequencies in this range are useful for BCIs, substantial evidence now suggests that the higher frequencies, which are easily accessible only with ECoG recording, may be even more useful for BCI development. The value of other physiological phenomena in ECoG (i.e., the LMP, cross-frequency or phase-amplitude coupling) for BCI purposes is currently unclear.

CURRENT ECoG-BASED BCIs

We now consider the methods by which ECoG signals are acquired, identified, and subsequently utilized for BCI applications in the current generation of ECoG-based BCIs. Although almost all ECoG-based BCI research to date has been in humans implanted with subdural electrode arrays for short periods prior to surgery, the results should be applicable to animals as well. This is particularly important because many issues critical to the development of ECoG-based BCIs are likely, for both practical and ethical reasons, to be addressed first in animals.

ECoG SIGNAL ACQUISITION

The current generation of ECoG recording devices has been used primarily in humans for clinical applications. As discussed in chapter 5, these devices usually consist of platinum electrodes that are embedded in a silastic base. In the newer generation of ECoG recording devices, small platinum electrodes are embedded on thin films made of biocompatible materials (e.g., polyimide, parylene, or silk). The choice of materials determines the ability of the recording device to

retain structural integrity and biocompatibility. It also constrains the possible implantation techniques. For example, very thin recording devices may provide optimal biocompatibility. However, due to their flexibility, it is difficult to push them to sites distant from the craniotomy during the implantation. On the other hand, it is difficult to implant relatively rigid devices in the sulci.

In addition to the choice of appropriate materials, acquisition of ECoG signals requires attention to several important properties of the ECoG signal. Because ECoG amplitude attenuates rapidly as frequency rises (Miller et al. 2009a; He et al. 2010) (e.g., from several hundred microvolts at low frequencies to several hundred nanovolts at higher frequencies), effective ECoG recording requires high-fidelity amplifiers/digitizers with sufficient resolution in time (i.e., adequate sampling rates) and with sufficient range and resolution in amplitude (i.e., adequate voltage range and resolution). In general, the sampling rate should be at least 1 kHz, the voltage range should be at least a few millivolts, and the resolution should be at least 16-bit or, better still, 24-bit. Moreover, any analog low- or high-pass filtering at the amplification stage should be able to accommodate the diverse physiological phenomena that are detected in ECoG. Ideally, there should be no high-pass filter, and the low-pass filter frequency should be less than half of the digitization rate (to satisfy the Nyquist-Shannon sampling theorem) (see chapter 7 in this volume). However, most clinical (and even some research) ECoG amplification/digitization systems do not at present meet these stringent requirements and thus may not be capable of acquiring ECoG signals with sufficient fidelity to capture all the information needed by a particular study.

Since at present most ECoG-based BCI research is performed in human subjects who have been temporarily implanted with an ECoG array for clinical reasons, substantial practical constraints and challenges are necessarily involved. Because of these difficulties, relatively few online ECoG-based BCI studies have been published to date (Leuthardt et al. 2004; Leuthardt et al. 2006a; Wilson et al. 2006; Felton et al. 2007; Schalk 2008; Hinterberger et al. 2008; Blakely et al. 2009; Rouse and Moran 2009; van Steensel et al. 2010; Miller, Schalk et al. 2010; Brunner et al. 2011).

ECoG-BASED BCI PROTOCOL DESIGN

The protocol of an ECoG-based BCI study usually has two parts. In the first part, the ECoG feature(s) to be used for BCI control are chosen. In the second part, the feature(s) are used for online BCI control of cursor movement or another output.

As in BCI studies with other kinds of signals, the first task is to select those signal features (e.g., gamma activity at a particular location) to be used for BCI control and to extract them from the complex raw signal data (see chapter 7). Typically, the criterion for this selection is that the particular ECoG feature shows a clear change from the resting state that is correlated with a motor action such as tongue or contralateral hand movement. Some studies have explored the use of features that change with sensory input (Wilson et al. 2006) or with specific cognitive functions (van Steensel et al. 2010). A different and as yet unrealized possibility is to select features that correlate with specific parameters of an action (e.g., velocity of hand movements). This approach is encouraged by recent animal (Mehring et al. 2004; Chao et al. 2010), and human (Leuthardt et al. 2004; Miller et al. 2007a; Leuthardt et al. 2007; Miller et al. 2007b; Schalk et al. 2007; Schalk et al. 2008; Pistohl et al. 2008; Sanchez et al. 2008; Kubánek et al. 2009; Miller et al. 2009b; Acharya et al. 2010) studies that indicate that ECoG can give detailed information about the kinematic parameters of a concurrent movement. Indeed, in properties relevant to BCI technology, ECoG can provide information comparable to (Schalk et al. 2007) or even exceeding (Kubánek et al. 2009) that provided by intracortical microelectrode recordings in nonhuman primates (Lebedev et al. 2005). This is probably due to the larger coverage of ECoG compared to microelectrode recordings, which perhaps compensates for ECoG's lower spatial resolution. Most important to BCI development, and not previously known or appreciated, is that signals recorded with ECoG contain a lot of information about movements. As yet, little is known about which brain functions (e.g., motor or sensory), which task-related parameters (e.g., hand movement vs. rest, hand velocity), and which corresponding ECoG features will prove to be the best basis for realizing BCI control.

In several studies (Leuthardt et al. 2004; Schalk 2008) the features to be used for control were selected by asking the subject to perform, or to imagine performing, various motor actions (e.g., opening and closing the hand contralateral to the electrode array, or protruding the tongue). First, the research subject engaged in the actual or imagined action during presentation of a visual cue. The cues, which lasted approximately 4 sec, were interspersed with rest periods of comparable duration. The different actions were interspersed randomly, and each was repeated at least 30 times. Offline analysis converted the raw ECoG data into the frequency domain using an autoregressive model (Pierce 1980; see chapter 7), and determined the ECoG features (e.g., amplitudes at specific frequencies and specific locations) that correlated with specific actual and/or imagined actions (i.e., that showed clear differences from the resting state). For a given ECoG feature and a given action, the strength of the correlation was measured as the coefficient of determination (r^2, [Wonnacott and Wonnacott 1977]) between the distribution of feature values for the action trials and the distribution for the interspersed rest periods. This measure indicated the fraction of the total variance of the feature that was accounted for by the action, and thus it indicated how much control the action had over the feature. The feature(s) with the highest r^2 values were chosen to be used for online BCI control.

In the second part of the typical ECoG BCI protocol, the subject is trained to operate the BCI by using the features chosen to control an output (e.g., usually a computer cursor). In work published to date, a linear combination of one or more of the chosen features controlled each dimension of movement. This approach is thus identical to that described in chapter 8 for EEG control of a computer cursor. After being set initially, the parameters of the linear transformation, such as offset (intercept), gain (slope), and coefficients for the features (independent variables) may remain constant throughout

performance, or they may be continually updated (adapted) on the basis of recent data, to adjust for ongoing changes in the features (e.g., as was done in Taylor et al. 2002 for single neuron-based control and in Wolpaw and McFarland 2004 and McFarland et al. 2010 for EEG-based control). Whereas such feature adaptations appear to be important for single neuron-based and EEG-based BCI movement control, they may be less important for ECoG-based movement. (Single-neuron-based BCI algorithms may require adaptations to adjust for changes in the sample of neurons recorded by the microelectrodes and/or in the activity of the individual neurons; EEG-based BCI algorithms may require adaptation to adjust for spontaneous changes in the features or changes due to adaptation [i.e., learning] by the user.) For ECoG, recent results (Blakely et al. 2009; Chao et al. 2010) suggest that cortical representations of function in ECoG are more stable than those detected with intracortical microelectrodes and that spontaneous signal fluctuations are less prominent than in EEG.

ECoG-BASED BCI CONTROL

Promising results from several laboratories have demonstrated online ECoG-based BCI control (Leuthardt et al. 2004; Leuthardt et al. 2006a; Wilson et al. 2006; Felton et al., 2007; Schalk 2008; Hinterberger et al. 2008; Blakely et al. 2009; Rouse and Moran 2009; van steensel et al. 2010; Miller, Schalk et al. 2010; Brunner et al. 2011). With one exception using nonhuman primates (Rouse and Moran 2009), these studies have been conducted with human volunteers. Almost all of them have used the highly flexible general-purpose BCI software platform BCI2000 (Schalk et al. 2004; Schalk and Mellinger 2010; see chapter 9).

Leuthardt et al. (2004) reported the first use of ECoG for BCI operation. Four people used different actual or imagined motor actions to move a cursor in one dimension (i.e. [up/down]) to reach a target located at the bottom or top of a computer screen. Over brief training periods of only 3–24 min, and using features associated with different actual or imagined actions, the four subjects achieved online success rates of 74–100% (with 50% expected by chance) (see fig. 15.8A for learning curves). Although the limited number of subjects and the limited number of study sessions do not permit meaningful quantitative (i.e., speed/accuracy) comparisons of the performance achieved with ECoG to that achieved with EEG-based or single neuron-based BCIs, the acquisition of control (see fig. 15.8A) appears to be faster than that typically achieved with EEG-based BCIs. For example, with less than 10 min of practice, one subject achieved an accuracy of 97% in controlling one-dimensional cursor movement by imagining (to move up) or not imagining (to move down) speaking the word "move." Offline analyses of data gathered from the four subjects while they were using a joystick to control two-dimensional cursor movement indicated that ECoG features at frequencies up to 180 Hz encode substantial information about both dimensions of movement (see fig. 15.5A).

The online one-dimensional BCI control reported in this initial report was confirmed and extended by several other studies using similar experimental protocols. Wilson et al.

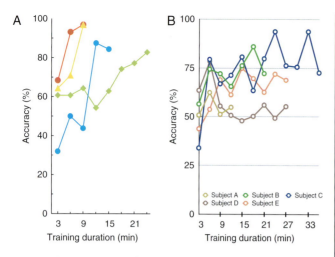

Figure 15.8 *(A) Learning curves for ECoG control of vertical cursor movement using motor imagery to move up and rest to move down. (Accuracy in absence of control would be 50%.) Patient B (green trace) imagined opening and closing the right hand, Patients C (yellow trace) and D (red trace) imagined saying the word "move," and Patient D (blue trace) imagined protruding the tongue. (From Leuthardt et al., 2004.) (B) Learning curves for ECoG control of two-dimensional cursor movement. (Accuracy in absence of control would be 25%.) (Modified from Schalk et al., 2008.)*

(2006) and Felton et al. (2007) reported comparable control using closer electrode spacing (i.e., 5 mm as opposed to 10 mm in Leuthardt et al. 2004) and ECoG features associated with sensory (rather than movement) imagery. van Steensel at al. (2010) showed that ECoG recorded over left dorsolateral prefrontal cortex, an area involved in working memory, can also support rapid acquisition of movement control. In work with a single subject, Blakely et al. (2009) found that an ECoG-based BCI with fixed parameters performed well over five days. Miller, Schalk et al. (2010) showed that motor imagery-based BCI control using locations in motor cortex can produce ECoG changes that exceed those produced by actual movements. Finally, in a study of potential importance for the development of practical long-term ECoG-based BCIs, Leuthardt et al. (2006a) found that an electrode placed epidurally (rather than subdurally) over premotor cortex also supported effective control (i.e., 100% accuracy).

In a study of item selection (rather than movement control), Hinterberger et al. (2008) showed that an ECoG-based BCI allowed subjects to select characters with motor imagery. In this study, the subjects imagined one of two movements (e.g., moving a hand or the tongue). The BCI detected which of these two imageries the subject was attempting and used the result in a multistep selection process to select a character. The best-performing subject spelled one character in approximately 3 min. In a more recent item-selection study involving a single test subject, Brunner et al. (2011) tested an ECoG-based matrix speller comparable to that developed for use with EEG (Schalk et al. 2004; Krusienski et al. 2006). The subject achieved spelling rates (i.e., 17 characters/min [69 bits/min]) sustained, 22 characters/min [113 bits/min] peak) several times higher than those reported for EEG (e.g., Serby et al. 2005; Sellers et al. 2006; Nijboer et al. 2008; Lenhardt et al. 2008; Guger et al. 2009; Sellers et al. 2010).

Schalk et al. (2008) extended the one-dimensional ECoG BCI results in a study showing that an ECoG-based BCI allowed five subjects to use imagined or actual motor actions to control a computer cursor in two dimensions. Over a brief training period of 12–36 min (see fig. 15.8B), each subject acquired substantial control of particular ECoG features recorded from several electrodes in a single array over one hemisphere (see fig. 15.9). After these few minutes of training, the ECoG features supported success rates of 53–73% in a two-dimensional, four-target, center-out task in which chance accuracy was 25%. In contrast, the somewhat higher levels of two-dimensional control that have been attained with EEG required three training sessions per week over at least 7 weeks (Wolpaw and McFarland 2004).

Whereas most ECoG-based BCI studies have been performed in human clinical patients, Rouse and Moran (2009) published the only online ECoG-based BCI study to date in monkeys. In this preliminary study with one monkey, ECoG features were used to control two different two-dimensional tasks: reaching and circle-drawing. For online control in either task, the authors used 65–100 Hz gamma activity in ECoG recorded from two arbitrarily selected epidural electrodes over primary motor cortex. The authors assigned gamma activity recorded from each of the two electrodes to horizontal or

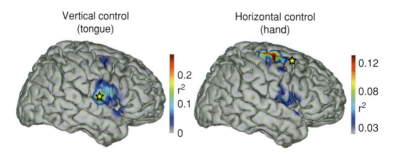

Figure 15.9 *Topographies of control of two-dimensional cursor movement for one subject, calculated for all locations and for the control signals provided by the ECoG features used online. These topographies show the color-coded correlation (as r² values) of the chosen ECoG features with vertical or horizontal movement and thus indicate the level of task-related control of different cortical areas. This subject used imagined tongue movements for vertical control and imagined hand movements for horizontal control. Yellow stars indicate the locations used for control online. These figures suggest that selection of different locations could have yielded better online performance, in particular for horizontal control. This demonstrates that appropriate feature selection is important. (Modified from Schalk et al., 2008.)*

vertical cursor movement control, respectively. Over the course of five recording days, the monkey was able to use gamma activity to achieve control of a cursor to successfully perform center-out reaching tasks as well as circle-drawing tasks. This study also suggested the particular gamma-frequency band that resulted in the best control.

In summary, the human and animal ECoG-based BCI studies to date show that ECoG recorded from different locations and in different experimental paradigms can support impressive BCI performance. ECoG might provide performance that exceeds that of EEG and that requires substantially less training to acquire. This probable superiority may be due largely to the ability of ECoG to record high-frequency (i.e., gamma) activity, which is minimal or entirely absent in EEG. Furthermore, ECoG may provide movement-related information comparable to that found in single-neuron activity and could prove more stable for long-term use.

LIMITATIONS

The ECoG-based studies reported thus far encourage further exploration of the value of research and development of ECoG-based BCIs. At the same time, it is important to consider at least three limitations to this technique.

The first limitation is that acquisition of ECoG signals for BCI research entails substantial practical obstacles, at least for recording in human subjects. Current human ECoG-based BCI research is limited almost exclusively to people who have been temporarily implanted (typically for only about 1 week) with an ECoG array, in order to localize a seizure focus and essential cortical functions prior to surgical resection for mitigation or cure of epilepsy or a tumor. When given the opportunity to participate in an ECoG study, most of the presurgical patients choose to do so. After the implantation and postoperative recovery (about 1–2 days), they are generally available for research only a few hours per day at most. These patients vary considerably in cognitive capacities (typically assessed by standard clinical neuropsychological testing), level of enthusiasm for participating, and clinical status (e.g., seizures, pain, nausea, medications). Their clinical needs necessarily take precedence over research interests. Thus, study schedules are often affected by their appointments for imaging, clinical tests (in particular electrical cortical mapping of function), medication regimens (e.g., pain medication), and personal visits. Furthermore, the ECoG recording is generally performed in a hospital room that has severe space constraints and may have considerable auditory and electromagnetic environmental noise (e.g., from electrical beds, pressurized stockings, or automated drug delivery systems) that may be difficult or impossible to reduce. In order to be successful in these studies, the research personnel must be highly trained and efficient, and should be ready to run experiments whenever the opportunity arises. The research system (both hardware and software) should be streamlined, robust, and always available.

The second limitation is related to ECoG's lower spatial resolution when compared to single-neuron recordings. ECoG's spatial resolution has been estimated to be around one mm (1.25 mm for subdural recordings [Freeman et al. 2000] and 1.4 mm for epidural recordings [Slutzky et al. 2010]). The spatial resolution of single-neuron recordings is approximately one order of magnitude higher. Thus, it will probably remain difficult or impossible to detect the firing of individual neurons from the cortical surface with ECoG. On the other hand, ECoG's larger coverage has been shown to compensate for this lower spatial resolution (Schalk et al. 2007; Kubánek et al. 2009). As yet it is unknown to what extent BCI performance depends on the ability to record activity from individual or very small assemblies of neurons. A related question is to what extent ECoG's limitation in spatial resolution will ultimately limit the degrees of freedom that can be extracted. Studies to date have demonstrated online two-dimensional BCI control (Schalk 2008) and offline decoding of five (Kubánek et al. 2009) and seven (Chao et al. 2010) different independent movement parameters.

The third limitation is that placement of ECoG recording electrodes requires an invasive (surgical) procedure. Although it is possible, or even likely, that invasive procedures for implantation of ECoG or single-neuron electrodes will eventually become as safe as many other invasive medical procedures, any invasive procedure will almost certainly entail greater risk and expense than noninvasive procedures, and thus it will likely be held to a higher standard of performance. Moreover, the need for surgical implantation of the electrodes will limit the practical utility of ECoG for nonmedical BCI applications such as gaming, artistic expression, and performance enhancement (see chapter 23).

IMPORTANT QUESTIONS AND AREAS FOR FURTHER RESEARCH

Studies published to date suggest that ECoG-based BCIs offer distinct advantages that could make them very useful to people with severe disabilities. At the same time, however, the work so far has barely begun to address the important questions that need to be answered if that promise is to be fulfilled. The questions to be addressed include: the best recoding locations; the best ECoG features (e.g., gamma vs. mu/beta vs. LMP); the best recording site and method (subdural/epidural/skull screws); the best electrode diameter and density (i.e., interelectrode distance); the best kinds of actual or imagined action (e.g., movements, sensations, cognitive functions); the best array designs for long-term biological impact and functional stability; and the realization of wholly implantable systems.

As is the case for BCIs that use other signals, online ECoG studies are essential for validating the systems and for developing optimal solutions. Although many issues can be explored through offline analyses, online testing is necessary to establish the validity of results. Human studies have been, and are likely to remain, largely confined to relatively short-term studies in people implanted temporarily for clinical purposes. Much of the essential research and development work can, and hopefully will, take place in animals (mainly monkeys and rats). This will be particularly true for issues that require long-term studies. Indeed, for many of the issues that must be resolved, there is no need or justification for human studies prior to satisfactory completion of animal studies to justify and guide the human studies. Animal studies are likely to yield a better understanding of the physiological bases of the different kinds of frequency-domain and time-domain features of ECoG (e.g., mu/beta, gamma, LMP, phase-amplitude coupling) that may enable informed choices for the configuration and implementation of ECoG-based BCI systems.

The current generation of ECoG implants, in particular those implanted prior to surgery (e.g., for epilepsy or tumors), are neither optimized nor even suitable for long-term BCI operation. The implant design (e.g., materials, electrode spacing) is generally determined purely by clinical needs and is suited only for relatively short-term use. These arrays are usually placed subdurally, cover areas up to 7×7 cm (thereby requiring a sizeable craniotomy), and have a percutaneous tethered connection to an external data-acquisition system. This placement and the percutaneous connection increase the risk for infection and for epidural or subdural hematomas. In contrast, ECoG-based BCI systems suitable for long-term use would be wholly implantable and might use arrays that cover relatively small areas of cortex and are placed epidurally. The work needed to develop the complete implants and establish their safety and effectiveness, first in animals and then in humans, has just begun.

Most of the components needed for a long-term ECoG-based BCI implant already exist. However, they have not yet received regulatory approval for human use. These components include ECoG implants that implement passive recording structures (J. Kim et al. 2007; Rubehn et al. 2009; see fig. 15.10A,B) or even active electronics on biocompatible substrates (D. H. Kim et al. 2010). These implants could be connected to amplification/digitization devices (Avestruz et al. 2008) and/or wireless transmission units (Anderson and Harrison 2010; Miranda et al. 2010; fig. 15.10C). With the addition of a battery (which could be implanted in areas distant from the ECoG implant, in the chest, for instance), these components could be combined into a fully and permanently implantable system, and could then be validated in animal and subsequent human studies.

It is worth noting that implantable ECoG-based BCI systems are likely to have two significant advantages over implantable intracortical (in particular single neuron-based) BCI systems. First, with ECoG arrays, it is more practical to record from larger areas of cortex than is practical with microelectrode implants, which record only from very small volumes of tissue. Thus, ECoG arrays may provide a more practical and comprehensive means to access the cortical networks that produce motor outputs. (On the other hand, minimizing an ECoG implant's invasiveness may require minimizing the size of the implant, thereby reducing this advantage.) Second, the power demands of ECoG recording are much more modest than those of single-neuron recording. This is a very important consideration for wholly implantable systems. Action-potential recording requires a digitization rate of >10 kHz per channel. With high numbers of channels, it is difficult to satisfy this requirement with wholly implanted low-power wireless-transmission systems without generating undue heat. In contrast, ECoG requires a digitization rate of only 500–1000 Hz per channel, more than an order of magnitude less. (On the other hand, LFP recordings from microelectrodes can also detect gamma activity, which can be satisfactorily recorded at sampling rates similar to those used for ECoG.) Furthermore, if a BCI relies on an ECoG feature such as gamma activity and an appropriate analog filter is employed, the digitization rate might be as low as 50 Hz per channel (Schalk 2008), more than two orders of magnitude less than that required for neuronal recording. In this case, a 1000-channel ECoG array would require a total digitization rate of only 50 kHz, the same rate required by only three to five microelectrodes. Whereas the requisite clinically approved devices are still in development, fully implantable devices capable of this digitization rate could readily be implemented using current technologies. Given the probable long-term stability of ECoG recordings (Chao et al. 2010; Schalk 2010), appropriate modification or extension of current technologies could lead to wireless ECoG implants that could transmit ongoing brain activity from many thousands of cortical sites and that could deliver robust signals over many years. Ideally, this system might consist of an epidural array that includes amplification/digitization/wireless electronics, is

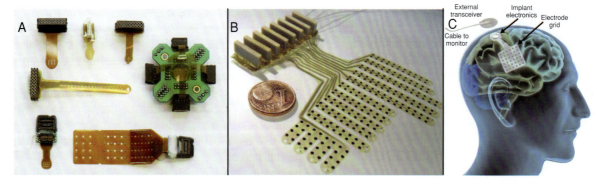

Figure 15.10 Emerging generation of ECoG recording devices. (A) Thin film-based ECoG devices and their connectors for recordings in different species. (Picture courtesy of Dr. Justin Williams.) (B) ECoG recording device for high-channel-number recordings in a monkey. (From Rubehn et al., 2009.) (C) Proposed ECoG grid with wireless interface. (Courtesy of Ripple, Inc.)

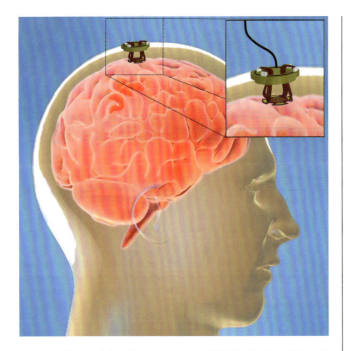

Figure 15.11 *Proposed clinical implementation of ECoG technology. Schematic illustration of micro-ECoG implant platform based on a standard 19-mm neurosurgical cranial trephine. The flexible electrode substrate is folded into a "leaf-spring" arrangement, allowing for the implant to flex and to accommodate relative motion between the brain and skull. (Image courtesy of Justin Williams and Joseph Hippensteel.)*

powered by a battery at a remote site (e.g., in the chest), and is permanently implanted through a small (e.g., 19-mm) burr hole in the skull (see simplified illustration in fig. 15.11).

SUMMARY

ECoG is generating strong and growing excitement for its potential as a clinically useful BCI signal modality. This interest is based on several highly advantageous characteristics of ECoG recording, as well as on recognition of the limitations of existing noninvasive and invasive signal types. ECoG has greater amplitude, higher topographical resolution, and a much broader frequency range than scalp-recorded EEG and is less susceptible to artifacts. With current and foreseeable recording methodologies, ECoG is likely to have greater long-term stability than intracortically recorded signals. Furthermore, it can more readily be recorded from larger cortical areas, and it requires much lower digitization rates, thus greatly reducing the power requirements of wholly implanted systems.

ECoG detects oscillations and evoked potentials with frequency contents from as low as direct-current frequencies and up to 500 Hz. It detects the mu- and beta-rhythm bands prominent in the scalp-recorded EEG and, most importantly, also detects higher-frequency gamma activity that is typically absent or minimally apparent in EEG. Gamma activity appears to have greater functional localization than lower-frequency activity and thus may be particularly useful for ECoG-based

BCI systems. In addition, ECoG also detects the LMP, which also displays high functional specificity.

Up to the present, ECoG-based BCI studies have been limited primarily to people temporarily implanted with ECoG recording arrays prior to surgery. Despite the many practical difficulties of such studies, the results are promising. They suggest that ECoG-based BCIs might provide control comparable to, or even superior to, that reported for EEG-based and single neuron-based BCIs. These results, combined with some likely practical advantages of ECoG methodology, are encouraging further efforts to develop ECoG-based BCI systems. Particularly important issues to be resolved include: determination of the best cortical locations (i.e., motor, sensory, cognitive); the best recording methods (i.e., epidural vs. subdural, cortical location, and electrode spacing); the optimal feature selection (i.e., mu, beta, gamma, LMPs); and the most effective algorithm designs. Many of these issues will be most readily addressed in animal studies.

ECoG-based BCI systems suitable for long-term human use must be wholly implantable and capable of performing reliably for many years. Although such systems have not yet been developed, the individual components that would comprise them do exist or are under active development. The extensive work needed to develop the complete systems and to validate them first in animals and then in humans has just begun. Its successful completion, combined with resolution of the other issues summarized here, could lead to ECoG-based BCI systems of great value to people with severe motor disabilities.

REFERENCES

Acharya, S., M. S. Fifer, H. L. Benz, N. E. Crone, and N. V. Thakor. Electrocorticographic amplitude predicts finger positions during slow grasping motions of the hand. *J Neural Eng*, 7(4):046002, 2010.

Allison, B. Z., D. J. McFarland, G. Schalk, S. D. Zheng, M. M. Jackson, and J. R. Wolpaw. Towards an independent brain-computer interface using steady state visual evoked potentials. *Clin Neurophysiol*, 119(2):399–408, 2008.

R. A. Andersen, S. Musallam, and B. Pesaran. Selecting the signals for a brain-machine interface. *Curr Opin Neurobiol*, 14(6):720–726, 2004.

G. Anderson and R. Harrison. Wireless integrated circuit for the acquisition of electrocorticogram signals. In *Proceedings of 2010 IEEE International Symposium on Circuits and Systems (ISCAS)*, pp. 2952–2955. IEEE, 2010.

F. Aoki, E. E. Fetz, L. Shupe, E. Lettich, and G. A. Ojemann. Increased gamma-range activity in human sensorimotor cortex during performance of visuomotor tasks. *Clin Neurophysiol*, 110(3):524–537, 1999.

A. Avestruz, W. Santa, D. Carlson, R. Jensen, S. Stanslaski, A. Helfenstine, and T. Denison. A 5 μw/channel spectral analysis IC for chronic bidirectional brain-machine interfaces. *IEEE J Solid State Circuits*, 43(12):3006–3024, 2008.

T. Ball, M. Kern, I. Mutschler, A. Aertsen, and A. Schulze-Bonhage. Signal quality of simultaneously recorded invasive and non-invasive EEG. *Neuroimage*, 2009.

N. Birbaumer, N. Ghanayim, T. Hinterberger, I. Iversen, B. Kotchoubey, A. Kübler, J. Perelmouter, E. Taub, and H. Flor. A spelling device for the paralysed. *Nature*, 398(6725):297–298, 1999.

T. Blakely, K. Miller, S. Zanos, R. Rao, and J. Ojemann. Robust, long-term control of an electrocorticographic brain-computer interface with fixed parameters. *J Neurosurg Pediatr*, 27(1):E13, 2009.

P. Brunner, A. L. Ritaccio, J. F. Emrich, H. Bischof, and G. Schalk. Rapid communication with a p300 matrix speller using electrocorticographic signals (ecog). *Front Neuroprosthet*, 5(5):1–9, 2011.

P. Brunner, A.L. Ritaccio, T.M. Lynch, J.F. Emrich, J.A. Wilson, J.C. Williams, E.J. Aarnoutse, N.F. Ramsey, E.C. Leuthardt, H. Bischof, G. Schalk, A Practical Procedure for Real-Time Functional Mapping of Eloquent Cortex Using Electrocorticographic Signals in Humans. *Epilepsy Behav*, 15(3):278–286, 2009.

L. A. Bullara, W. F. Agnew, T. G. Yuen, S. Jacques, and R. H. Pudenz. Evaluation of electrode array material for neural prostheses. *Neurosurgery*, 5(6): 681–686, 1979.

A. F. Calvet and J. Bancaud. Electrocorticography of waves associated with eye movements in man during wakefulness. *Electroencephalogr Clin Neurophysiol*, 40(5):457–469, 1976.

R. Canolty, M. Soltani, S. Dalal, E. Edwards, N. Dronkers, S. Nagarajan, H. Kirsch, N. Barbaro, and R. Knight. Spatiotemporal dynamics of word processing in the human brain. *Frontiers in Neuroscience*, 1(1):185, 2007.

R. T. Canolty, E. Edwards, S. S. Dalal, M. Soltani, S. S. Nagarajan, H. E. Kirsch, M. S. Berger, N. M. Barbaro, and R. T. Knight. High gamma power is phase-locked to theta oscillations in human neocortex. *Science*, 313(5793): 1626–1628, 2006.

R. T. Canolty and R. T. Knight. The functional role of cross-frequency coupling. *Trends Cogn Sci*, 14(11):506–515, 2010.

R. Caton. Electrical currents of the brain. *J Nerv Ment Dis*, 2(4):610, 1875.

E. F. Chang, E. Edwards, S. S. Nagarajan, N. Fogelson, S. S. Dalal, R. T. Canolty, H. E. Kirsch, N. M. Barbaro, and R. T. Knight. Cortical spatio-temporal dynamics underlying phonological target detection in humans. *J Cogn Neurosci*, 23(6):1437–1446, 2011.

Z. C. Chao, Y. Nagasaka, and N. Fujii. Long-term asynchronous decoding of arm motion using electrocorticographic signals in monkeys. *Front Neuroeng*, 3:3–3, 2010.

G. Chatrian. *Handbook of electroencephalography and clinical neurophysiology*. Amsterdam: Elsevier, 1976.

N. E. Crone, L. Hao, J. Hart, D. Boatman, R. P. Lesser, R. Irizarry, and B. Gordon. Electrocorticographic gamma activity during word production in spoken and sign language. *Neurology*, 57(11):2045–2053, 2001.

N. E. Crone, D. L. Miglioretti, B. Gordon, and R. P. Lesser. Functional mapping of human sensorimotor cortex with electrocorticographic spectral analysis. ii. Event-related synchronization in the gamma band. *Brain*, 121 (Pt 12):2301–2315, 1998.

N. E. Crone, D. L. Miglioretti, B. Gordon, J. M. Sieracki, M. T. Wilson, S. Uematsu, and R. P. Lesser. Functional mapping of human sensorimotor cortex with electrocorticographic spectral analysis. i. Alpha and beta event-related desynchronization. Brain, 121 (Pt 12):2271–2299, 1998.

F. Darvas, R. Scherer, J. G. Ojemann, R. P. Rao, K. J. Miller, and L. B. Sorensen. High gamma mapping using EEG. *Neuroimage*, 49(1):930–938, 2010.

K. Davids, S. Bennett, and K. M. Newell (Eds.). *Movement system variability*. Human Kinetics, Champaign, IL, 2005.

I. Dési, L. Nagymajtényi, and H. Schulz. Effect of subchronic mercury exposure on electrocorticogram of rats. *Neurotoxicology*, 17(3–4):719–723, 1996.

J. R. Dias-dos Santos and B. H. Machado. Cardiovascular and respiratory changes during slow-wave sleep in rats are associated with electrocorticogram desynchronization. *Braz J Med Biol Res*, 30(11):1371–1376, 1997.

J. Donoghue, A. Nurmikko, G. Friehs, and M. Black. Development of neuromotor prostheses for humans. *Suppl Clin Neurophysiol*, 57:592–606, 2004.

J. P. Donoghue, A. Nurmikko, M. Black, and L. R. Hochberg. Assistive technology and robotic control using motor cortex ensemble-based neural interface systems in humans with tetraplegia. *J Physiol*, 579(Pt 3):603–611, 2007.

E. Edwards, S. S. Nagarajan, S. S. Dalal, R. T. Canolty, H. E. Kirsch, N. M. Barbaro, and R. T. Knight. Spatiotemporal imaging of cortical activation during verb generation and picture naming. *Neuroimage*, 50(1):291–301, 2010.

L. A. Farwell and E. Donchin. Talking off the top of your head: toward a mental prosthesis utilizing event-related brain potentials. *Electroenceph Clin Neurophysiol*, 70(6):510–523, 1988.

E. A. Felton, J. A. Wilson, J. C. Williams, and P. C. Garell. Electrocorticographically controlled brain-computer interfaces using motor and sensory imagery in patients with temporary subdural electrode implants. Report of four cases. *J Neurosurg*, 106(3):495–500, 2007.

W. J. Freeman. Spatial properties of an EEG event in the olfactory bulb and cortex. *Electroencephalogr Clin Neurophysiol*, 44(5):586–605, 1978.

W. J. Freeman, M. D. Holmes, B. C. Burke, and S. Vanhatalo. Spatial spectra of scalp EEG and EMG from awake humans. *Clin Neurophysiol*, 114:1053–1068, 2003.

W. J. Freeman, L. J. Rogers, M. D. Holmes, and D. L. Silbergeld. Spatial spectral analysis of human electrocorticograms including the alpha and gamma bands. *J Neurosci Methods*, 95(2):111–121, 2000.

W. J. Freeman and W. Schneider. Changes in spatial patterns of rabbit olfactory EEG with conditioning to odors. *Psychophysiology*, 19(1):44–56, 1982.

W. J. Freeman and B. W. van Dijk. Spatial patterns of visual cortical fast EEG during conditioned reflex in a rhesus monkey. *Brain Res*, 422(2):267–276, 1987.

I. Fried, G. A. Ojemann, and E. E. Fetz. Language-related potentials specific to human language cortex. *Science*, 212(4492):353–356, 1981.

H. Fritz, R. Bauer, B. Walter, O. Schlonski, D. Hoyer, U. Zwiener, and K. Reinhart. Hypothermia related changes in electrocortical activity at stepwise increase of intracranial pressure in piglets. *Exp Toxicol Pathol*, 51(2):163–171, 1999.

C. Gaona, M. Sharma, Z. Freudenburg, J. Breshears, D. Bundy, J. Roland, D. Barbour, G. Schalk, and E. Leuthardt. Nonuniform high-gamma (60–500 Hz) power changes dissociate cognitive task and anatomy in human cortex. *J Neurosci*, 31(6):2091–2100, 2011.

A. Georgopoulos, A. Schwartz, and R. Kettner. Neuronal population coding of movement direction. *Science*, 233:1416–1419, 1986.

B. Graimann, J. E. Huggins, A. Schlögl, S. P. Levine, and G. Pfurtscheller. Detection of movement-related desynchronization patterns in ongoing single-channel electrocorticogram. *IEEE Trans Neural Syst Rehabil Eng*, 11(3):276–281, 2003.

C. Guger, S. Daban, E. Sellers, C. Holzner, G. Krausz, R. Carabalona, F. Gramatica, and G. Edlinger. How many people are able to control a P300-based brain-computer interface (BCI)? *Neurosci Lett*, 462(1):94–98, 2009.

T. Hata, Y. Nishimura, T. Kita, A. Kawabata, and E. Itoh. Electrocorticogram in rats loaded with SART stress (repeated cold stress). *Jpn J Pharmacol*, 45(3):365–372, 1987.

B. J. He, J. M. Zempel, A. Z. Snyder, and M. E. Raichle. The temporal structures and functional significance of scale-free brain activity. *Neuron*, 66(3): 353–369, 2010.

T. Hinterberger, G. Widman, T. Lal, J. Hill, M. Tangermann, W. Rosenstiel, B. Schölkopf, C. Elger, and N. Birbaumer. Voluntary brain regulation and communication with electrocorticogram signals. *Epilepsy Behav*, 13(2):300–306, 2008.

N. Hirai, S. Uchida, T. Maehara, Y. Okubo, and H. Shimizu. Enhanced gamma (30–150 Hz) frequency in the human medial temporal lobe. *Neuroscience*, 90(4):1149–1155, 1999.

L. R. Hochberg, M. D. Serruya, G. M. Friehs, J. A. Mukand, M. Saleh, A. H. Caplan, A. Branner, D. Chen, R. D. Penn, and J. P. Donoghue. Neuronal ensemble control of prosthetic devices by a human with tetraplegia. *Nature*, 442(7099):164–171, 2006.

J. Huggins, S. Levine, S. BeMent, R. Kushwaha, L. Schuh, E. Passaro, M. Rohde, D. Ross, K. Elisevich, and B. Smith. Detection of event-related potentials for development of a direct brain interface. *J Clin Neurophysiol*, 16(5): 448–455, 1999.

H. Jokeit and S. Makeig. Different event-related patterns of gamma-band power in brain waves of fast- and slow-reacting subjects. *Proc Natl Acad Sci USA*, 91(14):6339–6343, 1994.

F. Kasanetz, L. A. Riquelme, P. O'Donnell, and M. G. Murer. Turning off cortical ensembles stops striatal up states and elicits phase perturbations in cortical and striatal slow oscillations in rat in vivo. *J Physiol*, 577 (Pt 1):97–113, 2006.

D. H. Kim, J. Viventi, J. J. Amsden, J. Xiao, L. Vigeland, Y. S. Kim, J. A. Blanco, B. Panilaitis, E. S. Frechette, D. Contreras, D. L. Kaplan, F. G. Omenetto, Y. Huang, K. C. Hwang, M. R. Zakin, B. Litt, and J. A. Rogers. Dissolvable films of silk fibroin for ultrathin conformal bio-integrated electronics. *Nat Mater*, 9(6):511–517, 2010.

J. Kim, J. Wilson, and J. Williams. A cortical recording platform utilizing μECoG electrode arrays. In *Engineering in Medicine and Biology Society, 2007. EMBS 2007. 29th Annual International Conference of the IEEE*, pp. 5353–5357. IEEE, 2007.

H. Kornhuber and L. Deecke. Hirnpotentialänderungen bei willkürbewegungen und passiven bewegungen des menschen: Bereitschaftspotential und reafferente potentiale. *Pflugers Arch*, 284:1–17, 1965.

D. Krusienski, F. Cabestaing, D. McFarland, and J. Wolpaw. A comparison of classification techniques for the P300 speller. *J Neural Eng*, 3(4):299–305, 2006.

J. Kubánek, K. J. Miller, J. G. Ojemann, J. R. Wolpaw, and G. Schalk. Decoding flexion of individual fingers using electrocorticographic signals in humans. *J Neural Eng*, 6(6):066001, 2009.

A. Kübler, B. Kotchoubey, T. Hinterberger, N. Ghanayim, J. Perelmouter, M. Schauer, C. Fritsch, E. Taub, and N. Birbaumer. The Thought Translation Device: a neurophysiological approach to communication in total motor paralysis. *Exp Brain Res*, 124(2):223–232, 1999.

A. Kübler, F. Nijboer, J. Mellinger, T. M. Vaughan, H. Pawelzik, G. Schalk, D. J. McFarland, N. Birbaumer, and J. R. Wolpaw. Patients with ALS can use sensori-motor rhythms to operate a brain-computer interface. *Neurology*, 64(10):1775–1777, 2005.

J. P. Lachaux, P. Fonlupt, P. Kahane, L. Minotti, D. Hoffmann, O. Bertrand, and M. Baciu. Relationship between task-related gamma oscillations and bold signal: new insights from combined fmri and intracranial eeg. *Hum Brain Mapp*, 28(12):1368–1375, 2007.

M. A. Lebedev, J. M. Carmena, J. E. O'Doherty, M. Zacksenhouse, C. S. Henriquez, J. C. Principe, and M. A. Nicolelis. Cortical ensemble adaptation to represent velocity of an artificial actuator controlled by a brain-machine interface. *J Neurosci*, 25(19):4681–4693, 2005.

A. Lenhardt, M. Kaper, and H. J. Ritter. An adaptive P300-based online brain-computer interface. *IEEE Trans Neural Syst Rehabil Eng*, 16(2): 121–130, 2008.

E. Leuthardt, K. Miller, N. Anderson, G. Schalk, J. Dowling, J. Miller, D. Moran, and J. Ojemann. Electrocorticographic frequency alteration mapping: a clinical technique for mapping the motor cortex. *Neurosurgery*, 60: 260–270; discussion 270–1, 2007.

E. Leuthardt, K. Miller, G. Schalk, R. Rao, and J. Ojemann. Electrocorticography-based brain computer interface—the Seattle experience. *IEEE Trans Neural Syst Rehabil Eng*, 14:194–198, 2006a.

E. C. Leuthardt, G. Schalk, D. Moran, and J. G. Ojemann. The emerging world of motor neuroprosthetics: a neurosurgical perspective. *Neurosurgery*, 59(1):1–14, 2006b.

E. Leuthardt, G. Schalk, J. Wolpaw, J. Ojemann, and D. Moran. A brain–computer interface using electrocorticographic signals in humans. *J Neural Eng*, 1(2):63–71, 2004.

S. P. Levine, J. E. Huggins, S. L. BeMent, R. K. Kushwaha, L. A. Schuh, E. A. Passaro, M. M. Rohde, and D. A. Ross. Identification of electrocorticogram patterns as the basis for a direct brain interface. *J Clin Neurophysiol*, 16:439–447, 1999.

S. P. Levine, J. E. Huggins, S. L. BeMent, R. K. Kushwaha, L. A. Schuh, M. M. Rohde, E. A. Passaro, D. A. Ross, K. V. Elisevich, and B. J. Smith. A direct brain interface based on event-related potentials. *IEEE Trans Rehabil Eng*, 8(2):180–185, 2000.

G. E. Loeb, A. E. Walker, S. Uematsu, and B. W. Konigsmark. Histological reaction to various conductive and dielectric films chronically implanted in the subdural space. *J Biomed Mater Res*, 11(2):195–210, 1977.

J. Manning, J. Jacobs, I. Fried, and M. Kahana. Broadband shifts in local field potential power spectra are correlated with single-neuron spiking in humans. *J Neurosci*, 29(43):13613, 2009.

E. Margalit, J. Weiland, R. Clatterbuck, G. Fujii, M. Maia, M. Tameesh, G. Torres, S. D'Anna, S. Desai, D. Piyathaisere, A. Olivi, E. J. de Juan, and M. Humayun. Visual and electrical evoked response recorded from subdural electrodes implanted above the visual cortex in normal dogs under two methods of anesthesia. *J Neurosci Methods*, 123(2):129–137, 2003.

D. J. McFarland, D. J. Krusienski, W. A. Sarnacki, and J. R. Wolpaw. Emulation of computer mouse control with a noninvasive brain-computer interface. *J Neural Eng*, 5(2):101–110, 2008.

D. J. McFarland, G. W. Neat, and J. R. Wolpaw. An EEG-based method for graded cursor control. *Psychobiology*, 21:77–81, 1993.

D. J. McFarland, W. A. Sarnacki, and J. R. Wolpaw. Electroencephalographic (EEG) control of three-dimensional movement. *J Neural Eng*, 7(3):036007, 2010.

C. Mehring, M. Nawrot, S. de Oliveira, E. Vaadia, A. Schulze-Bonhage, A. Aertsen, and T. Ball. Comparing information about arm movement direction in single channels of local and epicortical field potentials from monkey and human motor cortex. *J Physiol (Paris)*, 98(4–6):498–506, 2004.

V. Menon, W. J. Freeman, B. A. Cutillo, J. E. Desmond, M. F. Ward, S. L. Bressler, K. D. Laxer, N. Barbaro, and A. S. Gevins. Spatio-temporal correlations in human gamma band electrocorticograms. *Electroencephalogr Clin Neurophysiol*, 98(2):89–102, 1996.

J. del R. Millán, F. Renkens, J. Mouriño, and W. Gerstner. Noninvasive brain-actuated control of a mobile robot by human EEG. *IEEE Trans Biomed Eng*, 51(6):1026–1033, 2004.

K. Miller. Broadband spectral change: evidence for a macroscale correlate of population firing rate? *J Neurosci*, 30(19):6477, 2010.

K. Miller, E. Leuthardt, G. Schalk, R. Rao, N. Anderson, D. Moran, J. Miller, and J. Ojemann. Spectral changes in cortical surface potentials during motor movement. *J Neurosci*, 27:2424–2432, 2007a.

K. Miller, G. Schalk, E. Fetz, M. den Nijs, J. Ojemann, and R. Rao. Cortical activity during motor execution, motor imagery, and imagery-based online feedback. *Proc Natl Acad Sci USA*, 107(9):4430, 2010.

K. Miller, L. Sorensen, J. Ojemann, and M. Den Nijs. Power-law scaling in the brain surface electric potential. *PLoS Comput Biol*, 5:e1000609, 2009a.

K. Miller, S. Zanos, E. Fetz, M. den Nijs, and J. Ojemann. Decoupling the cortical power spectrum reveals real-time representation of individual finger movements in humans. *J Neurosci*, 29(10):3132, 2009b.

K. J. Miller, M. Dennijs, P. Shenoy, J. W. Miller, R. P. Rao, and J. G. Ojemann. Real-time functional brain mapping using electrocorticography. *Neuroimage*, 37(2):504–507, 2007b.

K.J. Miller, D. Hermes, C.J. Honey, M. Sharma, R.P. Rao, M. den Nijs, E.E. Fetz, T.J. Sejnowski, A.O. Hebb, J.G. Ojemann, S. Makeig, E.C. Leuthardt, Dynamic modulation of local population activity by rhythm phase in

human occipital cortex during a visual search task. *Front Hum Neurosci*, 29(4):197, 2010.

H. Miranda, V. Gilja, C. Chestek, K. Shenoy, and T. Meng. HermesD: A high-rate long-range wireless transmission system for simultaneous multichannel neural recording applications. *IEEE Trans Biomed Circ Syst*, 4(3): 181–191, 2010.

K. Müller and B. Blankertz. Toward noninvasive brain-computer interfaces. *IEEE Signal Processing Magazine*, 23(5):126–128, 2006.

E. Niedermeyer and F. Lopes da Silva, Eds. *Electroencephalography. Basic Principles, Clinical Applications, and Related fields*. Baltimore: Williams & Wilkins, 1993.

J. Niessing, B. Ebisch, K. Schmidt, M. Niessing, W. Singer, and R. Galuske. Hemodynamic signals correlate tightly with synchronized gamma oscillations. *Science*, 309(5736):948, 2005.

F. Nijboer, E. W. Sellers, J. Mellinger, M. A. Jordan, T. Matuz, A. Furdea, S. Halder, U. Mochty, D. J. Krusienski, T. M. Vaughan, J. R. Wolpaw, N. Birbaumer, and A. Kübler. A P300-based brain-computer interface for people with amyotrophic lateral sclerosis. *Clin Neurophysiol*, 119(8):1909–1916, 2008.

G. A. Ojemann, I. Fried, and E. Lettich. Electrocorticographic (ECoG) correlates of language. i. Desynchronization in temporal language cortex during object naming. *Electroencephalogr Clin Neurophysiol*, 73(5):453–463, 1989.

X. Pei, E.C. Leuthardt, C.M. Gaona, P. Brunner, J.R. Wolpaw, G. Schalk, Spatiotemporal Dynamics of ECoG Activity Related to Language Processing, *NeuroImage*, 54(4):2960–2972, 2011.

B. Peruche, H. Klaassens, and J. Krieglstein. Quantitative analysis of the electrocorticogram after forebrain ischemia in the rat. *Pharmacology*, 50(4):229–237, 995.

G. Pfurtscheller and R. Cooper. Frequency dependence of the transmission of the EEG from cortex to scalp. *Electroencephalogr Clin Neurophysiol*, 38:93–96, 1975.

G. Pfurtscheller, D. Flotzinger, and J. Kalcher. Brain-computer interface—a new communication device for handicapped persons. *J Microcomp App*, 16:293–299, 1993.

G. Pfurtscheller, B. Graimann, J. E. Huggins, S. P. Levine, and L. A. Schuh. Spatiotemporal patterns of beta desynchronization and gamma synchronization in corticographic data during self-paced movement. *Clin Neurophysiol*, 114(7):1226–1236, 2003.

G. Pfurtscheller, C. Guger, G. Müller, G. Krausz, and C. Neuper. Brain oscillations control hand orthosis in a tetraplegic. *Neurosci Lett*, 292(3):211–214, 2000.

G. Pfurtscheller and C. Neuper. Simultaneous EEG 10 Hz desynchronization and 40 Hz synchronization during finger movements. *NeuroReport*, 3(12):1057, 1992.

J. R. Pierce. *An Introduction to Information Theory: Symbols, Signals and Noise*. New York: Dover Publications, 2nd ed, 1980.

W. Pilcher and W. Rusyniak. Complications of epilepsy surgery. *Neurosurg Clin North Am*, 4(2):311–325, 1993.

T. Pistohl, T. Ball, A. Schulze-Bonhage, A. Aertsen, and C. Mehring. Prediction of arm movement trajectories from ECoG-recordings in humans. *J Neurosci Methods*, 167(1):105–114, 2008.

S. Ray, N. E. Crone, E. Niebur, P. J. Franaszczuk, and S. S. Hsiao. Neural correlates of high-gamma oscillations (60–200 Hz) in macaque local field potentials and their potential implications in electrocorticography. *J Neurosci*, 28(45):11526–11536, 2008.

M. M. Rohde, S. L. BeMent, J. E. Huggins, S. P. Levine, R. K. Kushwaha, and L. A. Schuh. Quality estimation of subdurally recorded, event-related potentials based on signal-to-noise ratio. *IEEE Trans Biomed Eng*, 49(1): 31–40, 2002.

A. Rouse and D. Moran. Neural adaptation of epidural electrocorticographic (EECoG) signals during closed-loop brain computer interface (BCI) tasks. *31st Annual International Conference of the IEEE Engineering in Medicine and Biology Society*, Minneapolis, Minnesota, 5514–5517, 2009.

A. Royer, A. Doud, M. Rose, and B. He. EEG control of a virtual helicopter in 3-dimensional space using intelligent control strategies. *IEEE Trans Neural Syst Rehabil Eng*, 18(6):581–589, 2010.

B. Rubehn, C. Bosman, R. Oostenveld, P. Fries, and T. Stieglitz. A MEMS-based flexible multichannel ECoG-electrode array. *Journal of Neural Engineering*, 6:036003, 2009.

J. C. Sanchez, A. Gunduz, P. R. Carney, and J. C. Principe. Extraction and localization of mesoscopic motor control signals for human ECoG neuroprosthetics. *J Neurosci Methods*, 167(1):63–81, 2008.

G. Santhanam, S. I. Ryu, B. M. Yu, A. Afshar, and K. V. Shenoy. A high-performance brain-computer interface. *Nature*, 442(7099):195–198, 2006.

G. Schalk. *Towards a Clinically Practical Brain-Computer Interface*. PhD thesis, Rensselaer Polytechnic Institute, Troy, 2006.

G. Schalk. Brain-computer symbiosis. *J Neural Eng*, 5(1):1–1, 2008.

G. Schalk. Can electrocorticography (ECoG) support robust and powerful brain-computer interfaces? *Front Neuroeng*, 3:9–9, 2010.

G. Schalk, J. Kubánek, K. J. Miller, N. R. Anderson, E. C. Leuthardt, J. G. Ojemann, D. Limbrick, D. Moran, L. A. Gerhardt, and J. R. Wolpaw. Decoding two-dimensional movement trajectories using electrocorticographic signals in humans. *J Neural Eng*, 4(3):264–275, 2007.

G. Schalk, E. C. Leuthardt, P. Brunner, J. G. Ojemann, L. A. Gerhardt, and J. R. Wolpaw. Real-time detection of event-related brain activity. *Neuroimage*, 43(2):245–249, 2008.

G. Schalk, D. McFarland, T. Hinterberger, N. Birbaumer, and J. Wolpaw. BCI2000: a general-purpose brain-computer interface (BCI) system. *IEEE Trans Biomed Eng*, 51:1034–1043, 2004.

G. Schalk and J. Mellinger. *A Practical Guide to Brain-Computer Interfacing with BCI2000*. Springer, London, 2010.

G. Schalk, K. J. Miller, N. R. Anderson, J. A. Wilson, M. D. Smyth, J. G. Ojemann, D. W. Moran, J. R. Wolpaw, and E. C. Leuthardt. Two-dimensional movement control using electrocorticographic signals in humans. *J Neural Eng*, 5(1):75–84, 2008.

M. Schürmann, T. Demiralp, E. Basar, and C. Basar Eroglu. Electroencephalogram alpha (8–15 Hz) responses to visual stimuli in cat cortex, thalamus, and hippocampus: a distributed alpha network? *Neurosci Lett*, 292(3):175–178, 2000.

E. W. Sellers, A. Kübler, and E. Donchin. Brain-computer interface research at the University of South Florida Cognitive Psychophysiology Laboratory: the P300 Speller. *IEEE Trans Neural Syst Rehabil Eng*, 14(2):221–224, 2006.

E. W. Sellers, T. M. Vaughan, and J. R. Wolpaw. A brain-computer interface for long-term independent home use. *Amyotroph Lateral Scler*, 11(5):449–455, 2010.

E. W. Sellers, T. M. Vaughan, and J. R. Wolpaw. A brain-computer interface for long-term independent home use. *Amyotroph Lateral Scler*, 11(5):449–455, 2010.

H. Serby, E. Yom-Tov, and G. F. Inbar. An improved P300-based brain-computer interface. *IEEE Trans Neural Syst Rehabil Eng*, 13(1):89–98, 2005.

M. Serruya, N. Hatsopoulos, L. Paninski, M. Fellows, and J. Donoghue. Instant neural control of a movement signal. *Nature*, 416(6877):141–142, 2002.

W. Shain, L. Spataro, J. Dilgen, K. Haverstick, S. Retterer, M. Isaacson, M. Saltzman, and J. Turner. Controlling cellular reactive responses around neural prosthetic devices using peripheral and local intervention strategies. *IEEE Trans Neural Syst Rehabil Eng*, 11:186–188, 2003.

K. Shenoy, D. Meeker, S. Cao, S. Kureshi, B. Pesaran, C. Buneo, A. Batista, P. Mitra, J. Burdick, and R. Andersen. Neural prosthetic control signals from plan activity. *Neuroreport*, 14(4):591–596, 2003.

N. Shinozuka and P. W. Nathanielsz. Electrocortical activity in fetal sheep in the last seven days of gestation. *J Physiol*, 513 (Pt 1):273–281, 1998.

A. Sinai, C. W. Bowers, C. M. Crainiceanu, D. Boatman, B. Gordon, R. P. Lesser, F. A. Lenz, and N. E. Crone. Electrocorticographic high gamma activity versus electrical cortical stimulation mapping of naming. *Brain*, 128(Pt 7):1556–1570, 2005.

M. W. Slutzky, L. R. Jordan, T. Krieg, M. Chen, D. J. Mogul, and L. E. Miller. Optimal spacing of surface electrode arrays for brain-machine interface applications. *J Neural Eng*, 7(2):26004, 2010.

R. J. Staba, C. L. Wilson, A. Bragin, I. Fried, and J. Engel. Quantitative analysis of high-frequency oscillations (80–500 Hz) recorded in human epileptic hippocampus and entorhinal cortex. *J Neurophysiol*, 88(4):1743–1752, 2002.

E. E. Sutter. The brain response interface: communication through visually guided electrical brain responses. *J Microcomput Appl*, 15:31–45, 1992.

D. M. Taylor, S. I. Tillery, and A. B. Schwartz. Direct cortical control of 3D neuroprosthetic devices. *Science*, 296:1829–1832, 2002.

C. Toro, C. Cox, G. Friehs, C. Ojakangas, R. Maxwell, J. R. Gates, R. J. Gumnit, and T. J. Ebner. 8–12 Hz rhythmic oscillations in human motor cortex during two-dimensional arm movements: evidence for representation of kinematic parameters. *Electroencephalogr Clin Neurophysiol*, 93(5):390–403, 1994.

M. van Steensel, D. Hermes, E. Aarnoutse, M. Bleichner, G. Schalk, P. van Rijen, F. Leijten, and N. Ramsey. Brain–computer interfacing based on cognitive control. *Ann Neurol*, 67(6):809–816, 2010.

T. M. Vaughan, D. J. McFarland, G. Schalk, W. A. Sarnacki, D. J. Krusienski, E. W. Sellers, and J. R. Wolpaw. The Wadsworth BCI research and development program: at home with BCI. *IEEE Trans Neural Syst Rehabil Eng*, 14(2):229–233, 2006.

M. Velliste, S. Perel, M. C. Spalding, A. S. Whitford, and A. B. Schwartz. Cortical control of a prosthetic arm for self-feeding. *Nature*, 453(7198):1098–1101, 2008.

W. G. Walter, R. Cooper, V. J. Aldridge, W. C. McCallum, and A. L. Winter. Contingent negative variation: An electric sign of sensorimotor association and expectancy in the human brain. *Nature*, 203:380–384, 1964.

K. A. Waters, C. S. Beardsmore, J. Paquette, G. A. Turner, and I. R. Moss. Electrocorticographic activity during repeated vs continuous hypoxia in piglets. *Brain Res Bull*, 41(3):185–192, 1996.

J. Wilson, E. Felton, P. Garell, G. Schalk, and J. Williams. ECoG factors underlying multimodal control of a brain-computer interface. *IEEE Transactions Neural Syst Rehabil Eng*, 14:246–250, 2006.

J. R. Wolpaw, N. Birbaumer, D. J. McFarland, G. Pfurtscheller, and T. M. Vaughan. Brain-computer interfaces for communication and control. *Electroencephalogr Clin Neurophysiol*, 113(6):767–791, 2002.

J. R. Wolpaw and D. J. McFarland. Multichannel EEG-based brain-computer communication. *Electroencephalogr Clin Neurophysiol*, 90(6):444–449, 1994.

J. R. Wolpaw and D. J. McFarland. Control of a two-dimensional movement signal by a noninvasive brain-computer interface in humans. *Proc Natl Acad Sci USA*, 101(51):17849–17854, 2004.

J. R. Wolpaw, D. J. McFarland, G. W. Neat, and C. A. Forneris. An EEG-based brain-computer interface for cursor control. *Electroencephalogr Clin Neurophysiol*, 78(3):252–259, 1991.

T. H. Wonnacott and R. Wonnacott. *Introductory Statistics*, 3rd ed. New York: John Wiley & Sons, 1977.

T. G. Yuen, W. F. Agnew, and L. A. Bullara. Tissue response to potential neuroprosthetic materials implanted subdurally. *Biomaterials*, 8(2):138–141, 1987.

16 | BCIs THAT USE SIGNALS RECORDED IN MOTOR CORTEX

JOHN P. DONOGHUE

One useful way of categorizing a brain-computer inter-face (BCI) is by the location of its sensor. The type and site of the sensor are directly tied to the kinds of signals that can be obtained and enable or limit the fidelity or quality of the signal. *Intraparenchymal BCIs* (iBCIs) are those that acquire brain signals from electrodes implanted within brain tissue (i.e., parenchyma), usually cerebral cortex. These are also called *penetrating* or *intracortical BCIs*. These BCIs are distinguished from *extraparenchymal BCI* (eBCIs), which acquire signals from electrodes located outside brain tissue (e.g., those placed on the scalp or on the surface of the brain). eBCIs record field potentials (FPs), which are a complex prod-uct of activity in many synapses and neurons (see chapter 3 in this volume). Recording potentials on the scalp is called *elec-troencephalography* (EEG), whereas recording potentials on the surface of the brain is called *electrocorticography* (ECoG). iBCIs are unique in that they can record not only field poten-tials, but also *single-unit activity* (SUA) (i.e., the action poten-tials [also called *spikes*] that reflect the output of single neurons). Furthermore, if spikes of a cluster of neurons are combined, they produce what is called *multiunit activity* (MUA). Thus, in providing BCI control, an iBCI can use detailed information about *spiking patterns* within the nervous system, as well as detailed information about *local field potentials* (LFPs). The type of iBCI recording desired determines the sensor's design. An electrode with an appropriately small recording surface is needed for recording spikes (Lempka et al. 2006). A larger intraparenchymal electrode can record a more general field potential (FP) (sometimes called an iEEG). (Such large elec-trodes would typically not record distinct spikes, even though located in brain tissue.)

The first evidence that spikes recorded from cortical neu-rons were potentially useful as a BCI output signal came from the pioneering work of Eberhard Fetz and collaborators who showed in the late 1960s and in the years following that mon-keys could learn to use a single neuron to control a meter needle to achieve food rewards (Fetz 1969; Fetz & Finocchio 1972). These seminal studies provided critical initial evidence that signals from motor cortex could be used in real time to control physical systems, and thus presaged demonstrations of closed-loop, multineuron control a quarter of a century later. Later work, in turn, rekindled interest in learning how much control can be provided by one neuron alone (Moritz et al. 2008). A second landmark was the introduction of the concept of *population coding*, the power of populations of neurons in motor cortex to provide smooth control signals (Humphrey et al. 1970; Georgopoulos 1988).

Whether BCIs record FPs or spikes, they need to process (e.g., filter, amplify, etc.) the recorded signals and decode them into commands that can be used to control a device. Since iBCIs use signals acquired at their source (i.e., within the brain), the hope is that they will produce better device control than is possible for eBCIs: that iBCIs will achieve more com-plex control (i.e., more degrees of freedom); be able to control multiple body parts (e.g., multiple limbs); and be more natural to use. At the same time, however, the unique requirements for iBCI sensors and the nature of the signals they record create challenges that are in several ways distinct from the require-ments of eBCIs. Much progress has been made in achieving stable, reliable signals in iBCIs, and the results are encouraging. This chapter describes iBCIs developed to date and addresses the issues involved in their further development, issues con-cerning biocompatibility, design, reliability, and signal proper-ties. We also refer the reader to chapters 2 and 5 in this volume and to a number of reviews that cover various aspects of these issues more comprehensively than is possible here (e.g., Hatsopoulos & Donoghue 2009; Waldert et al. 2009; Andersen et al. 2004; Donoghue 2008; Donoghue et al. 2007; Nicolelis & Lebedev 2009; Ryu & Shenoy 2009; Schwartz 2004).

GOALS IN DEVELOPMENT OF iBCI SYSTEMS

Because iBCIs use sensors implanted in the brain and record activity from relatively small populations of neurons, some of the goals of iBCI research and development are unique to iBCIs. The goals of iBCI development include:

- to demonstrate the ability of signals recorded from limited neuronal populations to provide complex control (e.g., of cursor movements or limb movements)

- to establish the range of functionally useful actions that iBCIs can restore to people who are paralyzed

- to identify the advantages and benefits of iBCIs over eBCIs, which do not require that sensors be implanted in the brain

- to develop iBCIs that are safe for long-term use (i.e., years and decades)
- to develop iBCIs that can function reliably and stably for years

These goals are being addressed through studies in both animals (primarily monkeys and rats) and, in early-stage human clinical trials in people with severe motor disabilities. Animal models are important for development and testing of new sensor designs (including device-tissue interactions) and decoding algorithms, and they are also contributing to new understanding of the neuronal control of movement.

COMPLEX CONTROL FROM SMALL POPULATIONS OF NEURONS

Although iBCIs can record both LFPs and spikes, and although the potential for using both LFPs and spikes is currently being explored, most of the iBCI studies to date have emphasized the use of information from spikes. A major premise underlying this emphasis is that the signals (i.e., spikes) reflecting the activity of the individual neurons that normally generate movement commands (e.g., for the hand and arm) are likely to provide better control than more global EEG or ECoG signals or even LFPs. The hypothesis is that coupling to the brain's actual command-signal source will enable control that is natural to use and immediately available, with low demand for attention and low requirements for learning. At the same time, however, iBCIs can record signals from only a small sample of the extensive panoply of neurons engaged in performing even a simple voluntary action. Thus, one of the major challenges in iBCI development is to determine the amount of control that is possible from a limited sample of neurons. If it is found that use of small neuronal populations does limit control, it is possible that this limitation might be overcome by the user learning (i.e., to encode movement commands in the activity of these neurons) and/or by the iBCI software learning (i.e., to better decode the activity of these neurons). Although complete answers to such questions require understanding fundamental cortical information processing and neural coding, empirical solutions have already been found even without full understanding of the complex underlying mechanisms. Some of these will be described in this chapter.

FUNCTIONALLY USEFUL ACTIONS FOR PEOPLE WHO ARE PARALYZED

A major goal of all BCIs is to restore useful actions to people unable to move because of defects in the neuromuscular pathways that usually produce movement. This target user population could include not only people who are totally unable to move (i.e., as in the rare *totally locked-in syndrome*, as may occur in late-stage ALS), but also those with greatly impaired movement control because of paralysis from stroke or injury, or because of amputation. Preliminary data from a few humans

with nearly complete body paralysis (e.g., due to high-level spinal cord injury or stroke) engaged in pilot iBCI trials have found that spiking patterns from the arm area of the motor cortex can provide useful commands even years after injury (Hochberg et al. 2006; Kim et al. 2008; Truccolo et al. 2008; Simeral et al. 2011). People with tetraplegia have provided simple demonstrations of the ability to type and communicate through a computer interface, to control robotic limbs to reproduce arm actions, and to operate other potentially useful technologies. Up to the present, iBCIs are the only BCI systems to have demonstrated the ability of people with tetraplegia to achieve continuous control of a computer cursor or other devices (e.g., Hochberg et al. 2006).

These results constitute a proof-of-concept that iBCIs can be used by humans with longstanding tetraplegia from any of several causes (spinal cord injury, stroke, or ALS). More extensive animal studies have demonstrated iBCI ability to use decoded neural activity to perform two- and three-dimensional control of computer cursors, to operate robotic arms for self-feeding, and to move muscles through brain-activated electrical stimulators when nerve conduction is blocked (Serruya et al. 2002; Taylor et al. 2002; Moritz et al. 2008; Velliste et al. 2008). Other studies have also indicated that learning through use can enhance control (Ganguly & Carmena 2009). Most important, these studies have shown that small populations of neurons are capable of providing a rich signal source even in people with longstanding paralysis.

POSSIBLE ADVANTAGES OF iBCIs OVER eBCIs

At present, it remains to be determined what level of function an iBCI would need in order to justify the surgical procedure required to implant its sensors into the brain. As noted previously, the fact that iBCIs are the only modality that has access to signals reflecting the activity of the individual neurons that normally provide movement commands suggests that iBCIs should be able to provide substantially more complex, intuitive, and rapid control of output devices. Although it is difficult to directly compare the results reported for current iBCI and eBCI systems due to differences in sensors, signal processing, outputs, operating protocols, and assessment methods, more substantive and meaningful comparisons and value judgments should become possible in the coming years. At present, any claim of superiority must be examined skeptically.

Both iBCIs and eBCIs seem likely to lead to new classes of devices, each with the potential to help those with disabilities in various ways, but each with limitations. Knowledge gained from all of these systems will advance our understanding of neural function in health and disease and will probably make many other important and unexpected contributions to science and medicine. For example, the advances in implantable stimulators for cardiac disease contributed to the development of cochlear implants, which restore hearing; cochlear implants, in turn, have advanced understanding of auditory function in health and disease. In an analogous fashion, iBCI development may lead to a wide range of new devices that can take advantage of unique cellular-level signals to elucidate human disease or to ameliorate disorders such as epilepsy with closed-loop implantable systems (see chapter 22 in this volume).

SAFETY

Intracortical BCIs require sensors that are implanted in the cortex during a surgical procedure. This requirement for surgical implantation is what defines iBCI methods as *invasive*. The two major risks of surgically placed devices in general are infection and tissue damage that might produce long-lasting functional loss. Despite these risks, safety has been achieved for a variety of brain and nonbrain implantable technologies (e.g., cardiac pacemakers, cochlear implants, deep brain stimulators) and these devices are now widely used by hundreds of thousands of people with disease or disability.

The invasiveness of a BCI sensor is, of course, not unique to iBCIs: ECoG methods (see chapter 15) are also invasive since they require surgical implantation of the electrode array. The ECoG electrode arrays currently in use can be placed for <30 days only (by FDA rules), can require extensive surgery (i.e., wide skin incision and craniotomy), and entail a documented potential for serious adverse events (Wong et al. 2009). The development of smaller ECoG grids aims to reduce these problems while retaining selectivity in the recording areas targeted. Although ECoG methods do require surgery, the electrodes do not penetrate into the brain, but instead lie on the surface of the brain. By contrast, the electrodes used in iBCIs penetrate brain tissue. These iBCI electrodes are very small (<100 μm diameter). Although one might expect additional risk from the penetration of the electrodes into the brain, the somewhat limited human experience so far has provided no evidence for the risk of serious adverse events from these penetrating electrodes (Hochberg et al. 2006; Kennedy et al. 2000). Although there are few published data on the surgical risks for chronically implanted penetrating electrodes in humans (i.e., risks for deep-brain stimulators are reviewed in Clausen 2010), current versions of iBCIs have percutaneous connections (i.e., wires through the skin or cables to tether to external hardware) that risk the introduction of infection. For this reason, long-term safety of iBCIs (particularly safety from infection) will require fully implantable and wireless sensors. Devices of this kind require sophisticated electronics for signal processing that are unprecedented for long-term human application (Boviatsis et al. 2010). Current technological developments (e.g., microscale high bandwidth processors, signal transmission and powering methods) and initial animal and human data provide encouraging results, suggesting the eventual development of iBCIs that meet these goals (Song et al. 2009). At the same time, considerable work remains to be done to achieve and validate fully implantable, wireless iBCIs suitable for long-term human use over many years.

RELIABILITY

In addition to being safe, a practical iBCI must also provide reliable and stable long-term function. Lack of reliability and stability can introduce another level of risk in iBCIs, if further surgery is required to remove or replace nonfunctional devices. Thus, it is essential that, over many years, iBCIs be able to continue to record brain signals that can be reliably decoded into useful outputs. Variations in the signals, whether of technical or biological origin, must be minimized and must certainly not significantly impair iBCI performance. Although the animal and human results to date are generally encouraging (Suner et al. 2005; Simeral et al. 2011) and indicate that implanted microelectrodes can function reliably for several years, it is nevertheless clear that much remains to be done to fully address key issues, both technical (e.g., long-term encapsulant and mechanical robustness) and biological (e.g., the impact of tissue reactions). Such technical advances will help to achieve iBCIs suitable for life-long usage.

SIGNALS AVAILABLE TO iBCIs AND THE SENSORS THAT RECORD THEM

KEY FEATURES OF AN iBCI

Like all BCIs, iBCIs have three essential components: a sensor that records brain signals (see chapters 5 and 6 in this volume), a method of signal processing (i.e., feature extraction and translation) (see chapters 7 and 8) to decode the signals into commands, and an application device that implements the commands (see chapter 11). The most significant differences between iBCIs and eBCIs arise from their sensors. Whereas eBCIs use sensors located outside the brain (e.g., on the scalp as in EEG or on the cortical surface as in ECoG), iBCIs use sensors that penetrate into the brain (usually into the cerebral cortex). As a result, iBCIs can record two classes of signals: single-neuron action potentials (spikes); and field potentials (FPs). In contrast, eBCIs record only FPs. iBCI sensors can record both *field potentials* (FPs) and *action potentials* from the extracellular space simultaneously. Field potentials comprise 0–0.2 kHz potentials due to current flux through the somato-dendritic membranes of many neurons. In contrast, spikes are the brief (~1-msec) all-or-none impulses of higher frequency (~1 kHz) generated at the axon hillocks of individual neurons (figs. 16.1 and 16.2). Spikes are the measure of neuronal *output*, the neural information-carrying product of the neurons, which often passes over long distances to other brain areas. (It is important to note that the neuronal spikes recorded by iBCIs should not be confused with the spikes seen in EEG or ECoG in association with epileptic seizures. The latter spikes reflect the synchronized activity of many neurons.)

SIGNALS RECORDED BY iBCIs

An iBCI sensor can record three major types of signals:

- action potentials (also called spikes, single-neuron activity, or single-unit activity [SUA])
- multiunit activity (MUA)
- local field potentials (LFPs)

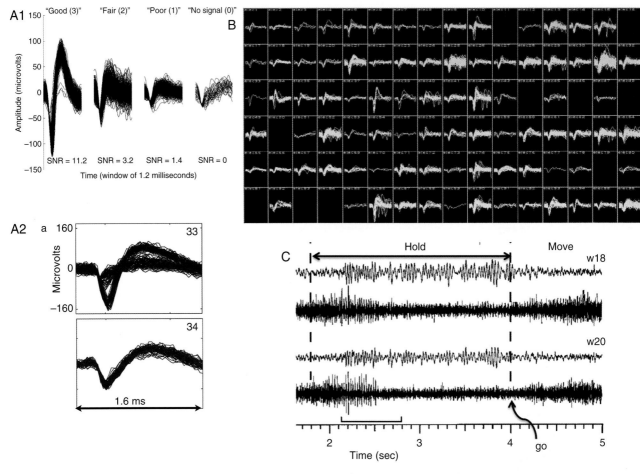

Figure 16.1 Action potentials (spikes) from motor cortex. *(A) Spikes from single neurons in primary motor cortex recorded by chronically implanted Si-platform multielectrode arrays (Blackrock Microsystems, Salt Lake City, UT). (A1) Waveforms from a monkey. (From Suner et al. 1999.) (A2) Waveforms from a human. (From Hochberg et al. 2006.) A1 shows the different quality of spiking signals (high to low) that can be detected from these arrays. A2 (top trace) illustrates two spikes simultaneously recorded on the same electrode, where the differences between the two neurons in spike shape as well as amplitude can be appreciated. (B) Simultaneous recordings from each of the 96 microelectrodes of a Si-platform array 23 months after implantation in the monkey primary motor cortex (Donoghue lab, unpublished data). Each box is the signal from a single electrode (channel). Spikes of various shapes and amplitudes are visible in many of the channels; about 150 total signals are present. The 9 (of 96 possible) channels with no visible traces may lack signal because the electrode is not close to a neuron, had noisy signals, or had nonfunctional connections. (C) Two types of electrical potentials (spikes and local field potentials (LFPs) are available from intraparenchymal microwires. (From Donoghue et al. 1999.) Each pair of traces shows recordings from microwires in monkey primary motor cortex derived from the same channel. The top trace of each pair is low-pass filtered (0.3–100 Hz) to show the LFP signal, while the bottom trace shows the same signal high-pass filtered (300–7.5 kHz) to show multiunit activity (MUA). Here, the monkey was motionless between the two vertical dashed lines in advance of a cue to move the wrist (i.e., "Go"). Note that the MUA has no predictable correlation with LFP, i.e., periods of spiking occur either with or without LFP oscillations, suggesting that they are separate information channels.*

ACTION POTENTIALS (SPIKES)

Neuronal spiking is of great interest as an iBCI signal source because it is likely to be a rich source of information. Spiking is generally assumed to be the major information output for long-distance, high-content communication for all neurons capable of spiking and to be a predominant form of coding in the nervous system (Shadlen & Newsome 1998). Spike *rate* (number of spikes in a specific interval or a related mathematical function) is generally considered to represent neural *output* information, although additional information may be available in the higher-order statistics of spike trains, such as their relative timing (e.g., a synchrony code [Singer 1999]).

The amount of movement information available from the spiking activity of even a single neuron is impressive: it includes information about future movements and movement parameters and also higher-order information about future movement sequences and goals. Hand velocity, position, forces, goals, and other variables can all be gleaned from single neurons in motor cortex, allowing accurate reconstruction of ongoing hand trajectories from populations of neurons recorded in able-bodied monkeys (Scott 2008; Kalaska et al. 1997; Georgopoulos 1988) (see chapter 2). Higher-level information, such as goals, plans for upcoming hand movement, as well as limb kinematics, can also be decoded from spiking in parietal and frontal areas that connect with primary motor cortex (M1 in fig. 16.3A) (Achtman et al. 2007; Pesaran et al. 2006; Scherberger & Andersen 2007) (see chapter 17).

The discrete nature of spikes, coupled with the need to discriminate among the spikes produced by different neurons (called *spike-sorting*), requires processing different from that

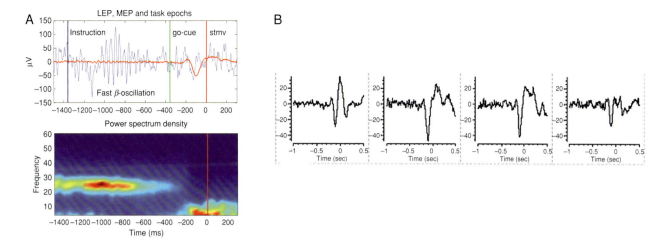

Figure 16.2 Local field potentials (LFPs) in motor cortex. (A, top) The raw (blue 0.3–100 Hz filtered) and multitrial averaged (red) LFP signals from one channel of a multielectrode array in monkey primary motor cortex (MI) show the premovement beta-band (~20–30 Hz) activity prior to the cue to move, as well as the motor event-related potential just prior to the start of the movement (time 0, red vertical line). (A, bottom) The spectrogram of the same LFP data shows prominent beta-band activity in the premovement delay period and lower-frequency activity around the time of arm movement onset. The color coding shows relative power (red = high, blue = low) (Truccolo and Donoghue, unpublished data). (B) Traces showing the low-frequency event-related potential (filtered 0.3–10 Hz) around the time of arm movement onset (time = 0) while a monkey reached in the horizontal plane to targets in each of four orthogonally positions (see fig. 16.3B). Differences in the form of the potential reflect directional tuning in this low-frequency LFP.

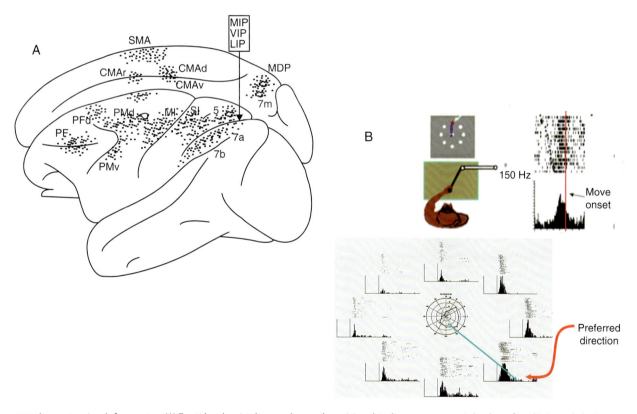

Figure 16.3 Arm motor signals from cortex. (A) Frontal and parietal areas where spike activity related to arm movements has been found in intact behaving monkeys. Stippling indicates the points in each cortical area (e.g., M1, PM) where single neurons have been recorded that modulate with movement kinematics (and, for some areas, forces, goals, plans, and other features as well). (From Kalaska & Crammond 1992.) (See chapter 2 this volume.) Each area is a potential source of BCI control signals. (B) Movement-related spiking activity in a monkey M1 during reaching. (Top left) Cartoon of monkey performing a "center out" reaching task; movement goals (all possible targets, white; current target, red) are presented on a vertically presented monitor. The monkey directs the cursor to the selected target by making arm movements from the center hold zone to one experimenter-selected target. (Top right) Raster plots and summary histogram show that spikes rates for this M1 neuron increase ~150 msec before movement and in association with movement. Each raster line is one trial; the trials are aligned on the start of movement (vertical bar is at 0, each time tick is 100 msec, y axis is spikes/sec). (Below) Directional tuning for one M1 neuron. Each raster plot and summary histogram shows the firing of a neuron during movement to one of eight targets (as shown in B, above). Note that this neuron is most active for movements that are down and to the right (i.e., its preferred direction) and that its activity diminishes as movement diverges from this direction. The smooth correlation of spike number with movement direction is well fit by a cosine function, which can be used as a model to predict the direction of movement from the firing rate (chapter 2). Populations of directionally tuned neurons provide a reliable estimate of the actual direction of movement that can be used as a control signal for iBCIs (unpublished data from Donoghue laboratory).

used for FPs, which are continuous lower-frequency signals. As described in chapter 7, spike data can be processed as discrete time series, using the armamentarium of methods for such analyses. At the same time, spike recording makes special demands on the sensors. They must be very small, they must remain intact and functional in an inhospitable (i.e., warm and ionic) environment for long periods, they must not produce infections, they must stay close to the neurons generating spikes, and they must not kill the neurons or induce scarring (i.e., gliosis) that degrades or prevents spike recording (see chapter 5). Whereas these stringent demands are not required for EEG electrodes (the major adverse issue of which may be skin irritation), ECoG sensors may evoke some of the adverse tissue responses encountered by the penetrating sensors of iBCIs. Moreover, since spike recording requires much higher sampling rates than FP recording, the digitization and power needs of iBCIs are substantial. This high power requirement increases the challenge of realizing the fully implantable systems essential for very long-term use. Nevertheless, rapid advances in miniaturized electronics are quickly diminishing the significance of this issue (chapter 5).

While a single neuron can provide substantial information, populations (or ensembles) of many single neurons can provide much more information and with greater fidelity (i.e., with higher signal-to-noise ratio) (Georgopoulos et al. 1986; Maynard et al. 1999). Neural populations can provide very accurate predictions of ongoing limb actions, such as the trajectory of the hand during a reach (fig. 16.3B). This collective information coding by populations of neurons is often called a *population* or *ensemble code*. It is this code that has the potential to provide real-time estimates of intended movements for iBCIs.

MULTIUNIT ACTIVITY

The neuronal spikes recorded extracellularly from different neurons usually differ from one another in shape and amplitude (fig. 16.1). The moveable microelectrodes used mainly in short-term laboratory settings can be adjusted to focus on a particular neuron and can thus maximize the signal-to-noise ratio and increase the certainty that the properties of that individual neuron are being evaluated. However, most iBCIs use microelectrodes that are in relatively fixed positions, the spikes they record are often small, and those of multiple neurons may be intermingled (fig. 16.1A). As a result, separating the spikes from different neurons is often difficult. Thus, sophisticated software is applied to extract specific features of the spike waveforms and use them to separate the spikes of different neurons. This is called *spike sorting* (see chapter 7 in this volume). Nevertheless, low-amplitude noise-ridden recordings may be difficult to process in this way, either manually or with automated software.

Alternatively, neuronal spiking can be treated as *multiunit activity* (MUA), without being sorted into individual neurons (fig. 16.1C). Although the complex mixtures of neurons that comprise MUA make it less useful for basic-science studies of neural information codes, it appears that effective iBCI operation may not require the careful spike-sorting that is essential for characterizing neural information processing

(Cunningham et al. 2009; Wood et al. 2004). Thus, for iBCIs, MUA may be an effective signal that is less prone to signal nonstationarities while preserving the unique information that is present in spiking signals.

LOCAL FIELD POTENTIALS

Field potentials (FPs) are signals that may reflect highly local or broadly distributed changes in electrical potential. Although the actual sources of FPs are complex, it is often convenient to think of them as a reflection of input to neurons (i.e., synaptic currents) (Nunez 1996) (see chapter 3). The FPs recorded by small sensors within brain tissue, such as the microelectrodes used by iBCIs, are LFPs, that is, they are FPs that are highly localized. A distinct advantage of electrodes placed within neural tissue is their ability to record LFPs and spikes simultaneously (fig. 16.1C). Although LFP signals are complex mixtures of activity from many sources (Bullock 1997), they capture local electrical-field changes originating close to the microelectrodes. In general, one expects electrodes with smaller recording surfaces to be relatively more sensitive to nearby activity than are electrodes with larger recording surfaces. FPs contain both rhythmic activity (sensorimotor rhythms [see chapter 13]) and potentials related to particular central or peripheral events (event-related potentials [see chapter 12]) (e.g., Colebatch 2007) (fig. 16.2).

It is generally agreed that three major frequency bands are readily evident in all types of FP recording from primary sensorimotor cortex in alert primates, including humans: a low-frequency (<8-Hz) band that can contain distinct movement- or event-related potentials (ERPs); a mid-frequency (8–30 Hz) band that contains mu- and beta-rhythm activity (see chapter 13); and a high-frequency (>30-Hz) gamma band (see chapter 15). Mu, beta, and gamma rhythms are collectively referred to as sensorimotor rhythms. (A good comparison of these signals is provided in Waldert et al. 2009 and Zhuang et al. 2010.) Although the exact relationships among these bands (and other bands within them) are a renewed area of intense inquiry, the low-frequency bands have been most correlated with synaptic input, high-frequency bands have been most correlated with spiking, and the mid-frequency bands seem to be related to attentional or other more global signals (Belitski et al. 2008).

Mu and beta rhythms recorded within or above primary sensorimotor cortex have been shown to change in association with movement and movement imagery (Shoham et al. 2001). They are of great interest as BCI control signals (see chapter 13), particularly because they can persist even in humans who are paralyzed, and are still capable of modulation in association with intended movement (Hochberg et al. 2006) (fig. 16.4) . All LFP bands have generated interest as possible independent or linked-control signals for iBCIs (Rickert et al. 2005; Waldert et al. 2009; Zhuang et al. 2010). iBCI sensors thus have a rich source of control signals that can be treated as information channels, including several LFP bands in addition to spikes.

Whereas FPs have traditionally been assumed to contain only low frequencies (i.e., from low direct-current frequencies to those up to about 100 Hz), ECoG can record signals at higher frequencies (e.g., 500 Hz [Gaona et al. 2011])

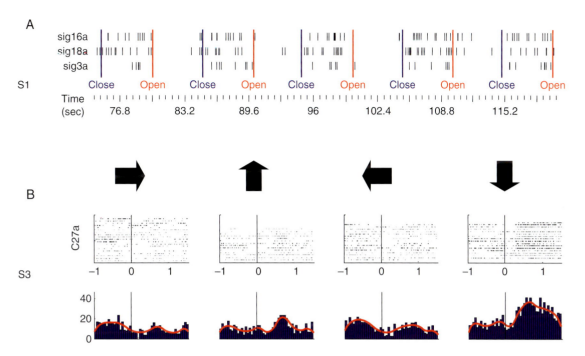

Figure 16.4 *Arm and hand neural activity from M1 cortex of humans with tetraplegia recorded with a chronically implanted multielectrode array during imagined upper-limb movements. (A) Raster plots of spikes from three M1 neurons during successive verbal requests to imagine closing or opening the hand (S1, spinal cord injury). Note the clear correlation of each neuron's spikes with the intention to close the hand. (From Hochberg et al. 2006.) (B) Directional tuning of an M1 neuron in a human with tetraplegia subsequent to a brainstem stroke (S3). The rasters show firing during repeated single trials when the participant is instructed to imagine right, up, left, or down arm movements as indicated by the arrows. The histograms show the summed activity of the trials for each direction (firing rate in hertz; time in seconds; 0 = time of verbal request; red line = smoothed rate). Note directional tuning to imagined arm reaches that resembles activity seen in able-bodied monkeys making reaching movements (compare with fig. 16.3) (also see chapter 2).*

(chapter 15). FP recordings that include such high frequencies may also include some neuronal spikes in addition to the FPs that they are traditionally thought to record. (Published reports are often lax in describing FP bandwidth and processing, which can have a major impact on BCI performance.) BCI research has launched a number of efforts to improve our understanding of the relationships between neuronal spiking and FPs, which may further our understanding of how information is processed in the brain (e.g., Zhuang et al. 2010; Moran & Bar-Gad 2010). Depending on the sensor used, the FP signal may reflect highly local or broadly distributed changes in electrical potential and can include spike activity, especially when spikes are highly synchronized.

TYPES OF iBCI SENSORS

Intraparenchymal recording is performed using a variety of electrode types. As illustrated in figure 16.5, these include:

- Multielectrode arrays (MEAs) (also called platform arrays or Utah arrays).
- Multisite electrodes (also called shank electrodes or Michigan electrodes)
- Microwire arrays
- Cone electrodes (also called neurotrophic electrodes)

For each of these types of recording sensor, several basic but challenging criteria must be met in order to successfully record from a population of neurons for long periods of time. First, the implanted device must be safe. Second, it must function reliably, ideally for decades. Third, it is desirable to incorporate more recording sites, since it is expected (although not yet fully validated) that a larger population of neurons will produce better iBCI performance. Fourth, the recording sites must be arranged in a geometry that minimizes tissue damage during insertion and during the sensor's subsequent residence in the tissue. To complicate matters further, the third and fourth criteria involve a trade-off: while larger numbers of recording sites impart an added benefit in the redundancy they provide in case the number of neurons recorded declines over time, too many electrodes will produce substantial tissue damage. The ideal balance between these competing factors is not yet known.

The electrodes developed for iBCIs vary greatly in materials and form. These are discussed in detail in chapter 5 and are briefly described here. At present, considerable controversy surrounds the relative merits of these various sensors, with strong claims made as to each one's ability to achieve long-term, reliable recording. Although there is strong evidence that electrode insertion causes tissue reaction and damage (Shain et al. 2003; Szarowski et al. 2003) (see chapter 5), long-term neuronal recording is nevertheless clearly possible with all of them. At the same time, no BCI sensor has yet been shown to provide reliable long-term recording in a large study.

MULTIELECTRODE ARRAYS

Multielectrode arrays (MEAs) (also called *platform arrays* or *Utah arrays*) have multiple microelectrodes protruding from a flattened superstructure that rests on the arachnoid membrane (i.e., below the dura). Each electrode has a sharp tip and is insulated except over the recording surfaces. For example, the array commercially available from Blackrock Microsystems (Salt Lake City, USA) has a flattened 4 × 4-mm platform with 100 metal or silicon 1.5-mm-long microelectrodes protruding from it. The platform sits against (i.e., floats on) the cortical surface (fig. 16.5A and 16.5B) (Donoghue 2008). Referred to as the *Utah array*, this design was originally developed by Richard Normann and his research group at the University of Utah (Campbell et al. 1991) and was further developed into a long-term implantable device suitable for iBCIs through a collaborative effort of the laboratories of Normann and John Donoghue (Maynard et al. 1999) (with support from Cyberkinetics Neurotechnology Systems). The electrodes of the array are inserted quickly through the arachnoid and pia via a custom pneumatically driven inserter (Rousche &

Normann 1992). As the *BrainGate neural interface system*, this array is currently under evaluation (limited to investigational use) for long-term use in people with tetraplegia, under an investigational device (FDA IDE) exemption (Hochberg et al. 2006) (see chapter 21). Other MEA platforms in which metal microelectrodes are fixed to platforms of various materials (Fofonoff et al. 2004; Musallam et al. 2007) are being used in animals for preclinical iBCI studies and other purposes.

The MEA platforms designed to date have the disadvantage of having only one recording site at the tip of each probe. Thus, recording from a neuron relies on the random chance that the tip's final position after insertion is close to the neuron's soma or major dendrites (i.e., within <~100 μm [Buzsaki 2004]). Since the array is fixed in place once inserted, there is no further opportunity for improving recording by moving the electrode. Fortunately, the high packing density of cortical neurons makes it highly probable that a tip is close enough to a neuron and that any tip is within recording distance of tens of neurons (Gold et al. 2006). Use of arrays with many electrodes (typically now~100) means that a considerable number

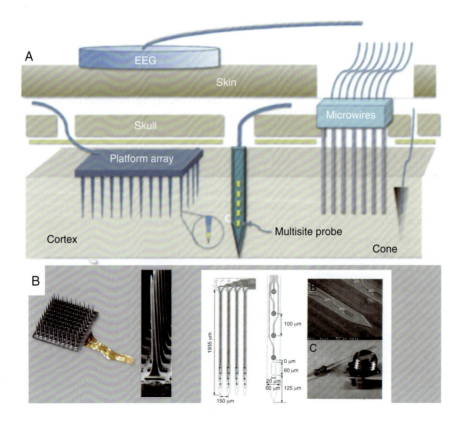

Figure 16.5 *iBCI sensors. Types of iBCI sensors for long-term neuronal (spike) and local field potential (LFP) recording. A platform array (A, left) has multiple electrodes protruding from a flattened superstructure that rests on the pia-arachnoid, with each electrode having a sharp tip and insulation except over the recording surface. (From Donoghue 2008.). (B, left) On the left is a 100-microelectrode array with a 4 × 4-mm platform and 1.0-mm electrodes, and on the right a scanning electron micrograph enlargement of one row of the microelectrodes illustrating their geometry (Blackrock Microsystems). The Multisite probes shown in A (center) and B (right) are flattened shanks with multiple exposed side ports that allow recording at multiple sites along their length (commercially available from Neuronexus, Ann Arbor, MI). Microwires, shown in A (right) are typically laboratory-fabricated arrays of fine (~50 μm) wires with only the ends exposed and are usually fixed to the skull. Cone electrodes (A, lower right) consist of 1–4 microwires encased in a glass pipette tip that contains growth factors. Neuronal processes (neurites) grow into the cone, and their spikes can then be detected by the wires. This sensor is essentially integrated into the cortex. (From Kipke 2004; Vetter et al. 2004.)*

of neurons are likely to be recorded. Particularly in motor cortex, the large apical dendrites of deeper neurons generate large fields; thus, there is a bias to detect these neurons, and they can be recorded over relatively longer distances than smaller neurons. This geometry strengthens the likelihood that neurons of interest could be recorded for long time periods. Moreover, in agranular cortex, which includes the motor cortex, the middle depths include the largest pyramidal neurons of deep layer III and layer V (see chapter 2) where movement-related activity is readily encountered (fig. 16.3); this zone is located at about 1–1.5 mm in depth (Meyer et al. 1996). (In monkeys, many pyramidal tract neurons are also encountered at a depth of ~1.5mm [Humphrey & Corrie 1978].)

It is not yet clear what the potential for long-term multi-electrode recordings in humans really is. However, it is encouraging that one person participating in a study in the laboratory of the author has an implanted array that, to date, has provided functional recording for over five years.

MULTISITE ELECTRODES

Multisite electrodes (also called *shank electrodes* or *Michigan electrodes)* are flattened shanks with multiple (~8–16) recording sites distributed along the length of a single flat narrow blade. The most prominent example of this type of electrode was developed from a silicon substrate by Daryl Kipke and his group at the University of Michigan and is thus called the *Michigan electrode* (Kipke 2004). These are commercially available from Neuronexus (Michigan, USA) (Kipke 2004; Vetter et al. 2004). When the shank is inserted into cortex, the multiple recording sites can provide recordings from multiple cortical levels. It is also possible to combine multiple shank electrodes into two-dimensional sets of parallel electrodes that provide a large number of recording sites distributed horizontally as well as vertically through a cortical area (Kipke 2004). Shank electrodes have been used in iBCI-related animal studies (Marzullo et al. 2006; Parikh et al. 2009), but they have not yet been applied in human studies. Other examples of shank electrodes have been made with ceramic (Moxon et al. 2004).

MICROWIRE ARRAYS

Microwire arrays are the third major form of multielectrode design. These are typically laboratory-fabricated arrays of fine (~50 μm diameter) rigid wires with only the ends exposed; they are usually fixed to the skull (e.g., Kralik et al. 2001; Schwartz 2004; Donoghue 2008). Microwire arrays can be fabricated inexpensively in the lab, making them valuable for many research applications. Although there is great diversity from one laboratory to another, microwire arrays for cortical recordings commonly consist of a set of uniform diameter, thin (10–70 μm diameter), insulated metal wires glued together in a regular pattern of any number (e.g., typically 8 or more). The wire tips, which may be blunt or tapered, are exposed and provide the recording surfaces. They are inserted into the cortex by a variety of methods particular to each laboratory. They have been used successfully for long-term iBCI studies in

rodents and monkeys (Porada et al. 2000), for recordings over at least a year (Nicolelis et al. 1997), and for recordings up to seven years (Kruger et al. 2010). In one case (Patil et al. 2004), with microwires inserted as a bundle through a cannula, they were used for an acute iBCI-related human study that recorded from basal ganglia. Overall, the long-term performance of microwire arrays has been mixed, with common reports of decline in signal quality over time for a significant percentage of the wires. Nevertheless, microwires have been and are being used in several laboratories for long-term recordings in monkey cortex (Kruger et al. 2010; Nicolelis et al. 2003; Donoghue et al. 1998; Taylor et al. 2002; Ganguly and Carmena 2009).

CONE ELECTRODES

Cone Electrodes (also called *neurotrophic electrodes*) are the fourth major type of electrode used within the brain. Kennedy and colleagues developed this intriguing modification of microwire design, in which the exposed end(s) of one to four microwires are housed in a short glass cone containing various neurotrophic (growth) factors (Kennedy 1989; Kennedy et al. 1992). As part of the tissue response to the insertion of the cone electrode and in response to the growth factors, neurites often grow into the cone so that they are close to the recording surfaces of the wires and their spikes can be detected. This sensor becomes essentially integrated into the cortex and can provide long-term recording (Kennedy 1989). The cone anchors the wire in the brain so that it moves with the brain (Kennedy 1989; Kennedy et al. 1992). This appears to reduce the recording disturbances caused by small brain movements.

iBCI STUDIES

SELECTION OF THE CORTICAL AREA FOR IMPLANTATION

Many iBCIs tested in monkeys have used neurons related to arm movements and recorded from the arm area of primary motor cortex (MI), the premotor area, and the parietal reach region (e.g., Serruya et al. 2002; Taylor et al. 2002 Carmena et al. 2003; Hatsopoulos et al. 2004; Shenoy et al. 2003; Andersen et al. 2010). This emphasis on arm areas may derive in part from the perceived importance of the arm in humans and monkeys and from the fact that, for people with tetraplegia, recovering arm function would be greatly enabling.

The anatomical location of the M1 arm area in humans is indicated by a distinct anatomical feature called the *knob*, which is part of the precentral gyrus and is readily seen in a standard MRI (Yousry et al. 1997), facilitating surgical implantation of the iBCI array. In iBCI studies in monkeys, the focus on neurons related to arm control arises mainly from the large literature on the relationship between skilled arm use and neuronal activity in cortical motor areas (see chapter 2). This literature is especially abundant on the role of primary motor cortex in arm function (e.g., neuronal population coding of multiple movement dimensions [Paninski et al. 2007]). Prior research also revealed the locations of other cortical areas important in arm control (e.g., fig. 16.3). In monkeys, more than 10 well-defined areas are known to be involved in the planning or generation of arm movements (Kalaska & Crammond 1992). The relative advantages and disadvantages of each of these areas as signal sources for iBCIs are still largely unexplored.

In contrast to the attention given to arm-movement control, much less attention has been paid to cortical control of the leg, perhaps due to the greater difficulty of experiments involving highly controlled leg movements and the poorer accessibility of the deeply situated midline cortical areas that are involved in leg movements. Nevertheless, Fitzsimmons et al. (2009) recently studied the decoding of leg movements in monkeys and showed the potential to decode aspects of these movements.

There is no consensus on what is the ideal anatomical source of control signals and if, in fact, there is an ideal source. Since many different brain areas interact in complex ways to produce output, signals from multiple areas are likely to be important, and each area can provide its own control signals and potentially make a unique contribution. Since the majority of iBCI studies to date use signals from M1 and closely related motor areas, we will focus on these. Use of the parietal cortex and other areas for iBCIs is discussed in chapter 17 of this volume.

iBCI STUDIES TO DATE IN NONHUMAN AND HUMAN PRIMATES

The increasing success of multielectrode arrays as chronic recording devices in the cortex of monkeys, the substantial knowledge regarding arm-movement coding by populations of neurons in primary motor cortex, and the anatomical and functional similarities between monkeys and humans, have all contributed substantially to the success of and interest in the development of iBCIs using recording from motor cortex. Emergent iBCI systems demonstrated to date differ from one another in the type of sensor they employ, in their decoding algorithms, and in the uses to which they put their outputs. Most of these efforts have focused on producing arm control or arm-like control. These systems have been applied in monkeys (e.g., Velliste et al. 2008) and in humans with tetraplegia (e.g., Hochberg et al. 2006). These research efforts have produced a range of closed-loop demonstrations of the ability of iBCIs to achieve continuous control of computer cursors, to operate physical robotic systems, and to control muscles.

iBCI STUDIES IN ABLE-BODIED MONKEYS

Monkeys have been the major model for human iBCIs. Fetz and colleagues (Fetz 1969; Fetz & Finocchio 1971) provided early demonstrations of a simple iBCI by showing that monkeys could adjust the firing rate of a single neuron in motor cortex when rewarded for doing so. Serruya et al. (2002) reported the first demonstration of iBCI control of a computer cursor in two dimensions in a closed-loop system. The monkey was initially trained to move a handle with its arm and thereby control movement of a cursor to reach targets randomly placed on a screen. Cortical neuron activity was recorded throughout this training. A linear decoding algorithm was developed based on the correlations between cortical-neuron activity and arm movements. Then, actual arm control of the cursor was replaced by the output of decoded neural signals as the control mechanism. The decoded neural signal was immediately effective as a substitute for arm movement: the monkeys continued to be able to perform the task of cursor control; although the monkeys could still move their arms, the cursor was actually controlled by the brain signals, not by arm movements. Importantly, this control continued for as long as the monkey was engaged in the task, without any need for resetting or recalibration. In one case, the monkey stopped moving its arm as its brain signals moved the cursor, indicating that it had uncoupled actual arm movement from the M1 neuronal activity.

Taylor et al. (2002) advanced this work further by showing that monkeys could use M1 activity to control three-dimensional cursor movement in a virtual-reality task. Carmena et al. (2003) subsequently showed concurrent continuous and discrete iBCI control, including control of both cursor position and target selection (i.e., grasp). Additional work has demonstrated the potential for iBCI control using neurons from non-primary motor cortical areas, including the premotor cortex (Santhanam et al. 2006) and the parietal cortex (Hwang & Andersen 2009) (see chapter 1).

These studies in monkeys have demonstrated iBCI control of a variety of outputs. Although most studies have involved a computer task (i.e., movement of a cursor and/or selection of an item on a computer screen), Schwartz and his colleagues have also demonstrated control of a multijoint robotic arm that emulates human reach and grasp actions (Velliste et al. 2008). This work is particularly significant in that it allows direct evaluation of the ways in which the brain changes to achieve direct control of complex mechanical devices (e.g., a multijointed robotic arm), that is, without the usual mediation by intervening brain and spinal cord connections and by muscles. In these studies, the monkeys fed themselves using the iBCI-controlled robotic arm, and their control improved with continued practice.

iBCI STUDIES IN PARALYZED MONKEYS

Whereas the iBCI studies described above involved able-bodied monkeys, BCI technology is intended to serve people who lack useful movement control due to a wide variety of neuromuscular disorders. Thus, it is important to determine whether long-standing paralysis interferes with the ability of the motor cortex to control a BCI. Humans unable to move their limbs could certainly benefit from the ability to control complex devices that mimic the actions of their own arms, and sophisticated robots are now available that might be controlled by a BCI. The amount of BCI control possible will depend on the user's ability to provide the brain signals needed to control the device. For an iBCI, the question is whether neuronal spiking patterns corresponding to movement *intention* are produced even in the absence of the *ability* to move. This is particularly important because, in most forms of paralysis, CNS motor pathways and/or neuronal areas are damaged (as in spinal cord injury or stroke) or have undergone pathological degeneration (as in ALS).

To create an experimental model of paralysis in monkeys, muscle activation can be prevented by a reversible pharmacological peripheral nerve block. In studies conducted by Moritz et al. (2008) and by Pohlmeyer et al. (2009), monkeys were able to create useful control signals despite such pharmacologically induced disconnection of the CNS from the muscles. When cortical neurons were used to control electrical stimulation of the muscles (i.e., the cortical neurons were essentially reconnected to their intended muscle targets), it was possible for these animals to learn to execute simple limb movements (Moritz et al. 2008; Pohlmeyer et al. 2009). Reminiscent of Fetz's work decades before, Moritz et al. (2008) also showed that activity from only one or two cortical neurons was sufficient to control simple actions. Thus, these iBCI studies in temporarily paralyzed monkeys suggest that paralyzed humans may be able to use cortical neurons to control the movements of devices such as robotic arms, or even the movements of their own limbs. At the same time, it is not yet known to what degree this model accurately captures the state of the nervous system for a human with long-term paralysis.

iBCI STUDIES IN PEOPLE WITH PARALYSIS

The long history of microelectrode studies in animals, the success in decoding the recorded cortical neuronal activity, and the iBCI demonstrations in monkeys all contributed to the launch of pilot clinical trials of iBCI systems in humans with tetraplegia. This provides a superb example of the ways in which years of fundamental research can lead to the development of technology with great potential to help humans with paralysis. As it turns out, the results in monkeys parallel the ongoing iBCI studies in humans with severe motor disabilities that impair the normal CNS output pathways (Hochberg et al. 2006).

The first studies of iBCIs in humans were begun in the late 1990s by Philip Kennedy and colleagues (Kennedy and Bakay 1998; Kennedy et al. 2000). Their first study showed that a person with ALS could intentionally modulate spiking activity recorded by two cone electrodes in motor cortex (Kennedy and Bakay 1998). In a second study, a person who was locked in by a brainstem stroke (i.e., totally paralyzed except for limited eye movements) used the spikes recorded by one cone electrode to move a cursor in one direction (i.e., 0.5-dimensional control) (Kennedy et al. 2000). (In this case, to demonstrate that neural control could be uncoupled from remaining movements, the participant first learned over a 4-month period to dissociate contraction of periorbital muscles from modulation of the spike rate.) This initial human iBCI trial demonstrated the ability to use neural signals to control a computer cursor.

The first pilot study of a human iBCI system that used populations of cortical neurons began in 2004 (Hochberg et al. 2006) and used the BrainGate iBCI sensor (consisting of a multielectrode platform array) implanted in the arm region of M1 (i.e., the knob) (Yousry et al. 1997). As of this writing, four people with tetraplegia have been implanted with this initial BrainGate System1 (which is approved for study as an investigational device by the FDA). Two of these people had high-cervical spinal-cord injury, one had ALS, and one had a pontine stroke. The results showed that both neuronal spiking and LFPs

persisted in the M1 arm areas of all four people even years after onset of paralysis (Hochberg et al. 2006, Truccolo et al. 2008; Kim et al. 2008; Simeral et al. 2011). Furthermore, and most importantly, the M1 neurons were immediately engaged by imagining limb actions: even in the absence of any actual movement, and without learning or practice, the act of imagining the action was immediately able to change cortical neuronal activity. This was remarkable since these individuals had not moved their arms voluntarily for 2–9 years. Despite the years of nonuse, the neuronal spiking and LFPs found in M1 bore many similarities to those that occur in the M1 arm areas of able-bodied monkeys. Cortical neurons well-tuned to the direction of imagined movement were readily detected (e.g., fig. 16.4).

BrainGate2, a second and larger trial involving up to 15 participants, began in 2009. It is designed to assess the long-term safety, stability, and reliability of the implanted array, the quality and quantity of the neuronal activity found following high-level spinal cord injury or brainstem stroke, or in a degenerative disorder (e.g., ALS), and the possibilities for controlling assistive devices, such as a typing interface or robotic assistant.

LONG-TERM PERFORMANCE OF iBCIs

A recent preclinical study (Suner et al. 2005) reported encouraging evidence of the possibility of good long-term performance by a platform array. This array was used to record signals from three monkeys over 514-, 154- and 83-day periods, respectively (fig. 16.6). The signals varied in number and form from day to day, but there was no evidence for a time-related

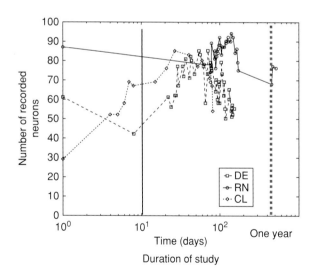

Figure 16.6 Number of neurons recorded in three monkeys by a multielectrode platform array over a period of 83, 154, or 514 days. Each monkey was recorded from for the defined duration (log scale of time), and then data collection stopped. Note that in the first weeks, both increases and decreases occurred in the numbers of neurons discriminated from the recordings and that fluctuations in the count on the order of 10% occurred regularly, with occasionally larger up or down changes. Also note that the numbers of neurons were about the same for the first and last sessions of the prolonged periods over which data were collected. This indicates that large numbers of signals can be recorded for lengthy periods by iBCI arrays in monkey cortex. (From Suner et al. 1999.)

decline in the number neurons recorded. Recordings were the most unreliable during the first few weeks, with one array increasing its reliability, one decreasing, and one remaining roughly stable. Useful spike recording continued through these periods, although the numbers of neurons recorded waxed and waned (i.e., for some electrodes, signals came and went), and the sizes and shapes of their spikes changed as well. One monkey was studied for an additional 3 years.

Experiences from the first BrainGate pilot clinical trial were consistent with the conclusion that platform arrays can perform reliably over long periods. All four of the participants in the trial (people with tetraplegia) had the platform array implanted in the arm region of motor cortex (Hochberg et al. 2006; Truccolo et al. 2008; Kim et al. 2008), and spikes were recorded for at least 10 months after implantation. As of this writing (nearly 5 years after implantation), one of the participants is still in the study (figs. 16.7B and 16.8), and spikes continue to be recorded. (Furthermore, over a total of >2800 days of implantation [7.7 years] in these four people, no infection has occurred, either in the CNS or in the skin.)

Kennedy's glass-cone electrodes (Kennedy & Bakay 1998) were also tested in humans and those results too supported long-term recording in humans.

Thus, only two iBCI sensor types have been tested in human for prolonged periods: the Si-platform array (Hochberg et al. 2006) and the glass-cone electrode (Kennedy et al. 2000). Both are in pilot trials under an Investigational Device Exemption (IDE) from the Food and Drug Administration

(FDA) (see chapter 21). Data from only a few humans, with only a few time points, are currently in the literature. Since iBCIs in humans are still in the investigational stage, no system has been fully validated and established. Testing and validation require a long process that is highly regulated to ensure sound clinical and ethical principles. For the same reasons the long-term reliability of ECoG sensors for BCI use has not yet been tried in human clinical trials. However, an early-stage study of the reliability of implanted ECoG grids for seizure monitoring in epilepsy is in progress (Van Gompel et al. 2008). The early stage of results coming from all of these studies makes it difficult to make substantive comparisons of the long-term biostability or biocompatibility of implanted sensors, whether they are intracortical and extracortical. Nevertheless, the data on safety of all these implanted devices seems encouraging.

Despite these promising successes, most iBCI investigators report that, after successfully recording for months, some arrays may fail within a year of implantation (e.g., Donoghue et al. 2004; Schwartz et al. 2006). Despite the temptation to attribute this failure to lack of biocompatibility, results from studies specifically examining tissue response indicate that injury-related changes appear to be largely complete within the first two months after implantation (Shain et al. 2003). It is thus probable that later device failure may be due to material degradation (e.g., issues of biostability) or mechanical factors, rather than issues of biocompatibility.

In summary, the results to date in animals and humans indicate that, although sensor movement relative to the brain

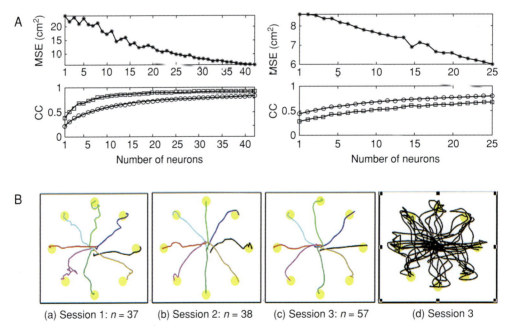

(a) Session 1: n = 37   (b) Session 2: n = 38   (c) Session 3: n = 57   (d) Session 3

Figure 16.7 Control using iBCI systems. (A) Decoding movement from small populations of M1 neurons (from Wu et al. 2006). Plots showing success in decoding of arm-reaching movement in center-out tasks (see fig. 16.3) for two monkeys as a function of the numbers of neurons used. The upper panel shows mean squared error deviation from an ideal (straight) path, and lower panels show cross-correlation coefficient as a function of number of neurons. Depending on the monkey, performance appears to asymptote with about 25–40 neurons. (B) Panels a–c show examples of average decoded trajectories from a population of M1 neurons for a human with tetraplegia in a center-out task that required moving the cursor from a center hold zone to a peripheral target. Actions were repeated continuously (without interruption) for all of the movements made, but only outward paths are shown for clarity. Panel d shows every path for one session. (Data and figures from Kim et al. 2008.)

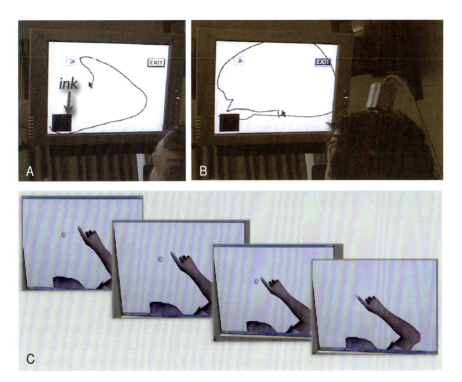

Figure 16.8 *Cursor control using the BrainGate neural interface system. (A, B) Two attempts by a human with tetraplegia to use imagined arm movement to draw a circle with a cursor (arrowhead). The cursor is controlled by neuronal activity recorded from a population of neurons in M1 cortex. The movement starts from the black square (which serves as an ink well) and is shown by the line ending in the cursor. In the first trial, the participant avoids moving the cursor to the eraser (upper left) but is unable to complete a circle. In a subsequent attempt in the same session, without additional practice, the subject avoids the eraser and succeeds in producing a full loop. (From Hochberg et al. 2006.) (C) Neurally controlled virtual functional electrical stimulation (FES) system. The panels illustrate the motions produced during neural control by a human with tetraplegia of a virtual FES system that models all features of a paralyzed arm controlled by a current FES system. In this case, the fingertip position is controlled by the simulated FES system that drives models of four shoulder and two elbow muscles, based on commands derived from neuronal activity in M1 of a human with tetraplegia. The user is able to move the fingertip to the red dot, which was placed at a random screen location. In the rightmost panel the target is reached and turns white. This demonstrates the possibility of using neuronal activity recorded by an iBCI array to drive an FES system that excites muscles that have been paralyzed by spinal cord injury, stroke, or other central lesions. (From Chadwick et al. 2011.)*

probably does affect the population of neurons recorded and although biocompatibility and biostability continue to be of concern, iBCI electrode arrays can continue to record neuronal spikes for long periods, even years (Bartels et al. 2008). The results suggest that long-term recordings are feasible for human iBCIs.

LONG-TERM RECORDING ISSUES

Since the surgical implantation of foreign objects always carries some amount of risk, invasive BCI devices, whether implanted within the brain itself or within the cranium, must last for many years without requiring replacement or repair. Furthermore, the long-term implantation itself must not entail significant risks of infection or tissue damage. These risks can be minimized by good choices as to the type and geometry of the implanted materials, by using proper surgical insertion techniques, by ensuring implant stability, and by continued monitoring of tissue responses and possible infection. Although these factors undoubtedly contribute to risk/benefit assessment and to the success of long-term recording, they have not been formally evaluated in a comprehensive fashion. Given the many variables that distinguish the various sensor approaches

from one another, it is difficult to make direct comparisons with compelling conclusions.

FACTORS THAT AFFECT RECORDING STABILITY

The variables that most affect long-term iBCI sensor performance can be grouped into three major classes:

- *Movement* (the extent to which physical forces cause motion of the electrodes relative to the surrounding brain tissue)
- *Biocompatibility* (the ability of the tissue to accept the device, i.e., the extent of tissue damage and/or tissue responses that encapsulate the electrodes and impair their recording capacity)
- *Biostability* (the ability of the implant to resist damage by the body's environment and to resist material failure during long-term use).

Movement of the sensors relative to the surrounding brain tissue is a key issue for iBCIs. iBCIs that use single-neuron spike detection require that the recording surface be very small and that it remain very close to the neuron. The best quantifications of this requirement indicate that a microelectrode tip must be less than ~100 μm from a neuron to detect its spike with a reasonable signal-to-noise ratio (Buzsaki 2004; Buzsaki & Kandel 1998; Henze et al. 2000). Fixation of the array to the skull (called *tethering*) may result in a disturbance of this crucial proximity as the brain moves within the skull (e.g., due to cardiac or respiratory pulsations, head or body movements, etc.). With such a small margin of allowable movement, it is impressive and encouraging that some laboratories describe years of recording with multielectrode arrays (Suner et al., 2005). In addition, several studies report that ~40% of the recorded neurons can be recorded stably for weeks in monkeys with microelectrode arrays (Ganguly & Carmena 2009; Dickey et al. 2009; Nicolelis et al. 2003).

The question of *biocompatibility* involves consideration of possible tissue reactions to an implanted device. These reactions might interfere with its function, and/or have other effects (e.g., infection) that put the patient's wellbeing at risk. Tissue reaction around an intracortical microelectrode may include the death of neurons near the electrode and the formation of a layer of glial cells around the electrode, commonly thought to be a major impediment to long-term recording (chapter 5). Although immediate and chronic tissue responses to specific electrode implants have been carefully delineated in several studies (Shain et al. 2003; Winslow & Tresco 2010), it is difficult to draw general conclusions because of substantial differences across iBCI sensors in size, shape (e.g., platforms vs. single probes), coating material, insertion technique, surgical procedure, manufacturing venue (lab or commercial), and quality control. Furthermore, understanding the long-term impact of tissue reaction on neuronal health and spike recording is complex. Nevertheless, although the effects of damage are debated, there is general agreement that most reactive processes stabilize within a few months of electrode implantation (Winslow and Tresco 2010). Moreover, those animal and human studies showing recordings lasting a year or more suggest that tissue reaction does not prevent long-term recording.

Whether on or in the brain, intracranial devices pose all the risks associated with neurosurgery and the introduction of a foreign material in the body. Most prominently, these include infection, bleeding, and mechanical damage to tissue. Most information concerning the biocompatibility of devices implanted in the brain comes from deep brain stimulating (DBS) electrodes (Awan et al. 2009; Seijo et al. 2007). These devices penetrate centimeters into the brain and are much larger in diameter than microelectrodes (1.27 mm vs. ~50 μm). Yet, DBSs have been implanted in more than 80,000 people and have functioned successfully for decades—and with no more than the typically low rates of complication found with other established neurosurgical procedures.

The available clinical data for brain implants of all types (i.e., epidural, subdural, penetrating) indicate that the overall complication rate is about 5% (Hamani & Lozano 2006). These complications include excessive bleeding, swelling, and/or acute skin, meningeal or (very rarely) brain infections after implantation. The vast majority of these complications resolve without long-term consequences, although a few serious adverse events have been reported. In evaluating these studies, it is important to recognize that, although infection is often listed as one of the more common events, clinical evaluations of devices often use the single label "infection" to describe a whole gamut of conditions of very different severity: superficial skin infections, infections along lead wires, or, of much greater concern, intracranial infections (i.e., infections that involve the meninges and/or the brain itself).

Biostability is the ability of implanted sensors to withstand the warm, relatively high-salt environment inside the body. Biostability is closely related to biocompatibility, and it is often difficult to differentiate their individual contributions to any observed loss in signal. Although very important, biostability has received less overall attention in the BCI field than biocompatibility. Many materials degrade after long-term exposure to the body's warm, ionic environment. Aging of materials, along with physical forces, may cause device failure due to broken connections, failed wire bonds, degraded electrode coatings, or leaks in insulating materials. Failure of the insulation along the electrical path causes shunting of the signals or *cross-talk* between different wires. Although it would clearly be advantageous to create signal processors that would last for decades and that would fit within or just above the skull, the goal of implantable electronics for iBCIs has not yet been reached. Development of such implantable electronics is challenging because of the possibility of exposure of the electronics to ionic fluids. Achieving this for iBCI devices is more challenging than for other sensors currently implanted in humans (Hsu et al. 2009; Song et al. 2005) because of the significantly greater complexity of the electronics capable of sampling small-amplitude brain signals at high rates across many channels.

All BCIs must address the issues of sensor movement, biocompatibility, and signal stability, but their importance is compounded when the sensors are implanted, especially when they are implanted in brain tissue. However, because of the number of characteristics that vary from one method to another, it is very difficult to directly compare different methods of recording with regard to these issues. Consider, for example, two different and well-known iBCI sensor designs: the Si-platform array (an MEA) and a microwire array. The Si-platform array produced by Blackrock Microsystems (Salt Lake City, UT) has a machine-fabricated 10×10 grid of 100 tapered silicon microelectrodes separated from one another by 400 μm (fig. 5). The electrode shanks are coated with parylene, and the tips are coated with platinum. During implantation, the array is inserted very rapidly into the cortex by a custom pneumatic inserter. The rigid platform, which floats on the brain's surface, is subject to tethering forces generated by a partially flexible cable that leads to a skull-mounted connector. This array has been implanted mainly in old-world monkeys but also in a few human study participants (Hochberg et al. 2006; Truccolo et al. 2008). It would be difficult to make a direct comparison of this array with a microwire array (Kralik et al. 2001). Microwire arrays may contain a variable number of blunt-tipped 45-μm-diameter tungsten wires in various spacing patterns. The wires (which are coated with isonyl) are inserted very slowly and glued to the skull, so that the brain and the wires move independently. Most tests of their function are in rats which have a thin skull and relatively little movement of the brain with respect to the skull. (In addition, it is not certain that tissue responses in rats are the same as in humans.) In sum, it is not possible to make meaningful comparisons between different arrays used in different species with different coating materials, different foreign body combinations, and different anchoring methods. Systematic methods and tools are needed to compare the individual contributions of the different factors that affect recording success and failure.

DECODING THE NEURONAL SPIKES RECORDED BY iBCIs

All BCIs need to translate the brain signals they record into command signals that will achieve the user's intentions, such as where or how to move a cursor, an arm, or a wheelchair. Thus, each BCI must determine the relationships between its brain signals and the user's intent (Donoghue et al. 2007; Serruya et al. 2003). As previously noted, iBCI sensors can record *both* neuronal spikes (single-unit activity) *and* local field potentials (LFPs). The methods for decoding both spikes and field potentials, including LFPs, are discussed extensively in chapters 7 and 8 of this volume. Although the possibility of using both neuronal spikes and LFPs from the same iBCI electrodes has been explored in monkeys (Hwang & Andersen 2009), most attention has been focused on spikes for iBCI control. Thus, in this section we review the methods used for decoding of spikes.

Spike decoding is somewhat different from the decoding of EEG, ECoG, and LFPs because the spikes consist of discrete events often including contributions from up to 100 or more individual neurons that can be combined to produce a useful output signal. Decoding spikes from motor cortex benefits greatly from an almost 50-year history of studies of the relationships between neuronal activity in primary motor cortex (i.e., MI) and arm movements in behaving monkeys (Kalaska & Crammond 1992) (e.g., fig. 16.3) (see chapter 2). Neuronal spike trains that display direction- and velocity-tuning to arm reaches are easily found in motor cortex. Thus, even random sampling of neurons by fixed, implanted electrode arrays can provide a rich sample of neurons that are cosine-tuned for direction and hand speed (Maynard et al. 1999) (chapter 2).

The spike trains of such neurons provide information that can be used to provide continuous reconstruction of hand position and/or velocity. Indeed, simple linear combinations of small groups of M1 neurons can produce accurate predictions of hand trajectory (direction and speed) in intact monkeys (e.g., Moran & Schwartz 1999) as well as of imagined movements in paralyzed humans (see Hochberg et al. 2006) (figs. 16.1 and 16.4). In addition, a vast literature of basic research shows that spikes from specific neurons can predict joint angles, muscle-contraction strengths, force levels, and individual or combined finger actions, as well as bimanual and unimanual actions. Furthermore, spikes from neurons in secondary motor areas (fig. 16.3A) can provide information about goals, as well as direction information during motor

planning (Santhanam et al. 2006). The well-known general topographic organization of motor areas (chapter 2) makes it possible in principle to decode actions for each of the limbs (left and right, leg and arm). The capacity for such localization appears to be an advantage of iBCIs: the spikes from different cortical areas could then be used as relatively independent output control channels. Of course, this would require implantation of multiple arrays.

Relating neuronal spikes to CNS outputs, such as hand motion, is of interest in basic neuroscience as well as in development of BCI technology. For both endeavors, decoding is based on understanding the fundamental principles of neural coding and information processing (Serruya et al. 2003; Tillery & Taylor 2004; Panzeri et al. 2002) (chapter 2). Knowledge about the operation of neurons in producing normal motor function can be applied in development of BCI systems. In addition, spikes may also be used for iBCI control in ways that are not used in normal CNS operation. For example, spikes from particular neurons might produce BCI outputs at time-lags different from those occurring in normal function, or the spike trains from different neurons might be combined in non-physiological ways to produce outputs. Since the goals of basic neuroscience and iBCI development overlap significantly in many of their objectives, the realization of optimal information-extraction methods has generated widespread interest.

In humans, spike decoding for BCI applications typically begins with the recording of spikes during an actual or imagined set of movements. With spike trains from multiple neurons, each neuron is a single channel of information, and together they comprise a multichannel signal, or *population source* that creates a vector of values that summarizes for each time point the information contained in the data from the population of neurons (chapter 7). The data are then used to select and parameterize a model (see chapter 8) that describes how the spikes are related to movements.

Since neuronal spiking can be considered a discrete process, decoding strategies typically use spike-counts in small time intervals, or *bins* (which can be as small as 1 msec, but are more typically 10–100 msec). The bins of spike trains serve as the data points that are the independent variables in the models; movements are the dependent variables. The model is the equation that relates the independent variable (the bins of spike trains) to the dependent variable (the movement). Bin length is usually defined empirically to optimize decoding or to reduce processing time. (It appears that the exact specifics of time-binning are not major factors in determining the outcome of the decoding process [Chestek et al. 2009a].) After binning, a spike train may be converted into a continuous function, or spikes may be used to compute an instantaneous rate and then decoded using methods appropriate for continuous functions. Such analyses are discussed in detail in chapters 7 and 8 of this volume.

Spike-decoding has used both linear and nonlinear models to relate spike trains to actual or intended actions. Model performance is typically measured by comparing the movement derived from the spike trains to the actual (or intended) movement and computing their difference in terms of mean-squared error (i.e., the closer to zero, the better) or a correlation coefficient (i.e., the closer to +1, the better) (fig. 16.7A). Multiple movement features, such as position and velocity, may be derived from the same spike trains. Opinions as to the most effective models differ considerably across research groups. Linear functions are the simplest models, and have been used with substantial success (e.g., Paninski et al. 2004). A number of other models have also been studied as possibilities for improving the accuracy with which trajectories can be reconstructed and for making iBCI movement control more like natural movements.

Bayesian models (see chapter 8) may improve the quality of iBCI decoding (Wu et al. 2004; Wu et al. 2006). The appeal of Bayesian models is that they are probabilistic, and, by setting model parameters according to the likelihoods of particular observations, they can reduce the influence of outlier spiking patterns (see chapter 8 for fuller discussion). That is, if a particular pattern of spike trains from the designated neuronal population (i.e., the neuronal ensemble) is highly unlikely, it is given less weight in calculating movement parameters. Models that incorporate Kalman filters (chapter 8) can be particularly effective. They can routinely achieve high correlations between the spiking signal and movement kinematics, and they consistently outperform purely linear models (Sykacek et al. 2004; Wu et al. 2006; Wu & Hatsopoulos 2008). At the same time, although decoding may be improved by various nonlinear models (Shoham et al. 2005; Pouget et al. 2000; White et al. 2010; Wu et al. 2009), the improvement is often small, and the computational overhead can be extremely high compared to linear models. Thus, such models may sometimes prove impractical for real-time operation.

Of particular concern in model selection are nonstationarities in the spike trains that degrade decoding accuracy because they change the relationships between spike trains and movement kinematics (Stevenson et al. 2011). Nonstationarities can arise from external events or from as yet largely unknown internal sources and are often encountered in iBCI performance. Nevertheless, as will be illustrated later, decoder performance can be remarkably good in spite of this problem. The extensive past work on spike decoding and the critical related issues are reviewed in detailed in several sources (Fagg et al. 2009; Wu & Hatsopoulos 2008; Wu et al. 2006; Truccolo et al. 2005; Serruya et al. 2003; Pouget et al. 2000; Paninski et al. 2009; Paninski et al. 2007; Sanger 2003).

For optimal decoding, one also needs to establish the time-lag, or delay, between the spike measures and the kinematic variable of interest (e.g., the delay between the spike measure and movement onset). Lags are typically defined on the basis of the recorded data so as to maximize the correlation between the measure and the kinematic variable. Lags are typically 100–150 msec; that is, spikes account best for movements that occur 100–150 msec in the future. This observation is consistent with the assumption that these spikes contribute to producing subsequent movements. At the same time, however, neurons differ in optimal lag times; for some the lag is negative, suggesting that they are responding to movement-related feedback from sensory receptors (Paninski et al. 2004) and may have sensory roles in addition to their roles in movement control.

Although most iBCI studies have focused on translating the spike trains produced by single neurons (or putative single neurons, given the frequent uncertainties in distinguishing between spikes from different neurons), *multiunit activity* (MUA) might also be used for iBCIs control. Use of MUA could impart some valuable advantages. First, using MUA avoids the need for spike discrimination. Second, it may simplify model parameterization. Third, and perhaps more important, MUA data may be less dependent on the precise placement of the implanted array and may be less affected by its subsequent small movements relative to the surrounding brain tissue. There is no established definition for the composition of an MUA signal: it may range from two fairly distinguishable neurons to an unknown, but presumably large, number of indistinguishable neurons. The differences between multiunit activity and single-unit activity in the kind and amount of information they provide, as well as their relative values for iBCI purposes, require further study.

OPEN-LOOP AND CLOSED-LOOP DECODING

As noted above, the single-neuron recording methods now being applied in iBCI development have been used for decades in basic neuroscience studies of cortical function. As used in basic neuroscience, single-neuron recording is a powerful observation method. It is used in an entirely passive, *open-loop* fashion: there is usually no feedback from the recording system to the nervous system. Use of iBCI sensors simply in this open-loop fashion, to examine the correlations between neuronal activity and actual movements (and to obtain results that have important implications for BCI development), does not, however, constitute a true BCI (see chapter 1).

True BCIs operate, by definition, in a *closed-loop* fashion: the recorded activity produces output (hopefully the action desired by the user) that is provided in real time as feedback (usually visual) to the user. Thus, the BCI output can affect subsequent neuronal activity, and the user has the opportunity to improve system operation through adaptive changes in that activity.

This opportunity to recruit the full resources of the brain for improving control may help account for the remarkable success of small numbers of neurons and simple linear models in closed-loop iBCI settings. Fortunately, these central adaptive capacities often remain intact even when the brain's normal output pathways are damaged (e.g., as in spinal cord injury). Closed-loop operation permits the user to learn how to provide brain signals that optimize the BCI's ability to recognize and implement the user's intent. In very early studies, Fetz and Finoccio (1971) showed that monkeys could modify the firing of single cortical neurons in response to feedback. Several iBCI studies of multidimensional cursor control in monkeys (e.g., Serruya et al., 2002) provide further evidence for adaptive changes in neuronal behavior and suggest that intermediary structures, such as the basal ganglia or cerebellum, may contribute by modifying the input-output relationships of the cortical neurons being recorded. Furthermore, monkeys can adapt when a decoding algorithm is deliberately scrambled, so that the relationships between activity in specific neurons and the

BCI's output are changed; that is, they learn to change neuronal firing to match the new decoder and to regain good control of the BCI output (Taylor et al. 2002; Helms Tillery et al. 2003; Jarosiewicz et al. 2008; Ganguly & Carmena 2009; Koyama et al. 2010).

CONTINUOUS DECODING AND DISCRETE DECODING

BCIs in general, and iBCIs specifically, have been used to provide one of two kinds of decoding: *continuous* or *discrete*. Continuous decoding is best described as real-time control of an ongoing movement, such as of a cursor or a robotic limb. Discrete decoding consists of the ability to classify specific events, as when a letter or icon is selected from among a set of possible choices. (These terms correspond to *process control* and *goal selection* protocols; see chapters 1 and 10.) In an example of discrete decoding, Santhanam et al. (2006) used neuronal activity recorded in premotor cortex while a monkey planned to reach to a goal (but did not actually move to select the goal). They calculated that the discrete goal-selection capacity demonstrated by the data could, if converted to keystrokes, be used to type up to 15 words/min (see chapter 17 of this volume for further discussion). Discrete and continuous decoding may also be combined.

It is possible to apply both continuous and discrete decoding to the neuronal activity recorded from a single array and to thereby achieve two different outputs concurrently (e.g., mouse control and keystroke control). A human with tetraplegia was able to move a cursor in two dimensions (through continuous decoding) and was also able to select targets (through discrete decoding) (Kim et al. 2007b). Such demonstrations reveal the richness of the information that can be decoded from the spikes of even a small neuronal population, and they thereby indicate the great potential of iBCIs for producing complex multichannel communication and control.

COMMUNICATION AND CONTROL APPLICATIONS OF iBCIs

People with severe paralysis could use an iBCI to control a variety of devices. People who are tetraplegic have used implanted cortical arrays to operate a computer, a robotic limb, a wheelchair, and various electrical or electromechanical assistive devices (Donoghue et al. 2007). All four of the participants in the first BrainGate study performed a two-dimensional task requiring movement of a cursor under continuous control to one of four targets placed at screen edges (Hochberg et al. 2006; Kim et al. 2008; Truccolo et al. 2008). They also used several different speller designs to type messages (Kim et al. 2008) (e.g., fig. 16.9). The reliability of this capability has not, however, been systematically evaluated in a rigorous quantitative manner. In addition to cursor control (fig. 16.8A), BrainGate participant S1 was able to open and close a myoelectric hand at will (one-dimensional control) and was able to reach and grasp objects with a robotic arm that was guided by a 5-target cursor interface, allowing him to grasp objects at one location

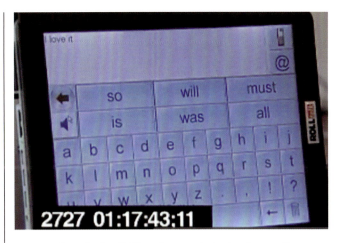

Figure 16.9 Example of an iBCI-based communication interface used by a human with tetraplegia. The computer displays an alphabetically organized keyboard and implements word prediction as letters are typed (Rolltalk system, Abilia, Sweden). Letter selections are made by moving the cursor to the letter or word using neural activity from M1 decoded while making imagined hand movement, then selecting this location with an imagined hand squeeze. The sentence "I love it" has been typed in response to a query about the user's opinion of the system. (From Hochberg laboratory, with permission.)

and deliver them to someone at another location (Hochberg et al. 2006).

BCIs seek to provide at least one, but preferably more, stable and reliable control channels. As discussed in chapter 11, a reliable control channel from any type of BCI could be coupled to nearly any application device, from a simple on/off switch to a fully functioning computer, robotic arm, or wheelchair. Although it is generally thought that control is limited by the richness of the BCI's input signal (i.e., the number of independently controllable dimensions), in reality it is often the application that is the critical limiting factor. Thus, on the one hand, by *goal selection* (see chapter 11), a robot can be designed to respond automatically to a switch input to open a bottle of water, pour it into a cup, and deliver it so that a person could drink from the cup; however, this requires custom software and hardware that is generally intolerant of significant changes in the circumstances of use (e.g., object locations, sizes, weights, etc.). On the other hand, by *process control* (see chapter 11), a very high-dimensional control signal could be adjusted by the user to accommodate altered circumstances: a glass of different shape, a bottle now nearly empty, or a cup at a different location. Such adjustments mimic those that the intact neuromuscular system routinely performs effortlessly. A major motivation behind iBCI development is the opportunity to engage the actual output circuitry of the cortical motor areas to capture the same signals that produce these natural actions and allow them to achieve these same flexible functions for people with motor disabilities. Because the range of assistive devices is covered in chapter 11, the discussion in this chapter is limited to the potential unique advantages of iBCIs and special cases where iBCIs may meet the goal of more fully replacing lost functions.

If properly developed, iBCIs might provide a wide range of uses with multiple potentially independent control signals that far exceed the limitations in speed and flexibility of any current assistive technologies. The small size of each sensor and the high information content of spikes might allow bilateral implants in both arm and leg areas that could simultaneously control both arms and legs. The potential to engage any cortical area as an additional control output (e.g., premotor and parietal areas), and the possibilities for using both spike trains and LFPs for control, suggest that iBCIs could provide very complex control approaching or even conceivably surpassing the normal highly flexible neuromuscular control of people without disabilities. Although these exciting speculations are as yet unrealized, recent data do show that even a single small array in one area of cortex can provide high-dimensional control of a limb. For example, Vargas et al. (2010) showed in monkeys that a single array can provide about 10 independent dimensions of control that can decode voluntary reaching and grasping actions performed by able-bodied monkeys. Applied to robotic arms, this control might provide highly flexible and very useful reach-and-grasp actions for people with upper-limb paralysis. Even more significantly, such a system might allow the reanimation of a person's own paralyzed muscles.

A long-range goal of neural engineering research is to recreate the connection between the brain and the muscles, thus circumventing the damage to pathways and structures that normally deliver motor commands from the brain to other areas of the body. Ideally, such a system would be fully internalized and as flexible as the intact system. Initial steps toward realization of such a system have provided promising results. First, functional electrical stimulation systems (FES) have been fully and permanently implanted to activate muscles with volitional control signals (Peckham & Knutson 2005; Hincapie & Kirsch 2009). About 600 people with incomplete paralysis (e.g., thoracic or mid- to low-cervical spinal cord injuries) currently have FES systems that allow them to control arm and hand muscles to reach and grasp, or to control trunk and leg muscles to maintain posture, or to sit or stand. The current systems use the activity of muscles that remain under voluntary control as control signals. However, these command signal sources are very limited in dimensionality, require mapping of one signal onto another, require significant remaining muscle control, and interrupt the normal functions of this remaining control. Command signals from iBCI implants could avoid some or all of these limitations.

iBCIs can be operated without initial learning and without undue attentional demands. For example, talking, head movements, and attention to other tasks can occur while engaging in BCI-controlled tasks (Hochberg et al. 2006). This suggests that reanimation of paralyzed muscles is feasible through iBCIs without interfering with concurrent control of unparalyzed muscles. Furthermore, the ability of iBCIs to tap into the brain's own independent control channels for both arms and legs also suggests that control of the entire body might one day be achieved. In a recent study, command signals from an iBCI implant in a person with tetraplegia were used to control a virtual arm by stimulating its virtual muscles with an FES system (Chadwick et al. 2011). The subject was able to move the arm immediately and continuously in a two-dimensional plane and flex the virtual finger with an imagined hand squeeze

(fig. 16.8C). This system could be implemented with FES technology already available to allow this person to reach and grasp an object.

iBCI USER POPULATION

As described in many chapters of this book, there are numerous disorders in which the brain's normal neuromuscular output pathways are interrupted or grossly disturbed in other ways. Spinal cord injuries, brainstem strokes, cerebral palsy, and many degenerative disorders can damage the corticospinal and other descending pathways carrying voluntary movement signals, thus preventing intentions generated in the brain and brainstem from acting on spinal motor control structures. Peripheral nerve disorders and muscular dystrophies can also prevent the brain's commands from producing movements. These conditions disconnect and/or destroy important motor structures, and in their most severe forms they can produce total paralysis, requiring assistive support for essentially all activities. An iBCI that restores only a fraction of the lost motor functions could have an enormous impact, restoring some independence in the activities of daily living, the ability to interact with others, and perhaps even the ability to work.

As iBCI technology advances and becomes more fully automated and easier to use, it may also have value for people with less severe disabilities. Thus, for example, in people who are paralyzed on one side due to a subcortical hemispheric stroke or traumatic injury, an iBCI might reconnect the cortex to the limbs and restore voluntary control of the contralateral arm and hand. Furthermore, iBCI systems could be useful to the many children and adults with cerebral palsy so severe that they have little or no useful motor control. Finally, with iBCIs that can provide sufficiently rich control signals, it might be possible for amputees to control a multidimensional artificial limb such as that recently developed by the DARPA Revolutionizing Prosthetics Initiative.

Developing iBCIs suitable for all these populations is an ambitious goal that requires progress in a number of critical areas. Achieving this goal could greatly benefit millions of people with movement disabilities from moderate to severe.

ADVANCES NEEDED TO ACHIEVE iBCI SYSTEMS PRACTICAL FOR LONG-TERM HUMAN USE

The studies to date in both animals and humans show that iBCIs have great promise for restoring useful function to people with severe neuromuscular disabilities. At the same time, however, it is equally clear that realization of this promise depends on advances in several crucial areas. These advances are needed to produce iBCI systems that are fully implantable, safe, and easy to use, that can function stably and reliably for decades, and that provide function substantially superior to that provided by noninvasive BCI systems.

FULLY IMPLANTABLE, SAFE, AND BIOCOMPATIBLE SYSTEMS

The iBCI systems used in human pilot trials to date have a number of shortcomings that make them impractical for long-term everyday home use. These include the use of percutaneous connectors, the tethering to cumbersome hardware, the need for on-site technician oversight of system calibration and operation, and the possibility of device failures that may necessitate repeated surgical repair or even device removal.

Percutaneous connectors constitute a continuing risk for infection. An obvious solution to this problem, as well as to that of tethering, is a fully implanted device, without percutaneous connections, that transmits the signals it records by telemetry. Such wireless iBCIs will need to satisfy high signal-processing and power requirements if they are to have the many electrodes and high bandwidth needed to record both spikes and LFPs and to transmit them to next-order processors inside or outside the body. An ideal wireless system would have all of the processing and communication electronics mounted on the array itself, so that after insertion, the dura and bone

could be closed. Although such a system would require exceptionally small components and very complex integration to fit in the minimal space between the cortical surface and the skull, such devices are being developed (e.g., Kim et al. 2009). Another alternative under development places most or all of the initial-processing electronics in a pad of electronics that sits below the skin and above the skull, with a cable through the bone that connects to the intracortical array. This design (fig. 16-10A) is now being tested in animals (Song et al. 2007). In addition, any such electronic implant must remain impermeable to the tissue fluids that would damage the electronics. Device encapsulation methods to provide the necessary protection for many years are still in the development stage.

The powering of implanted medical devices in general is a problem that has not been fully resolved. Some implanted devices are successfully driven with implanted rechargeable batteries or external induction coils. However, useful iBCI implants would have larger power demands than the implanted medical devices now commonly in use. Power consumption generates heat, and it has not yet been established how much heat the brain can tolerate (Kim et al. 2007a). Assessment of

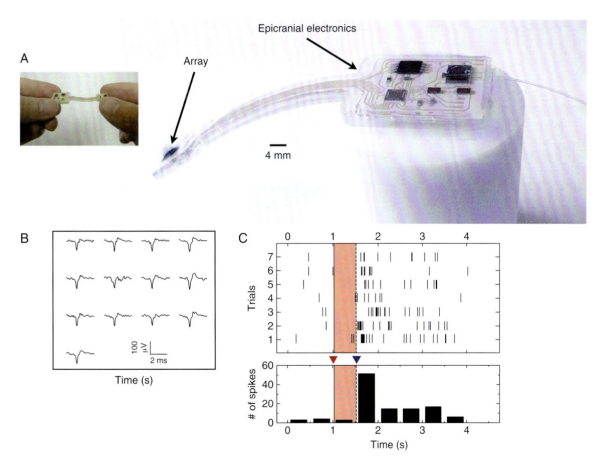

Figure 16.10 Prototype of fully implantable wireless iBCI array system for humans. (A) A 96- channel, chip-scale preamplifier and analog multiplexor mounted directly on the back of the platform base of the array (too small to be visible). Signals from 100 microelectrodes are carried via the ribbon cable to a pad of electronics that is mounted above the skull and under the skin (epicranial electronics). These components filter the signals to create a broadband multiplexed signal (both LFPs and spikes) and then transmit these digitized signals through the skin via an infrared laser mounted in one of the chips. (B) Spike waveforms recorded from monkey M1 cortex using this system. A receiver just above the skin detected these signals, which were further processed (demultiplexed, filtered, discriminated) using external software and hardware. (C) The rasters summarized in the histogram below show modulation of a spike train associated with arm movements initiated during the interval marked by the red and blue triangles. (From Borton et al. 2009; Patterson et al. 2004.)

this critical question is particularly challenging because each implant design is likely to have its own unique thermal consequences. In addition, the substantial space, coil alignment, and other engineering issues involved in providing power to an implant with a rechargeable battery or an induction coil have not yet been resolved.

Despite these complex challenges, some progress toward fully implantable iBCIs suitable for long-term use has been made (e.g., Song et al. 2005; Song et al. 2007; Chestek et al. 2009b; Kim et al. 2009), and continued progress is anticipated (see chapter 5). Although the technology necessary to solve the remaining problems exists, the design, fabrication, and validation of iBCIs suitable for decades-long use is a complex multifaceted problem that requires substantial further work.

EASE OF USE

To be truly practical, an iBCI system must be simple and reliable enough for users or their caregivers to set it up and run it quickly, easily, and without extensive training. Effective long-term independent operation depends largely on automation handled by the BCI's software. Some aspects of this necessary automation have already been achieved, but much remains to be accomplished and then validated in comprehensive clinical testing.

In addition, iBCI systems that are small and highly portable are particularly desirable, both because they can be more easily integrated into often complex and crowded environments and because they can more readily move with the user (e.g., by being mounted on a wheelchair). Thus, the large, cumbersome systems typical of pilot studies must be replaced with miniaturized systems. The continuing advances in microprocessors and other electronics have made such miniaturization possible, but these now need to be applied to and realized in practical iBCI systems.

SIGNAL STABILITY AND ALGORITHM ADAPTIBILITY

If iBCI systems are to be practical for long-term use, their sensors must provide reasonably stable signals from day to day. Signal instabilities can be a problem with all BCIs. For BCIs to be suitable for long-term independent use, fully automated software must diminish signal instabilities. Data available in iBCI studies to date indicate that further improvements are essential. For example, long-term iBCI studies in both monkeys and humans show that the number (although perhaps not the identities) of the recorded neurons varies from day to day (e.g., Ryu et al. 2009; Suner et al. 2005; Santhanam et al. 2007), although some remain stable (Dickey et al. 2009; Ganguly & Carmena 2009; Ganguly et al. 2011). Effective methods for dealing with instabilities are not yet well developed.

Day-by-day changes in the composition of the neuronal population are often addressed by modifying the parameters in the process that decodes the neural signals to produce output commands (see chapters 7 and 8). While this currently requires a skilled technician and takes tens of minutes, it could, in principle, be performed by automated software. Adaptive algorithms could adjust the composition of populations contributing to the control signal as well as the equations that use their information.

Adaptive algorithms might also encourage and facilitate the user in learning to control neuronal firing so as to improve the output commands. Studies to date provide impressive evidence that such learning can occur and can improve performance (e.g., Taylor et al. 2002; Ganguly & Carmena 2009; Ganguly et al. 2011). Concerted efforts to define the capacities and limitations of this learning and to develop methods for encouraging and guiding it are critical to the future success of iBCIs. Although these advances are certainly possible, they will require extensive development and fairly long-term studies in animals and humans.

AUGMENTED SENSORY FEEDBACK

The iBCI systems discussed so far have relied exclusively on visual feedback to close the loop between user and system. However, normal neuromuscular movements also depend to a large degree on complex somatosensory inputs (e.g., concerning grip force, object contact, movement velocity, etc.) that help to guide actions. Together, these inputs are much more rapid and informative than the simple visual feedback provided by current iBCIs. Thus, iBCI performance might be markedly improved if such normal somatosensory feedback modalities could be added. Romo et al. (1998) showed that low-level microstimulation by electrodes chronically implanted in monkey somatosensory cortex could provide perceptually useful sensory feedback. These results have been confirmed and extended in other studies (London et al. 2008; O'Doherty et al. 2009; Rebesco & Miller 2011). These findings suggest that intracortical arrays in somatosensory cortex could provide complex spatiotemporal patterns of stimulation that could substitute for the sensory inputs normally associated with movement. Advances of this kind might substantially augment the speed and precision of the control possible with iBCI systems and reduce the requirement for visual monitoring of movement.

OTHER POTENTIAL APPLICATIONS OF iBCI TECHNOLOGY

Although the primary goal of the development of BCIs, including iBCIs, is to restore communication and control to people with severe neuromuscular disabilities, this technology may have other important uses as well. As previously noted, iBCI sensors can provide an unprecedentedly detailed view of animal or human cortex at a neuronal level—and can do so continually over lengthy periods of time. Thus, iBCI sensors are a powerful new tool for basic-science investigations as well as for studies aimed at developing new understanding of, and hopefully new ways to diagnose and treat, a variety of devastating neurological disorders, such as stroke, traumatic brain injury, and degenerative diseases (Hatsopoulos & Donoghue 2009).

For example, as described earlier in this chapter, it has recently and surprisingly been learned that single neurons in human motor cortex can still be responsive to intended motor actions years after spinal-cord injury produces paralysis that prevents such actions (Hochberg et al. 2006; Kennedy et al. 2000; Kim et al. 2008; Truccolo et al. 2008). It appears that the plasticity that occurs after injury or disease does not necessarily lead to dramatic reorganization that abolishes such responsiveness (Sanes & Donoghue 1997). In the future, iBCIs should provide other important insights into cortical function in normal and pathological states. The ability to record both spikes and LFPs simultaneously will also allow direct analysis of the relationships between LFPs (which are thought to reflect mainly synaptic inputs) and spikes (which reflect neuronal output). The dynamics of this transformation are a key aspect of cortical information processing.

iBCI sensors have many other potential applications in diagnosing or treating human neural disorders. This technology is being explored with regard to its possibilities for restoring cognitive function (Serruya & Kahana 2008). iBCI sensors could also be used to detect changes in neural state that predict ensuing disruption of brain function, for example in epilepsy (see chapter 22). During seizures, the normally random Poisson distribution of neuronal spiking can become broadly periodic. The ability to detect this transition in firing pattern well in advance of an overt seizure might potentially be used as a seizure predictor that would warn the person or that would trigger interventions to prevent or abort the seizure. A seizure-prediction device might control the systemic or local release of pharmacological agents (Rohatgi et al. 2009) or initiate patterned electrical stimulation that blocks seizure development (Skarpaas & Morrell 2009; Berenyi et al. 2010). Similar approaches might conceivably be applied to a range of episodic neurological or psychiatric disorders. Such advances will require better understanding of the complex and poorly understood relationships between the information embodied in neuronal spike trains and abnormal human brain function.

SUMMARY

This chapter reviews the current state of intraparenchymal BCIs or iBCIs, neural interfaces based on sensors implanted in brain tissue and intended to restore control and independence for people with paralysis. Demonstrations of iBCI functionality have been carried out in able-bodied and paralyzed monkeys, and, importantly, in humans with severe paralysis. Results to date indicate that intracortical microelectrode implants are able to record neural signals safely and reliably for long periods and can provide potentially useful control. Data suggest that biocompatibility, biostability, and mechanical forces are not major impediments to creation of successful iBCI devices. Nevertheless, considerable additional work is needed to ensure stable materials, to create wireless and automated systems, and to develop adaptive algorithms that encourage and maintain reliable high-level performance.

The implanted sensors used in iBCIs can record both LFPs and spiking. Although most studies have examined the types of control possible from spiking, the ability to combine LFPs and spikes provides a rich additional source of signals yet to be fully explored.

Devices controlled by iBCIs include robot arms and computer cursors. Both of these applications have potentially great value for people unable to move, by enabling them to manipulate their environment for feeding or self-care, to communicate, or to pursue other productive activities prevented by paralysis.

Additional data concerning safety, reliability, longevity, and utility are essential for further development and eventual commercialization of these systems to make them available to the user population.

iBCI sensors provide a unique perspective on human brain function because they allow the properties of single neurons to be evaluated. They may also be useful for understanding other brain disorders at a resolution not previously attained and may lead to other related classes of devices that treat diseases such as epilepsy. Overall, the future prospects for iBCIs are very promising; they point to a continual series of advances that can help people with paralysis to lead more independent lives, can improve the treatment of neurological disease, and can increase basic understanding of brain function.

REFERENCES

Achtman N, Afshar A, Santhanam G, Yu BM, Ryu SI, Shenoy KV. 2007. Free-paced high-performance brain-computer interfaces. *J Neural Eng* 4:336–347.

Andersen RA, Hwang EJ, Mulliken GH. 2010. Cognitive neural prosthetics. *Annu Rev Psychol* 61:169–190, C1–3.

Andersen RA, Musallam S, Pesaran B. 2004. Selecting the signals for a brain-machine interface. *Curr Opin Neurobiol* 14:720–726.

Awan NR, Lozano A, Hamani C. 2009. Deep brain stimulation: current and future perspectives. *Neurosurg Focus* 27:E2.

Bartels J, Andreasen D, Ehirim P, Mao H, Seibert S, et al. 2008. Neurotrophic electrode: method of assembly and implantation into human motor speech cortex. *J Neurosci Methods* 174:168–176.

Belitski A, Gretton A, Magri C, Murayama Y, Montemurro MA, et al. 2008. Low-frequency local field potentials and spikes in primary visual cortex convey independent visual information. *J Neurosci* 28: 5696–5709.

Berenyi A, Belluscio M, Buzsaki G. 2010. Suppressing epileptic spike-and-wave discharges by extracranial alternating current stimulation. *Neuroscience Meeting Planner* Program No. 245.10.

Borton DA, Song YK, Patterson WR, Bull CW, Park S, et al. 2009. Wireless, high-bandwidth recordings from non-human primate motor cortex using a scalable 16-Ch implantable microsystem. *Conf Proc IEEE Eng Med Biol Soc* 2009:5531–5534.

Boviatsis EJ, Stavrinou LC, Themistocleous M, Kouyialis AT, Sakas DE. 2010. Surgical and hardware complications of deep brain stimulation. A seven-year experience and review of the literature. *Acta Neurochir (Wien).*152(12): 2053–62.

Bullock TH. 1997. Signals and signs in the nervous system: the dynamic anatomy of electrical activity is probably information-rich. *Proc Natl Acad Sci USA* 94:1–6.

Buzsaki G. 2004. Large-scale recording of neuronal ensembles. *Nat Neurosci* 7:446–451.

Buzsaki G, Kandel A. 1998. Somadendritic backpropagation of action potentials in cortical pyramidal cells of the awake rat. *J Neurophysiol* 79:1587–1591.

Campbell PK, Jones KE, Huber RJ, Horch KW, Normann RA. 1991. A silicon-based, three-dimensional neural interface: manufacturing processes for an intracortical electrode array. *IEEE Trans Biomed Eng* 38:758–768.

Carmena JM, Lebedev MA, Crist RE, O'Doherty JE, Santucci DM, et al. 2003. Learning to control a brain-machine interface for reaching and grasping by primates. *PLoS Biol* 1:E42.

Chadwick EK, Blana D, Simeral JD, Lambrecht J, Kim SP, Cornwell AS, Taylor DM, Hochberg LR, Donoghue JP, Kirsch RF. 2011. Continuous neuronal ensemble control of simulated arm reaching by a human with tetraplegia. *J Neural Eng* 8(3): 034003.

Chestek CA, Cunningham JP, Gilja V, Nuyujukian P, Ryu SI, Shenoy KV. 2009a. Neural prosthetic systems: current problems and future directions. *Conf Proc IEEE Eng Med Biol Soc* 2009:3369–3375.

Chestek CA, Gilja V, Nuyujukian P, Kier RJ, Solzbacher F, et al. 2009b. HermesC: low-power wireless neural recording system for freely moving primates. *IEEE Trans Neural Syst Rehabil Eng* 17:330–338.

Clausen J. 2010. Ethical brain stimulation–neuroethics of deep brain stimulation in research and clinical practice. *Eur J Neurosci* 32(7):1152–1162.

Colebatch JG. 2007. Bereitschaftspotential and movement-related potentials: origin, significance, and application in disorders of human movement. *Movement Dis* 22:601–610.

Cunningham JP, Gilja V, Ryu SI, Shenoy KV. 2009. Methods for estimating neural firing rates, and their application to brain-machine interfaces. *Neural Netw* 22:1235–1246.

Dickey AS, Suminski A, Amit Y, Hatsopoulos NG. 2009. Single-unit stability using chronically implanted multielectrode arrays. *J Neurophysiol* 102:1331–1339.

Donoghue JP. 2008. Bridging the brain to the world: a perspective on neural interface systems. *Neuron* 60:511–521.

Donoghue JP, Nurmikko A, Black M, Hochberg LR. 2007. Assistive technology and robotic control using motor cortex ensemble-based neural interface systems in humans with tetraplegia. *J Physiol* 579:603–611.

Donoghue JP, Nurmikko A, Friehs G, Black M. 2004. Development of neuro-motor prostheses for humans. *Suppl Clin Neurophysiol* 57:592–606.

Donoghue JP, Sanes JN, Hatsopoulos NG, Gaal G. 1998. Neural discharge and local field potential oscillations in primate motor cortex during voluntary movements. *J Neurophysiol* 79:159–173.

Fagg AH, Ojakangas GW, Miller LE, Hatsopoulos NG. 2009. Kinetic trajectory decoding using motor cortical ensembles. *IEEE Trans Neural Syst Rehabil Eng* 17:487–496.

Fetz EE. 1969. Operant conditioning of cortical unit activity. *Science* 163: 955–958.

Fetz EE, Finocchio DV. 1971. Operant conditioning of specific patterns of neural and muscular activity. *Science* 174:431–435.

Fetz EE, Finocchio DV. 1972. Operant conditioning of isolated activity in specific muscles and precentral cells. *Brain Res* 40:19–23.

Fitzsimmons NA, Lebedev MA, Peikon ID, Nicolelis MA. 2009. Extracting kinematic parameters for monkey bipedal walking from cortical neuronal ensemble activity. *Front Integr Neurosci* 3:3.

Fofonoff TA, Martel SM, Hatsopoulos NG, Donoghue JP, Hunter IW. 2004. Microelectrode array fabrication by electrical discharge machining and chemical etching. *IEEE Trans Biomed Eng* 51:890–895.

Ganguly K, Carmena JM. 2009. Emergence of a stable cortical map for neuroprosthetic control. *PLoS Biol* 7:e1000153.

Ganguly K, Dimitrov DF, Wallis JD, Carmena JM. Reversible large-scale modification of cortical networks during neuroprosthetic control. *Nat Neurosci* 14:662–667.

Georgopoulos AP. 1988. Neural integration of movement: role of motor cortex in reaching. *FASEB J* 2:2849–2857.

Georgopoulos AP, Schwartz AB, Kettner RE. 1986. Neuronal population coding of movement direction. *Science* 233:1416–1419.

Gold C, Henze DA, Koch C, Buzsaki G. 2006. On the origin of the extracellular action potential waveform: A modeling study. *J Neurophysiol* 95: 3113–3128.

Hamani C, Lozano AM. 2006. Hardware-related complications of deep brain stimulation: a review of the published literature. *Stereotact Funct Neurosurg* 84:248–251.

Hatsopoulos NG, Donoghue JP. 2009. The science of neural interface systems. *Annu Rev Neurosci* 32:249–266.

Hatsopoulos N, Joshi J, O'Leary JG. 2004. Decoding continuous and discrete motor behaviors using motor and premotor cortical ensembles. *J Neurophysiol* 92:1165–1174.

Helms Tillery SI, Taylor DM, Schwartz AB. 2003. Training in cortical control of neuroprosthetic devices improves signal extraction from small neuronal ensembles. *Rev Neurosci* 14:107–119.

Henze DA, Borhegyi Z, Csicsvari J, Mamiya A, Harris KD, Buzsaki G. 2000. Intracellular features predicted by extracellular recordings in the hippocampus in vivo. *J Neurophysiol* 84:390–400.

Hincapie JG, Kirsch RF. 2009. Feasibility of EMG-based neural network controller for an upper extremity neuroprosthesis. *IEEE Trans Neural Syst Rehabil Eng* 17:80–90.

Hochberg LR, Serruya MD, Friehs GM, Mukand JA, Saleh M, et al. 2006. Neuronal ensemble control of prosthetic devices by a human with tetraplegia. *Nature* 442:164–171.

Hsu JM, Rieth L, Normann RA, Tathireddy P, Solzbacher F. 2009. Encapsulation of an integrated neural interface device with Parylene C. *IEEE Trans Biomed Eng* 56:23–29.

Humphrey DR, Corrie WS. 1978. Properties of pyramidal tract neuron system within a functionally defined subregion of primate motor cortex. *J Neurophysiol* 41:216–243.

Hwang EJ, Andersen RA. 2009. Brain control of movement execution onset using local field potentials in posterior parietal cortex. *J Neurosci* 29: 14363–14370.

Jarosiewicz B, Chase SM, Fraser GW, Velliste M, Kass RE, Schwartz AB. 2008. Functional network reorganization during learning in a brain-computer interface paradigm. *Proc Natl Acad Sci U S A* 105:19486–19491.

Kalaska JF, Crammond DJ. 1992. Cerebral cortical mechanisms of reaching movements. *Science* 255:1517–1523.

Kalaska JF, Scott SH, Cisek P, Sergio LE. 1997. Cortical control of reaching movements. *Curr Opin Neurobiol* 7:849–859.

Kennedy PR. 1989. The cone electrode: a long-term electrode that records from neurites grown onto its recording surface. *J Neurosci Methods* 29: 181–193.

Kennedy PR, Bakay RA. 1998. Restoration of neural output from a paralyzed patient by a direct brain connection. *Neuroreport* 9:1707–1711.

Kennedy PR, Bakay RA, Moore MM, Adams K, Goldwaithe J. 2000. Direct control of a computer from the human central nervous system. *IEEE Trans Rehabil Eng* 8:198–202.

Kennedy PR, Bakay RA, Sharpe SM. 1992. Behavioral correlates of action potentials recorded chronically inside the cone electrode. *Neuroreport* 3:605–608.

Kim S, Bhandari R, Klein M, Negi S, Rieth L, et al. 2009. Integrated wireless neural interface based on the Utah electrode array. *Biomed Microdevices* 11:453–466.

Kim S, Tathireddy P, Normann RA, Solzbacher F. 2007a. Thermal impact of an active 3-D microelectrode array implanted in the brain. *IEEE Trans Neural Syst Rehabil Eng* 15:493–501.

Kim S-P, Simeral J, Hochberg L, DOnoghue J, Friehs G, MJ. 2007b. Multistate decoding of point and click control signals from motor cortical activity in a human with tetraplegia. *Proceedings of the 3rd International IEEE EMBS Conference on Neural Engineering* 2007:486–489.

Kim SP, Simeral JD, Hochberg LR, Donoghue JP, Black MJ. 2008. Neural control of computer cursor velocity by decoding motor cortical spiking activity in humans with tetraplegia. *J Neural Eng* 5:455–476.

Kipke DR. 2004. Implantable neural probe systems for cortical neuroprostheses. *Conf Proc IEEE Eng Med Biol Soc* 7:5344–5347.

Koyama S, Chase SM, Whitford AS, Velliste M, Schwartz AB, Kass RE. 2010. Comparison of brain-computer interface decoding algorithms in open-loop and closed-loop control. *J Comput Neurosci* 29:73–87.

Kralik JD, Dimitrov DF, Krupa DJ, Katz DB, Cohen D, Nicolelis MA. 2001. Techniques for long-term multisite neuronal ensemble recordings in behaving animals. *Methods* 25:121–150.

Kruger J, Caruana F, Volta RD, Rizzolatti G. 2010. Seven years of recording from monkey cortex with a chronically implanted multiple microelectrode. *Front Neuroeng* 3:6.

Lempka SF, Johnson MD, Barnett DW, Moffitt MA, Otto KJ, et al. 2006. Optimization of microelectrode design for cortical recording based on thermal noise considerations. *Conf Proc IEEE Eng Med Biol Soc* 1: 3361–3364.

London BM, Jordan LR, Jackson CR, Miller LE. 2008. Electrical stimulation of the proprioceptive cortex (area 3a) used to instruct a behaving monkey. *IEEE Trans Neural Syst Rehabil Eng* 16:32–36.

Marzullo TC, Miller CR, Kipke DR. 2006. Suitability of the cingulate cortex for neural control. *IEEE Trans Neural Syst Rehabil Eng* 14:401–409.

Maynard EM, Hatsopoulos NG, Ojakangas CL, Acuna BD, Sanes JN, et al. 1999. Neuronal interactions improve cortical population coding of movement direction. *J Neurosci* 19:8083–8093.

Meyer JR, Roychowdhury S, Russell EJ, Callahan C, Gitelman D, Mesulam MM. 1996. Location of the central sulcus via cortical thickness of the precentral and postcentral gyri on MR. *AJNR Am J Neuroradiol* 17: 1699–1706.

Moran A, Bar-Gad I. 2010. Revealing neuronal functional organization through the relation between multi-scale oscillatory extracellular signals. *J Neurosci Methods* 186:116–129.

Moran DW, Schwartz AB. 1999. Motor cortical representation of speed and direction during reaching. *J Neurophysiol* 82:2676–2692.

Moritz CT, Perlmutter SI, Fetz EE. 2008. Direct control of paralysed muscles by cortical neurons. *Nature* 456:639–642.

Moxon KA, Leiser SC, Gerhardt GA, Barbee KA, Chapin JK. 2004. Ceramic-based multisite electrode arrays for chronic single-neuron recording. *IEEE Trans Biomed Eng* 51:647–656.

Musallam S, Bak MJ, Troyk PR, Andersen RA. 2007. A floating metal micro-electrode array for chronic implantation. *J Neurosci Methods* 160: 122–127.

Nicolelis MA, Dimitrov D, Carmena JM, Crist R, Lehew G, et al. 2003. Chronic, multisite, multielectrode recordings in macaque monkeys. *Proc Natl Acad Sci USA* 100:11041–11046.

Nicolelis MA, Ghazanfar AA, Faggin BM, Votaw S, Oliveira LM. 1997. Reconstructing the engram: simultaneous, multisite, many single neuron recordings. *Neuron* 18:529–537.

Nicolelis MA, Lebedev MA. 2009. Principles of neural ensemble physiology underlying the operation of brain-machine interfaces. *Nat Rev Neurosci* 10:530–540.

Nunez PL. 1996. Spatial analysis of EEG. *Electroencephalogr Clin Neurophysiol Suppl* 45:37–38.

O'Doherty JE, Lebedev MA, Hanson TL, Fitzsimmons NA, Nicolelis MA. 2009. A brain-machine interface instructed by direct intracortical micro-stimulation. *Front Integr Neurosci* 3:20.

Paninski L, Ahmadian Y, Ferreira DG, Koyama S, Rahnama Rad K, et al. 2009. A new look at state-space models for neural data. *J Comput Neurosci* 29:107–126.

Paninski L, Fellows MR, Hatsopoulos NG, Donoghue JP. 2004. Spatiotemporal tuning of motor cortical neurons for hand position and velocity. *J Neurophysiol* 91:516–532.

Paninski L, Pillow J, Lewi J. 2007. Statistical models for neural encoding, decoding, and optimal stimulus design. *Prog Brain Res* 165:493–507.

Panzeri S, Pola G, Petroni F, Young MP, Petersen RS. 2002. A critical assess-ment of different measures of the information carried by correlated neu-ronal firing. *Biosystems* 67:177–185.

Parikh H, Marzullo TC, Kipke DR. 2009. Lower layers in the motor cortex are more effective targets for penetrating microelectrodes in cortical prosthe-ses. *J Neural Eng* 6:026004.

Patil PG, Carmena JM, Nicolelis MA, Turner DA. 2004. Ensemble recordings of human subcortical neurons as a source of motor control signals for a brain-machine interface. *Neurosurgery* 55:27–35.

Patterson WR, Song YK, Bull CW, Ozden I, Deangellis AP, et al. 2004. A microelectrode/microelectronic hybrid device for brain implantable neuroprosthesis applications. *IEEE Trans Biomed Eng* 51:1845–1853.

Peckham PH, Knutson JS. 2005. Functional electrical stimulation for neuro-muscular applications. *Annu Rev Biomed Eng* 7:327–360.

Pesaran B, Nelson MJ, Andersen RA. 2006. Dorsal premotor neurons encode the relative position of the hand, eye, and goal during reach planning. *Neuron* 51:125–134.

Pohlmeyer EA, Oby ER, Perreault EJ, Solla SA, Kilgore KL, et al. 2009. Toward the restoration of hand use to a paralyzed monkey: brain-controlled func-tional electrical stimulation of forearm muscles. *PLoS One* 4:e5924.

Porada I, Bondar I, Spatz WB, Kruger J. 2000. Rabbit and monkey visual cortex: more than a year of recording with up to 64 microelectrodes. *J Neurosci Methods* 95:13–28.

Pouget A, Dayan P, Zemel R. 2000. Information processing with population codes. *Nat Rev Neurosci* 1:125–132.

Rebesco JM, Miller LE. 2011. Enhanced detection threshold for in vivo cortical stimulation produced by Hebbian conditioning. *J Neural Eng* 8:016011.

Rickert J, Oliveira SC, Vaadia E, Aertsen A, Rotter S, Mehring C. 2005. Encoding of movement direction in different frequency ranges of motor cortical local field potentials. *J Neurosci* 25:8816–8824.

Rohatgi P, Langhals NB, Kipke DR, Patil PG. 2009. In vivo performance of a microelectrode neural probe with integrated drug delivery. *Neurosurg Focus* 27:E8.

Romo R, Hernandez A, Zainos A, Salinas E. 1998. Somatosensory discrimina-tion based on cortical microstimulation. *Nature* 392:387–390.

Rousche PJ, Normann RA. 1992. A method for pneumatically inserting an array of penetrating electrodes into cortical tissue. *Ann Biomed Eng* 20:413–422.

Rutten WL. 2002. Selective electrical interfaces with the nervous system. *Annu Rev Biomed Eng* 4:407–452.

Ryu SI, Shenoy KV. 2009. Human cortical prostheses: lost in translation? *Neurosurg Focus* 27:E5.

Sanes JN, Donoghue JP. 1997. Static and dynamic organization of motor cortex. *Adv Neurol* 73:277–296.

Sanger TD. 2003. Neural population codes. *Curr Opin Neurobiol* 13:238–249.

Santhanam G, Linderman MD, Gilja V, Afshar A, Ryu SI, et al. 2007. HermesB: a continuous neural recording system for freely behaving primates. *IEEE Trans Biomed Eng* 54:2037–2050.

Santhanam G, Ryu SI, Yu BM, Afshar A, Shenoy KV. 2006. A high-perfor-mance brain-computer interface. *Nature* 442:195–198.

Scherberger H, Andersen RA. 2007. Target selection signals for arm reaching in the posterior parietal cortex. *J Neurosci* 27:2001–2012.

Schwartz AB. 2004. Cortical neural prosthetics. *Annu Rev Neurosci* 27: 487–507.

Schwartz AB, Cui XT, Weber DJ, Moran DW. 2006. Brain-controlled inter-faces: movement restoration with neural prosthetics. *Neuron* 52:205–220.

Scott SH. 2008. Inconvenient truths about neural processing in primary motor cortex. *J Physiol* 586:1217–1224.

Seijo FJ, Alvarez-Vega MA, Gutierrez JC, Fdez-Glez F, Lozano B. 2007. Complications in subthalamic nucleus stimulation surgery for treatment of Parkinson's disease. Review of 272 procedures. *Acta Neurochir (Wien)* 149:867–875; discussion 76.

Serruya M, Hatsopoulos N, Fellows M, Paninski L, Donoghue J. 2003. Robustness of neuroprosthetic decoding algorithms. *Biol Cybern* 88: 219–228.

Serruya MD, Hatsopoulos NG, Paninski L, Fellows MR, Donoghue JP. 2002. Instant neural control of a movement signal. *Nature* 416:141–142.

Serruya MD, Kahana MJ. 2008. Techniques and devices to restore cognition. *Behav Brain Res* 192:149–165.

Shadlen MN, Newsome WT. 1998. The variable discharge of cortical neurons: implications for connectivity, computation, and information coding. *J Neurosci* 18:3870–3896.

Shain W, Spataro L, Dilgen J, Haverstick K, Retterer S, et al. 2003. Controlling cellular reactive responses around neural prosthetic devices using periph-eral and local intervention strategies. *IEEE Trans Neural Syst Rehabil Eng* 11:186–188.

Shenoy KV, Meeker D, Cao S, Kureshi SA, Pesaran B, et al. 2003. Neural prosthetic control signals from plan activity. *Neuroreport* 14:591–596.

Shoham S, Halgren E, Maynard EM, Normann RA. 2001. Motor-cortical activity in tetraplegics. *Nature* 413:793.

Shoham S, Paninski LM, Fellows MR, Hatsopoulos NG, Donoghue JP, Normann RA. 2005. Statistical encoding model for a primary motor cortical brain-machine interface. *IEEE Trans Biomed Eng* 52:1312–1322.

Simeral JD, Kim SP, Black MJ, Donoghue JP, Hochberg LR. 2011. Neural control of cursor trajectory and click by a human with tetraplegia 1000 days after implant of an intracortical microelectrode array. *J Neural Eng* 8:025027.

Singer W. 1999. Neuronal synchrony: a versatile code for the definition of rela-tions? *Neuron* 24:49–65, 111–125.

Skarpaas TL, Morrell MJ. 2009. Intracranial stimulation therapy for epilepsy. *Neurotherapeutics* 6:238–243.

Song YK, Borton DA, Park S, Patterson WR, Bull CW, et al. 2009. Active microelectronic neurosensor arrays for implantable brain communication interfaces. *IEEE Trans Neural Syst Rehabil Eng* 17:339–345.

Song YK, Patterson WR, Bull CW, Beals J, Hwang N, et al. 2005. Development of a chipscale integrated microelectrode/microelectronic device for brain implantable neuroengineering applications. *IEEE Trans Neural Syst Rehabil Eng* 13:220–226.

Song YK, Patterson WR, Bull CW, Borton DA, Li Y, et al. 2007. A brain implantable microsystem with hybrid RF/IR telemetry for advanced neu-roengineering applications. *Conf Proc IEEE Eng Med Biol Soc* 2007: 445–448.

Stevenson IH, Cherian A, London BM, Sachs NA, Lindberg E, Reimer J, Slutzky MW, Hatsopoulos NG, Miller LE, Kording KP. 2011. Statistical assessment of the stability of neural movement representations. J Neurophysiol, in press.

Suner S, Fellows MR, Vargas-Irwin C, Nakata GK, Donoghue JP. 2005. Reliability of signals from a chronically implanted, silicon-based electrode array in non-human primate primary motor cortex. *IEEE Trans Neural Syst Rehabil Eng* 13:524–541.

Sykacek P, Roberts SJ, Stokes M. 2004. Adaptive BCI based on variational Bayesian Kalman filtering: an empirical evaluation. *IEEE Trans Biomed Eng* 51:719–727.

Szarowski DH, Andersen MD, Retterer S, Spence AJ, Isaacson M, et al. 2003. Brain responses to micro-machined silicon devices. *Brain Res* 983:23–35.

Taylor DM, Tillery SI, Schwartz AB. 2002. Direct cortical control of 3D neuro-prosthetic devices. *Science* 296:1829–1832.

Tillery SI, Taylor DM. 2004. Signal acquisition and analysis for cortical control of neuroprosthetics. *Curr Opin Neurobiol* 14:758–762.

Truccolo W, Eden UT, Fellows MR, Donoghue JP, Brown EN. 2005. A point process framework for relating neural spiking activity to spiking history, neural ensemble, and extrinsic covariate effects. *J Neurophysiol* 93: 1074–1089.

Truccolo W, Friehs GM, Donoghue JP, Hochberg LR. 2008. Primary motor cortex tuning to intended movement kinematics in humans with tetraple-gia. *J Neurosci* 28:1163–1178.

Van Gompel JJ, Stead SM, Giannini C, Meyer FB, Marsh WR, et al. 2008. Phase I trial: safety and feasibility of intracranial electroencephalography using hybrid subdural electrodes containing macro- and microelectrode arrays. *Neurosurg Focus* 25:E23.

Vargas-Irwin CE, Shakhnarovich G, Yadollahpour P, Mislow JM, Black MJ, Donoghue JP. 2010. Decoding complete reach and grasp actions from local primary motor cortex populations. *J Neurosci* 30:9659–9669.

Velliste M, Perel S, Spalding MC, Whitford AS, Schwartz AB. 2008. Cortical control of a prosthetic arm for self-feeding. *Nature* 453:1098–1101.

Vetter RJ, Williams JC, Hetke JF, Nunamaker EA, Kipke DR. 2004. Chronic neural recording using silicon-substrate microelectrode arrays implanted in cerebral cortex. *IEEE Trans Biomed Eng* 51:896–904.

Waldert S, Pistohl T, Braun C, Ball T, Aertsen A, Mehring C. 2009. A review on directional information in neural signals for brain-machine interfaces. *J Physiol Paris* 103:244–254.

White JR, Levy T, Bishop W, Beaty JD. 2010. Real-time decision fusion for multimodal neural prosthetic devices. *PLoS One* 5:e9493.

Winslow BD, Tresco PA. 2010. Quantitative analysis of the tissue response to chronically implanted microwire electrodes in rat cortex. *Biomaterials* 31:1558–1567.

Wong CH, Birkett J, Byth K, Dexter M, Somerville E, et al. 2009. Risk factors for complications during intracranial electrode recording in presurgical evaluation of drug resistant partial epilepsy. *Acta Neurochir (Wien)* 151:37–50.

Wood F, Black MJ, Vargas-Irwin C, Fellows M, Donoghue JP. 2004. On the variability of manual spike sorting. *IEEE Trans Biomed Eng* 51:912–918.

Wu W, Black MJ, Mumford D, Gao Y, Bienenstock E, Donoghue JP. 2004. Modeling and decoding motor cortical activity using a switching Kalman filter. *IEEE Trans Biomed Eng* 51:933–942.

Wu W, Gao Y, Bienenstock E, Donoghue JP, Black MJ. 2006. Bayesian population decoding of motor cortical activity using a Kalman filter. *Neural Comput* 18:80–118.

Wu W, Hatsopoulos NG. 2008. Real-time decoding of nonstationary neural activity in motor cortex. *IEEE Trans Neural Syst Rehabil Eng* 16: 213–222.

Wu W, Kulkarni JE, Hatsopoulos NG, Paninski L. 2009. Neural decoding of hand motion using a linear state-space model with hidden states. *IEEE Trans Neural Syst Rehabil Eng* 17:370–378.

Yousry TA, Schmid UD, Alkadhi H, Schmidt D, Peraud A, et al. 1997. Localization of the motor hand area to a knob on the precentral gyrus. A new landmark. *Brain* 120 (Pt 1):141–157.

Zhuang J, Truccolo W, Vargas-Irwin C, Donoghue JP. 2010. Decoding 3-D reach and grasp kinematics from high-frequency local field potentials in primate primary motor cortex. *IEEE Trans Biomed Eng* 57:1774–1784.

17 | BCIs THAT USE SIGNALS RECORDED IN PARIETAL OR PREMOTOR CORTEX

HANSJÖRG SCHERBERGER

Chapter 16 focused on the primary motor cortex as a source of neuronal activity for BCIs. Two additional cortical areas are of particular interest for BCIs that use neuronal activity and have been fruitfully studied: the *parietal cortex* and the *premotor cortex*. Both of these regions contain specific areas that are involved in planning motor behaviors. These areas receive input containing sensory and volitional information, and they produce output that goes to the primary motor cortex, which in turn sends motor commands down the spinal cord for execution. Although the exact role of these parietal and premotor areas is not yet completely understood, it is clear that several distinct subregions in these areas are specialized for particular motor functions and are strongly involved in the transformation of sensory information into motor actions. As we know from many psychophysical and lesion experiments (Clower et al., 1996; Wise et al., 1998; Kurata and Hoshi, 1999), this mapping from sensory to motor coordinates is constantly updated. Whereas neural plasticity could improve the decoding performance of BCIs in general, it might be particularly effective in the parietal and premotor cortices because of the natural role of these areas in sensorimotor transformations. Thus, their use in BCIs is an attractive possibility. This chapter reviews the roles of the parietal and premotor cortices in motor planning and discusses BCI studies that have focused on these brain areas.

BCIs based on recordings from both parietal cortex and premotor cortex have the potential to benefit people with paralysis by providing high-level, goal-related information to drive movement of a computer cursor, a robotic arm, or a prosthesis (Andersen et al., 2010; Vansteensel et al., 2010; Green and Kalaska, 2011). Since we have a reasonable understanding of the principles of how movement intentions are represented in the premotor and parietal planning areas (see chapter 2 in this volume), it should be possible to decode them by recording simultaneously and in real time from a large number of neurons.

ANATOMY

Figure 17.1 shows the locations of *parietal* and *premotor cortices* and identifies several subregions of particular relevance to BCI development. The *parietal cortex* is located posterior to the primary somatosensory cortex, anterior to the visual

cortex, and medial to the auditory cortex (which is in the temporal lobe) (see chapter 2). It integrates sensory information from primary sensory areas and generates a representation of the outside world, particularly of objects and space. This information is further processed for the generation of specific actions. For example, neurons in the lateral intraparietal (LIP) area encode saccadic eye movements (rapid eye movements to a particular location). In contrast, neurons in the parietal reach region (PRR), located more medially and posteriorly in the intraparietal sulcus, encode the position, and to some extent the trajectories, of upcoming arm-reaching movements (Andersen et al., 1997; Andersen and Buneo, 2002; Scherberger and Andersen, 2003), whereas neurons in the anterior intraparietal (AIP) area are specifically active during the planning and execution of hand-grasping movements (Sakata et al., 1995; Baumann et al., 2009).

Similarly, the *premotor cortex*, located posterior to the prefrontal cortex and anterior to the primary sensorimotor cortex, integrates higher-order sensory and volitional information and generates specific movement intentions. Like parietal cortex, premotor cortex contains specialized subareas for eye-, arm-, and hand-movements (Rizzolatti et al., 1997; Rizzolatti and Luppino, 2001; Fluet et al., 2010). The frontal eye field (FEF) contains neurons that represent saccadic eye movements. More medially, the dorsal premotor area (PMd) encodes reach movements; and more laterally a rostral portion of the ventral premotor cortex (called area F5) is specifically active in hand-grasping movements. Given the typically close coordination of eye-, arm-, and hand-movements in everyday life, it is not surprising that these premotor areas are anatomically intimately interconnected. They also receive strong projections from the frontal cortex, which conveys volitional and motivational signals. Furthermore, these premotor areas are directly and reciprocally connected to their corresponding eye-, arm-, and hand areas in the parietal cortex: PMd with PRR, FEF with LIP, and F5 with AIP (see arrows in fig. 17.1). These connections thereby represent an action-specific network for sensorimotor transformation that spans the relevant brain areas and that is, as a result, able to combine volitional information from the frontal cortex with perceptional signals from the parietal cortex for the generation of high-level action plans. But how do the neurons in these areas actually represent movement intentions?

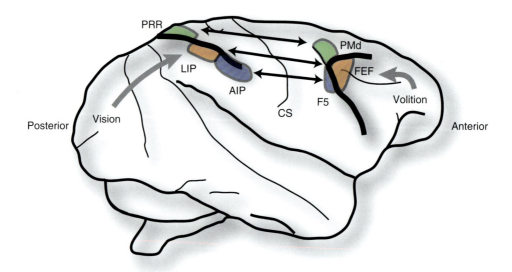

Figure 17.1 *Parietal and premotor brain areas related to action planning in the monkey brain. Parietal and premotor cortices are subdivided into specific areas with different functions. Parietal cortex areas: PRR, parietal reach region (green) (arm reaching); LIP, lateral intraparietal area (orange) (eye movements); AIP, anterior intraparietal area (purple) (hand grasping). Premotor cortex areas: PMd, dorsal premotor cortex (also green) (arm reaching); FEF, frontal eye field (also orange) (eye movements); F5, premotor area F5 (also purple) (hand grasping). Functionally related areas are connected with direct and reciprocal anatomical projections (bidirectional arrows, with like colors indicating related areas). Parietal areas receive strong sensory, in particular visual, input. Premotor areas receive volitional input. CS: central sulcus. Anterior: anterior pole of the brain. Posterior: posterior pole of the brain.*

ACTION PLANNING

EYE MOVEMENTS AND REACHING

Much of what is known about the representation of movements in the primate brain has been obtained by single-neuron recording in awake, behaving monkeys. In such studies, animals are first trained to perform a specific behavioral paradigm, and then microelectrodes are slowly lowered into the brain to record the neural activity of individual neurons while the animal performs the behavior. For example, the animal might be trained in a center-out movement task to look at, or reach toward, visually presented targets.

In figure 17.2A, the movement paradigm is a *delayed-saccade task*. (A *saccade* is a rapid eye movement to a target.) A delayed-saccade task requires that the animal waits a specified amount of time before making the saccade. Specifically, in the delayed-saccade task illustrated in figure 17.2A, a monkey first looks at and touches a central fixation light (i.e., typically a light-emitting diode [LED]). Then, a red target-cue light flashes briefly (~300 msec) at one of eight possible locations on the periphery of the screen. The monkey must then wait about one second until the central fixation light goes out, at which time it can look at the target (by making a saccade), but it must still continue to touch the central fixation light. Thus, during the waiting time between the brief flash of the red target light and the extinguishing of the central-fixation light, the animal must remember the location of the target and can plan the saccade, but it must withhold its execution. If the monkey is successful in the trial (i.e., if it waits the required time and then looks at the target while still touching the central-fixation light), it receives a reward consisting of a small amount of juice; no reward is given when the trial is not completed successfully.

In either case the animal can initiate the next trial by looking again at the central fixation light when it reappears after some delay (~1 sec).

A *delayed-reach task* can be constructed in an analogous fashion. In this case, the sequence of events is the same, except that the animal plans and executes a reach to the target while continuing to look at the center-fixation light. The monkey is informed of the type of task (i.e., delayed-saccade vs. delayed-reach) for any given trial by the use of two different target colors as cues (red for saccade, green for reach), such that delayed-saccade and delayed-reach trials can be randomly interleaved.

After the animal has learned these tasks, neural activity can be recorded from the brain with implanted microelectrodes while the monkey performs delayed-saccade and delayed-reach trials. The methodology for recording cortical neuronal activity in awake behaving monkeys has been well established for nearly 50 years (Cordeau et al., 1960; Evarts, 1965; Mountcastle et al., 1975). Figure 17.2B shows the activity of sample neurons in the parietal areas LIP (top row) and PRR (bottom row) during the two tasks (Snyder et al., 1997). In the saccade task the LIP neuron shows elevated activity during the target-cue itself, during the delay period, and during execution of the saccade; in the reach task the same neuron shows elevated activity only during the cue. In contrast, the PRR neuron shows the opposite effect: it is only transiently active during the saccade task and is strongly active during the cue, delay, and execution epochs of the reach task. From these representative examples, one can conclude that neurons in LIP and PRR are specifically active for saccades and arm movements, respectively (Snyder et al., 1997). The activity of these neurons during the intervening delay epoch suggests that

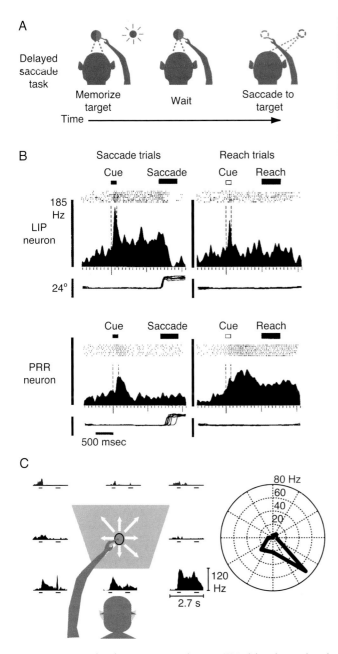

Figure 17.2 Action-related activity in parietal cortex. (A) A delayed-saccade task separates sensory from motor components of behavior. Animals memorized the location of a briefly flashed visual target, waited in complete darkness for a go signal, and then made an action (here a saccade) to the remembered target location. (B) Intention-specific neural activity in LIP and PRR during a delayed-saccade task and a delayed-reach task. An LIP neuron (top row, left) showed elevated activity during the delay period (150–600 msec after the cue) before a saccade but not before a reach movement (top row, right). In contrast, a PRR neuron (bottom row, left) showed no saccade-related activity but did show reach activity (bottom row, right). Each panel shows a spike raster (eight trials aligned on cue presentation, every third action potential shown) and the corresponding spike density histogram. The short horizontal bars indicate the timing of target flash (filled bar: saccade cue; open bar: reach cue); the long horizontal bars indicate the approximate time of motor response (saccade or reach). The thin horizontal plot (bottom of each panel) shows vertical eye position. Vertical scale bars: neuronal firing rate (Hz) and vertical eye position (degrees). (C) Directional tuning of a PPR cell with a right/down preferred direction. Left and center: Spike density histograms (as in B) for all reach directions (white arrows). Right: spatial tuning of the average firing rate during the delay period. For this neuron, reach activity was maximal in the right/down direction. (Modified from Snyder et al., 1997; Scherberger and Andersen, 2003.)

they play a role in remembering the target location and/or planning the movement. Presumably, they are involved in the sensorimotor transformation of behaviorally relevant sensory stimuli into a representation that encodes a specific motor action.

As the example in figure 17.2B illustrates, specific areas in parietal and premotor cortices are selectively active for particular types of actions (Rizzolatti and Luppino, 2001; Andersen and Buneo, 2002). But how are these actions represented in neuronal activity? Figure 17.2C shows the activity of a PRR neuron during the delayed-reach task for movements from the central fixation point to eight different peripheral targets. The neuron is strongly active in the cue, delay, and movement epochs when the animal reaches to the right-down target, is essentially silent when it moves to the opposite (left-up) target, and is somewhat active when it moves to targets between these two extremes. Such a movement preference is typical for parietal and premotor neurons, with many neurons having an individual preference (Mountcastle et al., 1975; Weinrich et al., 1984) and with all movement directions being represented in the overall neuronal population. Thus, each individual neuron in the population is essentially voting for (*tuned to*) a particular movement direction, and the overall movement appears to be determined by the combined activity of a large number of neurons.

As we know from our own everyday behavior, movements are not slavishly driven by external stimuli. We often select an action from a multitude of possible options, and we can act even in the absence of external stimuli. For such natural circumstances, one could ask whether parietal and premotor activity represents aspects of the sensory stimuli or the motor plan. Figure 17.3B shows the activity of a sample PRR neuron during a free-choice task, in which the monkey could freely select one of two stimuli as a reach target. This experiment also included control trials in which only a single target was offered (fig. 17.3A). In the control trials (fig. 17.3A), the PRR neuron was strongly active for a reach movement to the right and was inhibited for a movement to the left, indicating a preferred direction to the right. However, when both targets were presented and the animal was free to choose (fig. 17.3B), the neuron was active to some degree with both choices but was much more active when the choice was in its preferred direction (i.e., to the right). When the animal chose the right target, the neuron was active throughout the movement. In contrast, when the animal chose the left (nonpreferred) target, the neuron was active only briefly after target presentation and then quickly fell to an activity level below its pretarget baseline. Results of this kind indicate that neurons in parietal and premotor cortices are initially activated by sensory stimuli that represent potential movement targets but are then strongly modulated by the animal's choice and, eventually, reflect only the intended movement (Platt and Glimcher, 1999; Schall and Thompson, 1999; Scherberger and Andersen, 2007). Furthermore, as we will see (fig. 17.5B), activity can be modulated by the expected utility of, or reward for, the intended action. Thus, the parietal cortex and premotor cortex can be regarded as a network that integrates sensory and cognitive (e.g., intention-related) signals to generate motor actions.

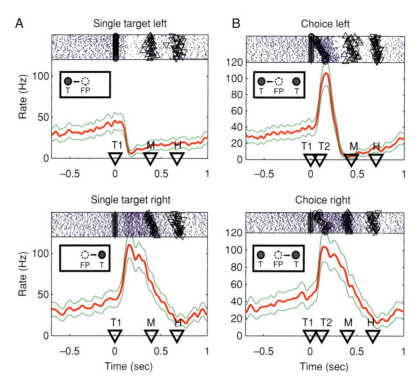

Figure 17.3 *Example of a neuron's activity during target selection for arm reaching. (A) Activity for single-target trials to the left or right (see insets). (B) Activity during choice trials, in which the animal selected either the left or right target (see insets). At the top of each panel is a spike raster with rows of dots indicating action potentials in single trials; and at the bottom is a peristimulus time histogram indicating the mean spike rate (red) and 95% confidence area (green). Time markers on the abscissa indicate the mean times of appearance of the first (T1) and second target (T2) and the mean times of the beginning (M) and end (H) of the movement. T2 appears with some delay to T1 to compensate for the animal's selection bias. Trials are aligned on the appearance of the first target (T1). (Modified from Scherberger and Andersen, 2007.)*

GRASPING

Primate hands are quite dexterous, and their movements are complex. One might therefore posit that more cognition is involved in these movements than in simpler reaching movements. Nevertheless, the neural mechanisms for the planning of hand movements seem to be organized in a fashion very similar to that for eye and arm movements (Baumann et al., 2009). Figure 17.4A shows the activity of a sample neuron in parietal area AIP during a *delayed-grasping task*, in which the animal grasped a handle using either a *precision grip* or a *power grip*. Typically, the monkey would use a power grip to hold a branch on a tree and a precision grip to pick up a raisin from the ground. In the experiment providing the data of figure 17.4 (modified from Baumann et al., 2009), the handle was positioned in various orientations (see rotatable handle positions at right in figure). During the cue epoch, a spotlight illuminating the handle revealed its orientation, while the color of an LED told the animal which grip to use (precision or power). In the subsequent delay epoch, the animal could prepare the grasping movement but had to wait until the dimming of the central fixation light to actually perform the grasp. Thus, this is a *delayed-grasping* task.

Figure 17.4A shows that after the start of the cue epoch, the firing rate of this neuron increased sharply and most strongly for power grips with handle orientation of +50°. Thus, this neuron was sensitive to the handle orientation as well as the grip type. In the overall population of the AIP neurons (fig. 17.4B),

many neurons were sensitive to other handle orientations and/ or grip types (Baumann et al., 2009). Many neurons represented the handle orientation from the cue epoch onward. In contrast, the number of neurons representing grip type increased during the task and peaked during movement execution. Similar grasp-related activity was also observed in premotor cortical area F5 which is closely related both anatomically and functionally to parietal area AIP (see fig. 17.1) (Fluet et al., 2010). In addition, other experiments have shown that AIP and F5 are sensitive to the visual presentation of objects even when no grasping actions are prepared (Murata et al., 2000; Raos et al., 2006).

These examples illustrate that the parietal and premotor cortices can be regarded as a network that integrates sensory and cognitive signals for the generation of actions. Whereas specific areas represent specific types of actions, individual neurons in these areas represent sensory stimuli as well as signals for planning and executing particular movements. Based on these findings, it is natural to ask whether such neuronal signals could be used for the decoding of specific intended actions for BCIs and what such BCIs might look like.

ACTION DECODING

REACH DECODING

Several research groups are currently developing BCIs for reaching that are based on signals from the parietal cortex or

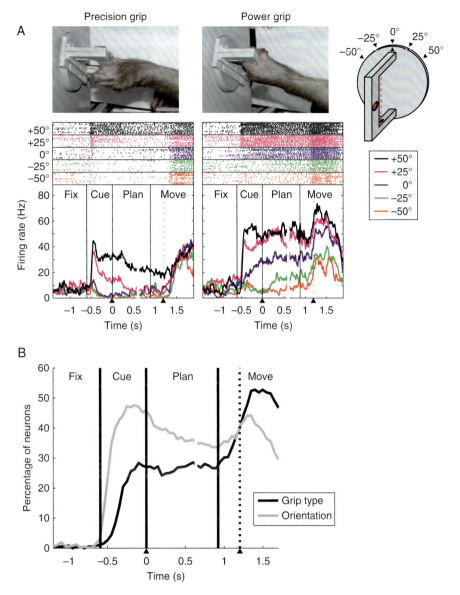

Figure 17.4 *Grasp-related activity in parietal cortex. (A) Activity of a single AIP neuron during a delayed-grasping task, in which a monkey grasps a rotatable handle (drawn at far right) either with a precision grip (left) or a power grip (right). Precision-grip trials are shown in the left column, and power-grip trials in the right column. Spike rasters and average firing rates are presented in different colors for each of the five handle orientations (key at far right). The neuron shown is tuned to (i.e., fires more with) the rightmost handle orientation (+50°) (black line in plot) and the power grip. (B) Orientation and grip-type tuning in the AIP neuronal population (571 single neurons). Curves show the percentages of neurons tuned to (i.e., the percentages for which firing rate is affected by) orientation (gray) or grip type (black) over the course of the trial (sliding window, 200-msec width, centered on each data point). Prior to 0.6 sec, the data curves are aligned to the end of the cue (t = 0 with arrowhead marker); after 0.6 sec, they are aligned to the start of movement (dotted line with arrowhead marker). This change in alignment is indicated by the break in the curves at 0.6 sec. (Modified from Baumann et al., 2009.)*

the premotor cortex (Musallam et al., 2004; Santhanam et al., 2006). Musallam and colleagues trained macaque monkeys first in a delayed-reach task and then in a brain-control task after they permanently implanted microelectrode arrays in parietal area PRR and premotor area PMd. Figure 17.5A shows the two tasks. In the reach task the animal first touched and looked at a central fixation spot on a touch-sensitive screen; then a visual cue was presented for several hundred milliseconds in one of up to eight possible locations in the periphery of the screen. Single- and multineuron activity was recorded simultaneously from many electrodes during the next period (called the *memory period*), and this activity was

then used to decode the intended reach location. The animal could plan the upcoming reach movement during the memory period but had to withhold execution until a signal was given that instructed the animal to reach to the target. Importantly, in the brain-control version of the paradigm, the animal was immediately rewarded if the neuronal activity during the memory period was correctly decoded (i.e., if it indicated the instructed reach direction correctly); but the animal did not actually have to reach to the target. Animals quickly adopted a strategy in which they planned, but did not execute, the intended reach movement. To provide additional feedback to the animal during these trials, a visual target

A

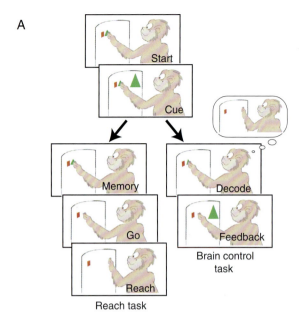

Reach task

Brain control task

B

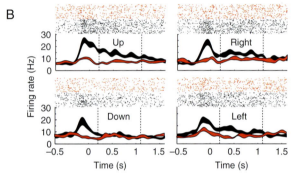

C

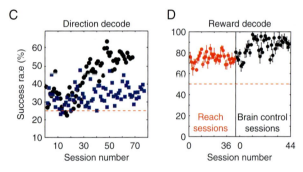

Figure 17.5 Cognitive control signals for neural prosthetics. (A) Delayed-reach task and brain-control task, as described in text. (B) Example of a neuron's activity during the brain-control task with instructions to the up, right, left, and down directions that were rewarded with either orange juice (black) or water (red). This neuron was more active for trials when the preferred reward (orange juice, black) was expected. (C) Overall success rate for decoding the intended movement from four possible targets in subsequent recording sessions of two animals (black and blue dots). Dotted line: chance level (25%). Both animals improve their performance with experience. (D) Success rate in the offline decoding of the reward expected (i.e., juice or water) in 36 reach (red) and 44 brain-control (black) sessions across three animals. Error bars indicate standard deviation obtained by cross-validation. Dotted line: chance level (50%). (Adapted from Musallam et al., 2004; with permission from AAAS.)

was placed on the screen to indicate the decoded target location.

Figure 17.5B shows data during the brain-control task from a sample neuron with a preferred reach direction up and to the right. Activity increased from baseline after cue onset and stayed elevated throughout the memory period (delineated by vertical dotted lines). However, the neural response was strongly modulated when different target-cue sizes were used to signal the type of reward (orange juice vs. water) to be expected for successful trial completion. Trials in which the animal knew in advance that it would receive a preferred reward (orange juice) produced a significantly stronger response (black curves and tick marks) than trials in which the animal received a less-preferred reward (water; red curves and tick marks). Notably, this was true independent of whether the preferred reward was indicated with the smaller or larger cue size. Similarly, activity was also stronger when the expected amount of reward (volume) was greater or when the reward probability was higher. This suggests that parietal and premotor neurons can reflect not only the intended target location but also the expected value of the intended action.

The decoding performance in the brain-control task gradually improved over the weeks and months of the ongoing experiment. Figure 17.5C shows the overall success rate for predicting the correct target position (one out of four possible positions) from 10–30 recording channels (single neurons and multiunits) in about 70 daily sessions of two animals (different colors). Whereas performance in the beginning was only slightly above chance (25%, dashed line), it gradually increased to about 55% in the first and 35% in the second animal. Similarly, figure 17.5D depicts the success rate for the offline decoding of the expected reward value (high or low) in a population of three animals (dashed line: chance level 50%). Interestingly, the mean decoding performance was significantly larger when the animals performed the brain-controlled task (85%) as compared to the reach task (75%).

These results indicate that the intended movement as well as the expected reward can be decoded simultaneously from neurons in PRR and PMd. Thus, signals from these areas might be useful for controlling movement of a cursor or a motor prosthesis. Certainly, as with signals from other brain areas, it will be important to identify those areas most suitable for decoding a specific motor function (e.g., hand grasp), particularly if the goal is to restore that function without interfering with other, still intact motor functions.

GRASP DECODING

Figure 17.6A shows the design of an experimental BCI for performing a hand-grasping task. This BCI is designed to decode intended hand movements from neuronal activity in parietal area AIP and premotor area F5. These areas receive sensory (particularly visual) information, and their neuronal activity is thought to represent intended hand movement. To test the hypothesis that signals from these areas can be used for decoding, 80 or 128 microelectrodes were implanted in AIP and F5 in two monkeys (Townsend et al., 2008 & 2011). Neuronal activity was recorded and sorted (to distinguish

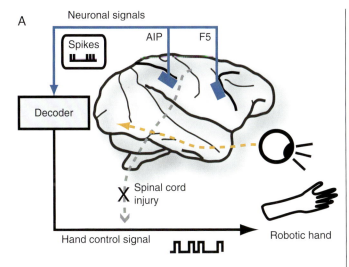

A

Neuronal signals

Spikes

AIP   F5

Decoder

Spinal cord
X injury

Hand control signal

Robotic hand

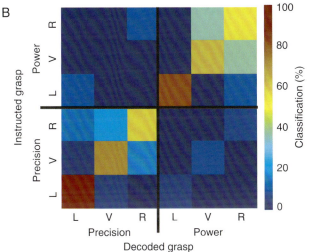

B

Instructed grasp — Power — R, V, L — Precision — R, V, L

Classification (%) — 100, 80, 60, 40, 20, 0

Decoded grasp — Precision (L, V, R) — Power (L, V, R)

Figure 17.6 Decoding of hand-grasping signals from neurons in AIP and F5 in a macaque monkey. (A) Decoding schematic. In paralyzed patients, motor commands can no longer pass from the brain to the motor effectors (dashed gray line). This deficit can be bypassed with neural recordings that are made directly in the brain (blue pads) and processed externally. (B) Confusion matrix (see text) indicating the performance in decoding the grip type (power vs. precision) and the grip orientation (leftward tilt [L], vertical [V], or rightward tilt [R]) from 80 permanently implanted electrodes in AIP and F5. Data show the results of one online decoding session with about 180 decoding trials. If decoding performance were perfect, 100% of the trials would align on the diagonal from the lower left to the upper right corner. Here, the diagonal shows an average performance of 72% across all six conditions. (Modified from Townsend et al., 2008 & 2011.)

among different neurons, see chapters 7 and 16 in this volume) in real time and subjected to a maximum-likelihood decoding analysis method (see e.g., Shenoy et al., 2003) that predicted the grip type (power vs. precision) and the hand orientation (left tilt, vertical, right tilt) from the activity during the delay epoch of the delayed-grasping task. The decoded grasp was then presented to the animal as a picture of a hand grasping an object. Importantly, for each correctly decoded grasp, the animal received a reward immediately without having to execute the movement. However, if the trial was not correctly decoded, the animal was not rewarded but instead had to execute the correct grasp movement in order to receive a reward.

Figure 17.6B shows the decoding results for a sample session. The overall correct decoding performance was about 50% (vs. 16.6% chance level). The matrix illustrated is a *confusion matrix* (i.e., a matrix of the six possible grasp instructions vs. the grasp-decoding results for each instruction). The matrix summarizes how each of the six possible grasp instructions was decoded. Most trials fell on the diagonal, indicating correct predictions (e.g., the precision grip with rightward orientation instruction was correctly decoded 59% of the time). Decoding errors occurred mainly for closely related grip orientations, while the grip type was almost never confused. These results provide proof of concept that grasp intentions can be decoded from these higher-order cortical areas, and they thus suggest that signals from these areas might be used to control a BCI.

FAST DECODING

As described throughout this book, both noninvasive and invasive recording methods are being applied in BCI research and development. It is often assumed, however, that the highest information transfer rates can be obtained with invasive methods, particularly those that record single-neuron (i.e., spike) activity. In a recent study Santhanam et al. (2006) used a 96-channel silicon electrode array implanted in PMd to explore particularly fast decoding strategies.

First, monkeys were trained in a delayed-reach movement task, from which a statistical description of the tuning properties of the recorded neurons (i.e., their correlations with reach direction) was obtained. Then, the paradigm was changed so that most of the trials were *prosthetic-cursor* trials, in which neuronal activity during the delay period was used to move the cursor to the target, so that no actual limb movement occurred. Figure 17.7A illustrates the prosthetic-cursor trials. Throughout the prosthetic-cursor trials, the animal continuously touched and looked at the central fixation spot (see fig. 17.7A, all boxes), while a visual cue (a yellow dot) appeared in the periphery of the screen to indicate the target (e.g., see fig. 17.7A, Trial 1). Data from the first 150-msec epoch following the cue presentation were ignored to avoid potential confounds related to the appearance of the visual stimulus. This first (cue) epoch was followed by a decoding epoch. After the decoding epoch, the target cue (the yellow dot of fig. 17.7A, Trial 1) disappeared, and the target location that was *decoded* was presented on the screen (dashed circle in fig. 17.7A, Trial 2); if the predicted location was correct (as it is in the figure), a new target location (yellow dot in fig. 17.7A, Trial 2) was then presented. Several such prosthetic trials (e.g., fig. 17.7A, Trial 1–3), each consisting of only these two epochs (cue plus decoding, totaling about 200–450 msec), were run in fast succession without rewarding the animal. Then a full delayed-reach task allowed the animal to reach toward the target and to receive a liquid reward if this reach trial and the preceding sequence of prosthetic trials were all successful.

Selection of the length of the decoding epoch clearly affected performance. Decoding from longer segments gave more accurate decoding because of reduced noise in the integrated signal. However, longer segments increased trial

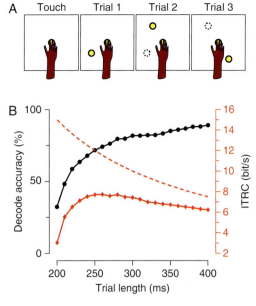

Figure 17.7 *Information-transfer rate capacity during fast prosthetic-cursor trials. (A) Sequence of three prosthetic-cursor trials. After the animal has placed its hand on the board (Touch), a target (solid circle) appears (Trial 1), the intended reach movement is decoded, and a cursor (Trial 2, dashed circle) is placed on the screen at the predicted location. If the predicted location is correct, the next cursor trial starts immediately, with a new target appearing at a new location (Trial 2, yellow dot). This process is repeated (e.g., Trial 3) for a total of three or more prosthetic-cursor trials, followed by a standard delayed-reach trial that allowed the animal to reach toward the target. The animal receives a liquid reward if this reach trial and the preceding sequence of prosthetic trials are all successful. In case of error, the trial sequence is aborted, and no reward is provided. (B) Decode accuracy (black curve) and information-transfer rate capacity (ITRC) (red solid curve) for different trial lengths, as assessed from an eight-target control experiment. Decoding accuracy increased with trial length (and begins to saturate at around 250 msec). ITRC was maximal for a trial length of about 260 msec and then declined. Theoretical ITRC (red dotted line) assumes 100% accuracy at all trial lengths. (Adapted from Santhanam et al., 2006.)*

duration and thereby decreased the number of trials per second and the maximum possible information-transfer rate. Thus, there was a fundamental speed–accuracy trade-off. Several different measures can be used to assess performance (fig. 17.7B). If performance was measured as the percentage of correctly decoded trials, it improved with increased trial duration but saturated for trials longer than 250 msec (black curve). A different measure of performance, the information transfer-rate capacity (ITRC) (solid red curve), reveals the rate at which information is transmitted: it is defined in bits/sec, and is a function of the decoding accuracy and the number of possible targets, divided by the trial duration (see chapter 8). The ITRC did not simply increase monotonically with trial duration but, rather, reached a peak of 7.7 bit/sec at a trial duration of 260 msec in an offline test dataset (red solid curve). As expected, this was lower than the theoretical maximal ITRC (red dotted curve), which assumes perfect decoding accuracy (100% correct) for all trial durations.

Using online sequences of prosthetic-cursor trials with a variety of possible numbers of targets (2, 4, 8, or 16), Santhanam et al. (2006) found maximal ITRCs in two animals of 6.5 bit/sec and 5.3 bit/sec, respectively, for the 8-target task. These rates

exceed those achieved to date by other, noninvasive and invasive, BCI studies. Thus, this new paradigm might enable high information transfer rates and support improved performance very useful for people who are paralyzed.

DECODING FROM LOCAL FIELD POTENTIALS

While spiking activity originates from a single neuron located close to the electrode tip, the *local field potential* (LFP) is the summation of excitatory and inhibitory dendritic potentials from a large number of neurons in the neighborhood of the recording site (see chapters 3 and 16 in this volume). Because of the larger volume from which it gathers electrical information, LFP activity is likely to be less affected by tissue reactions (see chapter 5) following electrode implantation. It is therefore logical to ask whether LFPs could be used to control a neural prosthetic device, and what kind of information might be carried by such signals. By similar reasoning, signals recorded from the cortical surface (i.e., electrocorticographic [ECoG] activity [Chapter 15]) might also be used to decode movement intentions.

LFP activity has been investigated in cortical and subcortical areas (Eckhorn et al., 1988; Gray et al., 1989; Buzsaki and Draguhn, 2004). Several studies that relate motor, parietal, and premotor cortex LFP activity to behavior in experimental animals show that LFP signals are modulated over the course of task performance as well as by different behavioral conditions (Murthy and Fetz, 1996; Donoghue et al., 1998; Baker et al., 1999; Pesaran et al., 2002). For example, in the parietal reach region (PRR), the power (i.e., amplitude squared) in specific LFP spectral bands is modulated during the planning and execution of a center-out reach or saccade task (Scherberger et al., 2005). Individual panels in figure 17.8A show the average LFP power spectrogram across 10–20 trial repetitions from a set of recording sites in PRR for reaches (left column) and saccades (right columns), and for movements in the preferred (top row) and nonpreferred (bottom rows) direction. (Preferred directions were determined for each recording site by the modulation in the 25–35 Hz frequency band.) The data shown in the figure indicate that low-frequency components (0–15 Hz) encoded the movement type (reach vs. saccade) during planning and execution independently from the movement direction (i.e., note the similarity at low frequencies between the spectrograms for preferred and nonpreferred directions). At higher frequencies (15–50 Hz), however, the LFP also reflected the movement direction (i.e., note the difference at high frequencies between the spectrograms for preferred and nonpreferred directions).

Simulations of decoding based on these sequentially recorded data showed that LFP activity from parietal area PRR could decode the movement direction as well as the animal's concurrent behavioral state (i.e., baseline fixation, reach planning, reach execution, saccade planning, saccade execution). To produce a simulation of this type, the data from subsequently acquired recording sites were treated as if they had been recorded simultaneously and subjected to a Bayesian

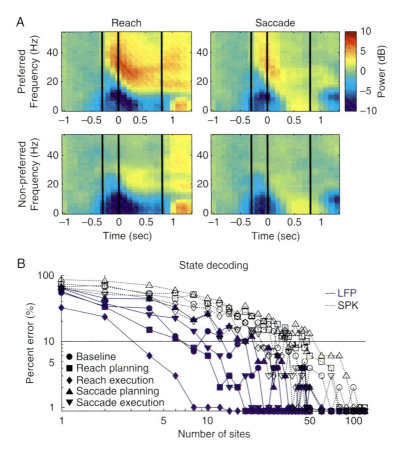

Figure 17.8 Reach-movement decoding from LFP activity in PRR. (A) Population spectrogram of LFP activity (10–20 trial repetitions from a set of recording sites in PRR) during delayed-reach (left column) and delayed-saccade (right column) movements in the preferred (upper row) and nonpreferred (lower row) directions. Color code indicates LFP power relative to baseline activity (in decibels). Vertical lines mark the starts of the cue, planning, and movement periods. (The preferred directions were determined for each recording site by the modulation in the 25- to 35-Hz frequency band.) The data shown in the figure indicate that low-frequency components (0–15 Hz) encoded the movement type (reach vs. saccade) during planning and execution independently from the movement direction (i.e., note the similarity at low frequencies between the spectrograms for preferred and nonpreferred directions). At higher frequencies (15–50 Hz), the LFP also reflected the movement direction (i.e., note the difference at high frequencies between the spectrograms for preferred and nonpreferred directions). (B) Decoding of five behavioral states using LFP (blue) or spiking activity (black). Behavioral states were baseline (circles), reach planning (squares), reach execution (diamonds), saccade planning (upward-pointing triangles) and execution (downward-pointing triangles). Decoding performance of behavioral states was consistently better (i.e., smaller percentage error) with LFP (blue) than with spiking activity (black). (Modified from Scherberger et al., 2005.)

decoder with cross-validation. Figure 17.8B illustrates the error rates for decoding these five behavioral states with a Bayesian classifier (see chapter 8) using various numbers of randomly selected recording sites. For LFP activity (blue), prediction errors were below 10% when 20 or more sites were used for decoding. In contrast, errors were much larger when the neuronal spiking activity recorded at the same sites was used for decoding (black).

LFPs from PRR also appear to be capable of predicting the movement direction with impressive accuracy: the overall decoding accuracy was 81% for reach direction and 40% for saccade direction (chance: 6.25%). Arm and eye movements were never confused. However, the accuracy of this decoding of direction with LFPs was lower than when neuronal spiking activity was used for decoding (97% for reach and 72% for saccade direction).

Taken together, these studies indicate that LFP activity in PRR can predict both behavioral state and planned reach direction. The lesser decoding accuracy of LFPs compared to spiking activity for the reach direction might be compensated for by employing a greater number of LFP recording sites (which is relatively easy to achieve). Results similar to these have also been obtained in other studies using LFP activity from primary motor cortex to predict reach movements and from the lateral intraparietal area (LIP) to predict saccades (Pesaran et al., 2002; Mehring et al., 2003). It therefore appears that the LFP is a suitable signal for decoding movement intentions and might be even better suited than spiking activity for some types of information, such as behavioral states. Moreover, LFP signals are relatively simple to record and potentially more robust than spiking activity during chronic recordings.

Other brain signals (e.g., ECoG [chapter 15]), might also play an important role in future BCI-controlled devices. ECoG is a cortical summation signal that is less localized than individual LFPs, but still has much greater topographical resolution, wider frequency range, and higher amplitude than scalp-recorded EEG (Slutzky et al., 2010). Since ECoG electrodes do not penetrate the brain (and may even be extradural), they are considered to be less invasive than intracortical electrode arrays. Because the performance of their electrodes does not depend on maintaining close proximity to individual cortical neurons, both ECoG and LFP signals might prove to be more robust and reliable for long-term use in BCI applications than neuronal-spiking activity. At the same time, the tuning properties of LFPs and ECoG (i.e., their correlations with movement intention) are just beginning to be explored and require substantial further investigation.

PERSPECTIVES

The *parietal cortex* and the *premotor cortex* play important roles in the generation of intentional movements. Both areas are intimately connected to the sensory system as well as to areas related to volition, motivation, and reward. This places the parietal and the premotor cortices at the center of sensorimotor transformation and decision-making related to planning and execution of actions. Brain-computer interfaces (BCIs) can take advantage of the activity in these areas by recording these signals and using them for device control.

In this chapter, we have reviewed the evidence that these two areas, the parietal cortex and the premotor cortex, contain information about the goal and the timing of intended actions. This evidence indicates that the physiological role of these areas is to prepare and plan intended actions on the basis of sensory and volitional information. In these roles the parietal and premotor cortices comprise distinctive subregions that are specialized for specific movement types. Thus, as with other cortical areas (primary motor cortex and subcortical areas) (see chapter 2), the parietal and premotor cortices also convey important timing information that may be useful for BCI methodology. These properties could make them attractive for chronic implantation of electrodes, in particular for decoding movement goals and movement timings. Since the coding schemes in these areas are reasonably well understood, it should be possible to develop decoding algorithms that are optimized for BCI use. It is likely that future BCI applications will combine information from several brain areas for the control of specific actions.

Current invasive BCI approaches, like the ones discussed in this chapter, still suffer from technical problems that need to be ameliorated in order to make today's BCI technology useful for tomorrow's users. One of the most pressing problems is the long-term stability of the signals derived from implanted electrodes. Typically, in the months and years after implantation, these electrodes gradually lose sensitivity to neuronal action potentials, presumably due to mechanical micromotion and foreign-body reactions that tend to encapsulate the electrodes (see chapters 5 and 16). The problem might be addressed with improvements in electrode technology and implantation technique and also by using alternative signals such as LFPs and ECoG, which are likely to be less affected by this encapsulation process. Further studies are needed to delineate and maximize the usefulness of spiking activity, LFPs, and ECoG for long-term BCI applications and to determine the circumstances in which these different signals might complement each other (and possibly noninvasive methods as well), so as to support long-term BCI performance of substantial value to people with severe disabilities.

What makes the parietal cortex and the premotor cortex interesting for BCI development is the fact that these areas are able to process action-related information in parallel to other actions. In everyday life, we are able to grasp a cup of coffee while reading the newspaper or while talking. The neural substrates for these capabilities are localized in the premotor and in particular the parietal cortices. Patients with lesions in parietal cortex quite often have deficits in performing such functions, either at all or without excessive cognitive effort (Perenin and Vighetto, 1988; Goodale and Milner, 1995). Such capabilities of these regions will also be important for tomorrow's BCI technology. An ideal BCI should operate effortlessly and should allow parallel activities such as listening and talking, attending to other objects, and even performing other movements simultaneously. The success of the future of a BCI will be measured not only by its capacity to perform the required movement, but also by its ability to do so without requiring excessive cognitive effort. Tapping into the networks dedicated to action-specific sensorimotor transformations in parietal and premotor cortices might therefore be particularly worthwhile.

REFERENCES

Andersen RA, Buneo CA (2002) Intentional maps in posterior parietal cortex. Annu Rev Neurosci 25:189–220.

Andersen RA, Hwang EJ, Mulliken GH (2010) Cognitive neural prosthetics. Annu Rev Psychol 61: 169–90, C1–3.

Andersen RA, Snyder LH, Bradley DC, Xing J (1997) Multimodal representation of space in the posterior parietal cortex and its use in planning movements. Annu Rev Neurosci 20:303–330.

Baker SN, Kilner JM, Pinches EM, Lemon RN (1999) The role of synchrony and oscillations in the motor output. Exp Brain Res 128:109–117.

Baumann MA, Fluet M-C, Scherberger H (2009) Context-specific grasp movement representation in the macaque anterior intraparietal area. J Neurosci 29:6436–6448.

Buzsaki G, Draguhn A (2004) Neuronal oscillations in cortical networks. Science 304:1926–1929.

Clower DM, Hoffman JM, Votaw JR, Faber TL, Woods RP, Alexander GE (1996) Role of posterior parietal cortex in the recalibration of visually guided reaching. Nature 383:618–621.

Cordeau JP, Gybels J, Jasper H, Poirier LJ (1960) Microelectrode studies of unit discharges in the sensorimotor cortex: investigations in monkeys with experimental tremor. Neurology 10:591–600.

Donoghue JP, Sanes JN, Hatsopoulos NG, Gaal G (1998) Neural discharge and local field potential oscillations in primate motor cortex during voluntary movements. J Neurophysiol 79:159–173.

Eckhorn R, Bauer R, Jordan W, Brosch M, Kruse W, Munk M, Reitboeck HJ (1988) Coherent oscillations: a mechanism of feature linking in the visual cortex? Multiple electrode and correlation analyses in the cat. Biol Cybern 60:121–130.

Evarts EV (1965) Relation of discharge frequency to conduction velocity in pyramidal tract neurons. J Neurophysiol 28:216–228.

Fluet MC, Baumann MA, Scherberger H (2010) Context-specific grasp movement representation in macaque ventral premotor cortex. J Neurosci 30:15175–15184.

Goodale MA, Milner AD (1995) The visual brain in action. New York: Oxford University Press.

Gray CM, Konig P, Engel AK, Singer W (1989) Oscillatory responses in cat visual cortex exhibit inter-columnar synchronization which reflects global stimulus properties. Nature 338:334–337.

Green AM, Kalaska JF (2011) Learning to move machines with the mind. Trends Neurosci 34: 61–75.

Kurata K, Hoshi E (1999) Reacquisition deficits in prism adaptation after muscimol microinjection into the ventral premotor cortex of monkeys. J Neurophysiol 81:1927–1938.

Mehring C, Rickert J, Vaadia E, Cardosa de Oliveira S, Aertsen A, Rotter S (2003) Inference of hand movements from local field potentials in monkey motor cortex. Nat Neurosci 6:1253–1254.

Mountcastle VB, Lynch JC, Georgopoulos A, Sakata H, Acuna C (1975) Posterior parietal association cortex of the monkey: command functions for operations within extrapersonal space. J Neurophysiol 38:871–908.

Murata A, Gallese V, Luppino G, Kaseda M, Sakata H (2000) Selectivity for the shape, size, and orientation of objects for grasping in neurons of monkey parietal area AIP. J Neurophysiol 83:2580–2601.

Murthy VN, Fetz EE (1996) Oscillatory activity in sensorimotor cortex of awake monkeys: synchronization of local field potentials and relation to behavior. J Neurophysiol 76:3949–3967.

Musallam S, Corneil BD, Greger B, Scherberger H, Andersen RA (2004) Cognitive control signals for neural prosthetics. Science 305:258–262.

Perenin MT, Vighetto A (1988) Optic ataxia: a specific disruption in visuomotor mechanisms. I. Different aspects of the deficit in reaching for objects. Brain 111:643–674.

Pesaran B, Pezaris JS, Sahani M, Mitra PP, Andersen RA (2002) Temporal structure in neuronal activity during working memory in macaque parietal cortex. Nat Neurosci 5:805–811.

Platt ML, Glimcher PW (1999) Neural correlates of decision variables in parietal cortex. Nature 400:233–238.

Raos V, Umilta MA, Murata A, Fogassi L, Gallese V (2006) Functional properties of grasping-related neurons in the ventral premotor area F5 of the macaque monkey. J Neurophysiol 95:709–729.

Rizzolatti G, Fogassi L, Gallese V (1997) Parietal cortex: from sight to action. Curr Opin Neurobiol 7:562–567.

Rizzolatti G, Luppino G (2001) The cortical motor system. Neuron 31: 889–901.

Sakata H, Taira M, Murata A, Mine S (1995) Neural mechanisms of visual guidance of hand action in the parietal cortex of the monkey. Cereb Cortex 5:429–438.

Santhanam G, Ryu SI, Yu BM, Afshar A, Shenoy KV (2006) A high-performance brain-computer interface. Nature 442:195–198.

Schall JD, Thompson KG (1999) Neural selection and control of visually guided eye movements. Annu Rev Neurosci 22:241–259.

Scherberger H, Andersen RA (2003) Sensorimotor transformations. In: The visual neurosciences (Chalupa LM, Werner JS, eds.), pp 1324–1336. Cambridge, MA: MIT Press.

Scherberger H, Andersen RA (2007) Target selection signals for arm reaching in the posterior parietal cortex. J Neurosci 27:2001–2012.

Scherberger H, Jarvis MR, Andersen RA (2005) Cortical local field potential encodes movement intentions in the posterior parietal cortex. Neuron 46:347–354.

Shenoy KV, Meeker D, Cao S, Kureshi SA, Pesaran B, Buneo CA, Batista AP, Mitra PP, Burdick JW, Andersen RA (2003) Neural prosthetic control signals from plan activity. Neuroreport 14:591–596.

Slutzky MW, Jordan LR, Krieg T, Chen M, Mogul DJ, Miller LE (2010) Optimal spacing of surface electrode arrays for brain-machine interface applications. J Neural Eng 7:26004.

Snyder LH, Batista AP, Andersen RA (1997) Coding of intention in the posterior parietal cortex. Nature 386:167–170.

Townsend B, Subasi E, Scherberger H (2008) Real time decoding of hand grasping signals from macaque premotor and parietal cortex. In: 13th Annual Conference of the International Functional Electrical Stimulation Society "From Movement to Mind" (Stieglitz T, Schuettler M, eds). Freiburg, Germany. Biomed Eng 53 supp. 1.

Townsend B, Subasi E, Scherberger H (2011) Grasp movement decoding from premotor and parietal cortex. J Neurosci, in press.

Vansteensel MJ, Hermes D, Aarnoutse EJ, Bleichner MG, Schalk G, van Rijen PC, Leijten FS, Ramsey NF (2010) Brain-computer interfacing based on cognitive control. Ann Neurol 67: 809–816.

Weinrich M, Wise SP, Mauritz KH (1984) A neurophysiological study of the premotor cortex in the rhesus monkey. Brain 107 (Pt 2): 385–414.

Wise SP, Moody SL, Blomstrom KJ, Mitz AR (1998) Changes in motor cortical activity during visuomotor adaptation. Exp Brain Res 121: 285–299.

18 | BCIs THAT USE BRAIN METABOLIC SIGNALS

RANGANATHA SITARAM, SANGKYUN LEE, AND NIELS BIRBAUMER

Most brain-computer interfaces (BCIs) currently under development use the brain's *electrical* signals. Nevertheless, nonelectrical *metabolic* signals also have potential for use in BCI development. Chapter 4 of this volume describes four methodologies currently available for measuring brain metabolic activity and focuses on the two of these methods that are of greatest immediate interest for BCI development: *functional near-infrared spectroscopy* (fNIRS) and *functional magnetic resonance imaging* (fMRI). fNIRS has the advantages of being noninvasive and inexpensive. fMRI has the advantages of being noninvasive and providing very high spatial resolution. However, as we will see in this chapter, both have the disadvantage of poor time resolution, which is a crucial element for real-time BCIs. Although BCIs based on these two methods are still in the earliest stages of development, significant recent advances have stimulated considerable attention to their potential value (Birbaumer, 2006; Birbaumer and Cohen, 2007; Sitaram et al., 2007; Sitaram et al., 2008; Sitaram et al., 2009; Weiskopf et al., 2007). In this chapter we focus on BCIs based on fNIRS and fMRI methods. We review the fundamental principles underlying their use, the factors important in their use for BCIs, the kinds of BCI applications that are most promising, and possible future directions and challenges.

Although both fNIRS and fMRI can in theory measure a wide variety of signals related to brain metabolism (see chapter 4 in this volume and Huettel, 2004), almost all current uses of these methods, including their BCI uses, are based on the measurement of task-induced blood oxygen level-dependent (BOLD) responses (Huppert et al., 2006; Ogawa et al., 1990; Villringer and Chance, 1997; Villringer and Obrig, 2002). The BOLD response reflects changes in blood flow and is an indirect measure of brain activity, but there is growing evidence that it is strongly correlated with the brain's electrical activity (Logothetis, 2007; Logothetis, 2008). Recent advances in fNIRS and fMRI technology have enabled real-time acquisition, decoding, and training of BOLD responses, leading to investigations of their behavioral correlates, and their application to restoring communication and control capacities to people with severe motor disabilities.

fNIRS-BASED BCIs

PRINCIPLES OF fNIRS METHODOLOGY

As discussed in chapter 4 of this volume, near-infrared spectroscopy is based on the Beer-Lambert Law which states that the attenuation or absorbance of light in a homogeneous medium, A, is proportional to the concentration of the absorbing molecule:

$$A = c \times \varepsilon \times l \tag{18.1}$$

where c is the concentration of the absorbing molecule, ε is a proportionality constant called absorptivity, and l is the optical path length. A change in the concentration of the absorbing molecule, Δc, will produce a proportional change in absorbance:

$$\Delta A = \Delta c \times \varepsilon \times l \tag{18.2}$$

This change can be detected by an fNIRS sensor. As described in chapter 4, fNIRS is based on the observations that near-infrared light (i.e., wavelengths of 700–1000 nm, the *near-infrared* [NIR] range of the electromagnetic spectrum) penetrates living tissue. This can be observed in everyday life when bright light is directed toward an open palm, and the light transmitted through the tissue causes a reddish glow on the back of the palm. The red color is due to the pigment hemoglobin in the blood. Since water molecules and hemoglobin absorb less NIR light than light of other wavelengths, NIR (red) light is transmitted through the tissue.

When placed on the scalp, pairs of optical sources and detectors can measure NIR transmission through layers of brain tissue. The light passing through the tissue is influenced by the functional state of the tissue. Brain activity is accompanied by changes in the components present in blood (e.g., changes in the concentrations of oxygenated and deoxygenated hemoglobin [Villringer and Obrig, 2002]). These changes can be detected as changes in the fNIR signal after transmission of near-infrared light through the brain tissue. Thus, fNIRS measurement allows for indirect detection and measurement of brain activation.

Although fNIRS spatial resolution (in the cm range) is lower than that of functional magnetic resonance imaging (fMRI) (in the mm range), fNIRS has significant advantages over other brain-imaging methods described in chapter 4. First, fNIRS is safe and it is noninvasive. It does not use potentially harmful radiation since it employs nonionizing near-infrared light. The intensity of light is maintained below safety limits to avoid thermal damage. fNIRS does not require the injection of contrast agents. With fNIRS, tissue function alone produces the signal that is imaged. fNIRS monitors changes in concentration of hemoglobin and changes in oxygen saturation of tissue and, from these measures, can calculate tissue perfusion and oxygen supply/demand. With recent advances in microelectronics, optical engineering, and computer technology, fNIRS systems can be relatively small and easily portable (especially in comparison to fMRI systems), and are much less expensive than other imaging modalities such as fMRI and positron emission tomography (PET).

In a typical fNIRS measurement of brain-tissue activity, an optical diode (called an *optode*) acts as a light source (or *emitter*). Light emitted by the optode passes through the intermediate layers of scalp and skull, enters cortical tissue, and then passes back out through the skull and scalp to one or more *detector(s)* located at fixed distance(s) from the source. The detector is typically a light-receiving optode connected to a photomultiplier or a charge-coupled device (CCD).

To explain how fNIRS detects changes in brain activity, we must first review two physiological changes that accompany changes in brain activity. As described more fully in chapter 4, these changes are responsible for what is called the BOLD response. Briefly, regional cerebral blood flow (rCBF) and regional cerebral oxygen metabolic rate (rCMRO$_2$) both increase when neuronal activity in that region increases. However, the increase in rCBF is greater than the increase in rCMRO$_2$; that is, the rCBF increase is greater than the increase needed to supply the extra oxygen required (Fox and Raichle, 1986). Thus, although both *total hemoglobin* and *oxyhemoglobin (oxy-Hb)* concentrations increase when neuronal activity increases, *deoxyhemoglobin (deoxy-Hb)* concentration decreases. Since oxy-Hb and deoxy-Hb absorb light at different near-infrared wavelengths, fNIRS can detect changes in their relative concentrations by measuring changes in the attenuation of light at specific frequencies and can then calculate the BOLD response, which is related to the concurrent changes in neuronal activity. Chapter 4 describes these events and methods in greater detail.

The three major types of spectroscopy used for fNIRS are continuous wave spectroscopy, time-resolved spectroscopy, and frequency-domain spectroscopy. These techniques are described in detail in Villringer and Obrig (2002). The continuous-wave (CW) approach is the one that is most widely used both in neuroimaging and in BCI studies. In commercially available CW fNIRS instruments, the light source is either a laser, a light-emitting diode (LED), or a simple halogen lamp that emits light at specific frequencies within the NIR spectrum. The advantages of the CW approach are its simplicity, flexibility, and potential for achieving a high signal-to-noise ratio. One disadvantage is that the CW approach cannot quantify the absolute values of oxy-Hb and deoxy-Hb but only their relative changes. Another disadvantage is that its measurements are susceptible to distortion by any concurrent changes in light absorption in superficial extracerebral tissues such as the scalp.

In most fNIRS applications, including BCI applications, the primary goal of data analysis is to detect differences in brain activity in specific areas as a function of different behavioral states. For example, the goal might be to detect differences between brain activity during rest versus during performance of a specific movement. In BCI usage in particular, the goal might be to detect differences in brain activity

between two task conditions: when a person wants to move a cursor to the left and when s/he wants to move it to the right.

fNIR-BCI STRUCTURE AND OPERATION

Like all BCI systems, an fNIR-BCI system has components for signal acquisition as well as components for signal processing (i.e., feature extraction and translation). It produces an output that gives a command to an application, and it provides real-time feedback to the user depending on the type of application. These components are depicted in figure 18.1.

fNIR SIGNAL ACQUISITION

Figure 18.2A illustrates the basic elements of an fNIRS measurement system. It includes: a light emitter (also referred to as an illuminator or a source); a detector; an amplifier; an analog-to-digital convertor; and finally the potentially usable fNIR signals. The emitter (red) and detector (blue) optodes are placed at specific alternating locations on the scalp (fig. 18.2B). The distance between the emitter and detector of each emitter/detector pair is 5–30 mm, depending on their arrangement on the scalp. A single emitter/detector pair is considered one *channel*.

Figure 18.2B shows an example of an optode configuration in which the emitter (red) and detector (blue) optodes are placed on the scalp over the left and right motor cortices (i.e., near the C3 and C4 locations [International 10–20 System]). The detector optodes are located 2 cm from the emitter optodes. As indicated by the dashed lines in figure 18.2B, any pair of emitter and detector optodes forms one channel. Thus, with its four emitters and four detectors, the optode arrangement shown in the figure results in 10 channels for each hemisphere. As indicated in figure 18.2A, near-infrared rays leave each emitter (only one shown in the figure), pass through the skull and the brain tissue of the cortex, follow a curvilinear path determined by the optical properties of the tissue, are reflected back out of the skull, and are received by one or more detector optodes. (Note the red photon banana [see chapter 4] representing the path of the photons.) The photomultiplier cycles through all the emitter-detector pairings to acquire data at every sampling period.

After the signals at each frequency are acquired and digitized, they are then preprocessed (e.g., to eliminate artifacts), are further processed to derive oxy-Hb and deoxy-Hb concentrations, and are finally stored on the hard-disk of the fNIRS-BCI workstation. For each time point the stored file typically includes: the raw signal intensities for each of the two or three wavelengths used; the Hb concentration changes calculated from these intensities; and codes indicating the current behavioral state of the subject (e.g., imagining moving the right hand, viewing an icon on a screen, etc.). If the system is operating in a real-time mode that controls an application and provides feedback to the subject, the data concurrently undergo further processing to produce the output feedback signals. Such real-time usage also typically entails a preliminary calibration procedure (and also perhaps periodic recalibrations) to define the parameters that are used to convert the measures of oxy-Hb and deoxy-Hb concentrations into the outputs.

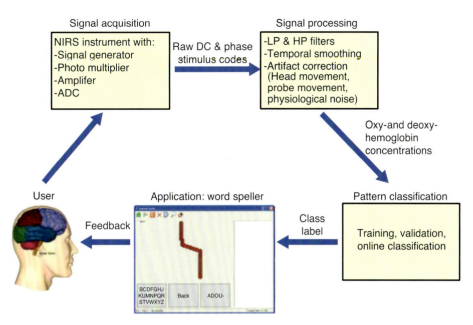

Figure 18.1 *Basic architecture of an fNIRS-based BCI. Single or multiple pairs of light sources and detectors (see fig. 18.2B) are positioned on the user's head in a configuration determined by the brain areas producing the signals to be used by the BCI. Direct-current (DC) amplitudes and phase values are acquired, amplified, and digitized by the fNIRS instrument, then preprocessed (i.e., by filtering and artifact-removal algorithms), converted into oxy-Hb and deoxy-Hb concentration values based on the Beer-Lambert Law, and finally translated (e.g., by simple thresholding, linear discriminant analysis, or pattern classification) into real-time output (e.g., to a spelling application or a device controller). Here the BCI output moves the descending red cursor in the Word Speller right or left to select the desired option at the bottom of the screen. (ADC is analog-to-digital converter; LP is low-pass; HP is high-pass.) (Modified and reprinted with permission from Sitaram et al., 2007a.)*

Secure connections between the optodes and the scalp are crucial for ensuring stable path lengths of the photons and for reducing movement artifacts. To maintain good contact between the optodes and the scalp and to reduce light attenuation, hair on the head must be kept out of the light path; this is usually accomplished by combing the hair, by using hair clips, or by some other means. Many types of headsets have been developed to keep the optode pairs in position and in good contact with the scalp. These include modified bicycle helmets, thermoplastic caps molded to the user's head, spring-loaded fibers attached to semirigid plastic forms, fibers embedded in rubber forms (Strangman et al., 2002), and a mechanical mounting system (Coyle et al., 2007).

fNIRS channel-placement schemes have not yet been standardized in a way comparable to that developed for EEG (e.g., the 10–20 system [Sharbrough, 1991]). Nevertheless, such standardization is essential for obtaining reproducible results from the same subject, for ensuring consistency across studies, and for comparing studies. Coyle et al. (2007) proposed an fNIRS polar-coordinate system derived from the EEG 10–20 system.

fNIR FEATURE EXTRACTION

Raw data acquired by an fNIRS instrument are typically contaminated by physiological noise such as cardiac pulsations, respiratory oscillations, and Mayer waves, which are spontaneous oscillations of arterial pressure occurring at a frequency lower than respiration. Arterial pulse oscillations cause fluctuations of fNIR signals across the whole brain and occur at frequencies of 1–2 Hz, depending on heart rate. Fluctuations caused by respiration occur at frequencies of 0.2–0.3 Hz,

depending on breathing rate. Mayer-wave fluctuations occur at ~0.1 Hz in conscious humans (Julien, 2006). Another confounding factor is the ongoing fluctuation of Hb oxygenation state, which occurs even during the resting state (Hoshi, 2007; Schroeter et al., 2004; Toronov et al., 2000). In addition, ongoing regional changes in brain activity cause slower (0.05 Hz) changes in Hb oxygenation state. These fluctuations are all superimposed on the signals associated with the behavioral states under study and thus add noise to the fNIRS data recorded. Moreover, additional contamination can result from movement artifacts, ambient light, and intensity variations due to obstructions from hair.

Although improved signal-correction and analysis techniques are needed to address these problems fully and to improve the signal-to-noise ratio, a number of corrections can be implemented to overcome or reduce some of these effects in order to extract the useful features from the raw signals. For example, Sitaram et al. (2007b) applied the following preprocessing steps in an offline analysis of their data. First, raw intensity data from all channels were normalized by dividing each value by the mean of all channels for all the time points. The intensity-normalized data were then low-pass filtered (see chapter 7) with a cutoff of 0.7 Hz. The rate of change of optical density, called delta-optical density, was then calculated for each wavelength as the negative logarithm of the normalized intensity. Following the calculation of the delta-optical density, two different principal component analysis (PCA) filters (see chapter 7) were applied to the data. The first PCA filter corrected for motion in the data (e.g., head movement). The second filter used the principal components of the baseline data (i.e., the data collected for 30 sec prior to the experimental

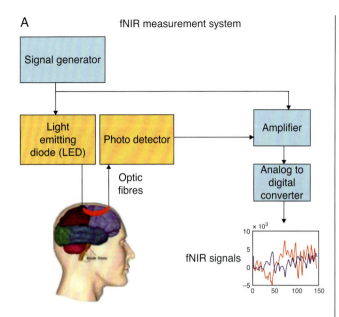

A   fNIR measurement system

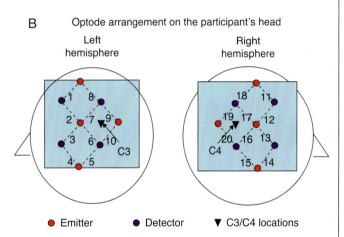

B   Optode arrangement on the participant's head

Left   Right
hemisphere   hemisphere

● Emitter   ● Detector   ▼ C3/C4 locations

Figure 18.2 (A) A continuous-wave (CW) fNIRS system in which light at two or more wavelengths (e.g., 700 nm and 805 nm) is generated constantly or is modulated at a low frequency (a few tens of kilohertz) by a signal generator. Light passes through the scalp and through a few millimeters of the upper layer of the brain in a curvilinear path, sometimes called the photon banana (see chapter 4). The light that emerges from the head is measured by a photodiode. Changes in the amplitude of the detected light at these wavelengths reflect changes in the concentrations of oxygenated and deoxygenated hemoglobin and are used to indicate the level of brain activity. The data shown in the example at bottom right in the figure (from Sitaram et al., 2007) were acquired by a multichannel fNIRS instrument (OMM-1000 from Shimadzu Corporation, Tokyo, Japan) operated at three different wavelengths (780, 805, and 830 nm), at a sampling rate of 14 Hz and were digitized by a 16-bit analog-to-digital converter during motor imagery (red is oxy-HB and blue is deoxy-Hb). (B) A multichannel fNIRS optode arrangement on the scalp. Optodes are arranged on the left and right sides of the subject's head, above the motor cortices (i.e., near the C3 [left hemisphere] and C4 [right hemisphere] locations of the International 10–20 System). A pair of adjacent emitter and detector optodes forms one channel (dotted lines). The four emitters and four detectors in the arrangement shown result in 10 channels on each side of the head (numbered 1–10 and 11–20). (Modified and reprinted with permission from Sitaram et al., 2007b.)

tasks) to remove physiological artifacts such as respiratory oscillations. The resulting covariance-reduced delta-optical density was used to calculate the change in concentration (i.e., the delta concentration) with a method based on the Beer-Lambert law (Villringer and Obrig, 2002).

A variety of other preprocessing procedures have been used. Naito et al. (2007) low-pass filtered their raw data with a cutoff of 0.1 Hz to remove the effects of respiration and other higher-frequency artifacts. Luu and Chau (2009) normalized each trial of raw intensity data by dividing it by the mean of the signal from the baseline period. The logarithm of the filtered signal was then subsampled to an effective sampling frequency of 3.125 Hz, based on the Nyquist criterion (chapter 7) that sampling rate should be two times the highest-frequency component of the signal.

Although used successfully in offline analyses of fNIRS data, these and other possible preprocessing techniques may or may not be directly transferable to online fNIR-BCI applications, as they require a large dataset for accurate and reliable computation or involve inordinately long processing times. Further work is needed to explore the adaptation of these methods for online, real-time usage.

Commercial manufacturers of fNIRS instruments provide custom-built analysis software packages. In addition, a program that provides basic signal processing, linear modeling, and image reconstruction of fNIRS data has been written by the Photon Migration Imaging Lab (Massachusetts General Hospital, Boston) and is freely available (http://www.nmr.mgh.harvard.edu/PMI/resources/homer/home.htm). Whereas these analysis methods have been developed mainly for offline analysis of fNIRS data, BCI use will require effective methods for real-time analysis and generation of appropriate outputs, including feedback to the BCI user. Better methods for eliminating the effects of spontaneous fluctuations in Hb oxygenation will be particularly important for such real-time applications.

fNIR FEATURE TRANSLATION AND OUTPUT

Feature translation converts the extracted features (i.e., the processed signals) into the BCI output commands that convey the user's intent (e.g., intent to move to the right or the left, intent to say "yes" or "no," etc.). The translation algorithm can distinguish among the signals representing different intents by using univariate statistical parametric mapping (SPM) (Hoshi, 2007) or several other methods such as a model-based analysis, an event-related analysis, or a combination of these two (Huppert et al., 2006; Schroeter et al., 2004) (see chapter 8).

Various methods have been used to translate the fNIRS measurements associated with specific cognitive or motor tasks into BCI output commands, such as those that control a spelling program, a cursor, or a wheelchair. These translation methods can be as simple as setting thresholds or ranges for the fNIRS measurements that identify different cognitive or motor states, or they can be more complicated, as in the use of sophisticated pattern-recognition algorithms. The choice of translation method should be based on the requirements of the application and the complexity and degrees of freedom of the fNIRS measurements. The choice may also be constrained by the need for online real-time processing and the capabilities of the computer software and hardware. Many of the translation methods used for fNIR are comparable to those used for translating other kinds of signals (e.g., electrical signals such as EEG or ECoG) (see chapter 8).

Support vector machines (SVM) (chapter 8) and hidden Markov modeling (HMM) (Rabiner, 1989; Rabiner and Juang, 1993) are two pattern-recognition methods that have been applied to fNIRS data to distinguish among different behavioral states. Sitaram et al (2007b) compared these two methods in classifying offline fNIRS data collected from 20 channels located over motor cortex, as subjects performed motor actions and motor imagery. Acquired signals were processed to remove artifacts produced by heartbeat and by muscle activity. For each trial, the investigators determined the changes in oxy-Hb and deoxy-Hb concentrations 2–10 sec after the stimulus that triggered the start of the motor or imagery task. After preprocessing, the data were classified by each of the two pattern-recognition methods, SVM and HMM. Most channels over the hemisphere contralateral to the task (fig. 18.3, upper right and lower left panels) showed increased oxy-Hb and decreased deoxy-Hb, indicating increased activity. In contrast, responses in channels over the ipsilateral hemisphere indicated either a smaller increase in activity (fig. 18.3, lower right panel) or

decreased activity (i.e., decreased oxy-Hb and increased deoxy-Hb) (fig. 18.3, upper left). Topographic images reconstructed from data of the 20 channels showed distinct patterns of activations with left hand and right hand motor imagery, although substantial intersubject differences were observed (Sitaram et al., 2007b). For both classification methods (SVM and HMM) and for all subjects, finger-tapping data were classified more accurately than motor-imagery data. In a direct comparison of the two pattern-classification techniques, HMM performed better than SVM for both finger-tapping and motor-imagery tasks.

Luu and Chau (2009) used a classifier based on Fischer linear discriminant analysis (chapter 8) of a two-dimensional feature space to decode subject preferences from fNIRS signals recorded from 16 channels over medial prefrontal cortex. They chose the medial prefrontal cortex as the target region of the study because this region had been previously implicated in subjective valuation and decision making (Luu and Chau, 2009). Images of two drinks were presented sequentially on the monitor, and the subjects were asked to view each drink as if it were being offered to them, to decide on a choice, and then to indicate their choice explicitly by clicking with a mouse on the graphical box corresponding to their choice. Analysis of the fNIRS signals during specific time periods produced the

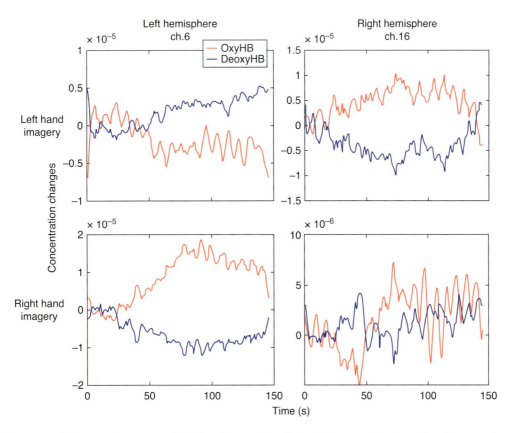

Figure 18.3 *The BOLD response during motor imagery over the ipsilateral (same side as the hand of movement) and contralateral motor cortices. The figure shows sample left- and right-hemisphere signals of average response from a subject performing left-hand and right-hand motor imagery. Channels over the side of the motor cortex contralateral to the motor imagery (upper right and lower left) show activation (i.e., increased oxy-Hb and decreased deoxy-Hb). Channels over the side of the motor cortex ipsilateral to the motor imagery (upper left and lower right) show either a similar but smaller response (lower right) or an opposite response (upper left). (Modified and reprinted with permission from Sitaram et al., 2007b.) The y-axes of all plots show change of molar concentration (red, oxy-Hb; blue, deoxy-Hb).*

features used by the classifier. Classification accuracy was evaluated by seven-fold cross-validation. Using simple features and a linear classifier, the authors demonstrated that it was possible to decode subject preference from a single presentation of each of the two choices with an average accuracy of 80%. If this paradigm can be adapted to online analysis, it could potentially be used in a BCI to provide communication and control.

Naito et al. (2007) tested an offline classifier with fNIRS signals recorded from a single channel over the left frontal lobe (an area known to be involved in cognitive tasks), while subjects were asked to answer simple questions with "yes" or "no" (fig. 18.4). They used a feature-extraction method based on

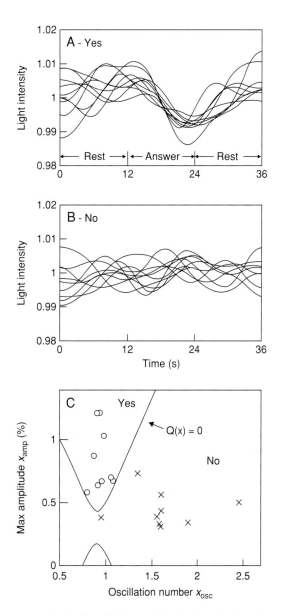

Figure 18.4 *Sample data from the first test of an fNIRS-based BCI in a large group of people with severe disabilities. Patients were asked to imagine singing a fast song to answer "yes" and to perform counting numbers in a reverse order to answer "no." (Top) Waveforms of "yes" responses. (Middle) Waveforms of "no" responses. Waves were low-pass filtered (0.1 Hz), and the response for each trial was normalized in terms of the average response. (Bottom) Linear discriminant analysis of "yes" and "no" waveforms (○ data for the answer "yes"; × data for the answer "no"). The analysis interval is 10–35 sec. (Reprinted with permission from Naito et al., 2007.)*

Hilbert transforms (King, 2009) to compute the instantaneous amplitude and phase values of the fNIRS signal at each time point. The values from a training data set (i.e., data for which the correct answers were known) were then used to define amplitude and phase vectors. A measure of Mahalanobis distance (an inverse measure of the covariance of a vector) (Mahalanobis, 1936) (chapter 7) was used to divide the two-dimensional plot of amplitude and phase vectors into two distinct regions, a "yes" region and a "no" region. When samples are normally distributed, the Mahalanobis distance is inversely proportional to the probability that a sample belongs to a given class. Mahalanobis distances for both "yes" and "no" vectors were separately computed. A discriminant function was subsequently determined from the training set as a difference of the square of the above two distances such that if the function was greater than zero, the sample belonged to the "yes" class and if it was less than zero it belonged to the "no" class (fig. 18.4, bottom panel). This function was then applied to test data to determine whether the subject's response was "yes" or "no." This method was found to perform well offline as indicated by the classification performance of above 70% (Naito et al., 2007). Whether it can be adapted to function effectively in an online BCI remains to be determined.

FEEDBACK TO THE BCI USER

During BCI operation, one or both of two kinds of adaptation may occur: the *system* may adapt to the user, and/or the *user* may adapt to the system (chapter 8). *System adaptation* involves changes in signal acquisition, feature extraction (chapter 7), and/or feature translation (chapter 8). *User adaptation* reflects changes in the signals that occur as the subject learns to use the system. In adapting to the system, the user may invoke a mental strategy to produce a suitable signal (e.g., motor imagery). Feedback to the user and reward for success are both generated by the system and are critical for enabling rapid and effective learning. Contingent feedback is known to help in the operant learning of control of brain activity for the successful operation of a BCI (e.g., Birbaumer et al., 2008). In the few online fNIR-BCI studies reported thus far, visual feedback has been used to indicate the degree of success of the subject's mental imagery in producing the target fNIR signal.

fNIRS-BCI IMPLEMENTATIONS TO DATE

Several laboratories have published studies describing fNIRS-based BCIs. The first such experiments were carried out with healthy subjects in separate efforts by Coyle and colleagues (Coyle et al., 2004; Coyle et al., 2007) and by Sitaram and colleagues (Sitaram et al., 2005). These studies took advantage of the observation that during motor imagery (as during actual movement), oxy-Hb concentration increases and deoxy-Hb concentration decreases in the contralateral hemisphere (as seen in figs. 18.3 and 18.5). Thus, they used fNIRS signals associated with various kinds of motor imagery.

Coyle et al. (2004) asked subjects to imagine continually clenching and releasing a ball with one hand while an fNIRS system recorded signals over the motor cortices of both hemispheres. They calculated average oxy-Hb concentration levels for successive 1-sec intervals from the data of two channels (i.e., two optode pairs), one over each motor cortex (near the C3 and C4 locations of the International 10–20 system). The data were acquired for 20 sec at a 100-Hz sampling rate. Visual feedback was provided by a circle on the screen that shrank and expanded with changes in oxy-Hb concentrations. To determine if the brain was in a state of rest or activation, they used a threshold of intensity of the oxy-Hb concentration at the contralateral motor cortex channel (i.e., they compared the measures from the right and left hemisphere channels). The reference level or threshold was set as the maximum amplitude during the first 10 sec of the window. An event was noted if the average oxy-Hb concentration was greater than the reference level.

Coyle et al. (2007) extended this study to develop a custom-built fNIRS-BCI system that they called the "Mindswitch." The Mindswitch operated in a synchronous mode (i.e., only during defined periods) with the objective of establishing a binary yes-or-no signal for communication (fig. 18.5). The authors compared the oxy-Hb concentration changes induced by motor imagery to drive a selection between two options provided by a visual interface. The option associated with a larger change in oxy-Hb was then chosen as the desired response. The fNIRS signal was derived from a single channel on the left motor cortex. The protocol consisted of two options alternately presented to the user and highlighted by the controlling software. When the desired option was highlighted, the users performed motor imagery (i.e., they were instructed to imagine clenching a ball with their right hand while attending to the kinesthetic experience of movement) to enhance the oxy-Hb signal in the motor cortex to indicate their choice. Experiments with healthy subjects showed that the signals were correctly classified in more than 80% of trials.

Sitaram et al. (2008) implemented an fNIRS-based online word speller as a potential means of communication for people who are locked-in. (Their system supports real-time data acquisition for two commercially available fNIR systems: OMM-1000 [Shimadzu Corporation, Tokyo, Japan] and Imagent System [ISS Inc., Champaign, USA]). The word-speller interface enables fNIRS responses created by left and right hand motor imagery to spell words by a two-choice cursor-control paradigm. The user employs left- or right-hand imagery to move the cursor to the left or right, respectively, to select a box that contains the letter of choice. Feature vectors of oxy- and deoxy-Hb values from all channels in a moving window of 4 sec are used as input to the pattern classifier to determine the brain state.

The study by Naito et al. (2007) was the first investigation of an fNIRS-BCI in a relatively large group of severely disabled people, 40 men and women with ALS, among whom 17 were in a completely locked-in state (see chapter 19). These investigators used a single forehead fNIRS channel with 30-mm source/detector spacing and two wavelengths of NIR emission (770 and 840 nm) to measure the BOLD response. The goal was to allow the subjects to express a simple yes-no response. The subject was asked a question. If the answer was "yes," the subject performed a mental calculation (e.g., multiplication of two big numbers) or imagined singing fast. If the answer was "no," s/he imagined relaxing. The amplitude and phase of the fNIRS signal for yes and no (fig. 18.4, top and middle panels) were calculated and analyzed by discriminant analysis to determine the person's answer. The average accuracy for the online operation of the BCI was 70% for the 23 people who were not completely locked-in, but only 40% (i.e., below the chance accuracy of 50%) for the 17 people who were completely locked-in. For the successful users, the average rate of correct detection was about 80%. The fNIRS signals of those who were completely locked-in showed only spontaneous low-frequency oscillations and no apparent responses to the questions. The authors suggest lack of motivation (i.e., as in learned helplessness), as well as low levels of brain activation as possible reasons for this observation.

These initial offline and online fNIRS-based BCI studies in people with and without disabilities suggest that a useful communication system might well be developed. However, its potential value for people with the most severe disabilities remains uncertain.

FUTURE PROSPECTS FOR fNIRS-BCI SYSTEMS

The principal advantages of fNIRS for BCI applications are that it is noninvasive and could readily be incorporated into relatively small, portable, inexpensive, and convenient systems. In these properties, it is clearly superior to other noninvasive imaging methods such as fMRI (see chapter 4 and discussion, this chapter), PET (chapter 4), and MEG (chapter 3), which are much more expensive and cumbersome and are thus largely confined to special laboratory environments (Hoshi, 2007). fNIR-BCI systems could prove to be more convenient than EEG systems that depend on wet electrodes. Further miniaturization using integrated optics and microelectromechanical

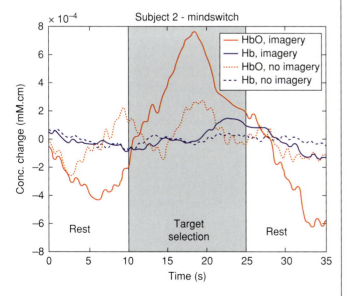

Figure 18.5 *fNIRS measurement of hemodynamic (BOLD) response from the right motor cortex during target selection by motor imagery in the "Mindswitch" system. The average response for 10 trials is shown. The subject's oxy-Hb (HbO) level increases during motor imagery. (HbO: oxy-Hb; Hb: deoxy-Hb) (Reprinted from Coyle et al., 2007, with permission.)*

(MEMS) devices could produce wearable fNIR-BCIs. In this regard portable instruments (e.g., HEO 200, from Omron Ltd., Tokyo, Japan) that allow users to move about during measurement have recently been developed.

Because NIR light penetrates only about 3.0 cm into the head, an fNIR-BCI is sensitive only to activity changes in superficial brain layers. Nevertheless, broad areas of cortex are accessible with this method. With further development of multichannel systems, fNIR-BCIs might enable increasingly complex real-time communication and control.

Although fNIRS *detection* has the advantage of good temporal resolution (i.e., <1 sec), the temporal resolution using this method is limited by the BOLD *response* itself, which is relatively slow (3–6 sec [Logothetis, 2003]), at least as measured by current imaging methods. Other optical signals, such as the event-related optical signal (EROS) (Gratton et al., 2006), have been reported to be faster; these offer the possibility of speedier activation and better control. For future use in BCI development, use of such signals needs to be replicated and confirmed, and signal acquisition and analysis methods need to be configured for real-time operation. Such developments could substantially increase the potential usefulness of fNIRS technology for BCI applications.

fMRI-BASED BCIs

Functional magnetic resonance imaging (fMRI) is another non-invasive imaging method based on *nonelectrical* brain signals that can be used for BCIs. As in fNIRS, fMRI also measures the BOLD effect: it infers changes in brain activity from the changes in blood flow that are calculated from changes in oxy-Hb and deoxy-Hb concentrations. Whereas an fNIRS system measures changes in oxy-Hb and deoxy-Hb based on their differing optical properties, fMRI detects changes in oxy-Hb and deoxy-Hb based on their differing *magnetic* properties. Because the hemodynamic response due to the BOLD effect lags behind neuronal activity by approximately 3–6 sec (Logothetis, 2003), hemodynamic signals acquired from fMRI, as is the case for fNIRS, have a relatively slow response time and low temporal resolution. On the other hand, fMRI offers very high spatial resolution and the possibility of complete brain coverage, including areas deep within the brain. Chapter 4 discusses the fundamental principles of fMRI operation. Here we discuss its use in a BCI.

The principal difference that distinguishes fMRI BCI applications from standard uses of fMRI is that the latter usually depend on offline analyses to produce the images, whereas BCI applications require rapid online analysis to enable real-time communication and control. Real-time fMRI was first reported by Cox and colleagues in 1995 (Cox et al., 1995). Since that time the development of fMRI-BCIs has been facilitated by several important advances: improved MRI scanners; faster data-acquisition sequences; better real-time preprocessing and statistical-analysis algorithms; improved methods for visualizing brain activation; and improved methods for providing feedback to the subject. This section reviews the basic principles of fMRI and discusses the architecture and components of an fMRI-based BCI, its applications to date, its strengths and weaknesses for BCI applications, and future developments that might be expected for this technology.

fMRI PRINCIPLES AND PRACTICE

MRI is based on the principles of nuclear magnetic resonance (NMR), a property of the quantum mechanical spin of atomic nuclei that was discovered in the 1940s. Although NMR has been used in chemical and biochemical research for many years, magnetic resonance imaging (MRI) is a more recent technology for generating detailed images of the human body. In the early 1990s, Ogawa and colleagues first reported the use of MRI to image the functional human brain in a completely noninvasive manner (Ogawa et al., 1990).

Brain function is known to involve many complex processes including changes in blood flow, blood volume, and blood oxygenation, and the production of metabolic by-products. fMRI has the capability to measure parameters related to several of these physiological functions. As discussed in chapter 4, the most common use of fMRI measures BOLD contrast (Bandettini et al., 1992; Kwong et al., 1992; Ogawa et al., 1990), which is based on the magnetic susceptibility of hemoglobin (Hb). Because deoxygenated-Hb (deoxy-Hb) is paramagnetic, its presence causes a distortion in the local magnetic field, which produces a local change in the magnetic resonance signal. Since brain activity changes deoxy-Hb concentrations in the blood, brain activity can be inferred by detecting changes in the magnetic resonance signal. The signal changes detected by fMRI are caused by the dominance of increased blood flow during brain activation relative to changes in blood volume and oxygen utilization (chapter 4). This constitutes the BOLD response that is also the basis for fNIRS methodology. Although details of the relationship between the BOLD signal and neural activity have not been completely established, accumulating evidence suggests that the BOLD signal is correlated with changes in local field potentials (LFPs) (Logothetis, 2003). With fMRI, measurement of the BOLD response allows the generation of detailed images of brain activity.

In a typical fMRI experiment, brain activity in a condition of interest (e.g., right-hand finger tapping) is determined by comparing functional images in this condition with images from a baseline condition in which the subject remains relaxed without performing the task. This is sometimes referred to as subtractive methodology. Only after generating an average subtraction image or a map of a statistical parameter (e.g., a pixel-by-pixel t-test comparison between the conditions), are the regions of activity discernible. These regions can be superimposed onto high-resolution anatomical images or rendered volumes in order to identify the structures in the brain that are activated. Real-time fMRI and later developments in fMRI-based BCI and neurofeedback have been enhanced by significant advances in several technical areas: higher-field magnets; multichannel receiver coils; improved techniques for signal preprocessing and artifact removal; improved analysis of functional images and statistical parametric mapping of brain activation; improved machine learning and pattern recognition techniques; and affordable high-performance computers. Moreover, with the advent of very rapid echo planar imaging (EPI) (Bandettini et al., 1992), fMRI captures fast changes in brain function with increased signal-to-noise ratios.

fMRI-BASED BCI STRUCTURE AND OPERATION

Like other BCI systems, an fMRI-based BCI system includes components for signal acquisition and signal processing (for feature extraction and translation) (fig. 18.6). It produces outputs for an application, and it must provide real-time feedback to the user. In present fMRI systems, these different components are typically handled by separate computers connected by a local-area network (LAN). Further details about the components and physical structure of fMRI-based BCI systems may be found in Sitaram et al. (2009) and Weiskopf et al. (2007).

fMRI SIGNAL ACQUISITION

An echo planar imaging (EPI) sequence (Bandettini et al., 1992) is used to acquire whole brain images from experimental subjects. With this technique, the three-dimensional brain is divided into a specified number of two-dimensional *slices* of

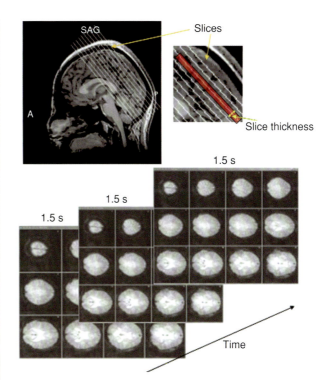

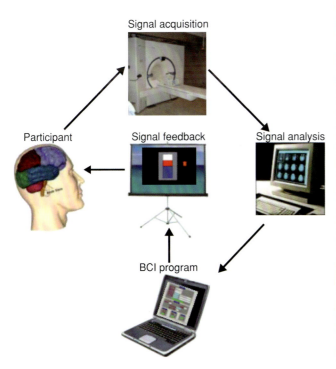

Figure 18.6 *An fMRI-based BCI system can be considered as a closed-loop control system. Whole-brain images from healthy subjects or patients are acquired employing a conventional Echo Planar Imaging (EPI) sequence or one of its variants. The measured hemodynamic response due to the BOLD effect is preprocessed for correction of artifacts (such as head motion). The signal analysis subsystem performs statistical analysis and generates functional maps. Feedback can be presented to the subject in different modalities (e.g., visual, acoustic) and with a variety of visualization methods (e.g., varying activity levels in one or more regions of interest [ROIs] using a graphical thermometer as shown in the figure, or with functional maps, continuously updated curves of the mean activity in one or more selected ROIs, or augmented interfaces such as Virtual Reality).*

Figure 18.7 *An illustration of slice positioning and image acquisition in a real-time fMRI measurement. Slices are positioned in an initial EPI reference scan of the subject. In this example, 16 slices are positioned in a sagittal view. Slice thickness and gap thickness between slices are shown. (Data from authors' laboratory.)*

specific thickness (e.g., 5 mm) and a specific gap (e.g., 1 mm) between the slices (fig. 18.7). More slices give better spatial resolution, but they also require more acquisition time. Thus, there is a trade-off between spatial and temporal resolution. This is important because a BCI functions in real time and thus depends on rapid signal acquisition, rapid signal processing, and rapid production of output and feedback to the user.

In fMRI-based BCI uses, each brain slice is typically about 5 mm thick and has 64×64 (i.e., 4096) pixels, giving 3–4 mm resolution in each dimension of the plane of the slice. For example, Caria et al. (2007) used 16 slices with 4096 pixels/ slice, providing a voxel size (i.e., the brain volume assesed by each data point) of ~54 mm^3 (i.e., ~3.3mm $\times$ ~3.3mm $\times$ 5mm), with each voxel containing millions of neurons. These parameters provided adequate spatial and temporal resolution to access the functional activation of a circumscribed region of the brain (e.g., the left anterior insula). Acquisition of whole-brain images is normally performed at intervals of 1–1.5 sec (deCharms et al., 2004; Weiskopf et al., 2003) using EPI.

fMRI SIGNAL PREPROCESSING AND FEATURE EXTRACTION

The real-time operation essential for an fMRI-based BCI requires that brain images be produced immediately after each set of whole-brain images is acquired for each *repetition time* (TR) (usually 1–1.5 sec). Because the standard MRI analysis options originally provided by manufacturers did not support such real-time image reconstruction, early developers of fMRI-based BCIs created their own sequences and image-reconstruction programs (see chapter 4). For example, Weiskopf and colleagues (Weiskopf et al., 2003; Weiskopf et al., 2004b) modified the Siemens (Siemens Medical Systems, Erlangen, Germany) scanner's software to reconstruct whole-brain images after each TR and to store these images in a folder that could be immediately accessed for further processing, analysis, output, and feedback by the fMRI-based BCI system. More recently, MRI manufacturers have upgraded their scanning software to enable real-time acquisition of whole brain images (e.g., Siemens 3T, Syngo version VB15).

After signal acquisition for each time point, the reconstructed images are transferred to another computer where the images are pre-processed to improve the signal-to-noise ratio (SNR). In general, the SNR of fMRI data increases with the strength of the main magnetic field and with more sophisticated MRI pulse sequences (chapter 4). Nevertheless, noise is inevitably present in the raw signal, and thus a variety of preprocessing procedures have been developed to remove it. One of the major sources of noise in fMRI data is head motion, which can interfere with detection of changes in brain activity or can even mimic them. Head padding or a bite bar can reduce head motion but cannot entirely eliminate it. Respiratory and cardiac artifacts are other sources of noise. Motion correction in real time requires efficient algorithms that can be executed on fMRI data sets within a single TR.

In addition to corrections for motion, preprocessing typically includes spatial smoothing (i.e., low-pass spatial filtering). It may also include averaging the data over specific brain regions of interest (ROI). These measures can further compensate for motion artifacts, minimize the impact of intersubject variability, and reduce data complexity (Weiskopf et al., 2004b).

fMRI FEATURE TRANSLATION AND OUTPUT

After the images are generated, the software performs statistical analysis and generates functional maps using such methods as: subtraction of active or rest conditions; correlation analysis; multiple regression; a General Linear Model (GLM); or pattern classification. Most fMRI-based BCI studies have used univariate signal-analysis methods to translate fMRI data into BCI output. A commonly used univariate method for detecting neuronal activity from fMRI time-series data is correlation analysis. This method computes correlation coefficients between the time series of the reference vector representing the change in the task conditions and the measurement vector of each voxel. For example, six alternating time blocks of motor imagery and rest conditions, each of 30-sec duration, with a 1-sec TR, could be a task protocol for an fMRI-based BCI experiment; in such a case, a reference vector could be produced by representing each scan of motor imagery with a value of 1 and each scan of the rest condition with a value 0.

Another common method is a general linear model (GLM), which provides a unified framework for univariate analysis of the fMRI data (Friston et al., 1995). A GLM can model multiple experimental and confounding effects simultaneously. Prior to actual online BCI use, an offline GLM analysis identifies the voxels that are significantly activated (i.e., show increased brain activity) in specific conditions (such as when a person performs motor imagery) and determines coefficients to be used to translate the data from these voxels into BCI output. Since the number of trials available for such preliminary analyses is usually limited, Bagarinao et al. (2003) developed a method for real-time GLM-coefficient estimation that can be updated as new data become available. Thus, this approach is adaptive (see chapter 8) and is suitable for fMRI-based BCIs. A similar approach is taken by the analysis software TBV (Brain Innovations, Maastricht, the Netherlands), which is employed in the data shown in figure 18.8. It uses the recursive least-squares regression algorithm (Pollock, 1999) to incrementally update the GLM estimates. In subsequent online operation the results of the updated GLM estimate (or the correlational analysis) are applied to the fMRI data from each successive time-point to determine the BCI output and provide feedback to the BCI user.

Up to the present, many fMRI-based BCI studies have employed univariate methods to focus on one or two ROIs. Although they measure brain activity repeatedly from many thousands of locations, univariate methods are limited because they analyze each location separately (Haynes and Rees, 2006). Recent work shows that the sensitivity of human neuroimaging may be improved by taking into account the spatial pattern of brain activity (Davatzikos et al., 2005; Mitchell et al., 2003; Norman et al., 2006; Polyn et al., 2005). A major argument for using more than single ROIs is that perceptual, cognitive, or emotional activities generally recruit a distributed network of brain regions. Pattern-based analysis methods recognize this and use not only the individual voxel values but also their spatiotemporal relationships. Many studies have reported offline classification of fMRI signals using various pattern-based methods, such as multilayer neural networks (Norman et al., 2006), Fisher Linear Discriminant (FLD) classifier (Mourao-Miranda et al., 2005), and Support Vector Machines (SVM) (Lee et al. 2010) (chapter 8). LaConte et al. (2006) and Sitaram et al. (2010) reported the implementation of real-time pattern-classification systems practical for BCI use.

Sitaram et al. (2010) implemented a real-time multi-class brain-state classification of fMRI signals using a support vector machine (SVM) to recognize discrete emotional states, such as happiness and disgust (as shown in fig. 18.9), on a scan-by-scan basis, in healthy individuals instructed to recall emotionally salient episodes from their lives. Real-time head-motion correction, spatial smoothing, and feature selection based on a new method of multivariate statistical mapping called *effect mapping* (Lee et al., 2010) reduced data dimension and improved prediction accuracy (Sitaram et al., 2010). The classifier showed robust prediction rates in decoding three discrete emotional states (happiness, sadness, disgust) in 16 participants. Subjective reports of the degree of emotional recall positively correlated with positive-affect scores and negatively correlated with negative-affect scores, indicating that the mood and motivational state of an individual determine his success at emotional imagery and regulation. Further research by this research group is in progress to apply the real-time pattern decoding of emotions to create an "affective BCI" for communicating with people with Alzheimer's disease.

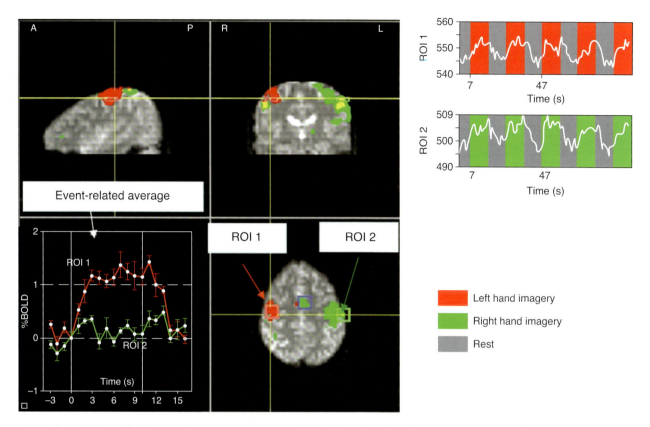

Figure 18.8 *Online generation of BOLD signal from two regions of interest (ROI): ROI1 (red) is in the right primary motor cortex and is activated by left-hand motor imagery (red time segments in top plot on upper right); ROI2 (green) is in the left primary motor cortex and is activated by right-hand motor imagery (green time segments in bottom plot on upper right). The subject used fMRI-based BCI feedback to acquire volitional regulation of the BOLD signal. The left side of the images is the right side of the brain (radiological orientation). A, anterior; P, posterior; R, right; L, left. (Data from authors' laboratory.)*

FEEDBACK TO THE BCI USER

People can learn to regulate brain activity when a measure of this activity, such as the BOLD signal, is provided as feedback (Schwartz and Andrasik, 1995). Learning is best if the feedback is accurate and occurs very quickly. With fMRI's high spatial resolution and whole brain coverage, it is possible to provide feedback from specific anatomical ROIs (Weiskopf et al., 2004a,b). A functional localization experiment (e.g., that presents a specific stimulus or asks the user to perform a specific mental task) is conducted to define the anatomical landmarks and identify the relevant activation, so that appropriate region-specific feedback can be provided. For example, overt

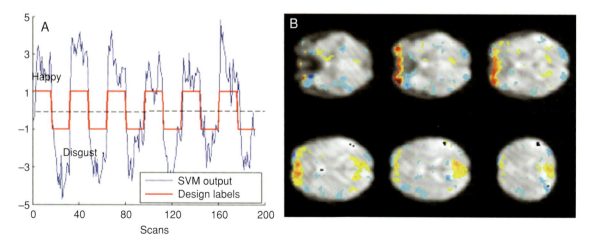

Figure 18.9 *Binary classification of two emotions (happiness and disgust) in one subject. (A) Online support vector machine (SVM) output. (B) Effect map, with yellow/red colors depicting pixels that discriminate for the happy condition and blue/green colors depicting pixels for the disgust condition. The six images represent brain slices from a single subject. The brain activations (in color) were the result of a multivariate analysis of fMRI signals acquired in multiple trials of emotional imagery. (Adapted from Sitaram et al., 2010.)*

finger tapping, movement imagery, or observing a particular action can activate specific brain regions. Pattern-based methods (Laconte et al., 2006) can identify patterns of activation in multiple spatially distributed ROIs that interact with each other, and these patterns can be used to control feedback.

After a specific ROI activation pattern to be used as feedback is identified, further processing is conducted to produce a representation of brain activity suitable for presentation as feedback. Feedback is most commonly presented visually and in a variety of forms including functional maps, continuously updated curves, graphical thermometers that display activity in one or more selected ROIs, or Virtual Reality (VR) displays (deCharms et al., 2004; Weiskopf et al., 2003; Sitaram et al., 2005; Sitaram, 2007). Feedback-presentation intervals cannot be less than the time needed for image acquisition and processing; this time depends on the speed of the computer hardware and the efficiency of the algorithms. The timing can directly affect system performance. If a user is to learn to control the activity in a particular ROI, it is important that feedback occur within 1–2 sec of the change in brain signal (Caria et al., 2007).

By conventional univariate methods, the signal change in an ROI is usually computed as a difference between the BOLD signal at that time-point and the BOLD signal during a baseline condition. The specificity of the feedback can be further improved by having it reflect both positive and negative changes in the activity in the ROI. Alternatively, some studies (e.g., Weiskopf et al., 2004b) have provided feedback that reflects the difference in activation between two ROIs. This method greatly reduces the nonspecific effects of global changes caused by factors such as arousal and attention due to the task or spontaneous changes in the user; it cancels out these nonspecific effects, leaving the effects specific to the task (i.e., imagining a right- or left-hand movement). Finally, correlation coefficients and effective connectivity measures might be used as feedback measures to train participants to regulate activation patterns in brain networks, rather than simply in individual circumscribed brain regions.

fMRI-BCI APPLICATIONS TO DATE

Due to the high expense, nonportability, and technical complexity of fMRI systems, fMRI has not been widely used in development of BCIs to provide communication and control for severely disabled people. Nevertheless, a few studies have determined that fMRI can enable BCI control. Lee et al. (2009) developed an fMRI-based BCI with which the user controlled the two-dimensional movement of a robotic arm. The users were able to regulate regional activation of the primary motor cortex with left- and right-hand motor imagery. The BOLD signal originating from the corresponding hand motor area was translated into horizontal or vertical robotic hand movement, and visual feedback was provided. Results with three participants demonstrated that brain activity associated with motor imagery was detected by fMRI and supported real-time control of the robotic arm.

Although fMRI has not been extensively used as a modality for BCIs for communication and control, fMRI-based BCIs

may have greater application as a tool in neuroscience research and in clinical treatment of neurological and psychiatric pathologies (Sitaram et al., 2007; deCharms et al., 2008; Ruiz et al., 2008).

Some recent studies (e.g., Boly et al., 2007) used fMRI to detect awareness in an unresponsive person with brain injury by detecting the brain activation produced by spatial navigation and motor-imagery tasks. Implementation of an online version of this protocol might enable the assessment of the state of consciousness in these individuals, and help medical personnel and caregivers to develop basic communication with them.

FUTURE PROSPECTS FOR fMRI-BCI SYSTEMS

In spite of its high cost and complex set-up, fMRI has distinct advantages for exploration and development of better BCI systems. Its high spatial resolution, whole-brain coverage, and anatomical specificity make it a potentially powerful tool for exploring novel BCI paradigms or for guiding the use of other BCI signal modalities. It could be useful for optimizing the placements of EEG, ECoG, or intracortical electrodes, or fNIRS optodes. Since technology for simultaneous acquisition of EEG and fMRI signals is already available, fMRI could help localize the sources of specific EEG features (e.g., specific evoked potentials or EEG rhythms). Furthermore, fMRI could be valuable in assessing the possible long-term effects of prolonged BCI use.

Beyond the practical considerations of the expense and size of the fMRI equipment, at present the major limitation of fMRI technology as a modality for BCI is its limited temporal resolution. This is due to the fact that, as now used, fMRI detects changes in brain activity by measuring changes in blood flow, which are relatively slow. However, methods are being developed for using MRI to directly measure changes in specific neurotransmitters and other chemical components, and to measure neuronal electrical processes. This technology, called *functional magnetic resonance spectroscopy* (fMRS), monitors the spectroscopic signals that reflect chemical processes associated with neural activity (see chapter 4). fMRS could directly measure metabolic activity involved in excitatory and inhibitory neurotransmission by following the concentrations and synthesis rates of metabolites involved in neuroenergetics, amino acid neurotransmission, and neuromodulation. Metabolites such as aspartate, gamma-amino butyric acid (GABA), glucose, glutamate, glutamine, and lactate could be measured within precisely defined regions in the brain.

Recently, Northoff et al. (2007) combined fMRI with fMRS measurements at rest to detect negative BOLD responses (i.e., reflecting decreased brain activity) and changes in the concentration of the neurotransmitter GABA in the right anterior cingulate cortex. With this approach they observed that the concentration of GABA in this region correlated with negative BOLD responses. Since it is not yet known whether humans can learn to control the concentrations of specific metabolites, online monitoring of metabolites by fMRS could provide important information about the underlying neurochemical processes during the learned control of brain activity. Such advances in fMRS methodology could also provide much more direct and precise measures of rapid changes in brain activity and thereby contribute to BCI development.

SUMMARY

BCIs that use metabolic signals (i.e., fNIR-based BCIs and fMRI-based BCIs) are still in the early stages of research and development compared to BCIs that use electrical signals recorded by EEG, ECoG, or intracortical methods. The fundamental limitation of these metabolic BCI methods is their dependence on the inherently slow BOLD response to measure brain activity. In the future this might be overcome by development of fNIRS and fMRI methods for more direct measurements of brain processes. In any case, with continued development, BCIs based on metabolic imaging are likely to contribute to BCI development in several important ways. With its high spatial resolution and whole-brain coverage, fMRI methodology could guide placement of recording electrodes and protocol design for BCIs that use EEG, ECoG or intracortical signals. fNIRS-based BCIs could be configured as inexpensive, convenient, and portable systems that could restore basic communication and control to people with severe disabilities.

REFERENCES

Bagarinao, E., Matsuo, K., Nakai, T., and Sato, S. (2003). Estimation of general linear model coefficients for real-time application. *Neuroimage, 19*(2 Pt 1), 422–429.

Bandettini, P. A., Wong, E. C., Hinks, R. S., Tikofsky, R. S., and Hyde, J. S. (1992). Time course EPI of human brain function during task activation. *Magn Reson Med, 25*(2), 390–397.

Birbaumer, N. (2006). Brain-computer-interface research: Coming of age. *Clin Neurophysiol., 117*(3), 479–483.

Birbaumer, N., and Cohen, L. G. (2007). Brain-computer interfaces: communication and restoration of movement in paralysis. *J Physiol, 579*(Pt 3), 621–636.

Birbaumer, N., Murguialday, A. R., and Cohen, L. (2008). Brain-computer interface in paralysis. *Curr Opin Neurol, 21*(6), 634–638.

Boly, M., Coleman, M. R., Davis, M. H., Hampshire, A., Bor, D., Moonen, G., Maquet, P. A., Pickard, J. D., Laureys, S., and Owenc, A. M. (2007). When thoughts become action: An fMRI paradigm to study volitional brain activity in non-communicative brain injured patients. *Neuroimage, 36*(3), 979–992.

Caria, A., Veit, R., Sitaram, R., Lotze, M., Weiskopf, N., Grodd, W., and Birbaumer, N. (2007). Regulation of anterior insular cortex activity using real-time fMRI. *Neuroimage, 35*(3), 1238–1246.

Cox, R. W., Jesmanowicz, A., and Hyde, J. S. (1995). Real-time functional magnetic resonance imaging. *Magn Reson Med, 33*(2), 230–236.

Coyle, S. M., Ward, T. E., and Markham, C. M. (2007). Brain-computer interface using a simplified functional near-infrared spectroscopy system. *J Neural Eng, 4*(3), 219–226.

Coyle, S., Ward, T., Markham, C., and McDarby, G. (2004). On the suitability of near-infrared systems for next generation brain computer interfaces. *Physiological Measurement, 25*(4), 815–822.

Davatzikos, C., Ruparel, K., Fan, Y., Shen, D. G., Acharyya, M., Loughead, J. W., Gur, R. C., and Langleben, D. D. (2005). Classifying spatial patterns of brain activity with machine learning methods: Application to lie detection. *Neuroimage, 28*(3), 663–668.

deCharms, R. C., Christoff, K., Glover, G. H., Pauly, J. M., Whitfield, S., and Gabrieli, J. D. (2004). Learned regulation of spatially localized brain activation using real-time fMRI. *Neuroimage, 21*(1), 436–443.

Fox, P. T., and Raichle, M. E. (1986). Focal physiological uncoupling of cerebral blood flow and oxidative metabolism during somatosensory stimulation in human subjects. *Proc Natl Acad Sci USA, 83*(4), 1140–1144.

Friston, K. J., Holmes, A. P., Poline, J. B., Grasby, P. J., Williams, S. C., Frackowiak, R. S., and Turner, R. (1995). Analysis of fMRI time-series revisited. *Neuroimage, 2*(1), 45–53.

Gratton, G., Brumback, C. R., Gordon, B. A., Pearson, M. A., Low, K. A., and Fabiani, M. (2006). Effects of measurement method, wavelength, and source-detector distance on the fast optical signal. *Neuroimage, 32*(4), 1576–1590.

Haynes, J. D., and Rees, G. (2006). Decoding mental states from brain activity in humans. *Nat Rev Neurosci, 7*(7), 523–534.

Hoshi, Y. (2007). Functional near-infrared spectroscopy: Current status and future prospects. *J Biomed Opt, 12*(6), 062106.

Huettel, S. A. (2004). Non-linearities in the blood-oxygenation-level dependent (BOLD) response measured by functional magnetic resonance imaging (fMRI). *Conf Proc IEEE Eng Med Biol Soc, 6*, 4413–4416.

Huppert, T. J., Hoge, R. D., Diamond, S. G., Franceschini, M. A., and Boas, D. A. (2006). A temporal comparison of BOLD, ASL, and NIRS hemodynamic responses to motor stimuli in adult humans. *Neuroimage, 29*(2), 368–382.

Julien, C. (2006). The enigma of Mayer waves: Facts and models. *Cardiovasc Res, 70*(1), 12–21.

King, F. W. (2009). *Hilbert Transforms: Encyclopedia of Mathematics and its Applications (Volume 1)*. Cambridge: Cambridge University Press.

Kwong, K. K., Belliveau, J. W., Chesler, D. A., Goldberg, I. E., Weisskoff, R. M., Poncelet, B. P., Kennedy, D. N., Hoppel, B. E., Cohen, M. S., and Turner, R. (1992). Dynamic magnetic resonance imaging of human brain activity during primary sensory stimulation. *Proc Natl Acad Sci USA, 89*(12), 5675–5679.

Laconte, S. M., Peltier, S. J., and Hu, X. P. (2007). Real-time fMRI using brain-state classification. *Hum Brain Mapp, 28*(10), 1033–1044.

Lee, J. H., Ryu, J., Jolesz, F. A., Cho, Z. H., and Yoo, S. S. (2009). Brain-machine interface via real-time fMRI: Preliminary study on thought-controlled robotic arm. *Neurosci Lett, 450*(1), 1–6.

Lee, S., Halder, S., Kübler, A., Birbaumer, N., and Sitaram, R. (2010). Effective functional mapping of fMRI data with support-vector machines. *Hum Brain Mapp, 31*(10), 1502–1511.

Logothetis, N. K. (2003). The underpinnings of the BOLD functional magnetic resonance imaging signal. *J Neurosci, 23*(10), 3963–3971.

Logothetis, N. K. (2007). The ins and outs of fMRI signals. *Nat Neurosci, 10*(10), 1230–1232.

Logothetis, N. K. (2008). What we can do and what we cannot do with fMRI. *Nature, 453*(7197), 869–878.

Luu, S., and Chau, T. (2009). Decoding subjective preference from single-trial near-infrared spectroscopy signals. *J Neural Eng, 6*(1), 016003.

Mahalanobis, P. C. (1936). *On the generalised distance in statistics*. Paper presented at the Proceedings of the National Institute of Sciences of India, *2*(1), 49–55. Retrieved 2008-11-05.

Mitchell, T. M., Hutchinson, R., Just, M. A., Niculescu, R. S., Pereira, F., and Wang, X. (2003). Classifying instantaneous cognitive states from FMRI data. *AMIA Annu Symp Proc*, 465–469.

Mourao-Miranda, J., Bokde, A. L., Born, C., Hampel, H., and Stetter, M. (2005). Classifying brain states and determining the discriminating activation patterns: Support vector machine on functional MRI data. *Neuroimage, 28*(4), 980–995.

Naito, M., Michioka, Y., Izawa, K., Ito, Y., Kiguchi, M., and Kanazawa, T. (2007). A communication means for totally locked-in ALS patients based on changes in cerebral blood volume measured with near-infrared light. *IEICE Trans. Inf. Syst., E90-D*(No. 7), 1028–1037.

Norman, K. A., Polyn, S. M., Detre, G. J., and Haxby, J. V. (2006). Beyond mind-reading: Multi-voxel pattern analysis of fMRI data. *Trends Cogn Sci, 10*(9), 424–430.

Northoff, G., Walter, M., Schulte, R. F., Beck, J., Dydak, U., Henning, A., Boeker, H., Grimm, S., and Boesiger, P. (2007). GABA concentrations in the human anterior cingulate cortex predict negative BOLD responses in fMRI. *Nat Neurosci, 10*(12), 1515–1517.

Ogawa, S., Lee, T. M., Kay, A. R., and Tank, D. W. (1990). Brain magnetic-resonance-imaging with contrast dependent on blood oxygenation. *Proc Natl Acad Sci USA, 87*, 9868–9872.

Pollock, D. S. G. (1999). *A Handbook of Time-Series Analysis, Signal Processing and Dynamics*. San Diego, CA: Academic Press.

Polyn, S. M., Natu, V. S., Cohen, J. D., and Norman, K. A. (2005). Category-specific cortical activity precedes retrieval during memory search. *Science, 310*(5756), 1963–1966.

Rabiner, L.R., (1989). A tutorial on hidden Markov models and selected applications in speech recognition. *Proc. IEEE, 77*, 257–286.

Rabiner, L., and Juang, B. H. (1993). *Fundamentals of Speech Recognition*. Englewood Cliffs, NJ: Prentice-Hall.

Schroeter, M. L., Bucheler, M. M., Müller, K., Uludag, K., Obrig, H., Lohmann, G., Tittgemeyer, M., Villringer, A., and von Cramon, D. Y. (2004). Towards a standard analysis for functional near-infrared imaging. *Neuroimage, 21*(1), 283–290.

Schwartz, M. S., and Andrasik, F. (Eds.) (1995). *Biofeedback: A Practitioner's Guide.* New York: Guilford Press.

Sharbrough, F. W. (1991). Advances in epilepsy surgery offer patients new hope. *Minn Med, 74*(10), 9–12.

Sitaram, R. (2007). *fMRI Brain-Computer Interfaces.* Paper presented at the 15th Annual Conference of International Society for Neurofeedback and Research, Current Perspectives in Neuroscience: Neuroplasticity and Neurofeedback, San Diego, CA.

Sitaram, R., Caria, A., and Birbaumer, N. (2009). Hemodynamic brain-computer interfaces for communication and rehabilitation. *Neural Netw, 22*(9), 1320–1328.

Sitaram, R., Caria, A., Veit, R., Gaber, T., Kuebler, A., and Birbaumer, N. (2005). *Real-time fMRI based Brain-computer Interface enhanced by Interactive Virtual Worlds.* Paper presented at the 45th Annual Meeting Society for Psychophysiological Research, 20–25, Lisbon, Portugal.

Sitaram, R., Caria, A., Veit, R., Gaber, T., Rota, G., Kuebler, A., and Birbaumer, N. (2007a). FMRI brain-computer interface: A tool for neuroscientific research and treatment. *Comput Intell Neurosci*, 25487.

Sitaram, R., Hoshi, Y., and Guan, C. (2005). *Near Infrared Spectroscopy based Brain-Computer Interface. Proc. SPIE* 5852, 434.

Sitaram, R., Lee, S., Ruiz, S., Rana, M., Veit, R., and Birbaumer, N. (2010). Real-time support vector classification and feedback of multiple emotional brain states. *Neuroimage.* Epub ahead of print, August 6.

Sitaram, R., Weiskopf, N., Caria, A., Veit, R., Erb, M., and Birbaumer, N. (2008). fMRI brain-computer interfaces: A tutorial on methods and applications. *IEEE Signal Processing Magazine, Special Issue on BCI. 25*(1), 95–106.

Sitaram, R., Caria, A., and Birbaumer, N. (2009). Hemodynamic brain-computer interfaces for communication and rehabilitation. Neural Netw. 22(9), 1320–1328.

Sitaram, R., Zhang, H., Guan, C., Thulasidas, M., Hoshi, Y., Ishikawa, A., Shimizu, K., and Birbaumer, N. (2007b). Temporal classification of multichannel near-infrared spectroscopy signals of motor imagery for developing a brain-computer interface. *Neuroimage, 34*(4), 1416–1427.

Strangman, G., Culver, J. P., Thompson, J. H., and Boas, D. A. (2002). A quantitative comparison of simultaneous BOLD fMRI and NIRS recordings during functional brain activation. *Neuroimage, 17*(2), 719–731.

Toronov, V., Franceschini, M. A., Filiaci, M., Fantini, S., Wolf, M., Michalos, A., and Gratton, E. (2000). Near-infrared study of fluctuations in cerebral hemodynamics during rest and motor stimulation: Temporal analysis and spatial mapping. *Med Phys, 27*(4), 801–815.

Villringer, A., and Chance, B. (1997). Non-invasive optical spectroscopy and imaging of human brain function. *Trends Neurosci, 20*(10), 435–442.

Villringer, A., and Obrig, H. (2002). Near infrared spectroscopy and imaging. In: *Brain Mapping: The Methods* (2nd ed.): Elsevier Science.

Weiskopf, N., Mathiak, K., Bock, S. W., Scharnowski, F., Veit, R., Grodd, W., Goebel, R., and Birbaumer, N. (2004a). Principles of a brain-computer interface (BCI) based on real-time functional magnetic resonance imaging (fMRI). *IEEE Trans Biomed Eng, 51*(6), 966–970.

Weiskopf, N., Scharnowski, F., Veit, R., Goebel, R., Birbaumer, N., and Mathiak, K. (2004b). Self-regulation of local brain activity using real-time functional magnetic resonance imaging (fMRI). *J Physiol (Paris), 98*(4–6), 357–373.

Weiskopf, N., Sitaram, R., Josephs, O., Veit, R., Scharnowski, F., Goebel, R., Birbaumer, N., Deichmann, R., and Mathiak, K. (2007). Real-time functional magnetic resonance imaging: Methods and applications. *Magn Reson Imaging, 25*(6), 989–1003.

Weiskopf, N., Veit, R., Erb, M., Mathiak, K., Grodd, W., Goebel, R., and Birbaumer, N. (2003). Physiological self-regulation of regional brain activity using real-time functional magnetic resonance imaging (fMRI): Methodology and exemplary data. *Neuroimage, 19*(3), 577–586.

19 | BCI USERS AND THEIR NEEDS

LEIGH R. HOCHBERG AND KIM D. ANDERSON

Brain-computer interfaces (BCIs) have captured the imagination of scientists and the public for many years. As described in other chapters in this book, hundreds of research laboratories around the world, as well as a handful of companies, are now focused on BCI research and development. This phenomenon stands in sharp contrast to the very small number of people actually using BCIs outside of a research environment. If we define a BCI as *a system that provides brain control of an external device for communication or control*, BCIs are currently in daily use by fewer than 10 people (primarily people with advanced amyotrophic lateral sclerosis [ALS]). (Note that this definition does not include the investigational responsive neurostimulation systems that are discussed later in this chapter or the various other types of systems discussed in chapter 1.) The public, scientific, and media interest in BCI research results not from its widespread achievements but, instead, from promising early demonstrations of the remarkable potential for BCIs to help people replace or restore functions that have been compromised by illness or injury.

Most of this book is focused on the "what" and "how" of BCIs. For the purposes of this chapter, we will assume that the challenges of BCI development will be overcome and that the BCIs currently being envisaged will become available to the people who want and need them. Here, we ask a more fundamental question: for whom, exactly, are these BCIs being developed? Whom will they serve and in what ways? To address these crucial questions, we have organized our discussion by describing the *functions* that BCIs may eventually serve, and we highlight particular clinical disorders that result in loss of these functions and the challenges that these disorders pose for BCI development. Commonly anticipated BCI functions fall into three categories: *communication, mobility,* and *autonomic function*. Following discussion of these three categories, we consider other possible BCI uses and then conclude by enumerating the properties that ideal BCI systems would need to possess. Although such systems are certainly not available at present, describing their essential attributes can serve to focus and inform development efforts.

RESTORING FUNCTIONS LOST DUE TO INJURY OR DISEASE

IMPAIRED COMMUNICATION

The ability to communicate—whether by speech, email, text message, or even a simple head nod or smile—is central to

human interaction. For people who have severe communication disabilities despite intact cognition, BCI technology is poised to have a profound impact. One clinical condition, *locked-in syndrome (LIS)*, is commonly identified as the most immediate target for BCI research. LIS was defined by Plum and Posner in 1966 as: "...a state in which selective supranuclear motor de-efferentation produces paralysis of all four limbs and the last cranial nerves without interfering with consciousness. The voluntary motor paralysis prevents the subjects from communicating by word or body movement" (Plum and Posner 1966). LIS can result from a variety of clinical etiologies, including: *acute events* such as ischemic or hemorrhagic infarction of the brainstem (particularly the ventral pons), or traumatic brain injury leading to torsion or compression of brainstem structures, basilar artery vasospasm, or central pontine myelinolysis; *subacute disorders* such as Guillain-Barré syndrome; or *slowly developing or chronic diseases* such as brainstem tumor or motor neuron disease, most notably amyotrophic lateral sclerosis (ALS). A *transient LIS* can also be induced by pharmacologic neuromuscular blockade (with mechanical ventilation) in the absence of adequate sedation (Topulos et al. 1993).

The BCI literature displays some understandable inconsistency regarding the meaning of the term LIS. Indeed, the Plum and Posner definition continues with: "*Usually, but not always,* the anatomy of the responsible lesion in the brainstem is such that locked-in patients are left with the capacity to use vertical eye movements and blinking to communicate their awareness of internal and external stimuli."[emphasis added] (Plum and Posner 1982). The principal inconsistencies in the use of the term LIS have thus concerned whether the person still retains some control of eye movements. Bauer (Bauer et al. 1979) (cf. Laureys et al. 2005) provided a useful advance in the definition by distinguishing among:

- *total LIS* (with the absence of all voluntary movement, including eye movements)

- *classical LIS* (with intact vertical eye movements or blinking, as exemplified by Jean-Dominique Bauby, who wrote the book *The Diving Bell and the Butterfly* [Bauby 1997] using eyeblinks alone)

- *incomplete LIS* (with retention of remnants of voluntary movement, such as a finger twitch)

For people with incomplete or classical LIS, early BCIs using evoked potentials to choose among items in a matrix or to provide unidirectional or unidimensional cursor control have already been shown to enable selection of letters or words on a screen. BCIs of this kind are currently in use by a small number of people with advanced ALS (e.g., Sellers et al. 2010). In addition, BCIs that provide two-dimensional point-and-click interfaces have already been demonstrated (Kim et al. 2007; McFarland et al. 2008) and could enable powerful and intuitive control over standard software. When combined with word-prediction algorithms and text-to-speech programs, and made generally available, these first-generation BCIs are expected to restore basic communication to people with incomplete or classical LIS.

For people with total LIS (e.g., some people with advanced ALS and on chronic mechanical ventilation), there has not yet been a successful demonstration of BCI use. Although it is possible that this reflects the limitations of BCI systems attempted thus far and/or the dearth of sufficiently meticulous studies, it has also been suggested that the complete LIS state, as defined above, exists only transiently, since the state of complete de-efferentation might quickly lead to diminished goal-directed behavior (Birbaumer et al. 2008). Further research will support or refute this hypothesis. In this research it will be essential to overcome the challenge of distinguishing an unconscious state from failure of the BCI to enable a totally locked-in person to communicate.

The emergence of BCIs as tools to maintain communication for people with ALS raises important questions for both BCI development and clinical decision making. Although the vast majority of those with ALS in the United States and elsewhere currently elect not to be placed on mechanical ventilation or other life-sustaining therapies, the availability of BCIs that could ensure continued communication with family members and friends may change this decision (Hochberg and Cochrane 2011). This issue is further complicated by the growing recognition that ALS can affect other aspects of cerebral function. Whereas some people with ALS retain intact cognition, others develop cognitive deficits consistent with the frontotemporal-lobar degeneration that often accompanies the disease (Geser et al. 2010; Merrilees et al. 2010). Such associated deficits may limit the types and locations of brain signals that might be used by BCIs, as well as the levels of concentration and attention that the BCI users can maintain.

Apart from LIS, other neurologic or head and neck injuries can result in *anarthria*—the inability to speak, despite intact language comprehension and cognition. This differs from *aphasia*, in which the *formulation* or *understanding* of language is affected. Studies are beginning to explore the possibility that intended speech or language might be decoded from neural signals in order to produce a so-called "speech prosthesis" (Brumberg et al. 2010).

IMPAIRED MOBILITY

Moving from one place to another, changing body position or configuration, and manipulating objects in the immediate environment, whether for activities of daily living (e.g., eating, bathing, dressing, brushing teeth, etc.), employment, entertainment, or education (e.g., turning the pages of a book), occupy a substantial proportion of the day for most able-bodied people. Many diseases and injuries interfere with mobility, and thus the restoration of mobility is a major goal of BCI research. It is important to realize that restoration of even small amounts of mobility (e.g., hand grasp) can markedly improve a person's daily functioning. Hence, it is not essential to restore total mobility, which would often be a formidable or insurmountable task, particularly for people with severe disabilities. By considering a series of impairments in mobility, we can begin to imagine how BCIs may eventually serve different populations of people with physical disabilities.

TETRAPLEGIA

The partial impairment or total loss of function in the arms, trunk, legs, and pelvic organs (e.g., bladder, bowel) is referred to as *tetraplegia* (preferred to "quadriplegia" by the American Spinal Injury Association, ASIA [Maynard et al. 1997]). Whereas ASIA applies this term specifically to people with injuries to neural elements within the spinal canal, people with any disease or disorder that produces a partial or complete paralysis of the arms and legs are commonly referred to as having *tetraparesis* or *tetraplegia*. Among the conditions that can lead to tetraplegia are cervical spinal-cord injury, brainstem stroke, ALS and other motor neuron diseases, Guillain-Barré syndrome, myasthenia gravis, muscular dystrophy, postpolio syndrome, neurofibromatosis, multiple sclerosis, spastic tetraplegia (a form of cerebral palsy), and "watershed" distribution bilateral strokes (so-called "man-in-the-barrel" syndrome [Olejniczak et al. 1991]) (cf. Christopher and Dana Reeve Paralysis Foundation Report Foundation [CDR 2009]).

For the disabilities produced by many of these diseases and injuries, currently available rehabilitative therapies and assistive technologies are, at best, only modestly effective; furthermore, continued access to them is often significantly restricted by insurance coverage, or the lack thereof. Given the hope that BCIs will help to restore mobility (and/or other) functions for people with tetraplegia, it is tempting to perform a market survey, asking people with tetraplegia what they might want from a BCI and whether they might want to use a BCI that promises to achieve a particular outcome. However, market surveys have limitations when applied to medical devices and perhaps even more so for emerging neurotechnologies.

When a medical device is not yet supported by substantial evidence of safety and effectiveness (indeed, when the device might not even yet exist), it is unrealistic to expect people to decide whether they would use it, particularly if it involves some consideration of risk (e.g., an implanted BCI system). Deep brain stimulation (DBS) for Parkinson's disease provides an excellent example. Imagine that in 1987 a research team had told 1000 patients with Parkinson's disease that they might be able to walk more quickly and steadily and their hands might not shake as much if they underwent a 7-hr brain surgery, during which they would be awake, in which an electrode

50–60 mm long would be inserted near the center of the brain, with wires from the electrode tunneled under the skin to a pacemaker-like battery and stimulator in the chest, after which the clinician would use a magnet to program the stimulator. It is unlikely that many people would believe that such a device could exist, much less that it could significantly reduce their disabilities, or that they would agree, even hypothetically, to undergo the procedure. Nevertheless, less than 25 years later, DBS has become a standard of care (DBS 2001; Pahwa et al. 2006), and more than 80,000 patients with movement disorders have received these implants (Medtronic 2010). Thus, for people with tetraplegia, a market survey asking what a BCI should do is unlikely to be a reliable guide for the scientists and engineers designing BCIs.

Far better is the simpler, more tractable question that was asked by Anderson (2004): "What gain of function would dramatically improve your life?" In a survey of 347 people with tetraplegia and without mention of how such functional gains would be achieved:

- 48.7% selected *arm and hand function* as their top priority from among the seven choices that were provided

- 13% selected *sexual function*

- 11.5% selected *upper-body/trunk strength and balance*

- 8.9% selected *bladder/bowel function and the elimination of autonomic dysreflexia* (i.e., a life-threatening condition resulting from abnormal regulation of the autonomic nervous system)

- 7.8% selected *regaining walking movement*

- 6.1% selected *regaining normal sensation*

- 4% selected *eliminating chronic pain.*

We believe that these responses will be useful in guiding the development of BCIs aimed at future users with tetraplegia. It is not surprising that restoration of arm and hand function was the first priority for about half of those with tetraplegia, since these abilities are crucial to enhancing functional independence and increasing participation in everyday life functions. Results similar to these were reported by Snoek et al. (2004) after surveying people with tetraplegia in the United Kingdom and the Netherlands. The growing power and ubiquity of computer-based communication (e.g., email, text messaging) is further augmenting the importance of arm and hand function. The possibilities for using computers to control the local environment (e.g., in the home or work place) also enhance their contributions to functional independence. Thus, it is understandable and appropriate that much current BCI research and development is focused on providing keyboard-like or mouse-like control of computers.

PARAPLEGIA

Paraplegia is the partial or complete loss of movement of the lower, but not the upper, extremities. It may also be accompanied by autonomic dysfunction (e.g., impairments of bladder and bowel control; regulation of heart rate, blood pressure, body temperature; and sexual function) and is caused most commonly by injury to the spinal cord. Thoracic/lumbar/sacral spinal-cord injuries, postpolio syndrome, multiple sclerosis, neurofibromatosis, artery of Adamkiewicz ischemia, spastic diplegia (a form of cerebral palsy), some types of muscular dystrophy, and bilateral anterior cerebral artery vasospasm can all result in the inability to move the legs as well as impairments in bladder, bowel, and sexual function. Of the 334 people with paraplegia due to spinal cord injury surveyed in the Anderson (2004) study:

- 26.7% selected *sexual function* as their top priority

- 18% selected *bladder/bowel function and the elimination of autonomic dysreflexia*

- 16.5% selected *increasing upper body/trunk strength and balance*

- 15.9% selected *regaining walking movement*

- 12% selected *eliminating chronic pain*

- 7.5% selected *regaining normal sensation*

- 3.4% selected *arm and hand function*

It is striking—and perhaps surprising to many people without disabilities—that *sexual* and *bowel/bladder/autonomic dysfunction* are the most common first priorities for people with paraplegia, and they have higher priority than does walking for people with tetraplegia. This finding and its implications will be discussed in this chapter's section on autonomic function.

Mobility, which is the most common priority for people with tetraplegia, is also the first priority for about one-third of those with paraplegia (Anderson 2004; Donnelly et al. 2004). BCIs might help to restore mobility in a variety of ways, such as providing control of powered wheelchairs, hand orthoses, robotic arms, or powered exoskeletons. Ultimately and most desirably, systems that combine BCI technology with implanted functional electrical stimulation (FES) devices that activate paralyzed muscles might restore mobility that approaches normal motor control in speed, reliability, and ease of use (Donoghue et al. 2007a; Donoghue et al. 2007b).

LIMB LOSS

Amputation of one or more limbs due to trauma, vascular disease, or for therapeutic purposes in the cases of some cancers or infections, is another cause of decreased mobility or decreased ability to manipulate the immediate environment. Prosthetic limbs have been available for thousands of years (e.g., an early prosthetic leg, the "Roman Capua leg," dates to 300 BCE, and the "Cairo toe" dates to 1295 BCE [Laferrier and Gailey 2010]), and the past decade has seen the creation of remarkable powered and unpowered upper- and lower-extremity prosthetics (Aaron et al. 2006; Adee 2008). However, the functionality of these prostheses, particularly those for the upper extremity, has been sharply limited by the controllers that are available. These controllers are generally slow, provide only simple, low-dimensional control, and require high concentration on the part of the user. BCIs might provide much more rapid and complex control and might thereby enable dexterous control of prosthetic limbs. Efforts to develop such systems have begun (Aaron et al. 2006).

IMPAIRED AUTONOMIC FUNCTION

In considering the functional losses incurred by people with severe motor disabilities, able-bodied people frequently focus on the deficits that are most visible, that is, on losses of mobility and communication. This focus is reflected in the fact that most research endeavors target these problems. However, for those actually living with such disabilities, losses of bladder, bowel, and sexual function are often far more distressing and their restoration is thus considered most desirable. This reality is illustrated by the Anderson (2004) survey. For 39.7% of people living with tetraplegia and for 38% of those living with paraplegia, the first or second-highest priority was *restoring bladder/bowel function and eliminating autonomic dysreflexia* (Anderson 2004). For 28.3% of people living with tetraplegia and 45.5% of those living with paraplegia, the first or second-highest priority was *restoring sexual function* (Anderson 2004). Similar results have been demonstrated by Widerstrom-Noga et al. (1999).

Loss of autonomic functions (e.g., bladder and bowel control, sexual function, regulation of heart rate, blood pressure, and body temperature) can have a major impact on an individual's health, causing, among other problems, chronic kidney infections, and contributing to severe ulcerations of skin and subcutaneous tissues. Nearly every level and severity of spinal injury is associated with some degree of autonomic dysfunction. People with spinal injuries at thoracic level 6 or above can also experience an additional problem known as *autonomic dysreflexia*, a dangerous increase (or, less commonly, decrease) in blood pressure, which can be life-threatening if not managed properly (Blackmer 2003). Bladder and bowel dysfunction are the two principal triggers of autonomic dysreflexia (Blackmer 2003). Bladder and bowel dysfunction and autonomic dysreflexia also impair sexual function in people with spinal cord injuries (Anderson et al. 2007a, 2007b, 2007c). The significant correlation between experiencing autonomic dysreflexia during bladder and bowel care and experiencing it during sexual activity (Anderson et al. 2007a) suggests that the restoration of one aspect of autonomic function could benefit several bodily systems.

In addition to their potentially serious health ramifications, losses of bladder and bowel control have tremendous social implications. Because they are socially unacceptable, these losses are devastating for those trying to participate in the community. Deficits in the maintenance of bowel and bladder function impair the ability to be in environments that lack toilet facilities for unpredictable amounts of time (e.g., in a vehicle when there may be traffic, in a friend's home that doesn't have accessible facilities, on an airplane for a long trip). The restoration of the ability to control autonomic functions—specifically, to ensure continence when needed, and to permit voiding when desired—is a potentially valuable future role for BCI technology. Restoration of sexual function is similarly important, since sexual function affects how people perceive themselves and how they believe others perceive them. This importance is reinforced by the great emphasis placed on sexual function by society (e.g., the extensive attention and resources devoted to treating impotence in aging men).

The key point is the need to recognize that a person experiencing lost function may have priorities for restoring function that are different from those expected by the able-bodied population. In order to make devices that will actually be used by the population for which the devices are intended, it is imperative to address the priorities of that population.

Because bladder and bowel control, sexual function, and other autonomic functions (e.g., blood pressure regulation) are in large part neurally based, BCI technology has the opportunity to contribute to their restoration. Furthermore, bowel, bladder, and sexual functions generally take place during brief and often selectable time periods. Thus, the development of BCIs that restore these functions may not need to overcome the difficult problems associated with BCIs that must be available at most or all times (e.g., BCIs that restore mobility) and that thus must avoid unintended or inappropriate outputs.

BCIs FOR REHABILITATION OF STROKE PATIENTS

In addition to their potential role in *replacing* lost functions, BCIs might also be useful in *supplementing* standard neurorehabilitation therapies so as to improve functional outcomes (discussed in greater detail in chapter 22 of this volume). Physical, occupational, and/or speech and language therapy are commonly used in stroke rehabilitation. Recognizing the brain's capacity for activity-dependent plasticity, newer rehabilitative therapies seek to modify injured brain areas or to encourage noninjured brain areas to assume the functions of injured areas (Bolognini et al. 2009; Dobkin 2008; Wolf et al. 2006). BCIs might contribute to these goals by encouraging the return of brain activity that can enable voluntary control of the limbs, and/or by strengthening existing functional neural pathways by pairing movement intentions (as perceived by the BCI) with actual movements (as assisted during therapeutic exercise).

In general, the beneficial effects of rehabilitation therapies are often limited by the amount of time that can be spent in the therapy clinics and the number of visits that are covered by insurance (Buntin 2007). Hence, if BCI technologies are to be effective in this arena, they should be suitable for home use and easy to use without extensive ongoing professional assistance or oversight. If these requirements are not met, the devices will not be readily accessible to many in the target population. Input from the target population during all stages of BCI development and testing in these areas will also be critical for success.

OTHER POTENTIAL BCI USERS

PEOPLE WITH EPILEPSY

BCIs might assist in the management of other neurological or psychiatric illnesses. For example, in people with epilepsy, cortical-surface recordings may be used to detect the abnormal activity associated with seizures and then trigger stimulators to suppress this activity before the seizure becomes clinically apparent (Sun et al. 2008). This is an example of a system that both directly *detects* and directly *affects* brain activity. A BCI of this kind that could reliably predict an impending seizure might provide a warning ahead of time (which would be extremely valuable) or even abort the seizure by producing appropriate stimulation. Intracortical recordings are now being employed to better understand the complex activities of individual neurons and neuronal networks during the initiation, maintenance, and conclusion of seizures (Truccolo et al. 2011). Early indications are that these rich signals may be valuable in the BCI-enabled prediction of impending seizures.

PEOPLE WITH COGNITIVE, MOOD, OR OTHER DISORDERS

BCIs might be combined with neural-stimulation technologies for a variety of closed-loop applications. As described above, a BCI might detect seizures before they become clinically evident and then suppress them through neurostimulation. A BCI might be used in conjunction with deep brain stimulation (DBS), which is being investigated for use in obsessive-compulsive disorder (OCD) and in major depression (Greenberg et al. 2010; Lozano et al. 2008; Malone et al. 2009). If it is possible for a BCI to detect the neurophysiologic signatures of pathologically compulsive behavior, or the impending onset of an episode of major depression, it might conceivably trigger stimulation that could dampen or eliminate these conditions. BCI technology might also provide advance warnings and enable rapid interventions in the acute management of traumatic brain injury, status epilepticus, cerebral vasospasm, and other life-threatening conditions treated in the intensive-care unit.

It is even conceivable that a BCI might be used therapeutically outside the realm of diseases usually associated with the central nervous system. For example, if morbid obesity results in part from absence or inadequate brain processing of satiety signals, could a closed-loop BCI use brain stimulation to induce such signals or to enhance their effect on behavior? The use of BCIs for treating such complex disorders may be far in the future, but applications of this kind may begin to emerge over the coming decade as neurotechnologies continue to be developed and combined.

A WISH LIST FOR BCI USERS

Although BCIs are likely to be customized to the needs of individual users, this chapter offers an opportunity to look well into the future and to imagine what the ideal BCI might provide for a person with locked-in syndrome, or how it might provide people with tetraplegia the ability to care for themselves independently, or how it might restore dignity to the millions of people living with incontinence. As discussed in Anderson (2009) and noted in this chapter, it may not be possible for able-bodied researchers to fully understand the experience of a person living with a serious disability. It is thus imperative to seek end-user input early in the process of developing BCIs to help people with disabilities (see also chapter 11, this volume). Waiting until the marketing stage means wasted research time and resources. Here, taking into account as much as possible the expressed desires of people with severe disabilities (see also chapter 11, this volume), is a Top-Ten Wish List for a Perfect BCI.

TOP-TEN WISH LIST FOR A PERFECT BCI

1. Safe

2. Affordable (and reimbursable)

3. Works all the time: when the alarm clock goes off, at the work-place (and on the commute), during Happy Hour, etc.

4. Does not require the assistance of a caregiver, technician, or scientist

5. Restores communication at the speed of normal speech or typing

6. Restores real-time, multidimensional, dexterous control of one's own limbs (both hands and both legs); or provides similar control of prosthetic limbs

7. Esthetically acceptable or invisible (e.g., fully implanted)

8. Restores normal bowel/bladder control and sexual function

9. Reliable, lasts several years between battery changes and 10 years between upgrades

10. Requires no more concentration than the same functions do for an able-bodied person

We propose this list as a challenge to BCI research and development. Realization of each item will require the continued engagement of multidisciplinary teams that will necessarily include neuroscientists, neurologists, computer scientists, engineers, applied mathematicians, surgeons, speech and mobility specialists, regulatory experts, and probably device manufacturers and corporate leaders as well as the end-user consultants. One of the most exciting aspects of the BCI field is its iterative nature—the interactions among the professionals and the crucial feedback from participants in clinical trials—as BCI systems move toward this ideal. In this effort, the users for whom these technologies are being developed are crucial contributors at all stages.

SUMMARY

The primary justification and impetus for BCI research and development are their potential for addressing the needs of people with severe motor disabilities due to neuromuscular disease, stroke, or trauma. These needs fall into three broad categories: communication, mobility, and autonomic function. BCIs could eventually have a major impact in all three areas. Currently available systems focus mainly on communication, and substantial research is targeting mobility. Nevertheless, autonomic deficits (especially loss of bladder and bowel control and sexual function) are of equal or greater concern to many prospective users, such as those with paraplegia due to spinal cord injury. BCI development efforts need to focus on producing devices that address the deficits that are of most concern to the prospective users rather than simply the deficits that are most apparent to able-bodied observers. Thus, the target users should be consulted at all stages of development and testing. The ultimate goal should be BCIs that are safe, affordable, easy to use, reliable, aesthetically pleasing, long-lasting, and capable of restoring normal communication, mobility, and autonomic function.

(Note: The contents do not represent the views of the Department of Veterans Affairs or the United States Government.)

REFERENCES

Aaron RK, Herr HM, Ciombor DM, Hochberg LR, Donoghue JP, et al. 2006. Horizons in prosthesis development for the restoration of limb function. *J Am Acad Orthop Surg* 14:S198–204.

Adee S. 2008 (February). Dean Kamen's "Luke Arm" prosthesis readies for clinical trials. IEEE Spectrum, available at http://spectrum.ieee.org/biomedical/bionics/dean-kamens-luke-arm-prosthesis-readies-for-clinical-trials.

Anderson KD. 2004. Targeting recovery: priorities of the spinal cord-injured population. *J Neurotrauma* 21:1371–1383.

Anderson KD. 2009. Consideration of user priorities when developing neural prosthetics. *J Neural Eng* 6(5):1–3.

Anderson KD, Borisoff JF, Johnson RD, Stiens SA, Elliott SL. 2007a. The impact of spinal cord injury on sexual function: concerns of the general population. *Spinal Cord* 45:328–337.

Anderson KD, Borisoff JF, Johnson RD, Stiens SA, Elliott SL. 2007b. Long-term effects of spinal cord injury on sexual function in men: implications for neuroplasticity. *Spinal Cord* 45:338–348.

Anderson KD, Borisoff JF, Johnson RD, Stiens SA, Elliott SL. 2007c. Spinal cord injury influences psychogenic as well as physical components of female sexual ability. *Spinal Cord* 45:349–359.

Bauby J-D. 1997. *The diving bell and the butterfly*. New York: A.A. Knopf, distributed by Random House.

Bauer G, Gerstenbrand F, Rumpl E. 1979. Varieties of the locked-in syndrome. *J Neurol* 221:77–91.

Birbaumer N, Murguialday A, Cohen L. 2008. Brain-computer interface in paralysis. Curr Opin Neurol 21:634–638.

Blackmer J. 2003. Rehabilitation medicine: 1. Autonomic dysreflexia. *Can Med Assoc J* 169:931–935.

Bolognini N, Pascual-Leone A, Fregni F. 2009. Using non-invasive brain stimulation to augment motor training-induced plasticity. *J Neuroeng Rehabil* 6:8.

Brumberg JS, Nieto-Castanon A, Kennedy PR, Guenther FH. 2010. Brain-computer interfaces for speech communication. *Speech Commun* 52:367–379.

Buntin MB. 2007. Access to postacute rehabilitation. *Arch Phys Med Rehabil* 88:1488–1493.

DBS fPSG. 2001. Deep-brain stimulation of the subthalamic nucleus or the pars interna of the globus pallidus in Parkinson's disease. *N Engl J Med* 345:956–963.

Dobkin BH. 2008. Training and exercise to drive poststroke recovery. *Nat Clin Pract Neurol* 4:76–85.

Donnelly C, Eng JJ, Hall J, Alford L, Giachino R, et al. 2004. Client-centred assessment and the identification of meaningful treatment goals for individuals with a spinal cord injury. *Spinal Cord* 42:302–307.

Donoghue JP, Hochberg LR, Nurmikko AV, Black MJ, Simeral JD, Friehs G. 2007a. Neuromotor prosthesis development. *Med Health Rhode Isl* 90:12–15.

Donoghue JP, Nurmikko A, Black M, Hochberg LR. 2007b. Assistive technology and robotic control using motor cortex ensemble-based neural interface systems in humans with tetraplegia. *J Physiol* 579:603–611.

Foundation CDR. 2009. *One Degree of Separation: Paralysis and Spinal Cord Injury in the United States* Short Hills, NJ, Eds. Christopher and Dana Reeve Foundation. 1–28.

Geser F, Lee VM, Trojanowski JQ. 2010. Amyotrophic lateral sclerosis and frontotemporal lobar degeneration: a spectrum of TDP-43 proteinopathies. *Neuropathology* 30:103–112.

Greenberg BD, Gabriels LA, Malone DA, Jr., Rezai AR, Friehs GM, et al. 2010. Deep brain stimulation of the ventral internal capsule/ventral striatum for obsessive-compulsive disorder: worldwide experience. *Mol Psychiatry* 15:64–79.

Hochberg LR, Cochrane TI. 2011. Implanted neural interfaces: ethics in research and treatment. In Chatterjee A, Farah M, (Eds.) *Neuroethics in Practice*, Oxford University Press.

Kim SP, Simeral JD, Hochberg LR, Donoghue JP, Friehs GM, Black MJ. 2007. Multi-state decoding of point-and-click control signals from motor cortical activity in a human with tetraplegia. *CNE '07. 3rd International IEEE/EMBS Conference on Neural Engineering, 2007*, 486–489.

Laferrier JZ, Gailey R. 2010. Advances in lower-limb prosthetic technology. *Phys Med Rehabil Clin N Am* 21:87–110.

Laureys S, Pellas F, Van Eeckhout P, Ghorbel S, Schnakers C, et al. 2005. The locked-in syndrome: what is it like to be conscious but paralyzed and voiceless? *Prog Brain Res* 150:495–511.

Lozano AM, Mayberg HS, Giacobbe P, Hamani C, Craddock RC, Kennedy SH. 2008. Subcallosal cingulate gyrus deep brain stimulation for treatment-resistant depression. *Biol Psychiatry* 64:461–467.

Malone DA Jr., Dougherty DD, Rezai AR, Carpenter LL, Friehs GM, et al. 2009. Deep brain stimulation of the ventral capsule/ventral striatum for treatment-resistant depression. *Biol Psychiatry* 65:267–275.

Maynard FM Jr., Bracken MB, Creasey G, Ditunno JF Jr., Donovan WH, et al. 1997. International standards for neurological and functional classification of spinal cord injury. American Spinal Injury Association. *Spinal Cord* 35:266–274.

McFarland, DJ, Krusienksi, DJ, Sarnacki, WA, and Wolpaw, JR. 2008. Emulation of computer mouse control with a noninvasive brain-computer interface, J Neural Eng 5:101–100.

Medtronic I. 2010. *Questions and Answers—DBS Therapy*. http://www.medtronic.com/your-health/parkinsons-disease/therapy/questions-and-answers.

Merrilees J, Klapper J, Murphy J, Lomen-Hoerth C, Miller BL. 2010. Cognitive and behavioral challenges in caring for patients with frontotemporal dementia and amyotrophic lateral sclerosis. *Amyotroph Lateral Scler* 11:298–302.

Olejniczak PG, Ellenberg MR, Eilender LM, Muszynski CT. 1991. Man-in-the-barrel syndrome in a noncomatose patient: a case report. *Arch Phys Med Rehabil* 72:1021–1023.

Pahwa R, Factor SA, Lyons KE, Ondo WG, Gronseth G, et al. 2006. Practice parameter: treatment of Parkinson disease with motor fluctuations and dyskinesia (an evidence-based review): report of the Quality Standards Subcommittee of the American Academy of Neurology. *Neurology* 66:983–995.

Plum F, Posner JB. 1966. *The diagnosis of stupor and coma*. Philadelphia: F.A. Davis.

Plum F, Posner JB. 1982. *The diagnosis of stupor and coma*. Philadelphia: F.A. Davis.

Sellers EW, Vaughan TM, Wolpaw JR. 2010. A brain-computer interface for long-term independent home use. *Amyotroph Lateral Scler* 11:449–455.

Snoek GJ, IJzerman MJ, Hermens HJ, Maxwell D, Biering-Sorensen F. 2004. Survey of the needs of patients with spinal cord injury: impact and priority for improvement in hand function in tetraplegics. *Spinal Cord* 42:526–532.

Sun FT, Morrell MJ, Wharen RE Jr. 2008. Responsive cortical stimulation for the treatment of epilepsy. *Neurotherapeutics* 5:68–74.

Topulos GP, Lansing RW, Banzett RB. 1993. The experience of complete neuromuscular blockade in awake humans. *J Clin Anesth* 5:369–374.

Truccolo W, Donoghue JA, Hochberg LR, Eskandar EN, Madsen JR, Andersen WS, Brown EN, Halgren E, C SS. 2011. Single neuron dynamics in human focal epilepsy. *Nat Neurosci* 14(5):635–641.

Widerstrom-Noga EG, Felipe-Cuervo E, Broton JG, Duncan RC, Yezierski RP. 1999. Perceived difficulty in dealing with consequences of spinal cord injury. *Arch Phys Med Rehabil* 80:580–586.

Wolf SL, Winstein CJ, Miller JP, Taub E, Uswatte G, et al. 2006. Effect of constraint-induced movement therapy on upper extremity function 3 to 9 months after stroke: the EXCITE randomized clinical trial. *JAMA* 296:2095–2104.

20 | CLINICAL EVALUATION OF BCIs

THERESA M. VAUGHAN, ERIC W. SELLERS, AND JONATHAN R. WOLPAW

Previous chapters in this book have discussed the technical principles and methods of BCI technology. These chapters show that, despite their current limitations, BCIs are fast becoming effective communication and control devices. However, the rapid growth of this research and its remarkable progress are still confined almost entirely to the cosseted environments of a multitude of laboratories throughout the world. Furthermore, most BCI experiments have been and continue to be conducted in able-bodied humans or animals rather than in the severely disabled people for whom this new technology is primarily intended.

Certainly, there are compelling theoretical and practical reasons for this overwhelming focus on laboratory studies in normal subjects: laboratories provide the strictly controlled environments and expert oversight conducive to the development and optimization of new technology; and able-bodied populations are more available and avoid the additional variables introduced by disease and injury that may vary widely across individuals.

Nevertheless, this focus leaves a major research gap that must be addressed if BCIs are to fulfill their primary purpose and justify the considerable support that their development receives from governments and other funding entities. That is, the BCIs that work well in the laboratory need to be shown to work well in real life, to provide people with disabilities new communication and other capabilities that improve their daily lives.

In some ways, this essential task is considerably more complicated and more demanding than the laboratory research that produces a BCI system. That original research has a single aim: to design and optimize a BCI that provides reliable and accurate communication or control in a carefully controlled and closely monitored laboratory setting. In contrast, research that seeks to establish the real-life usefulness of a BCI system has four different aims. They may be stated as a set of four questions:

- Can the BCI design be implemented in a form suitable for long-term independent use?

- Who are the people who need the BCI system, and can they use it?

- Can their home environments support their use of the BCI, and do they actually use it?

- Does the BCI improve their lives?

This chapter addresses each of these questions in turn. It considers the steps involved in answering each and the potential problems that must be overcome. Since the present peer-reviewed literature lacks any formal multisubject studies that address these questions (and indeed has few reports of any kind that are directly relevant to these questions), the discussion necessarily relies heavily on the authors' experience to date, which is primarily with a noninvasive EEG P300-based BCI system (see chapter 12 in this volume). Nevertheless, the chapter's overall intent is to provide information and insight that would apply to any effort to take any BCI system out of the laboratory and validate its effectiveness in the everyday lives of people with disabilities.

CAN THE BCI DESIGN BE IMPLEMENTED IN A FORM SUITABLE FOR LONG-TERM INDEPENDENT USE?

For some BCIs, this first question is readily answered in the negative. For example, the expense, size, and complexity of fMRI-based or MEG-based BCI systems confine them to laboratory settings, at least for the foreseeable future (Bradshaw et al. 2001; Buch et al. 2008; Cohen 1972; Kaiser et al. 2005; Lee et al. 2009; Mellinger et al. 2007; Tecchio et al. 2007; van Gerven and Jensen 2009). BCIs that rely on implanted devices (e.g., electrocortigraphy [ECoG], local field potentials [LFPs], or single units) have demonstrated impressive capacity both in animals and in humans. These BCIs face the same safety requirements as any device for clinical use, and, in addition, they must demonstrate that they are sufficiently reliable and effective to warrant human implantation (Donoghue 2008). At present, BCIs based on EEG (and possibly also those based on functional near-infrared spectroscopy [fNIRS]) are the best candidates for independent use (Bauernfeind et al. 2008; Coyle et al. 2007; Naito et al. 2007). Even so, their transition from the laboratory to the home, and to long-term everyday use, requires substantial reconfiguration of their components and consideration of issues that do not generally arise in the laboratory.

Any BCI system deployed for independent use must be safe to operate in the home environment without on-site technical support. Components should be few, small, portable, and relatively inexpensive; and the connections between them should be minimized (e.g., by use of telemetry) and extremely robust. They must be packaged in sturdy and configurable

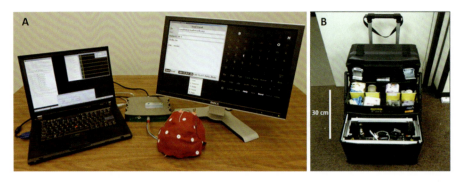

Figure 20.1 (A) The current Wadsworth P300-based BCI home system. The components include a laptop computer, an eight-channel EEG amplifier (Guger Technologies), an electrode cap (Electro-Cap International), a 20" monitor, and connecting cables. (B) A compact traveling BCI evaluation unit designed for easy setup, breakdown, and storage of all necessary hardware and supplies.

housing to provide flexible setup and easy storage and must be able to withstand potentially rough handling over many months. Ideally, the amplifiers should be insensitive to the many sources of electromagnetic noise present in home settings, and the electrodes and their mounting (e.g., for EEG, the electrode cap) should be capable of functioning safely and effectively for many hours per day over months without maintenance or replacement. The software should be easy to use and thoroughly tested (i.e., impervious to BCI user or caregiver error). Before attempting to take a BCI system out of the laboratory, investigators should meet these requirements to the greatest extent possible. At the same time, they should recognize that further changes are likely to be needed when the BCI is actually deployed in the home environment. In this regard the principles of modularity in the software (e.g., Schalk et al. 2004) and in the hardware (e.g., Cincotti et al. 2008) can expedite the implementation of improvements and upgrades, and the tackling of unexpected failures.

Figure 20.1A shows the current version of the P300-based BCI home system developed at the Wadsworth Center of the New York State Department of Health (Albany, NY); and figure 20.1B shows a compact traveling unit for evaluating this system's suitability for potential users who are homebound. Figure 20.2A shows the Wadsworth BCI home system in operation. This system has now been used by seven severely disabled people in their homes over months and years. It is managed by the caregivers in the users' homes, with internet oversight from the Wadsworth BCI laboratory and occasional home visits by technical personnel from the laboratory. The foreground of figure 20.2A shows the crowded environment of the user's room. It is typical of the technically challenging environments of people with severe disabilities.

WHO ARE THE PEOPLE WHO NEED THE BCI, AND CAN THEY USE IT?

Present-day BCIs have relatively modest capabilities. Thus, the communication and control applications they are able to provide are likely to be of significant value only to people with extremely severe disabilities that prevent them from using conventional assistive technologies (see chapter 11). Over the past decade a number of studies have begun to explore the BCI capacities of people who are severely disabled by disorders such as ALS or high-level spinal cord injury (e g , Bai et al. 2010; Birbaumer et al. 1999; Conradi et al. 2009; Farwell and Donchin 1988; Hochberg et al. 2006; Hoffmann et al. 2008; Ikegami et al. 2011; Kauhanen et al. 2007; Kennedy and Bakay 1998; Kübler et al. 2001; Kübler et al. 2005a; Kübler et al. 2009; McFarland et al. 2010; Miner et al. 1998; Mügler et al. 2010;

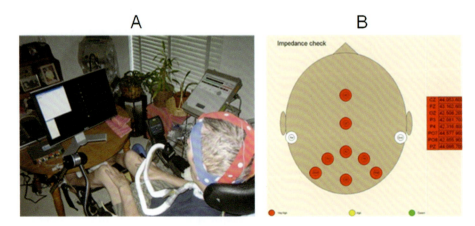

Figure 20.2 (A) A person severely disabled by amyotrophic lateral sclerosis (ALS) using the Wadsworth brain-computer interface (BCI) system in his home. He wears a modified eight-channel electrode cap. (B) Monitor display used by caregiver to check electrode impedance. Red dots are the locations of the eight recording electrodes. When all the locations become green, electrode impedance is sufficiently low, and the caregiver can initiate BCI use.

Müller-Putz et al. 2005; Nijboer et al. 2008; Pfurtscheller et al. 2000; Piccione et al. 2006; Pires et al. 2011; Sellers and Donchin 2006; Sellers et al. 2010; Silvoni et al. 2009; Townsend et al. 2010;). Although some subjects have been studied in their home environments, most of this work has generally consisted only of limited sessions with the experimenters closely over-seeing BCI operation. Nevertheless, the results to date are encouraging in that they indicate that many people with severe disabilities can use BCIs that could in theory help them in their daily lives.

These individuals are usually home-bound (or institution-bound) and attended by caregivers 24 hours per day (Albert et al. 2009). They comprise the target user population for the BCIs that are available now or likely to be available within the next decade.

DEFINING THE POPULATION OF PROSPECTIVE BCI HOME USERS

How does a BCI researcher find good subjects for studies testing the effectiveness and utility of BCI home use for people with severe disabilities? And how does he or she proceed with these subjects once they are identified? As in most clinical studies, subjects are selected according to a specific set of criteria. For the user population described above, the basic inclusion criteria would be:

- Little or no useful voluntary muscle control (e.g., people with late-stage ALS, muscular dystrophy, severe Guillain-Barré syndrome, brainstem stroke, severe cerebral palsy, high-level spinal cord injury, or a variety of other severe neuromuscular disorders). (For people with ALS or other progressive diseases, this criterion might be extended to include those who have not yet reached this level of disability but can be expected to do so eventually.)

- Conventional assistive (i.e., muscle-based) communication devices (e.g., eye-gaze systems, EMG switches) not adequate for their needs: they may be entirely unable to use these devices; their control may be inconsistent or they may fatigue quickly; they may not like the devices; or they may desire the additional communication and control capabilities that a BCI could provide.

- Medically stable, with the intent, and a reasonable expectation, of living for at least one year. If they have ALS, they have already begun artificial ventilation or have decided to do so when it becomes necessary.

- Able to follow spoken or written directions.

- Absence of any other impairment that would prevent BCI usage (e.g., extremely poor vision would prevent use of a BCI that uses visual stimuli).

- Stable living environment.

- Reliable caregivers (family members and/or professionals) possessing or capable of acquiring basic computer skills and committed to supporting the subject's BCI usage.

- Subject and caregivers able and willing to provide informed consent and clearly enthusiastic about participating in a research study that may have no lasting direct benefit to them (Vaughan et al. 2006).

Given the wide variety of disorders that can cause severe motor disability, the complexity of the disabilities they cause, and other variables associated with these disorders (e.g., medication, other medical problems), it may be difficult to determine whether a particular person satisfies these criteria (Kuebler et al. 2006). For example, aphasia, which occurs in over 25% of people with strokes, can interfere with the ability to understand instructions about how to use the BCI and/or with formulation of messages to be communicated with it (Pederson et al. 1995; Wade et al. 1986). On the other hand, a right or left hemianopsia (i.e., loss of the right or left visual field) produced by stroke would probably not interfere with BCI use if the screen is positioned in the remaining visual field. Since many prospective BCI users are older adults with ALS or strokes, age-related visual impairments (e.g., macular degeneration, glaucoma, and cataracts [Streiff 1967]) might also affect BCI capability. Appropriate assessment questions (e.g., can the person read text on a screen?) or a standard measure of visual acuity (e.g., Snellen test [Tucker and Charman 1975]) may evaluate this visual issue.

Another relevant factor includes current medications (e.g., sedatives) that may interfere with brain function or affect the EEG (Towler et al. 1962). Cognitive impairments (which occur in up to 40% of people with ALS [Woolley et al. 2010; Volpato et al. 2010]) and depression may also interfere with BCI use. Although the recent literature indicates that people with advanced ALS generally rate their quality of life as quite high, moderate depression is often present (Gauthier et al. 2007; Chio et al. 2004; Robbins et al. 2001; Simmons et al. 2006; Kübler et al. 2005b). As in other therapeutic endeavors (Kirchhoff and Kehl 2007) (as well as in most life endeavors), mood can affect motivation and play a significant role in BCI effectiveness (Kleih et al. 2010).

RECRUITING PARTICIPANTS FOR BCI HOME-USER STUDIES

Subject recruitment is a key part of any clinical study and often presents significant difficulties (e.g., Bedlack et al. 2010). Recruiting and retaining individuals who have entered the late stages of a progressive neurological disease can be particularly challenging (Shields et al. 2010). Hospitals, regional clinics, and medical specialists are traditional sources of subject referrals. However, many potential BCI home users no longer attend a clinic regularly or participate in routine rehabilitation services, and they may not be under the continuing care of medical specialists. On the other hand, many of these individuals are enrolled in programs that provide assistive technology (AT) for seating, mobility, and communication needs (Cotterell 2008). Thus, subject recruitment is often accomplished by contacting speech/language pathologists and/or physical therapists. Home-care physicians, rehabilitation hospitals, visiting-nurse services, and hospice providers can also be sources of potential BCI home users. Local school districts frequently have information on programs that serve people with extreme physical challenges. Finally, certain registries of patient populations can be useful in recruiting a clinical study cohort (e.g., the national registry of veterans with ALS developed by the Veterans Administration, National ALS Registry Home Page; Allen et al. 2008; Lancet Neurology Editorial 2009). Such registries can expand the number of potential contacts well beyond the immediate geographic region. Registries vary in the currency of their information and in the steps required to use them in subject recruitment (e.g., Registry board approval, local IRB oversight).

Whether a particular individual meets the inclusion criteria defined above can normally be determined from interviews with caregivers, medical personnel, and/or family members. Thus, in most instances, people who do not meet the criteria can be identified and excluded without actually testing them with the BCI. This can substantially reduce the time and effort the research group invests in testing people who do not turn out to be appropriate for the study. It may also substantially reduce the possibility that exclusion might greatly disappoint a prospective subject.

OBTAINING INFORMED CONSENT

The extremely disabled people who could benefit from current BCIs generally lack understandable speech. In many cases their communication depends entirely on subtle movements of the face, especially small movements of the eyes (Neumann and Kübler 2003). Thus, it may be difficult to obtain the subject's *informed consent* for participation in a BCI study. Nevertheless, individuals who retain a clear capacity to control such simple movements and to thereby communicate (e.g., via a letterboard held by a caregiver) can provide informed consent, although the process may require considerable time and effort for all concerned. Furthermore, for studies that are found to pose no significant risk (e.g., most noninvasive BCI studies), subjects may participate by providing *informed assent* (Black et al. 2010). Informed assent requires only that they be able to answer yes/no questions. Unlike informed consent, it does not require that they be able to ask questions.

For people in whom the capacity to provide informed consent (or assent) is uncertain, many locales have established procedures for permitting close relatives to act on behalf of an incapacitated person to provide informed consent for participation in a clinical trial. Although such surrogate approvals may be relatively straightforward for noninvasive minimal-risk BCI systems, they become more problematic for invasive BCI systems, which may entail significant risks (including possible discomfort) (see discussion in chapter 24). For people with progressive diseases such as ALS, informed consent may be obtained (and BCI use might be initiated) during earlier stages of the disease when adequate communication capacity is still present. (Early BCI use may also facilitate the transition to extensive BCI use when conventional communication is no longer possible.)

DETERMINING WHETHER A POTENTIAL STUDY SUBJECT CAN USE THE BCI

For each person who has met the inclusion criteria and provided informed consent (or assent), the next step is an evaluation of his or her ability to use the BCI. This evaluation represents a Go/No-Go decision for participation in the clinical study. In work to date by the Wadsworth BCI research group using a P300-based BCI, this evaluation has consisted of two or three 1–2 hour sessions. During each of these sessions the subject performs a cued letter-selection task referred to as copy spelling (Birbaumer et al. 1999). The goal is to collect data to parameterize the BCI so that the person can then use it to communicate intent (e.g., to spell freely, select icons, etc.). In most cases, as few as 21 copy-spelling selections (i.e., trials) are sufficient to parameterize the system (McCane et al. 2009). With the standard 6×6 P300 matrix (for which chance accuracy is 2.8%), accuracy of >70% is generally considered adequate for effective communication (Sellers et al. 2006).

McCane et al. (2009) used interviews to identify 25 people with ALS who appeared to be good candidates for use of a P300-based BCI. In subsequent testing with the BCI system, 17 of the 25 candidates (68%) achieved the requisite accuracy of >70% and were thus judged able to use the BCI. It is worth noting here that there was no correlation between the subjects' BCI accuracy and their disability level as measured with the ALS functional rating scale (Cederbaum et al. 1999). For the other eight people accuracy was <40%. Seven of these people had visual problems (e.g., ptosis, nystagmus, diplopia) that interfered with BCI use. (Such problems are common in people with late-stage ALS [Mizutani et al. 1990; Pinto and de Carvalho 2008]). These data further emphasize the importance of gathering relevant information prior to BCI testing.

The evaluation of a person's capacity to use the BCI may be particularly difficult with people who lack a clearly reliable means of basic communication (e.g., an eyeblink or muscle twitch). If an individual does not have an obvious and relatively fast way to ask and answer questions, the only way to know that he or she has understood the instructions is for the person to communicate using the BCI, and this requires and assumes that the BCI itself is working properly. The difficult issue of BCI use by people who lack any muscle-based communication (i.e., are completely locked-in) is addressed more fully in chapters 11 and 19 of this volume.

CAN THE HOME ENVIRONMENT SUPPORT BCI USE, AND IS THE BCI ACTUALLY USED?

ASSESSING THE ENVIRONMENT AND THE CAREGIVERS

Successful home use of current BCI systems requires a home environment that can support their use. Home environment assessment can be accomplished first by appropriate questions during telephone interviews and then during the initial BCI evaluation sessions. Home assessment includes evaluation of not only the physical environment but also the level of interest and ability of the users and their caregivers. The immediate environments of people with severe disabilities are often crowded with much essential equipment, including ventilators, mechanical beds, and wheelchairs. Thus, the placing of the BCI system and the positioning of the prospective user may be challenging, and significant sources of electrical noise and intermittent artifacts may be present. These factors, the difficulties they present, and the prospects for overcoming them can be initially assessed in the first home visits. These visits are also an opportunity to assess, at least in an informal fashion, the technical skills, learning capacities, interest, and motivation of the caregivers who will need to support BCI use. Without capable and motivated caregivers, long-term BCI home usage is not possible (Wilkins et al. 2009).

For subjects who have an adequate home environment and are able to use the BCI, the next step is to tell them and the caregivers who will support and oversee BCI use about the BCI applications available and about the time, effort, and specific tasks involved in BCI use. This will allow the level of motivation of both the subject and the caregivers to be further assessed. If they are motivated, a plan may then be formulated incorporating the purposes for which the user wants to use the BCI. For all users, particularly those who still retain some capacity for conventional (i.e., neuromuscular) communication, this planning step should involve both the user and the caregivers to the greatest extent possible. As described in chapters 11 and 19, the participants' involvement is a key factor in the success of testing new and/or old BCI applications. If the subjects and their caregivers are motivated and a good usage plan has been defined, the study can then move on to determine whether the person actually uses the BCI in daily life.

INITIATING AND EVALUATING BCI HOME USE

Initiation and evaluation of BCI home use includes five primary tasks:

- Configuring the BCI to satisfy the needs and preferences of the user

- Placing the BCI in the home

- Training the subject to use the BCI applications and the caregivers to support BCI use

- Providing ongoing technical support as needed

- Measuring the extent, nature, and success of BCI usage.

CONFIGURING THE BCI FOR THE USER

Before home use begins, the BCI should be configured for the individual user. For example, in the standard P300-based BCI, the numbers and sizes of the matrix items, as well as their brightness and flash-rate, can generally be adjusted according to the abilities and preferences of the user. Careful attention to each user's abilities and preferences is essential. Although speed is generally considered important in communication, it may or may not be of paramount importance to a user who has little or no remaining useful motor function (Millán et al. 2010). For these individuals, the restoration of some measure of independent communication may be more important than speed. They may prefer slower but more accurate output to faster but less accurate output. Indeed, one person severely disabled by ALS who uses a P300-based BCI in his daily life chooses to have a 9-sec pause inserted after each selection and thus communicates at a rate considerably slower than the maximum rate the BCI could provide (Sellers et al. 2010). When they become available for home use, BCI systems that use auditory stimuli or combined visual/auditory stimuli may be most appropriate for people who lack sufficient visual function (Farquhar et al. 2008; Hill 2005; Guo et al. 2010; Hinterberger et al. 2004; Klobassa et al. 2009; Sellers and Donchin 2006; Nijboer et al. 2008; Furdea et al. 2009; Kanoh et al. 2008; Schreuder et al. 2010).

BCI applications must also match their users' preferences. Carefully tailoring the application to the individual while working within the constraints of the system design will improve user acceptance and general satisfaction with the BCI. Since motivation is critical in ensuring subject participation, the choice of application is extremely important. For example, people with high spinal-cord injuries who are still able to speak, may not be interested in a BCI application that controls a speech-generating device, but may be very interested in an application that controls a computer mouse.

The BCI applications that have been tested thus far in home use are based mainly on selection of icons presented on a computer screen, and they often include sequential menu formats. They can provide a number of simple functions, including word processing, e-mail, environmental control, and Internet access (e.g., Sellers et al. 2010). Menu formats and sequences can be configured to match the capacities, needs, and preferences of each user. They can support important functions such as: requests for medical or other care; room temperature and other environmental controls; answering simple questions (in print or with a speech synthesizer); interactions with family members or friends; requests for food or drink; e-mail; word-processing; entertainment (e.g., TV access); Internet access; and others. Figure 20.3 shows an e-mail application that several users of the Wadsworth P300-based BCI home system are now employing to communicate with family and friends.

As discussed in detail in chapter 11, guidelines, standards, and examples abound in the field of AT, and BCI researchers

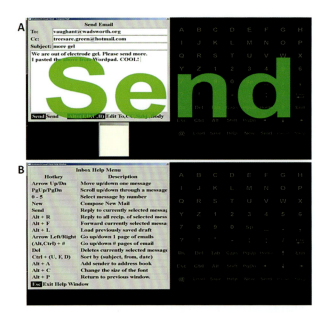

Figure 20.3 The e-mail application for the P300-based Wadsworth BCI home system. (A) On the right is the standard 8 × 9 matrix capable of controlling any Windows-based program that can be operated with a keyboard. On the left is an e-mail that the BCI user has just composed and sent. The green "Send" confirms to the user that the "Send" command has been recognized and executed. The small window below the message is an optional predictive speller feature that can increase writing speed. (B) On the left is the Help Menu, which can be accessed by selecting the word "Help" from the bottom row-fourth column of the matrix (right). This menu lists commands that can be executed through other matrix selections. (See chapter 12 in this volume for full explication of the P300-based BCI methodology used here.)

should avail themselves of the extensive technology, experience, and expertise available in that field. Indeed, BCI home systems are best viewed as technology that extends the spectrum of conventional (i.e., muscle-based) AT technology, and BCIs may be most effective when used as new control interfaces for existing AT devices (chapter 11). BCI clinical research can benefit from innovations in AT and in other areas of human-computer interface (HCI) research and development (e.g., Cook and Hussey 2002; Cremers et al. 1999). These can be as straightforward as language-prediction programs (Ryan et al. 2011) or as novel as the Hex-o-spell (Blankertz et al. 2007; Williamson et al. 2009).

PLACING THE BCI IN THE HOME

In the transition from the laboratory to the home, many new factors that can interfere with BCI use come into play (Sellers et al. 2003; Sellers and Donchin 2006; Neumann and Kübler 2003). Although the nature of their vulnerabilities varies with their methodology, all BCIs systems are likely to encounter a variety of difficulties in making the transition from the simple, highly controlled laboratory environment to much more variable, uncontrolled, and demanding home environments. This is likely to be the case for both noninvasive and invasive BCIs and for BCIs that use electrical or metabolic signals. Because most BCI types remain largely confined to the laboratory, the discussion here necessarily focuses on the problems encountered by the EEG-based BCIs now being tested in home use.

Figure 20.2A shows a person with ALS using a P300-based BCI. It is clear from the figure that, in addition to the BCI equipment, several other electronic and medical devices including a ventilator are in very close proximity. The clutter typical of the immediate home environment of severely disabled people (who are usually in a wheelchair or a bed with various medical equipment close by) requires that the BCI system be portable and sufficiently small to fit into this complex environment. The typical home also has other distractions (e.g., people entering and exiting the room, telephones ringing, dogs barking, etc.) that may interfere with the attention needed for BCI usage and that should also be considered in deciding where to place the BCI. Working together, the user, caregiver, and investigators should consider the setting(s) in which the BCI will be used, and decide how the user and the system components will be best situated.

The typical home has multiple sources of electromagnetic noise that can degrade the quality of EEG recording. In addition to generating ongoing 60-Hz (or 50-Hz) line noise, heating/cooling appliances (e.g., refrigerators) that cycle on and off and other appliances such as electric garage-door openers can produce severe transient artifacts. The ventilators essential to the survival of many prospective BCI users often cause high-frequency electromagnetic artifacts as well as low-frequency mechanical (i.e., movement) artifacts (Young and Campbell 1999). Such electromagnetic noise can be reduced by proper grounding and secure connection of the ground and reference electrodes and by such maneuvers as suspending the electrode cables or simply moving them away from the ventilator. Low-frequency mechanical artifacts caused by head movement with respiration may be reduced by simple solutions such as putting additional padding or pillows behind the user's head or dispensing with the sponge pads sometimes placed under EEG electrodes. Caregivers and others should be instructed to take care not to disturb system components or cables once they are properly placed. Furthermore, it may be necessary to eliminate remaining artifacts (e.g., 60-Hz line noise) with filtering methods (see chapter 7). Finally, in addition to addressing sources of artifacts, it is important to ensure that the electrical power in the home is sufficiently stable. In some situations, use of an uninterruptible power supply (UPS) may be necessary.

As each home environment is different, the various sources of interference must be addressed on a case-by-case basis (Sellers and Donchin 2006). To be suitable for home use, a BCI system must be robust enough to avoid or accommodate these problems. Determination of the extent to which a given system meets this requirement is one of the key goals of a home study.

Another important part of situating the BCI in the home is resolving how the daily data on system operation and other important data (e.g., periodic copy-spelling sessions for adjusting system parameters and/or measuring accuracy) can be transferred to the investigators remotely. Ideally, this can be accomplished in an automated fashion through an internet link. For example, this transfer may use remote desktop control (Cohen 2004). GoToMyPC® (Citrix Systems) is a service that provides secure access to remote sites and was used for transferring BCI data by Sellers et al. (2010). It supports data transfer as well as real-time interaction. A separate license is required for each site.

ENSURING SAFETY AND COMFORT

User safety and comfort and caregiver convenience are extremely important and require close and comprehensive attention. Many years of research and use in intensive care units, operating rooms, and emergency rooms show that long-term EEG use is compatible with ventilator technology (Friedman et al. 2009; Phillips et al. 2010; Tantum 2001). BCI clinical researchers must ensure that BCI presence and use does not affect the functioning of other important medical devices. Prior to home installation, each BCI home system, like all medical equipment, should undergo a formal safety evaluation by a hospital electronics support group or similar body.

Furthermore, users and caregivers need to understand that BCIs do not substitute for standard monitoring of the BCI user who has compromised pulmonary functions and thus that ventilator alarms and other safeguards must remain in place (Fludger and Klein 2008). In designing a BCI system and its clinical study, it is also important to eliminate to the greatest extent possible the chance that BCI (or user) malfunctions might compromise safety (see chapter 24). For example, studies that enable independent use of environmental controls should ensure that the BCI cannot produce outputs that could endanger the user (e.g., by setting the room temperature too high). All the tasks that the BCI enables should be structured to prevent their creation of safety hazards.

For EEG-based studies, there is an extremely small chance of skin abrasion. This risk depends on the particular sensor cap and gel. The Wadsworth Center BCI research group has used the Electro-Cap International™ cap system for 5000+ hours in the lab, has monitored 1000+ hours of its independent home use, and has not encountered a single incident of such abrasion. Despite this reassuring experience, researchers and caregivers must remain alert to the possibility, and caregivers should make regular scalp inspection part of their normal BCI routine.

TRAINING THE USER AND THE CAREGIVERS

In the course of the initial BCI evaluations and demonstrations of the available applications, the user typically becomes familiar with the basic features of BCI use. Nevertheless, to ensure that difficulties do not arise from simple misunderstandings or inadequate orientation, researchers should provide guided practice and well-documented help menus. The more challenging and complex requirement is training the caregiver to support BCI system use. It is essential to have a logical and complete caregiver training protocol. Caregivers must know how to initiate and oversee effective BCI operation. Since fully asynchronous BCIs are not yet available for home use (see chapter 10), the initiation of BCI usage requires substantial neuromuscular function, and thus it involves a caregiver.

The caregiver must learn how to: place the electrode cap on the user so that it is comfortable and properly positioned; add electrode gel; turn the BCI system on; check that all electrodes are recording good EEG signals and fix any that are not; initiate system use; monitor BCI operation; turn the system off; remove the cap and maintain the cap and electrodes in good working order; recognize technical problems or poor performance and request technical support as needed; ensure that data transfer to the research lab occurs as required; and ensure that periodic brief copy-spelling sessions for checking system parameters and/or measuring performance take place.

Typically, the caregiver's training will occupy two or three separate 1-hour sessions and will culminate with the investigator simply watching the caregiver go through the entire BCI usage process (i.e., placing the cap and starting the system, overseeing operation, removing and cleaning the cap), as well as the ancillary processes (e.g., data transfer, copy-spelling session).

Neither caregivers, users, nor other clinical personnel are likely to be trained researchers. Therefore, all information, even for routine tasks, should be carefully scripted. Each training objective (e.g., cap placement, skin preparation, gel application, electrode check, etc.) should be demonstrated and then practiced, with training objectives clearly described and proficiency for each task tested separately (Gursky and Ryser 2007). For the caregiver, the required objectives may include some that are seemingly obvious but nonetheless crucial (e.g., continuing to devote his or her attention to the user while following the instructions on the screen). In addition to initiating and stopping the BCI, the caregiver should also be able to pause and resume BCI operation for essential activities (e.g., tracheal suction for a user who is on a ventilator [C. Wolf, personal communication, 2011]).

Figure 20.2B displays a tool used to train the caregiver and to serve as a reminder that electrode impedances must be below an acceptable level prior to starting the BCI system. Eight circles representing the electrodes can be red, yellow, or green. Green indicates acceptable impedance. Yellow or red indicates that the electrode needs further attention (e.g., skin preparation, gel). Other screens provide guidance in placing the cap and in testing the connections between the computer and the amplifier and monitor. As a general rule, caregiver training is most likely to be successful when the complexity of the hardware and software are minimized to the greatest extent possible.

PROVIDING ONGOING TECHNICAL SUPPORT AS NEEDED

Once the BCI is placed in the home, and the user and caregiver(s) are adequately trained, independent daily use can begin. Throughout this use, and particularly in the initial weeks and months, the investigators should closely monitor operation remotely and be readily available to resolve any difficulties that arise. This oversight is essential for gathering the basic data of the study and also for maximizing the likelihood that the BCI will come to serve important purposes in the user's daily life. The system will be used only if it works reliably and with minimal difficulty. Thus, it is crucial, particularly in the early days, for the investigators to respond quickly to any problems that arise, and to be prepared to correct them immediately.

Many problems may be resolved remotely, through e-mail or phone discussions with the caregiver, analyses of data sent over the Internet, or real-time audiovisual interactions over the Internet. Others may require home visits, and (rarely) replacement of a system component. It is worthwhile, and might be considered a key aspect of a BCI home-use study, to employ a formal system for documenting problems and the time and effort involved in their solution. Such data are important in assessing the clinical (and ultimately the financial) practicality of the BCI system.

To a significant degree, problems may be reduced by careful selection of system components and prophylactic measures aimed at ensuring that they function satisfactorily as long as possible. For example, one of the most widely used EEG caps (ElectroCap, Inc.) has been estimated to have an average life span of 450 hours. This corresponds to 450 diagnostic sessions in a clinical EEG laboratory. However, a home BCI system might be used 5 hr/day, 7 days/week, which is 1820 hr/year (Sellers et al. 2010). Thus, several caps might be needed by an individual home user each year. Careful cleaning and regular cap rotation may extend cap and electrode life span and reduce the incidence of poor BCI performance caused by cap or electrode malfunction. Nevertheless, for a person who uses the BCI many hours per day, caps should be routinely replaced or refurbished every few months, rather than simply changed when they fail.

As time passes, and the skills and sophistication of the user and caregiver increase, problems are likely to arise less frequently. Nevertheless, it is prudent to continue periodic regular home visits, even if at relatively long intervals. During such visits, the user's physical state and environment may be reassessed, applications may be added or upgraded as appropriate, and adjustments may be made in the BCI hardware and configuration.

MEASURING THE EXTENT, NATURE, AND SUCCESS OF BCI USE

The automated transfer of complete data on BCI system operation should allow full quantification of the extent (i.e., days used, hours/day) and nature (i.e., specific applications) of daily BCI use. The measurement of performance, specifically accuracy, is more problematic because, for most routine usage, the actual intention of the user (i.e., the correct BCI output) is not known with certainty. Periodic brief copy-spelling sessions in which the system specifies the correct output are the most straightforward solution. Alternatively, or in addition, appropriate analysis programs (designed with appropriate attention to user privacy concerns [see chapter 24]) may detect errors (e.g., spelling mistakes in written text) and calculate accuracies.

It is also important to monitor other aspects of the user's state and environment for changes that may greatly affect BCI use. Disturbances such as intercurrent illnesses may interrupt the user's normal routine and can greatly reduce BCI use, at least temporarily. Other problems, such as the temporary absence or permanent departure of the caregiver who supports BCI use, and the need to train a replacement, may also reduce BCI use. Fluctuations or progression in the user's basic disease, particularly for users with ALS, may also affect BCI use. For people with ALS, monitoring of this progression may be accomplished with the revised ALS functional rating scale (ALSFRS R) which provides a succinct measure of disability (Cedarbaum et al. 1999). In addition to standard monitoring of these specific factors that may affect BCI use, caregivers and investigators should be alert to sudden changes in BCI use that might be caused by changes in the user's physical or mental state or other factors.

Finally, periodic questionnaire-based interviews of users, caregivers, and family members are useful ancillary tools for identifying system or procedure modifications that might improve BCI performance or usefulness and/or increase user or caregiver satisfaction and convenience.

DOES THE BCI IMPROVE THE USER'S LIFE?

Certainly, the simplest and most obvious measure of BCI usefulness is the extent to which it is used. No matter how simple and convenient, BCI use requires significant commitment on the part of both the user and the caregiver. Thus, frequent use is probably a good indicator that the user finds it worthwhile. At the same time, for scientific evaluation, the validation of a home BCI system requires more formal and substantive assessment of its impact on the lives of its users and their caregivers, as well as on their family and friends.

Recent studies indicate that, despite common assumptions, quality of life (QoL) can be quite good in people with severe motor disabilities (e.g., Kübler et al. 2005b; Nygren and Askmark 2006; Chio et al. 2004; Simmons et al. 2006). Indeed, this finding provides much of the impetus for BCI development. The measures developed for these QoL studies can also be used to evaluate the impact of BCI use.

One of the most important considerations in choosing an assessment instrument is its length. To ensure accurate and complete data collection from individuals who may have difficulty communicating, any instrument should be relatively brief. One such instrument is the McGill QoL questionnaire, which was designed for individuals with advanced disease (Cohen et al. 1995; Cohen et al. 1996). It is widely used as the basis for other, more elaborate questionnaires, including the Simmons scale designed specifically for ALS (Simmons et al. 2006). The McGill questionnaire consists of 17 questions in two parts. Part A consists of one comprehensive question asking the patient for an overall assessment of his/her quality of life (and is itself capable of providing a basic QoL measure). Part B includes 16 questions that cover physical, psychological, existential, and support domains. Answers are indicated on an 11-point Likert scale (0–10). Depending on practicality, additional more complex measures might be used to assess QoL in BCI users with severe disabilities (e.g., Chio et al. 2004; Kübler et al. 2007; Kurt 2007; Lulé et al., 2009; Mautz et al. 2010; Simmons et al. 2006).

In addition to the impact on the BCI users, comparable measures are available for evaluating BCI impact on others (e.g., caregivers, family members), as well for evaluating others' perceptions of how the BCI is affecting the user. These instruments (e.g., The Psychosocial Impact of Assistive Devices Scale [PIADS] [Derosier and Farber 2005; Giesbrecht et al. 2009; Scherer et al. 2010]) may be administered at the beginning of the study and at intervals of some months thereafter. Positive changes in these measures can constitute important evidence for the practical clinical value of a BCI system.

BCI efficacy may also be measured in other ways, such as by its ability to permit reductions in caregiver effort, or to increase the productivity of the user. For example, the independent communication enabled by present-day P300-based BCIs may free the caregiver from serving as a communication partner (and the user from the need to have a partner), or may even help the user to continue productive employment (e.g., Sellers et al. 2010).

DIFFICULT CHALLENGES IN BCI TRANSLATIONAL STUDIES

BCI translational studies confront five difficult challenges that arise from the nature of the user population. First, the users are typically extremely disabled and may have progressive diseases. Their highly compromised physical states, medication regimens, frequent intercurrent illnesses, and dependence on often transient caregivers mean that many factors unrelated to the BCI system itself may greatly affect its day-to-day usage and distort the data that quantify that use. Furthermore, for people with progressive disease (e.g., ALS, multiple sclerosis), their overall level of function and their need for and ability to use the BCI may change markedly over the course of the study. This may further complicate the task of assessing BCI impact. In the case of ALS particularly, a substantial number of users may die in the course of a long-term study (Murray 2006).

The second issue is that it is extremely difficult or even wholly impractical to conduct large-scale fully controlled studies that compare BCIs to conventional assistive technology. The number of appropriate subjects is limited and the participation of each one requires prolonged effort on the part of the investigators. Thus, studies implemented by a single laboratory will generally have small numbers of subjects. Although coordinated multicentered studies are a possible method for studying many subjects, they require an expensive and demanding second level of organization and oversight to ensure uniformity of subject selection, investigator training, and study execution across the multiple sites involved. Furthermore, controlled studies comparing BCI systems with other assistive technology (e.g., eye-gaze systems) introduce further complexity in terms of standardization of methods and uniformity of procedures. One potential response to this problem is a study design in which each subject serves as his or her own control (i.e., uses the BCI for 6 months, then an eye-gaze system or nothing for 6 months, etc.) However, such designs are likely to be difficult to justify ethically (much less implement) in extremely disabled users, and they may be essentially impossible in users with progressive disorders such as ALS.

The third issue concerns study duration and long-term commitment to the user. In general, formal studies usually specify a time period over which each subject is studied (e.g., 1 or 2 years in the case of home BCI use). However, if the BCI is successful, that is, if it substantially improves the user's life, he or she may very understandably want to continue to use it.

Indeed, this is particularly probable for the extremely disabled subjects who are the users of BCI systems now ready for clinical testing. Since these BCI systems are relatively inexpensive, simply allowing the user to keep the hardware past the end of the study may not be a major problem. However, the continuing need for technical support and supplies (e.g., electrode caps) requires continued funding as well as expertise that may be available only from the laboratory that conducted the study, which means that the laboratory personnel need to be available and able to provide the support. Although this problem will presumably be resolved when BCI systems ultimately become reimbursable medical devices, studies with currently nonreimbursable systems are needed to provide the data that will justify such reimbursement.

The issue of commitment is even more complex for subjects who have progressive disorders. The BCI may serve them well initially, but as their disease progresses the BCI may become ineffective. The subject, caregivers, or family members may then ask or expect the investigators to modify the system so that it can continue to function effectively. Although the investigators may indeed want to do this, they may lack the requisite resources or expertise. At this point no general solution is apparent for these very difficult situations, and acceptable courses of action must be developed on a case-by-case basis. It behooves the investigators to anticipate these situations as they design BCI studies and to consider how they might respond most effectively (see chapter 24 for further discussion).

The fourth issue concerns subjects who may well need a BCI, but who do not qualify for the study or cannot use the BCI system under study. The ad hoc development of new modifications to accommodate a single prospective user (beyond those possible in the existing system or readily implemented, such as covering one eye to prevent diplopia) is likely to divert investigator efforts and resources from the study itself and unlikely to be successful. Furthermore, such modifications may well constitute entirely new research endeavors that require their own IRB reviews and approvals. In general, if a clinical study is to be carried forward to completion and to yield substantive results, the range of possible subject-specific adjustments (e.g., matrix brightness, stimulus rate, etc.) should be defined from the start. Subjects who cannot achieve adequate accuracy within this range of adjustments should not be included in the study, difficult though this decision may be for all involved including the investigators. (At the same time, the investigators might still offer substantive help to such individuals as described in chapter 24.)

Finally, the need for initial and ongoing technical expertise often prevents the undertaking of BCI clinical studies altogether, or limits them to individuals or institutions with substantial resources and very strong commitments to the endeavor. The development of effective translational partnerships like that undertaken between the BCI research group at the Wadsworth Center and clinicians at the Helen Hayes Rehabilitation Hospital can enable BCI clinical studies (e.g., McCane et al. 2009). Such partnerships between researchers and clinicians may facilitate and accelerate the translation of BCI systems from the laboratory to successful long-term home use by those who need them.

FUTURE IMPROVEMENTS THAT WILL PROMOTE BCI CLINICAL TRANSLATION

The practicality and appeal of EEG-based BCI systems for home use should be greatly augmented by the continuing development both of more streamlined hardware and software and of applications that are useful to people with severe disabilities (e.g., Cincotti et al. 2008; Münßinger et al. 2010; Sellers et al. 2010). In addition, convenience and comfort can be increased by the development of dry or active electrode systems (e.g., Gargiulo et al. 2010; Popescu et al. 2007; Sellers et al. 2009; see also chapter 6 in this volume). Cosmesis can be improved with more attractive and/or inconspicuous electrode mountings (i.e., electrode caps that look like ordinary hats or helmets). Although the standard electrode cap with gel application functions adequately, gel-free electrodes and more comfortable caps are clearly important to many prospective users. Smaller more robust amplifiers and computers and replacement of wired connections with telemetry should further increase the convenience, cosmesis, portability, and durability of these systems. Decreases in the complexity of the system hardware (e.g., number of electrodes) and software, and increases in reliability, speed, and range of useful applications will also encourage BCI home use.

SUMMARY

BCIs are fast becoming effective communication and control devices. However, they are still confined almost entirely to the protected environments of a multitude of laboratories throughout the world. This focus leaves a major research gap that must be addressed if BCIs are to fulfill their primary purpose and justify the considerable support their development receives from governments and other funding entities. The BCIs that work well in the laboratory need to be shown to work well in real life and to provide to people with disabilities new communication and capabilities that improve their daily lives. To meet these requirements, they must be simple to operate, need minimal expert oversight, be usable by people who are extremely disabled, and provide reliable, long-term performance in complex home environments. Their capacity to satisfy these demanding criteria can be determined only through studies of their long-term performance in independent daily home use by the people with severe disabilities who constitute their target user population.

Once a BCI has proven itself in the laboratory, the translational research that seeks to establish its clinical usefulness must address four questions:

- Can the BCI be implemented in a form suitable for long-term home use?

- Who needs and can use the BCI?

- Can a user's home environment support the BCI usage and does she/he actually use it?

- Does the BCI improve his/her life?

This chapter reviews the multiple complex issues involved in addressing each of these questions. These include: BCI system robustness, convenience, and portability; subject inclusion criteria; informed consent; the suitability of the home environment; user and caregiver education and training; user-specific system configuration and applications; ongoing technical support; collection of data on amount, type, and success of BCI usage; complications by intercurrent illness and caregiver changes; and evaluation of impact on user quality of life. The chapter also addresses difficult issues particularly relevant to BCI studies, including disease progression, the practical limitations on controls and on the size of study populations, and the issues that may arise when time-limited studies end.

REFERENCES

Albert, S. M., A. Whitaker, J. G. Rabkin, M. del Bene, T. Tider, I. O'Sullivan, and H. Mitsumoto. 2009. Medical and supportive care among people with ALS in the months before death or tracheostomy. *J Pain Symptom Manage* 38(4):546–553.

Allen, K.D., E. J. Kasarskise, R. S. Bedlack, M. P. Rozear, J. C. Morgenlander, A. Sabetg, L. Sams, J. H. Lindquist, M. L. Harrelsona, C. J. Coffman, and E. Z. Oddone. 2008, The National Registry of Veterans with Amyotrophic Lateral Sclerosis. *Neuroepidemiology* 30:180–190.

Bai, O., P. Lin, D. Huang, D. Y. Fei and M. K. Floeter. 2010. Towards a user-friendly brain-computer interface: initial tests in ALS and PLS patients. *Clin Neurophysiol* 121(8):1293–1303.

Bauernfeind, G., R. Leeb, S. C. Wriessnegger, and G. Pfurtscheller. 2008. Development, set-up and first results for a one-channel near-infrared spectroscopy system. *Biomed Tech (Berl)* 53(1):36–43.

Bedlack, R.S., P. Wicks, J. Heywood, and E. Kasarskis. 2010. Modifiable barriers to enrollment in American ALS research studies. *Amyotroph Lat Scler* 11(6):502–507.

Birbaumer, N., N. Ghanayim, T. Hinterberger, I. Iversen, B. Kotchoubey, A. Kübler, J. Perelmouter, E. Taub, and H. Flor. 1999. A spelling device for the paralysed. *Nature* 398(6725): 297–298.

Black, B. B., P. V. Rabins, J. Sugarman, and J. H. Karlawish, 2010. Seeking assent and respecting dissent in dementia research. *Am J Geriatr Psychiatry* 18(1):77–85.

Blankertz, B., M. Krauledat, G. Dornhege, J. Williamson, R. Murray-Smith, and K.-R. Müller. 2007, A note on brain actuated spelling with the Berlin brain-computer interface. In C. Stephanidis (Ed.), *Universal Access in Human-Computer Interaction. Ambient Interaction*, Berlin: Springer-Verlag, 4555: 759–768.

Bradshaw, L. A., R. S. Wijesinghe and J. P. Wikswo, Jr. 2001. Spatial filter approach for comparison of the forward and inverse problems of electroencephalography and magnetoencephalography. *Ann Biomed Eng* 29(3):214–226.

Buch, E., C. Weber, L. G. Cohen, C. Braun, M. A. Dimyan, T. Ard, J. Mellinger, A. Caria, S. Soekadar, A. Fourkas, and N. Birbaumer. 2008. Think to move: a neuromagnetic brain-computer interface (BCI) system for chronic stroke. *Stroke* 39(3):910–917.

Cedarbaum, J. M., N. Stambler, E. Malta, C. Fuller, D. Hilt, B. Thurmond, and A. Nakanishi. 1999. The ALSFRS-R: a revised ALS functional rating scale that incorporates assessments of respiratory function. BDNF ALS Study Group (Phase III). *J Neurol Sci* 169(1–2):13–21.

Chio, A., A. Gauthier, A. Montuschi, A. Calvo, N. Di Vito, P. Ghiglione, and R. Mutani. 2004. A cross sectional study on determinants of quality of life in ALS. *J Neurol Neurosurg Psychiatry* 75(11):1597–1601.

Cincotti, F., D. Mattia, F. Aloise, S. Bufalari, G. Schalk, G. Oriolo, A. Cherubini, M. G. Marciani, and F. Babiloni. 2008. Non-invasive brain-computer interface system: towards its application as assistive technology. *Brain Res Bull* 75(6):796–803.

Cohen, D. 1972. Magnetoencephalography: detection of the brain's electrical activity with a superconducting magnetometer. *Science* 175(22):664–666.

Cohen, S. R., B. M. Mount, M.G. Strobel, and F. Bui. 1995. The McGill Quality of Life Questionnaire: a measure of quality of life appropriate for people with advanced disease. A preliminary study of validity and acceptability. *Palliative Med* 9(3):207–219.

Cohen, S R., B. M Mount, J. J. Tomas, and L. F. Mount. 1996. Existential well-being is an important determinant of quality of life. Evidence from the McGill Quality of Life Questionnaire. *Cancer*. 77(3):576–586.

Cohen, T. 2004. Medical and information technologies converge. *IEEE Eng Med Biol Mag* 23(3):59–65.

Conradi, J., B. Blankertz, M. Tangermann, V. Kunzmann, and Curio G. 2009. Brain-computer interfacing in tetraplegic patients with high spinal cord injury. *Int J Bioelectromag* 11(2):65–68.

Cook, A. M., and S. M. Hussey. 2002. *Assistive Technologies: Principles and Practice*. St. Louis: Mosby.

Cotterell, P. 2008. Striving for independence: experiences and needs of service users with life limiting conditions. *J Adv Nurs* 62(6):665–673.

Coyle, S. M., T. E. Ward, and C. M. Markham. 2007. Brain-computer interface using a simplified functional near-infrared spectroscopy system. *J Neural Eng* 4(3):219–226.

Cremers, G., H. Kwee, and M. Sodoe. 1999. Interface design for severely disabled people. In C. Buehler and H. Knops (Eds.), *Assistive Technology Research Series*. Washington, DC: IOS Press.

Derosier, R. and R. S. Farber. 2005. Speech recognition software as an assistive device: a pilot study of user satisfaction and psychosocial impact. *Work* 25(2):125–134.

Donoghue, J. P. 2008. Bridging the brain to the world: a perspective on neural interface systems. *Neuron* 60:511–521.

Farquhar, J., J. Blankespoor, R. Vlek, and P. Desain. Towards a noise-tagging auditory BCI-paradigm. *Proceedings of the 4th International Brain-Computer Interface Workshop and Training Course.* 2008:50–55.

Farwell, L. A., and E. Donchin. 1988. Talking off the top of your head: toward a mental prosthesis utilizing event-related brain potentials. *Electroencephalogr clin Neurophysiol* 70(6):510–523.

Fludger, S., and A. Klein. 2008. Portable ventilators. *Anaesth, Critl Care Pain* 8(6):199–203.

Friedman, D., J. Claassen, and L.J. Hirsh. 2009. Continuous electroencephalogram monitoring in the intensive care unit. *Anesth Analg.* 109(2):506–523.

Furdea, A., S. Halder, D. J. Krusienski, D. Bross, F. Nijboer, N. Birbaumer, and A. Kübler. 2009. An auditory oddball (P300) spelling system for brain-computer interfaces. *Psychophysiology* 46(3):617–625.

Gargiulo, G., R. A. Calvo, P. Bifulco, M. Cesarelli, C. Jin, A. Mohamed and A. van Schaik. 2010. A new EEG recording system for passive dry electrodes. *Clin Neurophysiol*, 121: 686–693.

Gauthier, A., A. Vignola, A. Calvo, E. Cavallo, C. Moglia, L. Sellitti, R. Mutani, and A. Chio. 2007. A longitudinal study on quality of life and depression in ALS patient-caregiver couples. *Neurology* 68(12):923–926.

Giesbrecht, E.M., J. D. Ripat, A. O. Quanbury and J. E. Cooper. 2009, Participation in community-based activities of daily living: comparison of a pushrim-activated, power-assisted wheelchair and a power wheelchair. *Disabil Rehabil Assist Technol* 4(3):198–207.

Guo, J., S. Gao, and B. Hong. 2010. An auditory brain-computer interface using active mental response. *IEEE Trans Neural Syst Rehabil Eng* 18(3):230–235.

Gursky B.S., and B. J. Ryser, 2007. A training program for unlicensed assistive personnel. J School Nurs 23:92–97.

Hill, N. J., T. N. Lal, K. Bierig, N. Birbaumer, and B. Schölkopf. 2005. An auditory paradigm for brain-computer interfaces. *Adv Neural Info Proc Syst* 17:569–576.

Hinterberger, T., N. Neumann, M. Pham, A. Kübler, A. Grether, N. Hofmayer, B. Wilhelm, H. Flor, and N. Birbaumer. 2004. A multimodal brain-based feedback and communication system. *Exp Brain Res* 154(4):521–526.

Hochberg, L. R., M. D. Serruya, G. M. Friehs, J. A. Mukand, M. Saleh, A. H. Caplan, A. Branner, D. Chen, R. D. Penn, and J. P. Donoghue. 2006. Neuronal ensemble control of prosthetic devices by a human with tetraplegia. *Nature* 442(7099):164–171.

Hoffmann, U., J. M. Vesin, T. Ebrahimi, and K. Diserens. 2008. An efficient P300-based brain-computer interface for disabled subjects. *J Neurosci Methods* 167(1):115–125.

Ikegami, S., K. Takano, N. Saeki, and K. Kansaku. 2011. Operation of a P300-based brain-computer interface by individuals with cervical spinal cord injury. *Clin Neurophysiol* 122:991–996.

Kaiser, J., F. Walker, S. Leiberg, and W. Lutzenberger. 2005. Cortical oscillatory activity during spatial echoic memory. *Eur J Neurosci* 21(2):587–590.

Kanoh, S., K. Miyamoto, and T. Yoshinobu. 2008. A brain-computer interface (BCI) system based on auditory stream segregation. *Conf Proc IEEE Eng Med Biol Soc* 2008:642–645.

Kauhanen, L., P. Jylanki, J. Lehtonen, P. Rantanen, H. Alaranta, and M. Sams. 2007. EEG-based brain-computer interface for tetraplegics. *Comput Intell Neurosci* Published online doi: 10.1155/2007/23864.

Kennedy, P. R., and R. A. Bakay. 1998. Restoration of neural output from a paralyzed patient by a direct brain connection. *Neuroreport* 9(8):1707–1711.

Kirchhoff, K. T., and K. A. Kehl. 2007. Recruiting participants in end-of-life research. *Am J Hosp Palliat Care* 24(6):515–521.

Kleih, S. C., F. Nijboer, S. Halder, and A. Kübler. 2010. Motivation modulates the P300 amplitude during brain computer interface use. *Clin Neurophysiol* 121(7):1023–1031.

Klobassa, D. S., T. M. Vaughan, P. Brunner, N. E. Schwartz, J. R. Wolpaw, C. Neuper, and E. W. Sellers. 2009. Toward a high-throughput auditory P300-based brain-computer interface. *Clin Neurophysiol* 120(7):1252–1261.

Kübler, A., A. Furdea, S. Halder, E. M. Hammer, F. Nijboer, and B. Kotchoubey. 2009. A brain-computer interface controlled auditory event-related potential (p300) spelling system for locked-in patients. *Ann N Y Acad Sci* 1157:90–100.

Kübler, A., B. Kotchoubey, J. Kaiser, J. R. Wolpaw, and N. Birbaumer. 2001. Brain-computer communication: unlocking the locked in. *Psychol Bull* 127(3):358–375.

Kübler, A., F. Nijboer, J. Mellinger, T. M. Vaughan, H. Pawelzik, G. Schalk, D. J. McFarland, N. Birbaumer, and J. R. Wolpaw. 2005a. Patients with ALS can use sensorimotor rhythms to operate a brain-computer interface. *Neurology* 64(10):1775–1777.

Kübler, A., S. Winter, A. C. Ludolph, M. Hautzinger, and N. Birbaumer. 2005b. Severity of depressive symptoms and quality of life in patients with amyotrophic lateral sclerosis. *Neurorehabil Neural Repair* 19(3):182–193.

Kürt, A., F. Nijboer, T. Matuz, and A. Kübler. 2007. Depression and anxiety in individuals with amyotrophic lateral sclerosis: epidemiology and management. *CNS Drugs.* 21.(4):279–291.

Lancet Neurology Editorial. 2009. National registry offers new hope for ALS. *Lancet Neurol.* 8:1.

Lee, J. H., J. Ryu, F. A. Jolesz, Z. H. Cho, and S. S. Yoo. 2009. Brain-machine interface via real-time fMRI: preliminary study on thought-controlled robotic arm. *Neurosci Lett* 450(1):1–6.

Lulé, D., C. Zickler, S. Häcker, M. A. Bruno, A. Demertzi, F. Pellas, S. Laureys and A. Kübler. 2009. Life can be worth living in locked-in syndrome. *Prog Brain Res* 177:339–351.

Matuz, T., N. Birbaumer, M. Hautzinger, and A. Kübler. 2010 Coping with amyotrophic lateral sclerosis: an integrative view. *J Neurol Neurosurg Psychiatry,* 81(8):893–898.

McCane, L.M., T. M. Vaughan, D. J. McFarland, D. Zeitlin, L. Tenteromano, J. Mak, E. W. Sellers, C. Townsend, C. S. Carmack, and J. R. Wolpaw. 2009. Evaluation of individuals with ALS for in home use of a P300 brain computer. In *Program No. 664.7/DD38. 2009 Neuroscience Meeting Planner*: Society for Neuroscience, Online (http://www.sfn.org/index.aspx?pagename=abstracts_am2009).

McFarland, D. J., W. A. Sarnacki, and J. R. Wolpaw. 2010. Electroencephalographic (EEG) control of three-dimensional movement. *J Neural Eng* 7(3):036007.

Mellinger, J., G. Schalk, C. Braun, H. Preissl, W. Rosenstiel, N. Birbaumer, and A. Kübler. 2007. An MEG-based brain-computer interface (BCI). *Neuroimage* 36(3):581–593.

Millán, J. del R., R. Rupp, G. Müller-Putz, R. Murray-Smith, C. Giugliemma, M Tangermann, C. Vidaurre, F. Cincotti, A. Kübler, R. Leeb, C. Neuper, K.-R. Müller, and D. Mattia. 2010 Combining brain-computer interfaces and assistive technologies: state-of-the-art and challenges. *Front Neurosci* 4:161.

Miner, L. A., D. J. McFarland, and J. R. Wolpaw. 1998. Answering questions with an electroencephalogram-based brain-computer interface. *Arch Phys Med Rehabil* 79(9):1029–1033.

Mizutani, T., M. Aki, R. Shiozawa, M. Unakami, T. Nozawa, K. Yajima, H. Tanabe, and M. Hara. 1990. Development of ophthalmoplegia in amyotrophic lateral sclerosis during long-term use of respirators. *J Neurol Sci* 99(2–3):311–319.

Mügler, E.M., C. A. Ruf, S. Halder, M. Bensch, and A. Kübler. 2010. Design and implementation of a P300-based brain-computer interface for controlling an internet browser. *IEEE Trans Neural Sys & Rehabil Eng* 18(6):599–609.

Müller-Putz, G. R., R. Scherer, G. Pfurtscheller, and R. Rupp. 2005. EEG-based neuroprosthesis control: a step towards clinical practice. *Neurosci Lett* 382(1–2):169–174.

Münßinger, J. I., S. Halder, S. C. Kleih, A. Furdea, V. Raco, A. Hösle, and A. Kübler. 2010. Brain painting: first evaluation of a new brain–computer interface application with ALS-patients and healthy volunteers. *Front Neurosci* 4:182, (http://www.frontiersin.org/neuroprosthetics/10.3389/fnins.2010.00182/full)

Murray B., Natural history and prognosis in amyotrophic lateral sclerosis. In H. Mitsomoto, S. Przedborski, and P. H. Gordon (Eds.), *Amyotrophic Lateral Sclerosis*. New York: Taylor & Francis, pp. 227–255.

Naito, M., Y. Michioka, K. Ozawa, Y. Ito, M. Kiguchi, and T. Kanazawa. 2007. A communication means for totally locked-in ALS patients based on changes in cerebral blood volume measured with near-infrared light. *IEICE Trans Inf Syst* E90-D(7):1028–1036.

National ALS Registry Home Page. https://wwwn.cdc.gov/ALS/ALSResources.aspx.

Neumann, N. and A. Kübler. 2003. Training locked-in patients: a challenge for the use of brain-computer interfaces. *IEEE Trans Neural Syst Rehabil Eng* 11(2):169–172.

Nijboer, F., A. Furdea, I. Gunst, J. Mellinger, D. J. McFarland, N. Birbaumer, and A. Kübler. 2008. An auditory brain-computer interface (BCI). *J Neurosci Methods* 167(1):43–50.

Nijboer, F., E. W. Sellers, J. Mellinger, M. A. Jordan, T. Matuz, A. Furdea, S. Halder, U. Mochty, D. J. Krusienski, T. M. Vaughan, J. R. Wolpaw, N. Birbaumer, and A. Kübler. 2008. A P300-based brain-computer interface for people with amyotrophic lateral sclerosis. *Clin Neurophysiol* 119(8):1909–1916.

Nygren, I., and H. Askmark. 2006. Self-reported quality of life in amyotrophic lateral sclerosis. *J.Palliative Med* 9:304–308.

Pedersen, P.M., H.S. Jørgensen, H. Nakayama, H. O. Raaschou, and T. S. Olsen. 1995 Aphasia in acute stroke: incidence, determinants, and recovery. *Ann Neurol* 38:659–666.

Pfurtscheller, G., C. Guger, G. Müller, G. Krausz, and C. Neuper. 2000. Brain oscillations control hand orthosis in a tetraplegic. *Neurosci Lett* 292(3):211–214.

Phillips, W., A. Anderson, M. Rosengren, J. Johnson, and J. Halpin. 2010. Monitoring sedation status over time in ICU patients: reliability and validity of the Richmond Agitation-Sedation Scale (RASS). *J Pain Palliat Care Pharmacother* 24(4):349–355.

Piccione, F., F. Giorgi, P. Tonin, K. Priftis, S. Giove, S. Silvoni, G. Palmas, and F. Beverina. 2006. P300-based brain computer interface: reliability and performance in healthy and paralysed participants. *Clin Neurophysiol* 117(3):531–537.

Pinto, S., and M. de Carvalho. 2008. Amyotrophic lateral sclerosis patients and ocular ptosis. *Clin Neurol Neurosurg* 110(2):168–170.

Pires, G., U. Nunes, and M. Castelo-Branco. 2011. Statistical spatial filtering for a P300-based BCI: tests in able-bodied, and patients with cerebral palsy and amyotrophic lateral sclerosis. *J Neurosci Methods* 195(2):270–281.

Popescu, F., S. Fazli, Y. Badower, B. Blankertz and K.-R. Müller. 2007. Single trial classification of motor imagination using 6 dry EEG electrodes. *PLoS One* 2:e637.

Robbins, R. A., Z. Simmons, B. A. Bremer, S. M. Walsh, and S. Fischer. 2001. Quality of life in ALS is maintained as physical function declines. *Neurology* 56(4):442–444.

Ryan, D.B., G.E. Frye, G. Townsend, D.R. Berry, S. Mesa-G., N.A. Gates, and E.W. Sellers. 2011. Predictive spelling with a P300-based brain-computer interface: Increasing the rate of communication. *Int J Hum Comput Interact* 27(1):69–84.

Schalk, G., D. J. McFarland, T. Hinterberger, N. Birbaumer and J.R. Wolpaw. 2004. BCI2000: a general-purpose brain-computer interface (BCI) system. *IEEE Trans Biomed Eng* 51:1034–1043.

Scherer, M. J., G. Craddock, and T. Mackeogh. 2011. The relationship of personal factors and subjective well-being to the use of assistive technology devices, *Disabil Rehabil* 33(10):811–817, Epub 2010 Aug 24.

Schreuder, M., B. Blankertz, and M. Tangermann. 2010. A new auditory multiclass brain-computer interface paradigm: spatial hearing as an informative cue. *PLoS One* 5(4):e9813.

Sellers, E. W., and E. Donchin. 2006. A P300-based brain-computer interface: initial tests by ALS patients. *Clin Neurophysiol* 117(3):538–548.

Sellers, E. W., D. J. Krusienski, D. J. McFarland, T. M. Vaughan, and J. R. Wolpaw. 2006. A P300 event-related potential brain-computer interface (BCI): the effects of matrix size and inter stimulus interval on performance. *Biol Psychol* 73(3):242–252.

Sellers, E. W., G. Schalk, and M. Donchin. 2003. The P300 as a typing tool: tests of brain computer interface with an ALS patient. *Psychophysiology* 42(S1):S29.

Sellers, E. W., P. Turner, W. A. Sarnacki, T. Mcmanus, T. M. Vaughan, and R. Matthews, R. 2009. A novel dry electrode for brain–computer interface.

In *Proceedings of the 13th International Conference on Human-Computer Interaction. Part II.* Berlin: Springer-Verlag, pp. 623–631.

Sellers, E. W., T. M. Vaughan and J. R. Wolpaw. 2010. A brain-computer interface for long-term independent home use. *Amyotroph Lat Scler* 11(5):449–455.

Shields, A. M., M. Park, S. E. Ward, and M. K. Song. 2010. Subject recruitment and retention against quadruple challenges in an intervention trial of end-of-life communication. *J Hosp Palliat Nurs* 12(5):312–318.

Silvoni, S., C. Volpato, M. Cavinato, M. Marchetti, K. Priftis, A. Merico, P. Tonin, K. Koutsikos, F. Beverina, and F. Piccione. 2009. P300-based brain-computer interface communication: evaluation and follow-up in amyotrophic lateral sclerosis. *Front Neurosci* 3:60. (http://www.frontiersin.org/neuroprosthetics/10.3389/neuro.20.001.2009/full)

Simmons Z., S. H. Felgoise, B. A. Bremer, S. M. Walsh, D. J. Hufford, M. B. Bromberg, W. David, D. A. Forshew, T. D. Heiman-Patterson, E. C. Lai, and L. McCluskey. 2006. The ALSSQOL: balancing physical and nonphysical factors in assessing quality of life in ALS. *Neurology* 67(9):1659–1664.

Streiff, E. B. 1967. Gerontology and geriatrics of the eye. *Surv Ophthalmol* 12(4):311–323.

Tatum, W. O. 2001. Long-term EEG monitoring: a clinical approach to electrophysiology. *J Clin Neurophysiol* 18(5):442–455.

Tecchio, F., C. Porcaro, G. Barbati, and F. Zappasodi. 2007. Functional source separation and hand cortical representation for a brain-computer interface feature extraction. *J Physiol* 580(Pt. 3):703–721.

Towler, M. L., B. D. Beall, and J. B. King. 1962. Drug effects on the electroencephalographic pattern, with specific consideration of diazepam. *South Med J* 55:832–838.

Townsend, G., B. K. LaPallo, C. B. Boulay, D. J. Krusienski, G. E. Frye, C. K. Hauser, N. E. Schwartz, T. M. Vaughan, J. R. Wolpaw, and E. W. Sellers. 2010. A novel P300-based brain-computer interface stimulus presentation paradigm: moving beyond rows and columns. *Clin Neurophysiol* 121(7):1109–1120.

Tucker, J., and W. N. Charman. 1975. The depth-of-focus of the human eye for Snellen letters. *Am J Optom Physiol Opt* 52(1):3–21.

van Gerven, M., and O. Jensen. 2009. Attention modulations of posterior alpha as a control signal for two-dimensional brain-computer interfaces. *J Neurosci Methods* 179(1):78–84.

Vaughan, T. M., D. J. McFarland, G. Schalk, W. A. Sarnacki, D. J. Krusienski, E. W. Sellers, and J. R. Wolpaw. 2006. The Wadsworth BCI Research and Development Program: at home with BCI. *IEEE Trans Neural Syst Rehabil Eng* 14(2):229–233.

Volpato, C., F. Piccione, S. Silvoni, M. Cavinato, A. Palmieri, F. Meneghello, and N. Birbaumer. 2010. Working memory in amyotrophic lateral sclerosis: auditory event-related potentials and neuropsychological evidence. *J Clin Neurophysiol* 27(3):198–206.

Wade, D. T., R. L. Hewer, R. M. David, and P. M. Menderby.1986 Aphasia after stroke: natural history and associated deficits. *J Neurol Neurosurg Psychiartry* 49:11–16.

Wilkins, V. M., M. L. Bruce, and J. A. Sirey. 2009. Caregiving tasks and training interest of family caregivers of medically ill homebound older adults. *J Aging Health* 21(3):528–542.

Williamson, J., R. Murray-Smith, B. Blankertz, M. Krauledat, and K.-R. Mueller. 2009. Designing for uncertain, asymmetric control: Interactions design for brain-computer interface. *Int J Hum Comput Stud* 67(10):827–841.

Wolf, C. 2011 Personal communication.

Woolley, S. C., M. K. York, D. H. Moore, A. M. Strutt, J. Murphy, P. E. Schulz, and J. S. Katz. 2010. Detecting frontotemporal dysfunction in ALS: utility of the ALS Cognitive Behavioral Screen (ALS-CBS). *Amyotroph Lat Scler* 11(3):303–311.

Young, G. B., and V. C. Campbell. 1999. EEG monitoring in the intensive care unit: pitfalls and caveats. *J Clin Neurophysiol* 16(1):40–45.

21 | DISSEMINATION: GETTING BCIs TO THE PEOPLE WHO NEED THEM

FRANCES J. R. RICHMOND AND GERALD E. LOEB

Brain-computer interfaces (BCIs) are medical devices developed to overcome functional deficits. The huge investment of time and resources needed to develop a BCI is justified only if these devices can ultimately serve people beyond the narrow confines of investigational trials. This would require commercialization of the BCIs developed in these investigational studies. However, there are major obstacles to the commercialization and market acceptance of any new medical product, and some of these obstacles are compounded for the specific case of BCI devices. Early in the development of such products, it is imperative to address questions related to business strategy and market entry with the same degree of rigor that is applied to questions of science and technology. This chapter presents the nontechnical issues and regulatory strategies from a United States (U.S.) perspective, with some consideration of key differences in Europe and Japan. (These countries are the usual locations for initial market entry since they have both the population and purchasing power to ensure a relatively high level of uptake and utilization.)

Commercial sustainability is a central and challenging issue for any new product, particularly one that serves a relatively small population of users. Even a highly effective technology cannot benefit patients unless it continues to be available from and supported by its manufacturer, prescribing physicians, and caregivers. In a capitalist society, this is normally the job of for-profit entities that expect a substantial return on investment to offset the risk of championing a new treatment or product. Occasionally, philanthropists with a specific interest or government agencies responsible for the common good are willing and able to shoulder at least some of this burden. Nevertheless, for medical devices, both the investment and the attendant risks are likely to be quite substantial. Whether the device is destined to be introduced in the environment of a profitable company or, alternatively, in some other venue, numerous questions concerning design, manufacture, safety, and efficacy must first be addressed before its use can be promoted to prospective prescribers or recipients. If the product and/or health services related to its use are to be paid for by public or private insurers, the advantages must be shown to outweigh the costs relative to the costs of alternative treatments that may be available. Once in use, income from all sources must cover the costs of manufacture, sales, distribution, technical support, and remediation of deficiencies. For any organization, survival depends on meeting its payroll and other expenses in a sustainable fashion. An organization that cannot do so is of no use to patients who rely on its products, especially if those products will need continuing service over time.

DESIGN CONSIDERATIONS— DO WE HAVE A PRODUCT?

SCIENTIFIC RESEARCH VERSUS ENGINEERING DEVELOPMENT

When an academic research team first tackles an unsolved clinical problem, the first step is normally a scholarly collection of the known facts regarding the normal and pathological anatomy and physiology and the details and results of any previous treatments that have been tried. The course of the project depends critically on whether there is sufficient scientific information available to proceed with the systematic engineering of a commercializable product. If not, then the knowledge base will have to be expanded through additional scientific research whose time-course and outcomes are likely to be far too uncertain to be attractive to investors or industrial partners. Thus, such research is typically funded by grants to academic institutions from government and/or philanthropic agencies.

The limited longevity of single-unit recordings from intracortical microelectrodes is a good example of a problem whose solution probably requires advancing our fundamental understanding of the processes involved in foreign-body reactions. At present, we have limited understanding of the extent of these processes (see chapter 5 in this volume), so it is impossible to put a schedule on the necessary discoveries to be made. As these processes are revealed, attempts will be made to target them through chemical, mechanical, or other means, but there is no way to know in advance if or when those attempts will be successful. Researchers may stumble on a quick fix, or progress may be incremental over many years before clinically viable interfaces are available. On the other hand, for signals such as field potentials (FPs) and electrocorticograms (ECoG), clinically viable interfaces do exist and are already in use for other purposes. These may be practical for BCI use within a shorter period of development and might prove to have sufficient bandwidth to support many of the applications originally envisioned for single-unit recordings. Government agencies are willing to support myriad research groups and methodologies in all of these areas and at any level of development because they do not care which one of them succeeds. In contrast, business investors need defined schedules and teams for actual product development and success by their own company. As described in the next section of this chapter, the process and management of this product-oriented engineering and clinical research are rather different from what goes on in most academic research laboratories.

DESIGN CONTROLS

When the knowledge base is sufficient to permit scientists and engineers to start developing a novel medical product, the first steps are relatively unstructured to enable relatively unconstrained experimentation with different methods and designs. The medical device regulations of the U.S. Food and Drug Administration (FDA) designate this as the *concept phase*. The goal is to obtain proof of principle that the application is feasible. The process is exempt from the procedures and documentation of design controls. Human experimentation would be unlikely at this point and would be subject to the usual review by an institutional review board (IRB). At some point in this process the ideas generated in a research lab must be formalized in order to ensure that the product can be made consistently and safely for patients. Before such a product is used in systematic clinical research, its design must be fixed, documented, and carefully scrutinized for potential problems that might lead to unexpected adverse outcomes. This is the process of *design controls*.

It is an oft-quoted observation that nearly half of all problems encountered by medical products can be attributed to errors in design, as opposed to defects in manufacture. Medical products are complex assemblages, and the systems that will be used to derive and use signals from the brain are especially challenging. This challenge is well recognized by regulatory agencies, which now insist that products with significant risk to patients (so-called Class II and III products) (see *Product Classification* in this chapter) must implement a well-controlled system of design steps. These so-called design controls must be applied quite early in the design process—after the concept for the product has been developed but before clinical trials commence and preferably before significant work has been done on how the product will actually embody the concept.

As illustrated in figure 21.1, design controls constitute an orderly method to identify product *requirements*, or *inputs*, in order to meet all of the needs of all product users. These inputs are then translated into engineering language by identifying the product *specifications*. These specifications are, in turn, translated into one or more *implementations/prototypes*. The specifications and implementations form the *design output* of the system. The inputs and outputs are linked by review steps that are mandatory and that must be documented when the product is eventually submitted for regulatory approval. The purpose of this process is to assure that the requirements are well considered and to examine broadly the suitability of the design in meeting the needs of patients, caregivers, healthcare personnel, and society. The design inputs serve as the framework

against which the specifications and prototypes can be verified to assure that the design meets the requirements of the users. The process of *verification* includes the systematic series of tests performed to evaluate the match between requirements and specifications, or between specifications and implementation. Such tests might include bench tests and animal tests. After a prototype has been built, a second step of testing, called *validation*, is performed to check that the prototype meets user needs. Validation is typically accomplished by involving users in the target population in the testing, through clinical trials, focus groups, or human-factors experiments. After all of these steps are completed, the design can finally be transferred to manufacturing, with appropriate ongoing reviews to ensure that the design can be manufactured correctly.

In the United States, the FDA requires manufacturers of Class II and III medical devices (including all invasive devices and other products entailing significant risk to the user) to adhere to *quality systems* regulations that are codified in the Code of Federal regulations (CFR; Title 21, Part 820; typically cited as 21 CFR 820). Quality systems include design controls (21 CFR 820.30) and are inspected for compliance by the FDA. In the European Union (EU) the quality of devices is described in one of two principal Directives (the Active Implantable Medical Device Directive [90/385/EEC] and the Medical Device Directive [93/42/EEC]) that outline similar approaches to conformity to quality systems that are enunciated in the U.S. regulations. However, the primary standard for quality systems in the EU and in Japan is based on an international standard, ISO 13485 (ISO, 2003), and will be audited not by the relevant government agency but by a third-party auditor called a "notified body," with which the company will work closely.

It is important to note that the details of the quality-system implementation in any jurisdiction are the responsibility of the *manufacturer*. In the design-control process itself, the manufacturer must identify what constitutes the design input

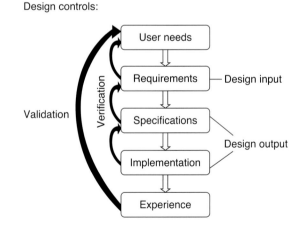

Figure 21.1 *Design control schema (Loeb and Richmond, 2003, adapted from Design Control Guidance for Medical Device Manufacturers, 1997). The boxes at top (User Needs) and bottom (Experience) reflect the external realities that the design-control process attempts to capture. The three intervening boxes represent the results of the design process that must be documented according to design controls defined by the developer's Quality Systems Manual.*

and what constitutes the design output. The manufacturer must also develop a Quality Systems Manual that details the steps it requires to design, build, and demonstrate the quality of its products, and the documents that will demonstrate compliance with those steps (21 CFR 820.40). Much of the manufacturer's documentation regarding the verification and validation of the device would be submitted with regulatory submissions for product testing (Investigational Device Exemption [IDE] in the United States) or with equivalent regulatory submissions in jurisdictions elsewhere. Additional information including the Quality Manual would be submitted as part of submissions for market approval. The FDA or notified body would likely audit the records of the manufacturer for compliance with its own Quality Systems Manual. Companies already in the medical-device business typically have a Quality Systems Manual. Research institutions that intend to develop and test functional prototypes of Class II and III medical devices will need to develop their own Quality Systems Manual—usually from templates and advice provided by industrial consultants.

Design-control principles look forbidding, but they are important for giving structure and documentation to an iterative and complex process. Design control is the mechanism by which the details of the medical product are communicated to others. Because the design-control system forms a solid structural framework for the activities of inventors and developers as the process matures, it is most useful if it is implemented early in the evolution of the project. The relationship between design controls and the research and development process is discussed in more detail in Loeb and Richmond (2003).

RISK MANAGEMENT

In addition to the design-control process in development of a medical product, it is also necessary to engage in a formal process of *risk management*. Risk management is typically implemented at several stages during the life cycle of the product, according to an internationally recognized risk management standard, ISO 14971 (ISO, 2007). As illustrated in figure 21.2, this standard enunciates a step-wise approach to identify, evaluate, control, and monitor risk. Risk-management activities typically include the use of one or more tools familiar to most engineers (Ozog, 1997). For example, failure modes and effects analysis (FMEA) starts with the ways in which each component can fail and considers the consequences of such failures. Fault tree analysis starts with actual harm that could occur and works backwards to all of the factors that could cause or contribute to the harm. Hazards and critical control point (HACCP) analysis looks at processes in the manufacture and use of a product to identify where hazards arise and how they might be minimized. The goal of the risk management exercise is to evaluate and rank the severity and frequency of each identified risk, so that resources and attention are directed toward the most significant risks. In addition, as new risks become apparent, analyses are updated so that the evolving history of the product's development can be documented systematically. This is important because this risk analysis will

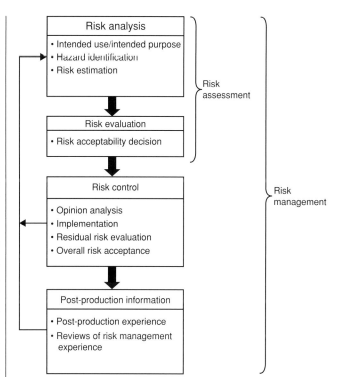

Figure 21.2 *Risk Management Framework from ISO 14971. The evaluation of risk is intended to achieve an appropriate balance between the benefits of the product itself and the various problems that might arise from its use (ISO, 2007).*

form an important part of the investigational device exemption (IDE) application (discussed below) when first approval is sought for clinical trials of new devices that are considered to have significant risk (which will be the case for some types of BCIs).

REGULATORY CONSIDERATIONS—ARE WE ALLOWED TO SELL OUR PRODUCT?

Once it is determined that a product can function as predicted and that its risks are not unacceptable, approval must be obtained from the relevant regulatory authority in the country where the device will be disseminated. In any country the sale of medical devices requires satisfying the requirements of its regulatory authority: in the United States, the FDA; in Europe, the governmental bodies of individual countries that enforce the Medical Device Directives generated by the European Commission; and in Japan, the Ministry of Health, Labor, and Welfare. There are broad philosophical and legislative differences between the United States and the EU. In the United States, regulation of medical products is an outgrowth of consumer protection and truth-in-advertising: the FDA often requires clinical evidence demonstrating that products actually provide the medical benefit that is claimed as part of their promotion. In the EU, the emphasis is largely on documentation of safety, but some risk can be deemed acceptable by a concomitant consideration of offsetting benefits. Clinical trials of an as yet unapproved medical device, or for a new indication for an approved device, require specific permission (called an IDE in the United States; see below) that is highly circumscribed in order to obtain exactly the data required to apply for permission to market the device.

For clinical trials and/or for general marketing, the application and approval process is complicated by differences between jurisdictions in the specific requirements for obtaining approval. For example, in the United States, application is made directly to a division of the FDA's Center for Devices and Radiological Health. In contrast, the EU typically engages a third party auditor/intermediary called a "notified body" to manage the evaluation of the design dossier and the ongoing quality audits that are needed to commercialize a product with the CE Mark (see below). Despite these differences in the formalities of documentation and review for approval of the device, there is a strong trend toward "harmonized standards" in most countries (see Global Harmonization Task Force, www. ghtf.org). For most devices that interface with the nervous system, three types of documentation are required: a technical dossier; a preclinical testing dossier; and a clinical dossier. Together, they are used to demonstrate that the product is designed appropriately and that it performs safely and consistently under certain defined conditions of use.

The product-development process is sufficiently complicated that great care should be used in mapping out a strategy to gain market approval without wasting large amounts of time and money unnecessarily. Several factors must be considered:

- In what country(s) will the product be introduced, and in what sequence? For some types of products, the regulatory pathway in the United States is simpler than that in the EU, whereas the opposite is true for other product types.

- Who is the target audience and how will the product be introduced to this audience? All product safety and efficacy regulations are viewed from the perspective of the intended patient population and conditions of use. Product labeling (a broad regulatory term that encompasses essentially all information provided in advertising, on packaging, in instruction manuals, and on the device itself) must be designed and approved from this perspective.

- What are the associated features of the product? Particularly in the United States, any claims regarding anticipated benefits for high-risk devices must be supported by clinical-trial data and approved by the FDA as part of the labeling. The company must restrict its advertising and promotion to the specific patient population and circumstances of use of those trials, even though individual clinicians

are free to prescribe what are called "off-label" applications of the product.

- What is the product distribution and support system? Most companies producing products for rehabilitation are relatively small and work through distributors, a strategy that may be inappropriate for products that present significant risks and/or require direct training of prescribers, caregivers, or users.

For the purposes of simplicity here, we will explore the very different routes to market that might be taken by a typical noninvasive BCI that records brain signals at the scalp versus that for an invasive BCI using implanted intracranial electrodes.

PRODUCT CLASSIFICATION AND REGULATORY STRATEGY

In the United States, as in other industrialized countries, medical devices are classified according to risk. The U.S. classification system specifies three classes in its Code of Federal Regulations (21 CFR 860):

- Class I devices are relatively safe and require only minimal controls, mostly over manufacturing quality.

- Class II devices have medium risk; quality, design control, and performance standards are set to minimize these risks.

- Class III devices have the greatest risk; they have additional requirements related to clinical performance and safety testing.

All currently marketed medical devices are classified within this structure and there are particular regulatory requirements for devices in each class (see also Kaplan et al., 2004). The appropriate class for a given medical device can usually be determined by comparison with similar or related products already on the market. For example, EEG equipment is covered in 21 CFR 882.1400 and is generally in Class II. There is an approved cortical electrode (21 CFR 882.1310) in Class II, but it is for temporary use. Chronically implanted electrical devices such as implanted intracerebral stimulators (21 CFR 882.5840) are in Class III, suggesting that a long-term, invasive BCI would probably be determined to be Class III by the FDA. Class I devices may not need to be submitted for approval if they are exempted by their low classification. Most products with which this book is concerned will be in Class II or above. In general, devices that are intended for long-term (>30 days) implantation or that emit energy into the body (e.g., stimulators) are in Class III, but they may be down-classified if actual clinical experience suggests that they pose little risk. Class III also includes all devices that are so novel that similar products are not yet on the market, unless the developer can reclassify the device to a lower class at the time of marketing submission, as described below.

TWO ROUTES FOR FDA SUBMISSION

The U.S. FDA has two principal routes for submission for marketing approval:

- the pre-market notification process [often called the 510(k) process, referring to section 510(k) of the 1976 amendment to the Food, Drug and Cosmetic Act]: this is available for products that are substantially equivalent to existing products (i.e., *predicate products*) already in Class II.

- the pre-marketing approval process (PMA): this is required for all products already in Class III or for which there is no *predicate product* (see below) in a lower class.

FDA 510(K) SUBMISSION

The 510(k) is the simpler process, and it relies on the ability to prove *substantial equivalence* between the product under consideration and a *predicate product*, another similar and already approved product that is on the market for the same use. In practice the required level of similarity depends on the perceived risks. For example, an EEG-based BCI used to operate a message service on a computer monitor would probably be accepted as similar to other Class II EEG equipment, whose classification in 21 CFR 882.1400 does not specify or delimit any actual use of the EEG information. In contrast, a similar interface used to control a powered wheelchair might well be considered to be Class III because it poses new safety concerns.

The submission package for the 510(k) product will be on the order of 30–100 pages and should include a relatively simple set of tests to prove comparability to a previously commercialized *predicate* product. Note that the new device need only be as safe and effective as the predicate device; it will not be compared to other, more recently approved technologies or products that may be safer or more effective. Because of the abbreviated path, the 510(k) product is generally considered to be *cleared* rather than *approved* by the FDA.

The reader might wonder how a new device can be considered different enough to have market viability and still qualify for substantial equivalence. The 510(k) process was originally introduced to "grandfather" the approval of all medical devices on the market in 1976 except those then deemed to pose particularly significant risks (which were specified to be Class III). The approved patient populations and uses for these older predicate devices tend to be quite broad or even unspecified (e.g., EEG equipment cited above). It is not uncommon for new devices to incorporate entirely new technologies (e.g., integrated circuits) and cosmetic form factors (e.g., molded packaging) and still be considered to be *substantially equivalent* to the predicate device as long as they introduce no new technical or safety issues. Furthermore, the 510(k) process can be used if the new device marries features of two different predicate products as long as both are already approved and fall into 510(k) or exempted categories (but see Footnote 1 below).

Submission via the 510(k) process is simpler because it reduces the amount of testing required for the new device, relying on the fact that the predicate(s) on the market is(are) already considered to be evidence that such products can be used safely under the same conditions of use. The file itself takes relatively little time to develop and often requires no new clinical data; the FDA typically reviews the file within about 90 days. Thus, a 510(k) submission means that new products can enter the market in relatively short order.[1]

FDA PRE-MARKETING APPROVAL

The more complicated FDA *Pre-Marketing Approval* (PMA) process is required for Class III products because they are considered to have substantial risks that are not adequately addressed by comparison to previously approved products. The PMA process requires a much lengthier submission to allow evaluation of the design, manufacture, safety, and efficacy of the new product without reference to a predicate. Even for a case in which a similar product is on the market, the new product must go through an independent review based on thorough testing of the product under both bench and clinical conditions. Preparation of the PMA submission is arduous, and FDA review and approval of the file typically take up to a year or more.

APPROVAL IN THE EU AND JAPAN

In the EU, a risk-based approach similar to the FDA's is used, although products are divided into four classes (Class I, IIa, IIb, and III), based on escalating risk, and are classified according to one of the Medical Device Directives. A general guidance for risk-based classification can be found in the GHTF Document, Principles of Device Classification (SG1-N15:2006). In the European system, market readiness is indicated by affixing a *CE* (Communauté Européenne) mark, after a notified body has evaluated the technical dossier, the clinical trials where needed, and the company's conformance with a quality system.

In Japan, a separate quasigovernmental agency called the Pharmaceutical and Medical Devices Agency (PMDA) is responsible for assessment of market readiness using a system similar to that in other countries, with final marketing permission recommended to the Ministry of Health, Labor and Welfare (MHLW) that approves the product registration.

---

1. At the time of this writing, the 510(k) process is under scrutiny by the FDA and the Institutes of Medicine. The FDA internal 510(k) working group released a preliminary report on August 4, 2010. Some of the recommendations of that report might affect a 510(k) strategy as outlined above. For instance, higher risk devices, such as those now regulated by Special Controls may eventually be grouped into what may be called "Class IIb," and subject to increased regulatory requirements. Devices that are regulated by "Special Controls," such as the EEG devices, may see increased regulatory scrutiny in the future. Additionally, the multiple predicate pathway, as defined above, has been criticized in the FDA's preliminary report. The reader is encouraged to research the most recent FDA policy on the 510(k) process when developing a 510(k) regulatory strategy for a BCI. See FDA News Release, August 4, 2010, FDA Issues Assessment of the 510(k) Program and Use of Science in Decision-Making: http://www.fda.gov/NewsEvents/Newsroom/PressAnnouncements/ucm221166.htm.

See also Draft Guidance for Industry and FDA Staff: Class II Special Controls Guidance Document: Cutaneous Electrode http://www.fda.gov/MedicalDevices/DeviceRegulationandGuidance/GuidanceDocuments/ucm199247.htm

SEEKING APPROVAL FOR A BCI

APPROVAL IN THE UNITED STATES

For FDA submissions, some of the novel devices developed by BCI researchers will be difficult to classify because they have no predicates. Because devices without predicates have traditionally been classified as Class III, the approval path for such BCI devices will almost always be long. However, if the new device does not pose substantial risks to patients (i.e., as in the case of a noninvasive BCI used for communication), then it may be eligible for a route called *de novo reclassification*. In this strategy, the new device is submitted under the 510(k) approval route, where it will be denied "substantial equivalence" designation (since there is no predicate device). The manufacturer then has 60 days to petition for reclassification of the device from Class III to Class II. This petition for reclassification is more demanding than a typical 510(k) submission, but it is worthwhile for two important reasons. First, the reporting requirements after commercialization are less onerous for Class II than for Class III. Second, the lower classification may help later iterations of the same product reach the market more quickly.[2]

Despite such advantages of the lower classification, there are also some significant disadvantages. Reclassification will mean that the application is not reviewed in the kind of detail that would constitute an approval of the underlying technology and design. The FDA instead notifies the applicant that it accepts the applicant's assurance that the product is "as safe and efficacious as" a predicate product. This *notification* (rather than *approval*) provides less protection from liability: because the FDA has not actually reviewed the product, the product does not benefit from the *safe harbor* presumption available to products that have gone through an approval process and received *approval* from the regulatory authority. In addition, *down-classification* opens the door for the product to be used as a predicate for competing products that can enter the market more easily by the 510(k) route, thereby simplifying their development path. This is an advantage or disadvantage depending on the goal of the inventor. It is a disadvantage if the goal is to establish a profit-making product because it helps competitors. It is an advantage if the inventor's goal is to encourage and expedite innovation in the field without regard to profit considerations.

The box entitled *Regulatory Process of a Class II Non-Invasive BCI* provides an example of the regulatory process for a noninvasive EEG-based BCI. The box entitled *Regulatory Process of a Class III Invasive BCI* provides an example of the regulatory process for a BCI based on electrodes implanted on the surface of the brain (as in electrocortigraphy [ECoG]; see chapter 15 of this volume) or within the brain (as in intracortical recording; see chapter 16).

---

2. Note that the FDA's internal 510(k) working group has recommended that the de novo process be streamlined to be faster and more effective. This recommendation has received favorable comment from industry. See CDRH Preliminary Internal Evaluations http://www.fda.gov/AboutFDA/CentersOffices/CDRH/CDRHReports/ucm220272.

ALTERNATIVE PATHWAYS FOR LABORATORY PROTOTYPES, ORPHAN PRODUCTS, AND CUSTOM DEVICES

LABORATORY PROTOTYPES

Noninvasive BCIs (likely be in Class II in the United States, as approved medical products) may well be considered to be *nonsignificant risk* devices when used as laboratory prototypes in a research setting [see 21 CFR 812.2(b), 21 CFR 812.3, 21 CFR 56]. In this case, the researcher need only convince his/her local IRB to accept that designation and to approve the research protocol and informed consent process (21 CFR 50); neither notification of nor approval by the FDA is required. Later, if a manufacturer eventually wants to commercialize the technology, some of this clinical research experience may provide useful supportive data; nevertheless, the manufacturer will have to generate complete regulatory submissions including documentation of any redesign and required preclinical and clinical data for the actual product. The FDA publishes an Information Sheet Guidance for IRBs, Clinical Investigators, and Sponsors; Significant Risk and Nonsignificant Risk Medical Device Studies (Good Clinical Practice Program, January 2006; http://www.fda.gov/downloads/ScienceResearch/Special Topics/RunningClinicalTrials/GuidancesInformationSheets andNotices/UCM118082.pdf).

ORPHAN PRODUCTS

The U.S. Congress has recognized that the high regulatory hurdles faced by low-risk medical devices can inhibit research and development of products for small markets. Thus, they empowered the FDA to establish a modified approval route specifically for medical devices when no current product satisfactorily treats a serious illness in a small population of patients (defined as incidence less than 4000 patients per year with the condition). These devices are referred to as *orphan products* (21 CFR 814, Subpart H). In this approval path, the first step is to gain designation as a *humanitarian-use device* (HUD). This is accomplished through application to the Office of Orphan Products in the FDA, in a letter outlining the particulars of the device and its manufacturer and arguing persuasively that the population is sufficiently small to warrant this classification. The primary hurdle in achieving HUD status is convincing the regulators that the intended user population is in fact small and is seriously impaired without such a device. For BCIs, this argument is probably straightforward. Classification as a HUD abbreviates the submission path because the sponsor of a HUD device is not required to demonstrate effectiveness (a requirement for PMAs). This may shorten the clinical-trial process considerably. The manufacturer must prove that the device is safe for its intended use and that it offers probable benefit for its intended patient population. Generally, this route is used only for Class III devices.

It may be possible to obtain an orphan-product designation for a noninvasive BCI that would be eligible for Class II designation (based on predicates) as long as no suitable product is currently available commercially, but this would have to be negotiated with the FDA. If a new device has a predicate in

BOX 21.1 REGULATORY PROCESS FOR A CLASS II NON-INVASIVE BCI

Obtaining a Class II designation for a non-invasive BCI depends on identifying one or more acceptable predicate Class II devices from the listing in 21 CFR Parts 870-890 (covering a wide range of electrodiagnostic and rehabilitative devices). The selection will depend on the technologies employed by the new device's interface (electrodes, telemetry, etc.), signal processing and other interactions with the user and his/her environment.

Once a possible predicate device and its associated 510(k) number are identified, it is possible to obtain that redacted application through Freedom of Information, and to identify what elements of the device would need to be replicated or shown to be substantially equivalent to those of the new BCI device. Furthermore, for more recently approved devices there is often a summary of features on the website that is sufficient to begin a design comparison. The predicate device may have its own predicate, in which case a comparison of the two applications can instruct someone new to this process about how the two devices were compared for regulatory purposes.

The following is a list of some Class II devices that may provide useful predicates.

- **Electroencephalograph 21 CFR Sec.882.1400).** *An electroencephalograph is a device used to measure and record the electrical activity of the patient's brain obtained by placing two or more electrodes on the head*

- **Electroencephalogram (EEG) telemetry system (21 CFR Sec. 882.1855).** *An electroencephalogram (EEG) telemetry system consists of transmitters, receivers, and other components used for remotely monitoring or measuring EEG signals by means of radio or telephone transmission systems.*

- **Biofeedback device (21 CFR Sec. 882.5050):** *A biofeedback device is an instrument that provides a visual or auditory signal corresponding to the status of one or more of a patient's physiological parameters (e.g., brain alpha wave activity, muscle activity, skin temperature, etc.) so that the patient can control voluntarily these physiological parameters.*

- **Single-function, preprogrammed diagnostic computer (21 CFR 870.1435):** *A single-function, preprogrammed diagnostic computer is a hard-wired computer that calculates a specific physiological or blood-flow parameter based on information obtained from one or more electrodes, transducers, or measuring devices.*

Once an acceptable predicate has been identified, the manufacturer can proceed with a 510(k) regulatory submission. This will typically include bench and perhaps animal testing to demonstrate substantial equivalence of the new product to the predicate product. If accepted, the FDA will issue a clearance permitting the new product to be marketed and sold for the predicate indications.

BOX 21.2 REGULATORY PROCESS FOR CLASS III INVASIVE BCI

Relatively few Class III invasive BCIs are available on the market currently, and most are under humanitarian device exemptions (see text). Previously classified products that would probably be deemed to pose similar risks include:

- Implanted cerebellar stimulator (21 CFR 882.5820): *An implanted cerebellar stimulator is a device used to stimulate electrically a patient's cerebellar cortex for the treatment of intractable epilepsy, spasticity, and some movement disorders. The stimulator consists of an implanted receiver with electrodes that are placed on the patient's cerebellum and an external transmitter for transmitting the stimulating pulses across the patient's skin to the implanted receiver.*

- Implanted intracerebral/subcortical electrical stimulator for pain relief (21 CFR 882.5840): *An implanted intracerebral/subcortical stimulator for pain relief is a device that applies electrical current to subsurface areas of a patient's brain to treat severe intractable pain. The stimulator consists of an implanted receiver with electrodes that are placed within a patient's brain and an external transmitter for transmitting the stimulating pulses across the patient's skin to the implanted receiver.*

Nearly all Class III devices enter the market through the PMA process whereby each device is evaluated on its own merits without primary reference to a predicate device. Although a Class III device cannot be approved on the basis of a predicate, it is often useful to examine the documentation of the approval application for a device with similar safety considerations. For example, although deep brain stimulators are not BCIs, they do involve many of the same safety considerations as BCIs that use implanted electrodes. Thus, the experience and testing of such Class III products as deep brain stimulators can help to guide an inventor in understanding what will need to be done to gain market approval. In this regard, there are a couple of important caveats. First, the bar for establishing safety and efficacy changes with time, better science, and regulatory experience, so what might work for submissions in one decade may not be adequate in another. Consultation with the FDA at an early stage is essential in ensuring that planning is appropriate and that time is not lost with inappropriate testing strategies.

Class II that is substantially equivalent, then the presumption is that the market is already adequately served.

A number of incentives are provided for the development of an orphan product. The applicant is eligible for R01 research grants up to $400,000/year total cost for four years that are awarded competitively to applicants in a special research competition that is reviewed through the FDA Office (currently RFA-FD-09–001). There are also helpful tax breaks and arrangements to waive certain aspects of Good Manufacturing Practices (referred to as "GMP"). Devices that are sold under HUD rules must not charge more for the products than is invested in the development and manufacture, but within this limit they have no required price controls. For pediatric devices, even this limit on price caps is waived.

Several provisos must be kept in mind before pursuing the HUD route. The labeling on the product must specify that the product has not been reviewed for its efficacy. Perhaps more importantly, the product cannot be sold freely like a typical commercially approved device. Instead, the device can be used only under the oversight of the IRB of a particular treatment center. The IRB determines the particular conditions under which the device can be used within that institution. Unlike in the case of an investigational device, the recipients are not part of a clinical trial with all of its attendant protocols and oversight. The treated patients do not have to sign an informed consent form as in a clinical trial, although they will almost certainly sign the usual surgical consent form and perhaps other documentation required by the institution's legal advisors. If the manufacturer later elects to pursue Pre-Market Approval for general marketing, clinical experience accrued during the HUD phase may provide useful supportive data regarding safety, but demonstration of efficacy will almost certainly require an investigational device exemption (IDE) and controlled clinical trial. Similar humanitarian-use systems are also in place in the EU and Japan.

CUSTOM DEVICES

Custom devices, designed for a specific patient and essentially prescribed by a physician, provide an even simpler route for providing Class II or III medical devices to individual patients (21 CFR 812.3). This path may be useful for designing one-of-a-kind interfaces for early-stage research. However, the IRB needs to review the research protocol separately for each patient and for each device, and this route cannot be used for similar implants in a series of patients. The field of orthopedics often uses custom orthoses designed on a patient-by-patient basis. If an implanted BCI is fitted to a particular patient and is essentially not marketed in a usable out-of-the-box form, it is possible that the single device might be made and even sold as a custom device. The manufacturer can be an academic or commercial enterprise. However, the custom-device approach has several important implications. Because such a device is considered to be part of the practice of medicine, the physician is involved in the specifications for the individual patient for which it is designed. The device goes through no formal submission process with the FDA. The physician and the institution thus implicitly accept much greater liability for the use of a custom device than for one that has been reviewed by a

regulatory authority. If publishable research uses data from a patient who has received such a device, the research protocol (but not the prescription of the device itself) will need the usual review by an IRB.

REIMBURSEMENT CONSIDERATIONS— WILL ANYONE PAY FOR OUR PRODUCT?

A device that is approved by the FDA by any of the routes outlined above is certainly not guaranteed to gain market acceptance. In most developed countries, few individual patients are willing or able to afford expensive medical devices such as BCIs. Costs of the device and attendant treatment are typically paid not by the patient but by a government-run or private medical insurance plan. The viability of these insurance plans requires that they keep costs down. One way to keep costs down is to minimize expenditures on expensive medical technologies. Thus, a key but often neglected area of the regulatory strategy for approval of a new device is the development of a reimbursement approval plan (Raab and Parr, 2009).

ELEMENTS OF THE REIMBURSEMENT STRATEGY

In the United States, obtaining reimbursement for a product first involves assuring reimbursement by the Center for Medicare and Medicaid Services (CMS) (http://www.cms.hhs. gov/Reimbursement), which is the biggest insurer by virtue of its responsibilities for most coverage of seniors, low-income families, and individuals with certain life-threatening problems such as kidney failure. Other insurers often look to Medicare decisions to guide their reimbursement decisions, so CMS decisions have far-reaching implications for market acceptance. CMS approves a new product through a submission process somewhat similar to that of the FDA. However, for CMS, the arguments do not hinge on claims of *safety and efficacy* but rather on claims of *reasonable and necessary* (Scherb and Kurlander, 2006).

For a medical device company to survive on insurance reimbursement for its product, three conditions must be met:

- a coverage decision must be in place
- a code for the procedure or device must exist (or be created)
- payment for the product must be adequate to justify manufacture and sales.

COVERAGE

First, the product must be *covered* by the insurer. Medical devices are often part of omnibus coverage of a procedure listed as a *diagnosis related group* (DRG), and the cost of the product is included in the total amount given for the covered procedure. However, insurance plans often require that very expensive devices be bought separately; and in this event, the insurance plan must make a coverage decision. In the case of Medicare, if the product is sold in too small a volume to justify seeking a national coverage decision, this decision can be made case-by-case. In this instance, the insurer can make a negative or positive decision, according to the judgment of the administering organization, which is often a contractor such as a private insurance company. However, to ensure that coverage will be granted to all individuals who are prescribed a device under the Medicare plan, it is necessary to seek a national coverage decision by formal application to CMS. This process entails some risk: if CMS does support coverage, then all appropriate patients become eligible for reimbursement, no matter where they live in the United States; if CMS does not support coverage, the device will not be reimbursed by CMS in any constituency.

The process to gain approval for coverage is lengthy. It requires submission of substantial clinical data beyond the clinical data normally required by the FDA. The clinical evidence to support coverage must also include information about pricing and cost-savings relative to other forms of medical care, such as reductions in hospital stay or caregiver support. If a new product is not covered by CMS by the time of FDA approval, there will be a delay of at least another year, and more commonly two years, before a coverage decision can be secured. In any case, coverage is not automatic even if the device is FDA-approved. A recent case involving Cyberonics (a manufacturer of an implanted vagus-nerve stimulator that was approved for the treatment of intractable epilepsy) is instructive. The company was able to obtain FDA approval for its implanted vagus-nerve stimulator as a therapeutic intervention for the treatment of depression. The company then applied for coverage to CMS, but coverage was denied because the clinical outcomes data were not sufficiently compelling for the higher threshold of *reasonable and necessary* as opposed to *safe and effective*.

CODING

When a healthcare facility or physician attempts to obtain payment for a covered device, it is essential that the appropriate *code* for the device be entered into the billing system. Without this code, the process to gain reimbursement is long and frustrating. A favorable decision on insurance coverage does not automatically result in an assigned code. If a code does not already exist, then it must be sought and approved. This takes substantial time. Thus, a company developing a medical device should seek expert guidance about the existence of coverage and coding for the device. Some devices will fall under existing codes for similar devices so that this process will be relatively painless. However, a novel device with no marketed precedents could face substantial and unpredictable delays before it obtains a coding decision.

PAYMENT

Even if coverage and coding decisions are in place, the level of reimbursement for a particular product under a preexisting code may be too low for commercial success. Thus, it is critical to gain a coverage decision that ensures adequate payment for the product. If the new product replaces another product that is more expensive, then the new product can profit from the generous reimbursement already established for the product. However, if the new product is more expensive than competing products or treatments, a readjustment of the payment schedule is needed. In the past, this has been a major impediment for new, relatively costly products with small target markets. However, a new scheme called the *new technology add-on payment (NTAP)* scheme was introduced in 2000. Although it has been further developed in recent years to address this problem, the program has not been very successful to date. Clyde et al. (2008) reported that 28 applications had been filed for consideration under this program, but only seven met the appropriate criteria and were approved.

PROVING REASONABLE AND NECESSARY

The notion that a product is *reasonable and necessary* is a central tenet of reimbursement by a healthcare insurer. Satisfaction of the criteria for *reasonable* requires clinical evidence that the product is not unreasonably expensive for the benefit that it provides. Satisfaction of the criteria for *necessary* requires clinical evidence that the product is therapeutically important.

First, insurers will ask: Are BCI devices *necessary* for the patients targeted? Insurers might argue that such patients have been managed in other ways for a long time and that such interfaces will not substantially improve health outcomes and may, in fact, add risks and costs to the health care of the individuals. If the devices can return patients to work, or decrease their utilization of hospital or health-provider services, it may be to the insurer's benefit to cover the technology. To provide such information for a new device, it is important to define very early what data will be needed to make the relevant arguments to CMS. This will allow the necessary data to be collected from the same clinical trials that are undertaken for the FDA submission. Of particular note is the fact that obtaining the data needed for CMS submission often necessitates following patients for a longer period of time than that needed for FDA submissions. A typical FDA pre-market trial seldom requires more than one year of follow-up for an individual patient, although patients are usually consented for follow-up until the end of the trial. Therefore, the first patients to be enrolled in the trial are generally followed longer than the last patients to be enrolled. For studies assessing the economic impact of the technology, clear documentation of net cost savings may need data collected over several years, effectively spreading out over several years the high initial costs associated with providing the system.

Second, insurers will ask: Are the costs of BCIs *reasonable* for the assistance that they provide to patients? To assess this, CMS requires documentation of *all* costs associated with long-term use, including service, repair, follow-up expenses, and management of any adverse events. Furthermore, the costs for recipients of the treatment who cease to benefit as a result of death or deterioration secondary to their underlying pathology must be included in the total costs. Obtaining sufficient clinical data from a small and widely scattered population of potential users generally requires recruitment at multiple centers beyond the institution that pioneered the new technology. This may result in poorer patient selection, increased adverse events, or reduced retention for long-term follow-up, all of which can make the case for reimbursement weaker than it appeared to be during the original pilot studies.

For an implanted BCI, it may be a challenge to make the case for satisfaction of the *reasonable* criterion. For example, if an implanted BCI were priced at $25,000–$40,000 (the price range for a cochlear implant), this cost would be substantial for an insurance company and would not currently be on their payment schedule for the kinds of conditions considered here. The case would depend on careful documentation of the current costs of care for the patient, including the significant costs of healthcare delivery to a patient with poor mobility and communication capabilities, which might be reduced by utilizing the new device.

WORKING WITH INSURERS

Although CMS is an important source of reimbursement for medical devices, BCI manufacturers may still have to assist their individual client patients and healthcare facilities in obtaining reimbursement from individual insurance plans. This battle is often more political than medical. Patient advocacy groups and philanthropic foundations can be critical allies, particularly in a field such as spinal cord injury. The opinions of physicians and therapists will also be important, but it is important to remember that they are also business proprietors. If the prescription and management of new technology reduce their costs or increase their billable procedures, they are more likely to engage in the often tedious process of securing reimbursement on a case-by-case basis after the basic coverage decisions are in place.

GLOBAL MARKETING

Medical-device marketing is seldom limited to a single country. Thus, for any product, an analysis such as that outlined above for the United States should also be mapped out for other countries where the product will ultimately be sold. The data required for regulatory and reimbursement approval in other countries will vary according to the classification and specific risks and benefits of the product.

There has been a fairly successful international effort to harmonize many aspects of the regulatory process. With proper planning, data collected for the U.S. FDA can support global applications. Conversely, clinical trial data from other countries can generally be used for the FDA. Nevertheless, reimbursement decisions and procedures remain highly balkanized (Simoens, 2008). Each country in Europe, each province in Canada, and each public and private insurer in the United States makes its own decisions based on financial considerations as well as on its own perception of the political climate among the local constituencies, healthcare professionals, and business associations. In many European countries, individual hospitals or healthcare districts may have fixed annual budgets for a large class of services and devices. Their decisions to provide a particular technology may depend on timing in the fiscal year and the influence of individual practitioners. In any venue, partnerships with other companies or with local distributors

can often facilitate the understanding and navigation of complicated systems of reimbursement.

FINANCIAL CHALLENGES— IS THE ENDEAVOR SUSTAINABLE?

The following analysis assumes that BCI technology will at least eventually be manufactured and supported by a commercial entity. This is the general route for making products available in a capitalist economic system such as now prevails in virtually all industrialized nations. Experience with similar products and endeavors provides a basis for rational analysis of the opportunities and challenges. It is also possible that a private philanthropist, or society in general, would decide to endow a noncommercial entity, based on the particularly compelling circumstances of typical candidates for BCIs. Given their unique nature, a formal analysis of such options based on precedents is not possible, but we will consider some potential scenarios here.

FUNDING A START-UP COMPANY

VENTURE CAPITAL AND ANGEL INVESTORS
The decision to start a for-profit business to build a new medical product is necessarily driven by the anticipated return on investment, prorated by the probability of success and discounted according to the delay until profitability. Professional investors known as *venture capitalists* (VCs) or *angels* are early-stage investors who appropriately use such a dispassionate analysis as the basis for deciding to invest in a device. Inventors and pioneers of new treatments may also be investing their own money in the start-up company; since they are also investing professional time (*sweat equity*), the decisions are more complicated. A company must generate a profit if it is to survive and make its products available to patients. If it cannot generate a profit, the products, no matter how effective they may be, will not be available. Investors also want to have a defined *exit strategy*—the mechanism and schedule by which they will be able to liquidate their original investment times a substantial multiplier (~10×) for the risk that they have taken with their money. This usually involves building the company to sufficient size and profitability that it can be sold to a larger entity or to the general public through an initial public offering of common stock. The box entitled *Building a Technology Start-Up Company Box* describes a typical scenario.

As the scenario described in the box shows, it is likely to be difficult to convince investors to initiate commercial development of even noninvasive BCI devices from scratch. One powerful way to make a risky business proposition more attractive is to leverage a small investment into a larger effort by taking advantage of research grants from government agencies and charitable foundations. This is particularly important for a field like BCI technology where the risks are high and the market is likely to be modest at best. As shown in the scenario described in the box, equity investment dilutes ownership, reducing the already limited upside potential of the original investors. By contrast, grants and contracts represent operating revenue, reducing the "burn rate" at which the original capital investment is consumed and thus making the balance sheet much more attractive to new investors or potential acquirers of the business.

FEDERAL GRANTS IN THE UNITED STATES

The appropriations legislation for most federal agencies in the United States now includes the requirement that a minimum percentage of their extramurally directed funding (called a *set-aside*) be allocated to U.S. small-business entities, defined as companies with less than 500 employees. Two types of small-business grants are available.

Small Business Technology Transfer (STTR) grants require a partnership with a nonprofit research institution that will perform at least 30% of the funded research. The STTR set-aside is currently only 0.3%, and these grants are reviewed by the usual mechanisms (e.g., NIH Study Sections), resulting in fairly low success rates. *Small Business Innovative Research* (SBIR) grants have a set-aside of 2.5% and are often reviewed by special panels with greater focus on product development and business opportunities. SBIR grants can be spent entirely by the small business, or they can include an academic subcontract

(not to exceed 30% of the awarded funds). The principal investigator (PI) for an STTR can have primary employment at either the business or the academic entity, whereas the PI for an SBIR must be employed primarily by the small-business entity.

Both STTR and SBIR grants are applied for and awarded in phases. Phase 1 pilot-study grants are small ($75–100K) and brief (~6 months). Phase 2 development awards are substantial ($750K–1M) and longer (2 years). An additional Phase 3 is also available in some programs but only with substantial cost-sharing by the small business. The rules and procedures for the STTR and SBIR grant applications are surprisingly similar to those for regular academic grants: scholarly reviews of the literature, detailed research plans, forms to complete, limited submission dates, and a long delay to review and award. The result is that these programs are relatively unattractive and relatively inaccessible to typical small businesses, which usually need to make rapid, incremental changes to existing products using staff engineers unfamiliar with academic research. In contrast, start-up companies with academic roots enjoy relatively high success rates, particularly in the well-funded SBIR program. Since the SBIR requires that the PI be employed

---

BOX 21.3 BUILDING A TECHNOLOGY START-UP COMPANY

- The inventors of a novel treatment raise $5M capital to start their business by selling 50% of their company to VCs. This deal implicitly values the intellectual property (patents, copyrights, experience, expertise, etc.) at $5M and the total company worth at $10M.

- At the end of 2 years, the $5M has been spent and the initial clinical trial data are encouraging, but the company is not yet turning a net profit, so more capital must be sought to keep business development going or everything invested to date will be lost.
  - If the results are very strong and a substantial market appears to be imminent, it may be possible to raise another $5M by issuing new shares equal to 20% of the value of the company. This implicitly values the company at $25M and causes a small dilution in percentage ownership by the original investors to 40%, now worth $10M (on paper).
  - If the results are modest and the remaining course appears lengthy, the company may have to raise $10M by issuing new stock representing 80% of the recapitalized company, effectively diluting the original investors to 10% ownership of a company worth only $12.5M. This represents a paper loss of $3.75M of their original investment, hence the term "down round" for such a second stage of financing.

Throughout these ups or downs, the only way the investors can recover their investment is to sell their shares to someone else; liquidating the company's assets will return only pennies on the dollar. The average success rate for technology start-ups is about 10% with profitability after 2-3 years; it is probably lower and much longer for novel medical devices because of the large regulatory and reimbursement risks. For this reason, VCs generally operate as pooled investment funds, with many concurrent projects in the hope that at least one will succeed.

- Just to break even (and not counting the cost of tying up their capital for several years), the VC doing first-round investments of $5M in 10 different companies would have to sell its share of one company for $50M, representing a corporate valuation of well over $100M, depending on dilution subsequent to the first round.

- Companies in the medical device sector can expect price:earnings ratios of 15:1 up to 50:1 depending on prospects for further growth. At a P:E of 20, a $100M company would have to generate $5M in net profits after all expenses.
- The selling price for a typical medical product will probably allow 10% profits, with 20% for cost-of-goods, 20% for management and infrastructure, and 50% for cost-of-sales (advertising, distributor's mark-ups, clinician training, technical support, etc.).
- So the company will need at least $50M/yr in sales when the original investors are ready to exit.
- That sales target would represent 5000 units/yr at $10K/unit, a challenging goal for most BCI applications currently under development.

at least 50% by the small-business entity, it has given rise to companies that are essentially SBIR-mills whose revenue is derived from such grants rather than from sales of actual products. When such efforts do not result in sales of actual products, they do not in the end satisfy the original intent of the law.

FINDING AND WORKING WITH BUSINESS PARTNERS
Business Partner Expertise

The doctoral-level scientists, engineers, and physicians who are the likely inventors of new medical technologies typically acquire deep but narrow expertise about a particular field of science or technology and are usually not well versed in fields such as business and law. When such inventors start a business based on their technical expertise, they often fail to perceive this shortcoming, ultimately dooming the enterprise regardless of its technical merit. The process of seeking and involving investors in a new business should be seen as an opportunity to rectify this problem, not limited just to the matter of acquiring working capital. Both the scientists and investors need to see this process as an opportunity to learn and assess. In the end, the success of the enterprise depends at least as much on fully utilizing the capabilities of both sides as on the amount of capital actually raised. If the investors are too inexperienced or emotionally involved to see that an enterprise is not commercially viable, an inevitable failure is simply postponed and magnified, valuable time is wasted, and a history is created that may poison the climate for future investment in related products and markets.

When outside investors are brought into a small business, the inventors must recognize that the investors will necessarily be sharing in ownership and control of the company, all according to the contractually agreed terms. Those terms are often rather complex because they must anticipate a huge range of contingencies in the development of new technologies, products, and markets. The development process almost inevitably takes longer and costs more than originally anticipated, leading to the need for multiple rounds of funding and further sharing of ownership and control (see box entitled *Building a Technology Start-Up Company*.) At the outset, it is important for researchers contemplating such a transfer to examine their personal motives. If the goal is to amass personal wealth or to realize their personal vision of the final product, they are likely to be disappointed. Surprisingly often, the product or market that actually results in commercial success is rather unlike the one that the researchers originally sought to develop. Much of the credit for and the profit from a success will go to those who correctly perceive, invest in, and exploit "market pull" rather than "technology push," and these people are often not the inventors of the original technology. In the long run, it is important that business-oriented individuals have some control for the company to succeed, because they provide not only capital, but also essential expertise to the company.

Reversion Rights

In setting the terms for the contract between investors and inventors, it is also important for the inventors to have some *reversion rights* to the technology if the enterprise fails (as most technology start-ups actually do). Without such reversion rights, any assets including intellectual property (IP) licensed to or owned by the company will be held by the receiver in the event of a bankruptcy, and the receiver could retain these indefinitely in the hope of a windfall through licensing to or infringement by a future entity. Reversion of IP to the nonprofit institution in which it was originally developed will at least make it possible to start again with another commercial or noncommercial attempt at developing the technology.

POSSIBLE ALTERNATIVE OPTIONS FOR DISSEMINATING AND SUPPORTING BCIs

An objective analysis of the commercial opportunities for present BCI technologies and markets reveals substantial challenges. The rate, accuracy, and reliability of the command signals currently obtainable from both transcutaneous and implanted BCIs are still relatively low, thus limiting their immediate appeal to a relatively small population of patients for whom there are essentially no other communication alternatives (e.g., people locked-in by brainstem strokes or by late-stage ALS; see chapter 19). Providing even a slow communication channel to such patients may greatly improve their quality of life, but it will not necessarily reduce their cost to insurers. Furthermore, the initial prescription and calibration, and the ongoing maintenance, of a BCI system, even a noninvasive system, are likely to involve additional professional services and may increase the required sophistication and daily workload of the caregivers.

These considerations, and the relatively small numbers of such severely disabled individuals, may discourage commercial entities' interest in present-day BCI systems. Thus, BCIs are in danger of becoming an *orphan technology*, a technology that is effective but that lacks viable commercial avenues for its dissemination to people who need it. Nevertheless, dissemination might be enabled by special strategies that circumvent or overcome this practical problem.

Given the extreme need and limited numbers of potential BCI users, it may be possible to induce a philanthropic foundation to guarantee a market base by agreeing to purchase, distribute, and support a certain number of units, thereby reducing the costs of marketing, sales, and distribution, and also thereby mitigating reimbursement risk, at least initially. Alternatively, it might be possible for a nonprofit foundation dedicated to such dissemination and support to establish itself as a permanent self-sustaining entity. Its income might come from grants (public or private), donations, and limited fees, and, if it also supports further BCI research and development, from licensing BCI-related intellectual property to commercial entities. One effort to develop such a foundation has recently begun (see www.braincommunication.org). It remains to be seen whether this alternative to commercial dissemination and support of BCI systems can be effective and sustainable.

Another possible alternative to dissemination of BCIs as medical products is to focus research and development on simplifying noninvasive BCI systems so that they can be priced and used as consumer "lifestyle" products, similar to a specialized mouse or computer game (e.g., "Brainwave Pong" toys now available commercially). If no medical claims were made in their promotion and they could be purchased and used without involving a prescribing physician, these BCIs might not be classified as regulated medical devices. This strategy could substantially reduce development time and expense, and it might greatly enhance market size, and thus commercial viability. At the same time, of course, the systems would need to incorporate capabilities and practicality suitable for the extremely disabled people who constitute the original target population.

The ultimate solution to the problem of BCIs potentially becoming orphan technology will be the realization of BCI systems that are far more capable, more practical, and more easily maintained. With such improvements in BCI capabilities and convenience, BCI technology could expand into much larger clinical markets and perhaps even to important nonmedical applications. This market expansion would make this technology more appealing to commercial entities. Military research has long been interested in BCIs for hands-free communication and control, and some promising applications in rapid image classification that are relevant to military needs have emerged recently (see chapter 23, this volume). Although such applications do not directly serve disabled people, their development could provide the critical incentive for the commercialization of BCIs that can then be adapted and approved for clinical markets.

TRENDS AND CONCLUSIONS

The present climate for developing novel medical devices is a rapidly evolving mix of both positive and negative factors. Most of the mature and profitable neural devices currently in use (particularly implanted devices such as cochlear implants, deep brain stimulators, and spinal cord stimulators) are based on foundational development in academia that occurred 20–30 years ago. At that time, there were fewer regulations on investigational use of medical devices, and insurance reimbursement was readily obtained based on largely anecdotal evidence. Today, regulatory processes present substantial barriers to both academic research on and commercialization of new technologies such as BCIs. On the positive side, successful products have spawned a sophisticated medical-device industry that now includes suppliers of high-tech, high-reliability components, consultants, and service organizations that can handle the bureaucratic tasks, and well-capitalized companies actively seeking opportunities to expand their product lines and markets. The stakes are higher, and the players are more sophisticated than they were in the past. In order to participate meaningfully in these endeavors, academic researchers need to understand more than just the science and technology (Zenios et al., 2010).

The first place to start is with careful, objective analysis of the risks and rewards of any proposed development effort. From their scientific research, academicians are already familiar with systematic collection of data, projection and analysis of trends, and logical deduction. They need to apply these analytic capabilities to business-related considerations: size of markets, cost of goods, regulatory and reimbursement risk, cost of sales and support, and return on investment. If the academic researcher does not have the knowledge or tools to evaluation these factors, the input of a business-knowledgeable partner becomes even more essential. In any case, the academic researcher needs to consider these factors at the outset, to inform decisions such as whether to proceed with a particular research project, how to design a prototype product, and how to collect the data about clinical applications that will spark interest in potential investors and business partners. The typical academic endeavors of securing grant funds and publishing journal articles may advance the basic knowledge needed to develop a product, but these alone will not directly benefit patients who need the new medical devices.

At least for the immediate future, BCI systems are likely to be orphan technology with limited commercial appeal. Their dissemination to the small populations of severely disabled individuals who need them may require special strategies including (but not limited to) philanthropic support or efforts that combine their development with that of BCI systems for use by people without disabilities.

REFERENCES

Clyde AT, Bockstedt L, Farkas JA, Jackson C (2008) Experience with Medicare's New Technology Add-on Payment Program. *Health Affairs* 27(6): 1632–1641.

ISO 13485:2003 Medical devices—Quality management systems—Requirements for regulatory purposes. http://www.iso.org/iso/iso_catalogue/catalogue_tc/catalogue_detail.htm?csnumber=36786

ISO 14971:2007 Medical devices—Application of risk management to medical devices. http://www.iso.org/iso/iso_catalogue/catalogue_tc/catalogue_detail.htm?csnumber=38193).

Kaplan AV, Baim DS, Smith JJ, Feigal DA, Simons M, Jefferys D, Fogarty TJ, Kuntz RE, Leon MB (2004) Medical device development: From prototype to regulatory approval. *Circulation* 109:3068–3072.

Loeb GE, Richmond FJR (2003) Making design controls useful for research and development. *Medical Device and Diagnostic Industry* 25(4):63–68.

Ozog H (1997) Risk management in medical device design. *Medical Device and Diagnostic Industry* 19(10):112.

Raab G, Parr D (2009) From medical invention to clinical practice: The reimbursement challenge facing new device procedures and technology–Part 2: Coverage. *J. Am. Coll. Radiol.* 3(10):772–777.

Scherb ER, Kurlander SS (2006) Requirements for Medicare coverage and reimbursement for medical devices. In Becker KM, Whyte JJ, Eds. *Clinical Evaluation of Medical Devices,* 2nd ed., Totowa, NJ: Humana Press.

Simoens S (2008) Health economics of medical devices: Opportunities and challenges. *J Med Econ* 11(4):713–717.

Zenios S, Makower J, Yock PG, Brinton TJ, Kumar UN, Denend L, Krummel T (2010) *Biodesign: The Process of Innovating Medical Technologies,* Cambridge: Cambridge University Press.

22 | BCI THERAPEUTIC APPLICATIONS FOR IMPROVING BRAIN FUNCTION

JANIS J. DALY AND RANGANATHA SITARAM

Brain-computer interfaces (BCIs) have been widely studied for their ability to facilitate communication and control. They have not been widely studied for their ability to facilitate or *induce recovery* of function. The exploration of BCI uses for inducing or facilitating recovery of motor, cognitive, or emotional function has just begun, and it is the subject of this chapter.

This chapter describes ways in which BCIs might be used as therapeutic tools to restore more normal motor control and more normal cognitive and emotional function to people with disabilities, and it reviews the exploratory studies to date. This is an important endeavor because conventional rehabilitation methods are often ineffective, or only minimally effective, in restoring these functions to people with neurological injury or disease. The persistence of motor and cognitive impairments in many of these people has made it imperative to investigate promising new methods and technologies of all kinds.

As described in previous chapters, many studies have shown that BCIs can provide communication and control capabilities to people who are paralyzed. These BCI applications *substitute* for lost neuromuscular functions. They are not intended or expected to change the nervous system so as to restore normal function. In contrast, the BCI applications described in this chapter are intended to help people *regain* normal functions lost due to injury or disease. Since the development of BCI applications of this kind is just beginning, most of the studies that have been reported are only preliminary and involve only small numbers of human subjects. Nevertheless, they are worthy of discussion because, in some cases, they provide promising results that justify further study.

Although their purpose is different from that of BCIs for communication and control, BCIs for these therapeutic purposes possess the essential properties of any BCI: they measure the user's brain signals and convert them into an output that provides immediate feedback to the user. That is, they establish a real-time, closed-loop interaction between the user and the BCI system. What differs in the use of BCIs for therapeutic purposes is that the feedback is designed to modify the brain activity in order to improve some aspect of motor or cognitive function, either by altering ongoing brain activity and/or by inducing and guiding long-term plasticity. This chapter reviews the present status, key problems, and future prospects of noninvasive BCIs with such therapeutic aims. It focuses on the use of electroencephalography (EEG) and functional magnetic resonance imaging (fMRI): to abort or prevent seizures; to improve

motor recovery after stroke; to improve attention, emotional reaction, and other cognitive processes; and to manage pain.

BCI-BASED FEEDBACK AS A POSSIBLE THERAPEUTIC TOOL

Central nervous system (CNS) plasticity encompasses the structural and functional neuronal and synaptic CNS changes that occur during learning of new information and during acquisition of new cognitive or motor skills. These changes can occur throughout the CNS, from the cortex to the spinal cord. Induced and guided by CNS activity, such plasticity occurs during development and throughout life (e.g., Wolpaw 2001; Ziemann 2004; Kempermann 1997; Foster 2001). These normal and continual adaptations in the CNS affect the cognitive processes and motor behaviors that are the manifestations of personal intent and behavior (e.g., conversing, eating, painting a picture, etc.). Studies in both animals and humans reveal that similar activity-dependent plasticity can occur after stroke or after other CNS trauma or disease (Umphred 1995; Nudo 1996; Traversa 1997; Liepert 1998; Jones 1999; Neumann-Haefelin 2000; Chu 2000; Marshall 2000; Foster 2001; Biernaskie 2001; Nelles 2001; Liepert 2001; Carey 2002; Newton 2002; Johansen-Berg 2002;; Nudo 2006).

Biofeedback is a training technique that enables an individual to gain some element of control over physiological processes such as blood pressure, heart rate, or brain activity that are not normally volitionally controlled. Biofeedback is based on the principle that a desired response can be learned, during training which provides information that illuminates whether or not a specific thought complex or action has produced the particular desired physiological response. It can be used as an intervention method to guide a person to improve function by modifying his/her own physiological processes. Stroke survivors can learn to modify electromyographic (EMG) signals from paretic muscles to guide recovery of some voluntary muscle activation (Dogan-Aslan 2010). Heart rate and other signals can be used to guide relaxation in individuals with anxiety (Elkins 2010). Feedback of various physiological signals can be used to guide reduction of pain (Kayiran et al. 2010), migraine headaches (Nicholson 2010), high or low blood pressure (Wang 2010), cardiac arrhythmias (Mikosch 2010), and Raynaud's disease (Karavidas 2006); and biofeedback using electroencephalographic (EEG) signals has been used in treating epilepsy (Walker 2005; Monderer 2002; Sterman 2006; Strehl 2006), attention deficit/hyperactivity disorders (Monstra 2005), and other cognitive impairments (Angelakis 2007).

These studies suggest that BCI-based feedback might provide a powerful tool for enabling people to modulate brain activity in a therapeutic manner. BCI-based feedback might be used to produce more normal cognitive processes and motor control after CNS damage or disease (Daly and Wolpaw 2008; Grosse-Wentrup et al. 2011).

THERAPEUTIC USES OF EEG-BASED BCIs

REDUCING SEIZURE FREQUENCY

EEG signals have been used for clinical diagnosis and investigation of brain function since 1929 (Berger 1929). The use of EEG feedback to reduce seizure frequency in people with epilepsy has been explored over several decades (e.g., Sterman 1972; Monderer 2002). Two approaches have yielded promising results: regulation of sensorimotor rhythms (SMRs) (see chapter 13); and regulation of slow cortical potentials (SCPs) (see chapter 14).

As described in chapter 13, *sensorimotor rhythms* (SMRs) are frequency–domain features from EEG recorded over sensorimotor cortex; their most prominent components are 8–12 Hz mu rhythms and 18–30 Hz beta rhythms. Several studies have shown that, after a series of BCI-based training sessions, people with epilepsy can learn to modify SMR amplitude and reduce seizure frequency (Andrews 1992; Lantz 1988; Sterman 2006). A meta-analysis of studies that included a total of 174 drug-refractory patients showed significantly improved seizure control (defined as a minimum of 50% reduction in seizure incidence) in response to SMR training for 82% of the study participants (Sterman 2000). The American Academy of Child and Adolescent Psychiatry (AACAP) has determined that use of such training to treat a seizure disorder meets its clinical guidelines for evidence-based practice and should thus be considered by clinicians (Sterman 2000).

Several other studies have examined intentional modulation of brain signals for epilepsy intervention. Ayers (1995) described a study involving simultaneous up-regulation of 15–18 Hz activity and down-regulation of 4–7 Hz activity in signals recorded over the sensorimotor cortex. A 10-year follow-up of 10 patients who had been otherwise medically intractable showed that they had become and remained seizure-free in response to this training. Walker et al. (2005) used a somewhat different approach, combining regulation of signal amplitude and coherence. Drug-refractory epilepsy patients were successfully trained to modify EEG signals toward normal, using the EEG signal features of power and coherence. These patients were able to reduce coherence across the two hemispheres. In one case, seizures resolved and medication was discontinued; in a second case, seizures were resolved, and the patient began driving and resumed his normal life activities. Although limited in scope, such studies provide encouraging results on which to base a possible new therapeutic protocol for epilepsy management.

Slow cortical potentials (SCPs) (chapter 14) are time-domain event-related EEG features that occur at predictable times before, during, or after specific events. SCPs from EEG recorded over sensorimotor cortex typically consist of negative potentials that precede actual or imagined movement or cognitive tasks (e.g., mental arithmetic). SCPs reflect changes in polarization of apical dendritic trees in superficial cortical layers that result mainly from changes in synaptic inputs from thalamocortical afferents (Birbaumer 1999). Negative SCPs indicate dendritic depolarization, which reduces the threshold for paroxysmal neuronal firing and is associated with seizure occurrence (Birbaumer 1990). Several studies have shown that SCP-based BCI training to suppress negative SCPs can decrease seizure frequency (Rockstroh et al. 1993; Kotchoubey et al. 1996; Kotchoubey et al. 1999; Kotchoubey et al. 2001).

In sum, EEG biofeedback training based on either SMRs and SCPs shows promise as a therapeutic tool for controlling seizures. SMR-based training has produced results sufficiently encouraging to be included in some clinical guidelines for epilepsy control. However, only single-site randomized control trials have thus far been conducted, and no direct comparison between SMR and SCP training has been carried out. Additional well-controlled studies, with more subjects and directly comparing control and study populations (perhaps through large, multicenter trials) could further validate these therapies and their respective advantages (Ramaratnam 2008).

TREATING ATTENTION-DEFICIT DISORDER AND IMPROVING COGNITIVE PROCESSING

EEG feedback and training have also been studied in people with attention-deficit hyperactivity disorder (ADHD) (Monastra et al. 2005) and in older adults with impaired cognitive function (Angelakis 2007). In a review of the ADHD treatment literature, Monastra et al. (2005) assessed the empirical evidence for treatment efficacy and found significant clinical improvement in approximately 75% of the subjects in each study evaluated. Using the efficacy guidelines jointly published by the Association for Applied Psychophysiology and Biofeedback (AAPB) and the International Society for Neuronal Regulation (ISNR), Monastra et al. (2005) concluded that EEG biofeedback was probably effective for the treatment of ADHD.

Several studies (reviewed in Angelakis 2007) have shown that some characteristics of EEG features are correlated with age and with cognitive performance in older adults. Beatty (1974) found that vigilance activity during a monitoring task improved after EEG training that resulted in augmented occipital theta (3–7 Hz) activity relative to the sum of theta, alpha (8–12 Hz), and beta (13–30) activity. In contrast, vigilance decreased after training that resulted in suppression of occipital theta. EEG training to increase parietal-occipital alpha (8–13 Hz) amplitude increased cognitive processing speed and function when training increased the frequency at which alpha was greatest (Angelakis, 2007), or it increased performance on a mental rotation test when training selectively increased the amplitude of higher-frequency, but not lower-frequency, alpha (Zoefel et al. 2011)

These illustrative studies indicate that EEG feedback training can have beneficial effects on attentional and cognitive behaviors and might be useful as a therapeutic intervention.

IMPROVING RECOVERY OF MOTOR FUNCTION

EEG-based BCI training can also be applied to the problem of motor recovery after neural injury. While conventional therapies for treating motor impairments after stroke, other CNS trauma, or disease rely on *exercise of the limbs*, BCI-based training offers a different approach to motor-recovery therapy.

BRAIN PLASTICITY AFTER NEURAL INJURY

Extensive brain plasticity can occur during natural recovery after stroke. For example, in animals, motor recovery after stroke is associated with structural changes in the brain such as neural outgrowth in the intact area around the infarction (Ng 1988; Stroemer 1995), increased synaptogenesis (Stroemer 1995), and increased axonal sprouting (Carmichael 2001) (even in older animals [Li 2006]). Evidence for functional brain changes includes increased excitability (Scheine 1996) and sequential expression of growth-promoting genes (Carmichael 2005). Human studies have also provided evidence of brain changes during natural recovery of motor function after stroke (Cramer 2006; Cramer 1997; Teasell 2005; Jaillard 2005). Even in regions distant from the infarction, Redecker (2000) reported changes such as hyperexcitability of neurons in both lesioned and nonlesioned hemispheres. There is also evidence for other kinds of changes during natural recovery, including reorganization of cortical sensory and motor maps (Frost 2003; Gharbawie 2005), sprouting of abnormal connections and new connections between cortical areas (Dancause 2005), and rerouting of normal intrahemispheric and interhemispheric connections between motor regions (Napieralski 1996).

In addition to the plastic changes occurring during natural motor recovery, several studies have demonstrated activity-dependent brain plasticity resulting from specific training after neural injury (e.g., animal model studies including Nudo 2006, Foster 2001, Chu 2000, Nudo 1996, Jones 1999, Nelles 2001, Biernaskie 2001; and human studies including Umphred 1995, Traversa 1997, Carey 2002, Newton 2002, Marshall 2000, Liepert 2001, Johansen-Berg 2002, and Neumann-Haefelin 2000). Taken as a whole, these studies provide abundant evidence of the extent and complexity of plasticity associated with recovery after injury. It is thus intriguing to consider that, by focusing training directly on brain activity, BCIs might induce or guide plasticity that results in the recovery of motor control.

Frequently repeated, skilled motor actions, particularly those employing precise temporal coordination of multiple muscle activations and joint movements, can induce changes in sensorimotor areas of the brain (Nudo 2007). Current therapeutic methods based on such repetition focus on improving limb movements, and any associated induced brain plasticity occurs ostensibly in response to the limb motor practice and

the sensory afferent input it induces. Notably, many studies in both humans and animals indicate that training based on feedback of EEG or other brain signals can markedly change brain activity (e.g., Fetz 1969; Taylor 2002; Carmena 2003; Leuthardt 2004; Daly 2006; Jackson 2006). Thus, BCIs, which can focus on changing brain activity itself, may offer a more direct and effective avenue for inducing brain plasticity that improves motor function. BCIs might provide a powerful new approach to improving motor function after CNS trauma or in disease.

STRATEGIES FOR USING BCIs IN MOTOR REHABILITATION

Two distinct strategies have been suggested for applying BCI-based feedback of brain signals to rehabilitation of motor function (Daly and Wolpaw 2008).

The first strategy focuses on changing the brain activity that occurs in the damaged brain area during the actual or imagined performance of a motor action. The goal is to make this brain activity more like the brain activity that would normally occur during the motor task; the expectation is that the production of more normal brain activity will improve execution of the motor task itself. This strategy is illustrated in figure 22.1A.

The second strategy uses brain activity to improve the practice of a motor action that has been impaired (e.g., by using the brain activity to control a movement-assist device that helps move the limb). The goal is to provide practice of the motor task in a movement pattern that is as close to normal as possible; the expectation is that the practice of a more normal movement pattern, with more normal sensory feedback, will encourage beneficial activity-dependent brain plasticity and will thereby gradually improve motor performance. This strategy is illustrated in figure 22.1B.

These two strategies, and the initial efforts to apply them, are addressed in the following two sections.

Improving Motor Function by Training More Normal Brain Activity

The goal of training people to generate brain activity that is more normal, and that thereby drives more normal movement, is analogous to the therapeutic approaches used in EEG training aimed at reducing seizure frequency (see above). If it proves effective, it would constitute a novel use of BCI technology. Such a BCI-guided rehabilitation approach seeks to engage the damaged area of the brain by asking the person to attempt or imagine movement that would normally depend on the damaged area specifically and by providing feedback about the activity in the damaged area. Thus, if the goal of treatment is to retrain impaired wrist extension, then the BCI feedback depends on the brain signal in the damaged brain area directly involved in wrist extension. (In targeting control of a specific brain area, this approach differs significantly from typical BCI applications in which the activity from *any* brain area may be used to control the output device [e.g., the brain signal generated from an imagined foot, arm, or facial movement might be used to activate a light switch.])

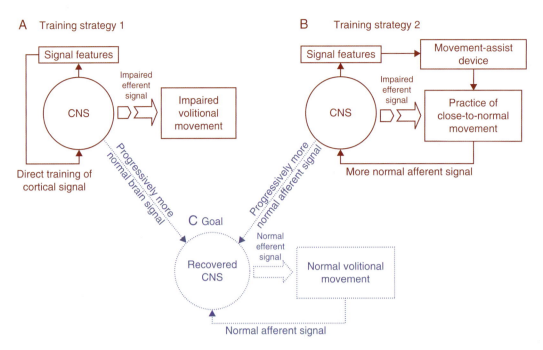

A   Training strategy 1

B   Training strategy 2

C Goal

Figure 22.1 *Two BCI-based strategies to encourage and guide CNS plasticity that improves motor function. (A) Training Strategy 1 translates specific features of brain signals into an action (e.g., cursor movement) and uses that action as feedback to train patients to produce more normal brain signals. The hypothesis is that the plasticity that produces these more normal signals will also restore more normal CNS function and will therefore improve motor control (C). (B) Training Strategy 2 engages specific features of brain signals to activate a movement-assist device that can compensate for the patient's impaired neuromuscular control during motor tasks. The hypothesis is that, by improving motor performance, this assistance will produce more normal sensory input that induces CNS plasticity that restores more normal motor control (C). In sum, Strategy 1 tries to normalize brain signals with the expectation that such normalization will be accompanied by improved motor function, whereas Strategy 2 uses brain signals to assist neuromuscular control with the expectation that the resultant more normal sensory input produced by the better motor performance will induce plasticity that improves neuromuscular control. (Modified from Daly and Wolpaw 2008.)*

It is not yet definitively known whether a person can actually learn to control the activity generated in a specific damaged area. As yet, only a few studies have addressed this question with the stroke population, and the results are mixed, but encouraging. Using feedback from magnetoencephalography (MEG) imaging in 20 training sessions, Buch et al. (2008) showed that patients were able to control brain signals related to a wrist-movement task with an accuracy of 72.48 ± 18.36% (the level of control achieved during the last of 20 sessions).

Daly (2008) showed that with feedback from an EEG-based BCI, three study subjects who had had strokes prior to BCI training and could not extend the wrist or move individual fingers, were able to gain control of brain signals (SMR frequency bands of 9–24 Hz) from the arm/hand region of cortex by attempting or imagining wrist or finger movement. They were trained to decrease (i.e., desynchronize) this SMR activity (which is indicative of volitional control of movement) by imagining or attempting movement and to increase (i.e., synchronize) this signal (which is indicative of a resting brain state) by imagining or attempting relaxation of the same muscles. Over nine training sessions (three weeks, with three sessions per week), they consistently achieved accuracies of 80–100%. These results are summarized in figure 22.2.

Ang (2010), also using an EEG-based BCI, showed that 48 of 54 stroke survivors (89%) could control a brain signal for a shoulder/elbow task with accuracies of 60–99%. In both this

and the Daly (2008) study, many subjects achieved good initial accuracies even in the first one or two sessions. The three subjects in the Daly (2008) study achieved impressive initial brain-signal control (80–99% in the first training session) (fig. 22.2A,B). In the study by Ang (2010), 11 subjects achieved initial accuracies ranging from 70–90% in the first two sessions. However, these two reports of high accuracies in the early session(s) contrast with others (Buch et al. 2008; Hill et al., 2006) that reported the need for more training sessions to achieve greater accuracies. The difference in these results might be due to differences in study design (e.g., signal processing methods, training paradigm) or in the severity and location of stroke damage in the study subjects.

While these preliminary studies provide some encouraging insights, additional larger studies are needed to establish that people can learn to control signals generated in damaged areas of brain and that they can use this control to produce signals similar to those associated with normal movements. It will then remain to be determined whether these more normal signals are associated with improved motor performance.

Improving Motor Function by Enabling More Normal Performance during Practice

In conventional motor rehabilitation, movement training should include practice of progressively more normal movement since practice of abnormal movement merely reinforces

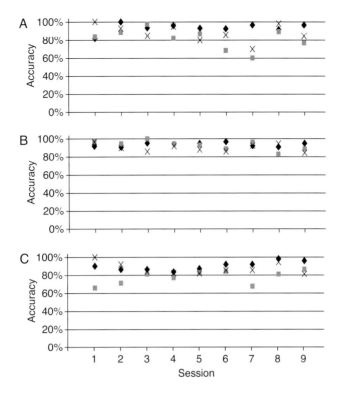

Figure 22.2 *Accuracy of sensorimotor rhythm (SMR) control across nine training sessions for three subjects performing the imagined wrist/hand task (A), the attempted wrist/hand task (B), or the relaxation task (C). In A and B, accuracy is high throughout, almost always falling in the range 80–100%. In C, it is slightly lower but remains in the range 70–100% throughout (except for 2 of the 27 sessions). (Modified from Daly et al. 2008.)*

the abnormal movement. After stroke, some people are unable to produce voluntary movements that are sufficiently close to normal movement to serve as useful motor practice. Clinical studies have shown that in such cases, a movement-assist device that enables close-to-normal movements during practice can enhance the eventual restoration of more normal movements (Daly 2005; Alon 2003; Lo 2010). The value of this strategy is supported by evidence from basic-neuroscience studies showing: that synchronous neural activity supports axon sprouting (Carmichael 2002); that sensory-afferent information from movement interacts in the temporal sulcus with the encoded observed or conceptualized movement which subjects are attempting to imitate (Iacoboni 2001); and that visual-perception information regarding observed movement is mapped in the primary motor region (Rizzolatti 2001).

A BCI that uses signals from relevant brain areas (either those damaged by a stroke or related intact areas) to control a movement-assist device might further increase the value of the therapy provided by the assist device (fig. 22.1B). Moreover, the addition of BCI output to movement-assist device therapy may increase the number of repetitions that can be tolerated, as well as the duration of practice. Finally, the addition of a BCI to the movement-assist system might reduce the need for the constant participation of a therapist for many hours during therapy (a requirement of conventional and emerging intensive therapies that is a major expense in rehabilitation).

Two types of movement-assistive devices are currently in use: functional electrical stimulators (FES) and robots. FES

devices have been used effectively for upper-limb movement-assisted practice for people mildly to moderately impaired after stroke (Ring 2005; Alon 2003) and for people severely impaired (Daly 2005). Daly (2008) trained three stroke survivors to use brain signals from the sensorimotor region of the lesioned hemisphere to activate an FES-assist device for practice of wrist/finger-extension movement. As noted above and illustrated in figure 22.2, they achieved high accuracy (80–100%) even in the first session and remained accurate over nine sessions.

In another case study of a stroke survivor, Daly et al. (2009) tested an EEG-based BCI system that was integrated with an FES movement-assist device. Training consisted of brain-signal feedback directed toward gaining control of signals recorded near the region of brain infarction, an area important for finger movement (fig. 22.3). Prior to the BCI-based FES training, the subject was unable to perform isolated index-finger metacarpal phalangeal (MCP) extension. After nine 1-hour BCI-based FES training sessions, the subject was able to produce 26° of isolated MCP index finger joint extension (fig. 22.4).

BCI systems for motor training with robotic devices have also been tested with stroke survivors. Using an MEG-based BCI, Buch (2008) showed that six of eight patients could activate a robotic wrist movement-assist device achieving an accuracy of 72.48 ± 18.36% by the last of 20 sessions. In another study, a large trial using an EEG-based BCI, Ang et al. (2009) reported that subjects could activate a shoulder/elbow robot with brain signals. For 89% of the subjects, accuracy ranged from 60% to 99% across subjects. These investigators

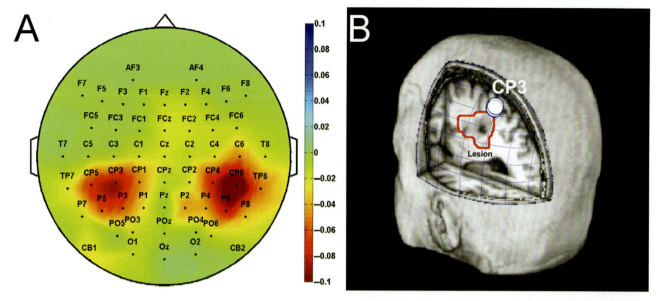

Figure 22.3 (A) Topographical distribution of the change in amplitude of 21–24 Hz sensorimotor rhythm (SMR) activity that occurs when the subject attempts to extend the right index finger. The change is shown as signed R^2 (the percentage of the total variance of the amplitude that is accounted for by attempting to extend the finger). The change is sharply focused over the hand regions of both the lesioned (left) and unlesioned (right) hemispheres (the CP3 and CP6 electrodes, respectively). The negative R^2 values indicate that amplitude at these locations decreases markedly with attempted finger extension. (B) Relationship of the CP3 electrode to the left hemisphere lesion (outlined region). The electrode is directly over the lesioned area. (Reproduced with permission from Daly et al. 2009.)

(Ang et al. 2009) also examined the value of adding BCI training to robotics training of shoulder/elbow movement. They did not find a statistically significant improvement in motor recovery for robotics+BCI training versus robotics training alone.

In another case study of a participant 14 months poststroke (Broetz 2010), goal-directed physical therapy was supplemented by a BCI that used signals from the motor cortex on the side of the stroke to drive movement of an orthosis and a robot attached to the upper extremity. The BCI used MEG and then EEG to measure brain signals. At the end of one year, hand function had improved according to motor function tests, although it is not possible to determine the extent to which BCI use improved the benefit of normal physical therapy. Leamy and Ward (2010) have begun to investigate the usefulness in neurorehabilitation of combining near infrared spectroscopy (NIRS)-based and EEG-based BCI control. Using an overt finger-tapping task in healthy adults, they found that the combination of NIRS and EEG activity at seven sites over the motor cortex provided better BCI performance than either method alone. The usefulness of this combined BCI approach for neurorehabilitation has not yet been determined. In sum, while encouraging early data have been obtained, it is not yet clear whether and how BCI-based methods might contribute to motor relearning and whether BCIs can use signals originating in damaged brain areas for this purpose.

KEY ISSUES FOR FUTURE RESEARCH IN BCI-BASED MOTOR REHABILITATION

Exploration of the potential role of BCI methods in motor training requires resolution of a number of issues. Who are the best candidates for BCI-based motor training or for BCI-based movement-assisted practice? How would BCI treatment outcome be influenced by characteristics such as etiology, location, nature, and severity of CNS injury or disease? Which brain signal features are most useful for motor relearning or for control of a learning-assist device? Which electrode locations are best for recording these signals, and which signal locations and features can be most readily controlled? In addition, it will be important to ascertain whether the brain-signal features used by the BCI change during recovery of motor function. If so, what are the implications for BCI use and for the motor learning process?

Finally, of greatest overall importance, the studies addressing these questions should include enough subjects and appropriate controls so that they can adequately test the basic hypothesis that BCIs can improve motor rehabilitation beyond that possible with current methods.

PRACTICAL ISSUES FOR INCORPORATING BCI-BASED MOTOR REHABILITATION INTO THE CLINICAL ENVIRONMENT

In the event that EEG-based BCIs can be effective in therapeutic motor-recovery applications, issues concerning their incorporation into clinical practice will become important. First, as discussed in chapter 19, the amount of time needed for set-up and clean-up should be minimized. Use of the minimum number of channels (i.e., electrodes) that give adequate brain-signal information for the application is desirable. If and when effective dry electrodes (i.e., not requiring gel) (chapter 6) are available, they should make a big contribution to EEG-based motor rehabilitation or any clinical application using EEG-based BCI methods.

Second, in a hospital setting, an electrically shielded room for motor therapy may help protect the EEG-based BCI from

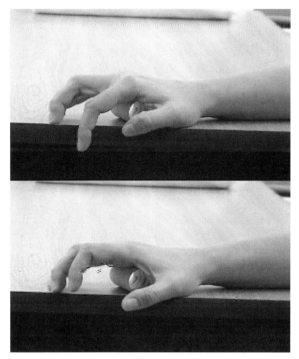

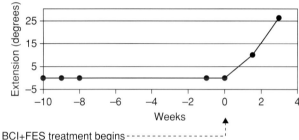

Figure 22.4 Capacity for volitional right index finger extension before and after nine sessions of BCI+FES training of the subject in figure 22.3. (A) Prior to training, the subject could not extend the finger. (B) After training, the subject could extend the metacarpal phalangeal (MP) joint of the finger 26°. (BCI and FES were not used during this test.) (C) Capacity for right index finger MP extension over 14 weeks. For 10 weeks prior to BCI+FES training, no MP extension occurred. After 3 weeks (nine sessions) of training, the subject had recovered 26° of MP extension. (Modified from Daly et al. 2009.)

electrical signal noise arising from other rehabilitation equipment or building electrical systems. Third, motor-rehabilitation personnel will require training in patient screening, decision-making, BCI set-up, and BCI training protocols. Fourth, an EEG-based BCI motor-assist system might be developed for home therapy performed by a stroke survivor alone or with the help of a caregiver. For this kind of application, the BCI must be noninvasive, the electrodes easy to don, and the software user-friendly (Li 2010). Finally, health care insurance reimbursement approval for BCI-assisted motor rehabilitation should be obtained.

THERAPEUTIC USES OF fMRI-BASED BCIs

BCIs may also use metabolic rather than electromagnetic signals produced by brain activity (see chapters 4 and 18). As discussed in chapter 4, magnetic resonance imaging (MRI) is a method for generating images of the brain, and *functional* MRI (fMRI) uses MRI to identify regions of the brain that are active during specific functions such as motor actions or emotional states (Logothetis 2008). In recent years, preliminary studies have been conducted to test the feasibility of using fMRI-based BCI technology for therapeutic purposes. In this vein, people with (or without) disabilities have been trained using fMRI feedback to *self-regulate* the brain activity associated with specific aspects of sensory processing, motor function, cognition, and emotion.

IMPROVING EMOTION PROCESSING AND CONTROL

Recent studies have tested the feasibility of an fMRI-based BCI for training people to regulate brain regions related to emotion. Caria et al. (2007) demonstrated the possibility of regulating the blood oxygenation-dependent (BOLD) signal (chapter 4) in the anterior insula in healthy participants (experimental group, $n = 15$; control group, $n = 6$) through fMRI-based BCI training. A follow-up study ($n = 27$) (Caria et al. 2010) showed that voluntary modulation of activity in the anterior insula induced changes in the subjective response to emotional stimuli (fig. 22.5). During the fMRI-based BCI training, study participants were asked to observe and assess emotional pictures after every time block of self-regulation of activity in the anterior insula. Increase in the BOLD response in the anterior insula correlated with a more negative emotional valence rating for pictures that evoked fear. This effect was not only area-specific, but also specific to the effect of the picture. That is, a BOLD increase in the anterior insula reduced the valence (i.e., made the perception more negative) only for pictures that evoked fear. These findings might conceivably be applied in protocols for treating people with posttraumatic stress syndrome (PTSD), anxiety, obsessive compulsive disorder, or other disorders.

Other studies suggest that fMRI-based BCI training might be used to improve the efficiency of the neuronal networks that produce behavioral responses. Lee and colleagues (2010, 2011) examined changes in functional connectivity between brain areas induced by training to regulate activity in the insular cortex. They used fMRI-based BCI training and data from an earlier study (Caria et al. 2007) to conduct a multivariate analysis. As illustrated in figure 22.6, connectivity analysis revealed that self-regulation training caused an initial increase and subsequent partial pruning in network density, and a strengthening of presumably important connections.

Another aim of current research on brain self-regulation using fMRI-based BCI is to improve understanding and treatment of mental disorders. Several studies have involved subjects with schizophrenia or sociopathic disorders to see if they could acquire self-regulation of brain regions responsible for emotion and to determine whether such learned regulation could affect their behavior. Sitaram et al. (2009) used contingent feedback, in conjunction with images associated with negative emotions taken from previous episodes in the lives of these subjects, to see if they could learn volitional regulation of the left anterior insula. Although the study was limited to a few

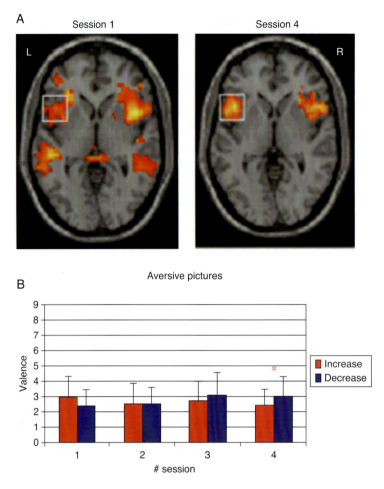

Figure 22.5 (A) Group statistical parametric maps for first and last sessions of fMRI-based BCI training of the BOLD signal in the left anterior insula in healthy participants. (B) Comparative ratings (mean and standard deviation) of valence (a value between 1 and 7 denoting the aversiveness of the picture) for aversive pictures. Red bars are ratings during upregulation training blocks, and blue bars during downregulation training blocks. (Modified from Caria et al. 2010.)

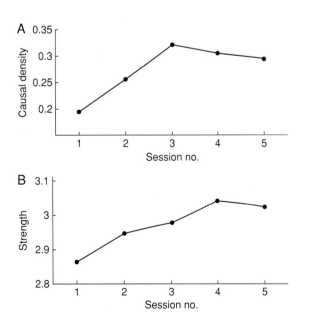

Figure 22.6 Functional interaction of brain regions as revealed by effective connectivity analysis of the fMRI signals acquired during fMRI-based BCI training of the anterior insular cortex. (A) Change in causal density across training sessions. (B) Average connection strength between connections across the training sessions. (Modified from Lee et al. 2011.)

subjects ($n = 5$) due to the difficulty in recruiting people from this special population, the results indicated that those with more severe disease evidenced poorer self-regulation of the brain signals. This finding supports the idea that these individuals have deficits in emotional processing.

Connectivity analysis (i.e., analysis of the functional interactions among brain areas) (Sitaram et al., unpublished data) showed that learning to regulate the signals of the anterior insula increased the number of causative connections (i.e., causal density) in the network of areas involved in emotion and also increased the difference between the number of outgoing and incoming connections. The number of outgoing connections from the left insula was greater than the number of incoming connections to it both before and after training, but time after training increased this difference. In another study, Ruiz et al. (in press) trained (>20 sessions) nine patients with DSM-IV schizophrenia (American Psychiatric Association 1994) to control the BOLD signal of left and right anterior insula. Their control of the BOLD signal increased over sessions. Increased control was accompanied by an increase in the causal density of the functional connections of the network involved in self-regulation of emotions. The changes involved many brain areas: insula; superior medial frontal gyrus (i.e., cognitive control area); anterior cingulate cortex (i.e., attention area); and cuneus (i.e., visual perception and mental imagery area). Participants were administered emotion-recognition tests. Those who had completed BOLD control training and were successful in up-regulation of the BOLD signal were able to more accurately recognize the "disgust" faces after training. These results suggest that fMRI-based BCIs may have a useful role in learned modulation of brain activation that has behavioral consequences in people with psychopathologies.

Rota and colleagues (2009) used an fMRI-based BCI to train healthy individuals to change activity in the right inferior frontal gyrus (rIFG), known to be involved in processing the emotional value of auditory stimuli (Dogil et al. 2004). As illustrated in figure 22.7, the results indicated progressive learning in response to training across the sessions. Improved control of the BOLD signal appeared to be associated with improved ability to detect and identify emotional speech. In contrast, syntactic processing ability, used as a control measure, did not show any change. Functional and effective connectivity analysis of the brain signals revealed strengthening of the connections of the rIFG with the prefrontal cortex and the bilateral precentral gyri (Rota et al. 2010). These findings suggest that functionally specific changes in connectivity may play an important role in the enhancement of speech processing.

IMPROVING RECOVERY OF MOTOR FUNCTION

Several studies provide preliminary information that may guide the use of fMRI-based BCI training for regulation of motor function. As noted earlier in this chapter, despite the availability of various conventional options for movement restoration in stroke patients, some patients show little or no functional

recovery of upper-limb or other motor function. fMRI-based BCIs might serve as an additional and novel tool for learning and consolidating specific motor-task strategies by people with movement disabilities. Numerous studies showing plasticity during motor recovery provide a theoretical basis for this expectation (e.g., after ischemic damage to the primary motor area [M1], secondary motor areas such as the ventral premotor cortex [PMv] may reorganize to promote functional recovery of the motor system [Ward and Cohen 2004; Gerloff et al. 2006]). It has been suggested that fMRI-based BCI may offer a potentially powerful tool for the systematic development of functional cortical reorganization (Ward and Cohen 2004), wherein intact brain areas assume the functions of the damaged areas.

In a pilot study, Sitaram et al. (2011) assessed the feasibility of fMRI-based BCI feedback training of poststroke patients to regulate brain activity in the PMv. This secondary motor area is involved in observation, imagery, and execution of movement (Grezes and Decety 2001) and has extensive anatomical connections with the primary motor cortex (M1). The effect of learned modulation of the PMv BOLD response was evaluated with transcranial magnetic stimulation (TMS). Four healthy adults and two people with chronic subcortical strokes without residual movement were trained for 3 days to regulate the BOLD response in the PMv. The results showed that the BOLD signal in the PMv increased significantly over training sessions. The participants' ability to learn this BOLD control correlated directly with intracortical facilitation and correlated negatively with intracortical inhibition (both measured by TMS) prior to feedback training. After training increased the BOLD response in the PMv, intracortical inhibition decreased significantly, indicating a beneficial effect of self-regulation training on motor cortical output. Although these results need to be confirmed with a larger sample population, this initial study suggests that fMRI-based BCIs may have a potentially important role in stroke rehabilitation.

PAIN MANAGEMENT

DeCharms et al. (2005) tested the ability of fMRI-based BCI feedback training to modulate pain perception, and showed that perception of a noxious stimulus could be modified with simultaneous up- or down-regulation of brain activity in the right anterior cingulate cortex (rACC). Patients with chronic pain who gained control of the rACC-activity level reported subsequent decrease in pain after training. These results are encouraging and merit further study with training paradigms designed to tightly correlate the region-specific training with the measured motor, cognitive, or emotional effects. In addition, further studies are needed to determine the most effective protocol parameters, such as the optimal timing of stimulus presentation or task performance (i.e., whether it should occur during BOLD control, or before or after).

FUTURE WORK IN fMRI-BASED BCIs

Prediction of cognitive, emotional, perceptual, and motor states from fMRI signals constitutes a possible future direction of research in this field. Recent advances in multivariate pattern

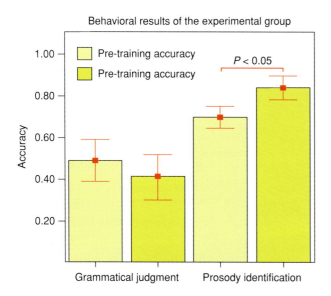

Figure 22.7 Behavioral effects of upregulation of the BOLD signal in right inferior frontal gyrus (rIFG) (Brodman area 45). The figure shows mean (±1.0 SE) levels of accuracy for grammatical judgments and prosody identifications before and after BOLD-feedback training. Significant improvement was observed only for prosody identification (i.e., identification of affective intonations) (two-sided Wilcoxon signed-rank test, p < 0.05). (Modified from Rota et al. 2009.)

classification of fMRI signals have made significant contributions to this potential by enabling it to capitalize on the high spatial resolution, whole brain coverage, and noninvasiveness of fMRI. Haynes and Rees (2006) have noted that multivariate approaches, which can integrate spatial and temporal information from different regions of the brain, are better able to decode brain states than univariate statistical parametric mapping, which analyses the information from each brain location in isolation.

Recent studies (Laconte et al., 2007; Sitaram et al., 2010) have demonstrated that brain states can be classified from fMRI signals online (with a time interval of about 1 sec) from spatially distributed patterns of brain activity and that this classification can be used for the development of fMRI-based BCI feedback training. However, the methods that are currently in use were developed specifically for individual subjects and need sample brain signals from each subject for pattern-classifier training. Further research may develop subject-independent classifiers that could be used in clinical rehabilitation. When this is achieved, patients with brain abnormalities pertaining to motor, cognitive, or emotion processing might be trained to achieve a normal level of functioning by providing BCI-based feedback from a real-time pattern classifier that has been trained on healthy subjects. By repeated operant training with contingent reward from the classifier, patients might learn to mimic the brain activation of healthy individuals and thereby mitigate their impairments.

Finally, to successfully move the predominantly laboratory-based systems of today to the practical applications of tomorrow, the possibilities for using more portable and affordable methods for measuring metabolic brain signals, such as functional near-infrared spectroscopy(fNIRS)-based BCIs (chapter 4) need to explored (Sitaram et al., 2009).

SUMMARY

Basic neuroscience provides fundamental knowledge about the principles underlying the production of brain signals, and the clinical literature provides evidence of the usefulness of learned regulation of EEG signals for reduction of seizure frequency. This background has prompted investigation of the application of BCI-based training to other impairments and dysfunctions.

Although preliminary, and in most cases conducted in small populations, the studies described in this chapter suggest that EEG-based and fMRI-based BCIs may prove useful in motor relearning, in improving cognitive function and emotional regulation, and in pain management. Thus, the use of EEG-based and fMRI-based BCIs to improve many aspects of CNS function constitutes a new and exciting research area. Furthermore, well-controlled demonstrations of efficacy in improving motor and other important functions would greatly increase the numbers of people who could benefit from BCI technology.

REFERENCES

Alon G, Sunnerhagen KS, Geurts AC, Ohry A. A home-based, self-administered stimulation program to improve selected hand functions of chronic stroke. *Neuro Rehabil* 18(3) (2003): 215–225.

Andrews DJ, Schonfeld WH. Predictive factors for controlling seizures using a behavioral approach. *Seizure* 1(2) (1992): 111–116.

Ang KK, Guan C, Chua KS, Ang BT, Kuah C, Wang C, Phua KS, Chin ZY, Zhang H. A clinical study of motor imagery-based brain-computer interface for upper limb robotic rehabilitation. Conference Proceedings of the IEEE Eng Med Biol Soc. 2009: 5981–5984.

Ang KK, Guan C, Chua KSG, Ang BT, Kuah C, Wang C, Phua KS, Chin ZY, Zhang H. Clinical study of neurorehabilitation in stroke using EEG-based motor imagery brain-computer interface with robotic feedback. 32nd Annual International Conference of the IEEE EMBS, Buenos Aires, Argentina, 2010: 5549–5552.

Angelakis E, Stathopoulou S, Frymiare JL, Green DL, Lubar JF, Kounios J. EEG neurofeedback: a brief overview and an example of peak alpha frequency training for cognitive enhancement in the elderly. *Clin Neuropsychol* 21(1) (2007): 110–129.

Beatty J, Greenberg A, Deibler WP, O'Hanlon JF. Operant control of occiptial theta rhythm affects performance in a radar monitoring task. *Science* 183 (1974): 871–873.

Berger H. Über das electrenkephalogramm des menchen. *Arch Psychiatrie Nervenkr* 87 (1929): 527–570.

Biernaskie J, Corbett D. Enriched rehabilitative training promotes improved forelimb motor function and enhanced dendritic growth after focal ischemic injury. *J Neurosci* 21(14) (2001): 5272–5280.

Birbaumer N, Cohen LG. Brain-computer interfaces: communication and restoration of movement in paralysis. *J Physiol* 579 (2007): 621–636.

Birbaumer N, Elbert T, Canavan AG, Rockstroh B. Slow potentials of the cerebral cortex and behavior. *Physiol Rev* 70(1) (1990): 1–41.

Birbaumer N, Ghanayim N, Hinterberger T, Iversen I, Kotchoubey B, Kübler A, et al. A spelling device for the paralysed. *Nature* 398(6725) (1999): 297–298.

Broetz D, Braun C, Weber C, Soekadar SR, Caria A, Birbaumer N. Combination of brain-computer interface training and goal-directed physical therapy in chronic stroke: a case report. Neurorehabil Neural Repair. 24 (2010): 674–679.

Buch E, Weber C, Cohen L, Braun C, Dimyan MA, Ard T, Mellinger J, Caria A, Soekadar S, Fourkas A, Birbaumer N. Think to move: A neuromagnetic brain-computer interface (BCI) system for chronic stroke. *Stroke.* 39 (2008): 910–917.

Carey JR, Kimberley TJ, Lewis SM, Auerbach EJ, Dorsey L, Rundquist P, et al. Analysis of fMRI and finger tracking training in subjects with chronic stroke. *Brain* 125 (2002): 773–788.

Caria A, Sitaram R, Veit R, Begliomini C, Birbaumer N. Volitional control of anterior insula activity modulates the response to aversive stimuli. A real-time functional magnetic resonance imaging study. *Biol Psychiatry* 68(5) (2010): 25–32.

Caria A, Veit R, Sitaram R, Lotze M, Weiskopf N, Grodd W, et al. Regulation of anterior insular cortex activity using real-time fMRI. *Neuroimage* 35(3) (2007): 1238–1246.

Carmena JM, Lebedev MA, Crist RE, O'Doherty JE, Santucci DM, Dimitrov DF, et al. Learning to control a brain-machine interface for reaching and grasping by primates. *PLoS Biol* 1(2) (2003): E42.

Carmichael ST, Archibeque I, Luke L, Nolan T, Momiy J, Li S. Growth-associated gene expression after stroke: evidence for a growth-promoting region in peri-infarct cortex. *Exp Neurol* 193(2) (2005): 291–311.

Carmichael ST, Chesselet MF. Synchronous neuronal activity is a signal for axonal sprouting after cortical lesions in the adult. *J Neurosci* 22(14) (2002): 6062–6070.

Carmichael ST, Wei L, Rovainen CM, Woolsey TA. New patterns of intracortical projections after focal cortical stroke. *Neurobiol Dis* 8(5) (2001): 910–922.

Chu CJ, Jones TA. 2000. Experience-dependent structural plasticity in cortex heterotopic to focal sensorimotor cortical damage. *Exp Neurol* 166(2) (2000): 403–414.

Cramer SC, Nelles G, Benson RR, Kaplan JD, Parker RA, Kwong KK, et al. A functional MRI study of subjects recovered from hemiparetic stroke. *Stroke* 28(12) (1997): 2518–2527.

Cramer SC, Shah R, Juranek J, Crafton KR, Le V. Activity in the peri-infarct rim in relation to recovery from stroke. *Stroke* 37(1) (2006): 111–115.

Daly JJ, Cheng RC, Hrovat K, Litinas KH, Rogers JM, Dohring ME. Development and testing of non-invasive BCI + FES/robot system for use in motor re-Learning after stroke. 13th International Functional Electrical Stimulation Society, Freiburg, Germany, 2008, Paper 5–5, at http://www.ifess2008.de/NR/rdonlyres/31C92C70-AAB8-4A0E-AF21-828F81251C8D/27648/IFESS_2008_final.pdf.

Daly JJ, Cheng R, Rogers J, Litinas K, Hrovat K, Dohring M. Feasibility of BCI training after stroke; a case study. *J Neurol Phys Ther* 33 (2009): 203–211.

Daly JJ, Fang Y, Perepezko E, Yue G. Prolonged brain motor planning time and elevated cognitive effort during a linear movement task following stroke. *IEEE Trans Neural Syst Eng* 14(2) (2006): 168–171.

Daly JJ, Hogan N, Perepezko EM, Krebs HI, Rogers JM, Goyal KS, et al. Response to upper-limb robotics and functional neuromuscular stimulation following stroke. *J Rehabil Res Dev* 42(6) (2005): 723–736.

Daly JJ, Wolpaw JR. Brain-computer interfaces in neurological rehabilitation. *Lancet Neurology* 7 (2008): 1032–1043.

Dancause N, Barbay S, Frost SB, Plautz EJ, Chen D, Zoubina EV, et al. Extensive cortical rewiring after brain injury. *J Neurosci* 25(44) (2005): 10167–10179.

deCharms RC, Maeda F, Glover GH, Ludlow D, Pauly JM, Soneji D, et al. Control over brain activation and pain learned by using real-time functional MRI. *Proc Natl Acad Sci USA* 102(51) (2005): 18626–18631.

Dirckx JH. (Ed.). *Stedman's Concise Medical Dictionary for the Health Professional*, 3rd Ed, 1997. Baltimore: Williams & Wilkins.

Doğan-Aslan M, Nakipoğlu-Yüzer GF, Doğan A, Karabay I, Ozgirgin N. The effect of electromyographic biofeedback treatment in improving upper extremity functioning of patients with hemiplegic stroke. *J Stroke Cerebrovasc Dis* 2010 [Epub ahead of print].

Dogil G., Frese I, Haider H, Röhm D, Wokurek W. Where and how does grammatically geared processing take place—and why is Broca's area often involved. A coordinated fMRI/ERBP study of language processing. *Brain Lang.* 89(2) (2004): 337–345.

Elkins G, Fisher W, Johnson A. Mind-body therapies in integrative oncology. *Curr Treat Options Oncol* 11(3–4) (2010): 128–140.

Fetz EE. Operant conditioning of cortical unit activity. *Science* 163(870) (1969): 955–958.

Foster TC, Dumas TC. Mechanism for increased hippocampal synaptic strength following differential experience. *J Neurophysiol* 85(4) (2001): 1377–1383.

Frost SB, Barbay S, Friel KM, Plautz EJ, Nudo RJ. Reorganization of remote cortical regions after ischemic brain injury: a potential substrate for stroke recovery. *J Neurophysiol* 89(6) (2003): 3205–3214.

Gerloff C, Bushara K, Sailer A, Wassermann EM, Chen R, Matsuoka T, et al. Multimodal imaging of brain reorganization in motor areas of the contralesional hemisphere of well recovered patients after capsular stroke. *Brain* 129 (2006): 791–808.

Gharbawie OA, Gonzalez CL, Williams PT, Kleim JA, Whishaw IQ. Middle cerebral artery (MCA) stroke produces dysfunction in adjacent motor cortex as detected by intracortical microstimulation in rats. *Neuroscience* 130(3) (2005): 601–610.

Grezes J, Decety J. Functional anatomy of execution, mental simulation, observation, and verb generation of actions: a meta-analysis. *Hum Brain Mapp* 12(1) (2001): 1–19.

Grosse-Wentrup M, Mattia D, Oweiss K. Using brain-computer interfaces to induce neural plasticity and restore function. *J Neural Eng* 8(2) (2011): 025004. Epub 2011 Mar 24.

Hill NJ, Lal TN, Schroder M, Hinterberger T, Wilhelm B, Nijboer F, Mochty U, Widman G, Elger C, Schoelkopf B, Kübler A, Birbaumer N. Classifying EEG and ECoG signals without subject training for fast BCI implementation: comparison of nonparalyzed and completely paralyzed subjects. *IEEE Trans Neural Syst Rehabil Eng* 14(2) (2006): 183–186.

Iacoboni M, Koski LM, Brass M, Bekkering H, Woods RP, Dubeau MC, et al. Reafferent copies of imitated actions in the right superior temporal cortex. *Proc Natl Acad Sci USA* 98(24) (2001): 13995–13999.

Jackson A, Mavoori J, Fetz EE. Long-term motor cortex plasticity induced by an electronic neural implant. *Nature* 444(7115) (2006): 56–60.

Jaillard A, Martin CD, Garambois K, Lebas JF, Hommel M. Vicarious function within the human primary motor cortex? A longitudinal fMRI stroke study. *Brain* 128 (2005): 1122–1138.

Johansen-Berg H, Dawes H, Guy C, Smith SM, Wade DT, and Matthews PM. Correlation between motor improvements and altered fMRI activity after rehabilitative therapy. *Brain* 125(Pt 12) (2002): 2731–2742.

Jones TA, Chu CJ, Grande LA, Gregory AD. Motor skills training enhances lesion-induced structural plasticity in the motor cortex of adult rats. *J Neurosci* 19(22) (1999): 10153–10163.

Karavidas MK, Tsai PS, Yucha C, McGrady A, Lehrer PM. Thermal biofeedback for primary Raynaud's phenomenon: a review of the literature. *Appl Psychophysiol Biofeedback.* 31(3) (2006): 203–216.

Kayiran S, Dursun E, Dursun N, Ermutlu N, Karamürsel S. Neurofeedback intervention in fibromyalgia syndrome; a randomized, controlled, rater blind clinical trial. *Appl Psychophysiol Biofeedback* (2010) 35(4): 293–302.

Kempermann G, Kuhn HG, Gage FH. Genetic influence on neurogenesis in the dentate gyrus of adult mice. *Proc Natl Acad Sci USA* 94(19) (1997): 10409–10414.

Kotchoubey B, Schneider D, Schleichert H, Strehl U, Uhlmann C, Blankenhorn V, Fröscher W, Birbaumer N. Self regulation of slow cortical potentials in epilepsy: a retrial with analysis of influencing factors. *Epilepsy Res* 25(3) (1996): 269–276.

Kotchoubey B, Strehl U, Holzapfel S, Schneider D, Blankenhorn V, Birbaumer N. Control of cortical excitability in epilepsy. In: Stephan H, Chauvel P, Andermann F, Shovron SD (eds.) *Plasticity in Epilepsy: Dynamic Aspects of Brain Function. (Advances in Neurology*, Vol. 81). Philadelphia: Raven Press (1999): 281–290.

Kotchoubey B, Strehl U, Uhlmann C, Holzapfel S, König M, Fröscher W, Blankenhorn V, Birbaumer N. Modification of slow cortical potentials in patients with refractory epilepsy: a controlled outcome study. *Epilepsia* 42(3) (2001): 406–416.

LaConte SM, Peltier SJ, Hu XP. Real-time fMRI using brain-state classification. *Hum Brain Mapp* 28 (2007): 1033–1044.

Lantz D, Sterman MB. Neuropsychological assessment of subjects with uncontrolled epilepsy: Effects of EEG biofeedback training. *Epilepsia* 29 (2) (1988): 163–171.

Leamy DJ and Ward TE. A novel co-locational and concurrent fNIRS/EEG measurement system: design and initial results. Conference Proceedings, Annual International Conference of the IEEE Engineering in Medicine & Biology Society. 2010: 4230–4233, 2010.

Lee S, Halder S, Kübler A, Birbaumer N, Sitaram R. Effective functional mapping of fMRI data with support-vector machines. *Hum Brain Mapp* 31(10) (2010): 1502–1511.

Lee S, Ruiz S, Caria A, Birbaumer N, Sitaram R. Detection of cerebral reorganization induced by real-time fMRI feedback training of the insular cortex: a multivariate investigation. *Neurorehabil Neural Rep* 25 (2011): 259–267.

Leuthardt EC, Schalk G, Wolpaw JR, Ojemann JG, Moran DW. A brain-computer interface using electrocorticographic signals in humans. *J Neural Eng* 1(2) (2004): 63–71.

Li S, Carmichael ST. Growth-associated gene and protein expression in the region of axonal sprouting in the aged brain after stroke. *Neurobiol Dis* 23(2) (2006): 362–373.

Liepert J, Miltner WH, Bauder H, Sommer M, Dettmers C, Taub E, et al. Motor cortex plasticity during constraint-induced movement therapy in stroke patients. *Neurosci Lett* 250 (1998): 5–8.

Liepert J, Uhde I, Graf S, Leidner O, Weiller C. Motor cortex plasticity during forced-use therapy in stroke patients: a preliminary study. *J Neurol* 248(4) (2001): 315–321.

Lin CT, Ko LW, Chang MH, Duann JR, Chen JY, Su TP, Jung TP. Review of wireless and wearable electroencephalogram systems and brain-computer interfaces--a mini-review. *Gerontology* 56(1): 112–119, 2010.

Lo AC, Guarino PD, Richards LG, Haselkorn JK, Wittenberg GF, Federman DG, Ringer RJ, Wagner TH, Krebs HI, Volpe BT, Bever CT Jr, Bravata DM, Duncan PW, Corn BH, Maffucci AD, Nadeau SE, Conroy SS, Powell JM, Huang GD, Peduzzi P. Robot-assisted therapy for long-term upper-limb impairment after stroke. *N Engl J Med.* 362(19) (2010): 1772–1783.

Logothetis NK. What we can do and what we can not do with fMRI. *Nature* 453(7197) (2008): 869–878.

Marshall RS, Perera GM, Lazar RM, Krakauer JW, Constantine RC, DeLaPaz RL. Evolution of cortical activation during recovery from corticospinal tract infarction. *Stroke* 31(3) (2000): 656–661.

Mikosch P, Hadrawa T, Laubreiter K, Brandl J, Pilz J, Stettner H, Grimm G. Effectiveness of respiratory-sinus-arrhythmia biofeedback on state-anxiety in patients undergoing coronary angiography. *J Adv Nurs* 66(5) (2010): 1101–1110.

Monastra VJ, Lynn S, Linden M, Lubar JF, Gruzelier J, LaVaque TJ. Electroencephalographic biofeedback in the treatment of attention-deficit/hyperactivity disorder. *Appl Psychophysiol Biofeedback* 30(2) (2005): 95–114.

Monderer RS, Harrison DM, Haut SR. Neurofeedback and epilepsy. *Epilepsy Behav* 3(3) (2002): 214–218.

Napieralski JA, Butler AK, Chesselet MF. Anatomical and functional evidence for lesion-specific sprouting of corticostriatal input in the adult rat. *J Comp Neurol* 373(4) (1996): 484–497.

Nelles G, Jentzen W, Jueptner M, Muller S, Diener HC. Arm training induced brain plasticity in stroke studied with serial positron emission tomography. *Neuroimage* 13(6 Pt 1) (2001): 1146–1154.

Neumann-Haefelin T, Moseley ME, Albers GW. New magnetic resonance imaging methods for cerebrovascular disease: emerging clinical applications. *Ann Neurol* 47(5) (2000): 559–570.

Newton J, Sunderland A, Butterworth SE, Peters AM, Peck KK, Gowland PA. A pilot study of event-related functional magnetic resonance imaging of monitored wrist movements in patients with partial recovery. *Stroke* 33(12) (2002): 2881–2887.

Ng SC, de la Monte SM, Conboy GL, Karns LR, Fishman MC. Cloning of human GAP-43: growth association and ischemic resurgence. *Neuron* 1(2) (1988): 133–139.

Nicholson RA, Buse DC, Andrasik F, and Lipton RB. Nonpharmacologic treatments for migraine and tension-type headache: how to choose and when to use. *Curr Treat Options Neurol* 13(1) (2011): 28–40. [Epub ahead of print].

Nudo RJ. Mechanisms for recovery of motor function following cortical damage. *Curr Opin Neurobiol* 16(6) (2006): 638–644.

Nudo JR. Stem cells and stroke recovery: Introduction to postinfarct cortical plasticity and behavioral recovery. *Stroke*. 38 (2007): 840–845.

Nudo RJ, Wise BM, SiFuentes F, Milliken GW. Neural substrates for the effects of rehabilitative training on motor recovery after ischemic infarct. *Science* 21; 272(5269) (1996): 1791–1794.

Ramaratnam S, Baker GA, Goldstein LH. Cochrane database systematic review. 3 (2008): CD002029.

Redecker C, Luhmann HJ, Hagemann G, Fritschy JM, Witte OW. Differential downregulation of GABA$_A$ receptor subunits in widespread brain regions in the freeze-lesion model of focal cortical malformations. *J Neurosci* 20(13) (2000): 5045–5053.

Ring H, Rosenthal N. Controlled study of neuroprosthetic functional electrical stimulation in sub-acute post-stroke rehabilitation. *J Rehabil Med* 37(1) (2005): 32–36.

Rizzolatti G, Fogassi L, Gallese V. Neurophysiological mechanisms underlying the understanding and imitation of action. *Nat Rev Neurosci* 2(9) (2001): 661–670.

Rockstroh B, Elbert T, Birbaumer N, Wolf P, Dutching-Roth A, Recker M, et al. Cortical self-regulation in patients with epilepsies. *Epilepsy Res.* 14 (1993): 63–72.

Rota G, Handjaras G, Sitaram R, Birbaumer N, Dogil G. Reorganisation of functional and effective connectivity during fMRI-BCI modulation of prosody processing. *Brain Lang* 117(3) (2011):123–132. Epub 2010 Oct 2.

Rota G, Sitaram R, Veit R, Erb M, Weiskopf N, Dogil G, Birbaumer N. Self-regulation of regional cortical activity using real-time fMRI: the right inferior frontal gyrus and linguistic processing. *Hum Brain Mapp* 30(5) (2009): 1605–1614.

Ruiz S, Lee S, Soekader S, Caria A, Veit R, Birbaumer N, Sitaram R. Learned self-regulation of anterior insula in schizophrenia: effects on emotion recognition and neural connectivity. Hum Brain Mapp (in press).

Schiene K, Bruehl C, Zilles K, Qu M, Hagemann G, Kraemer M, et al. Neuronal hyperexcitability and reduction of GABAA-receptor expression in the surround of cerebral photothrombosis. *J Cereb Blood Flow Metab* 16(5) (1996): 906–914.

Sitaram R, Caria A, Birbaumer N. Hemodynamic brain-computer interfaces for communication and rehabilitation. *Neural Network* 22(9) (2009): 1320–1328.

Sitaram R, Caria A, Gaber T, Veit R, Birbaumer N. Volitional control of anterior insula in psychopathic criminals, (unpublished data).

Sitaram R, Lee S, Ruiz S, Rana M, Veit R, Birbaumer N. Real-time support vector classification and feedback of multiple emotional brain states." *Neuroimage* 56(2) (2010): 753–765. Epub 2010 Aug 6.

Sitaram R, Veit R, Stevens B, Caria A, Gerloff, C, Birbaumer N, Hummel F. Learned self-regulation of ventral premotor cortex facilitates motor output: An exploratory real-time fMRI and TMS study. *Neural Rehabil Neural Repair* (in press).

Sterman MB. Basic concepts and clinical findings in the treatment of seqizure disorders with EEG operant condition. *Clin Electroencephaolgr* 31 (2000): 45–55.

Sterman MB, Egner T. Foundation and practice of neurofeedback for the treatment of epilepsy. *Appl Psychophysiol Biofeedback* 31(1) (2006): 21–35.

Sterman MB, Friar L. Suppression of seizures in an epileptic following sensorimotor EEG feedback training. *Electroencephalogr Clin Neurophysiol* 33 (1972), 89–95.

Strehl U, Trevorrow T, Veit R, Hinterberger T, Kotchoubey B, Erb M, et al. Deactivation of brain areas during self-regulation of slow cortical potentials in seizure patients. *Appl Psychophysiol Biofeedback* 31(1) (2006): 85–94.

Stroemer RP, Kent TA, Hulsebosch CE. Neocortical neural sprouting, synaptogenesis, and behavioral recovery after neocortical infarction in rats. *Stroke* 26(11) (1995): 2135–2144.

Taylor DM, Tillery SI, Schwartz AB. Direct cortical control of 3D neuroprosthetic devices. *Science* 296(5574) (2002): 1829–1832.

Teasell R, Bayona NA Bitensky J. Plasticity and reorganization of the brain post stroke. *Top Stroke Rehabil* 12(3) (2005): 11–26.

Traversa R, Cicinelli P, Bassi A, Rossini PM, Bernardi G. Mapping of motor cortical reorganization after stroke. A brain stimulation study with focal magnetic pulses. *Stroke* 28(1) (1997): 110–117.

Umphred DA. *Neurological Rehabilitation*. St. Louis: Mosby (1995).

Walker JE, Kozlowski GP. Neurofeedback treatment of epilepsy. *Child Adolesc Psychiatr Clin North Am* 14(1) (2005): 163–176, viii.

Wang SZ, Li S, Xu XY, Lin GP, Shao L, Zhao Y, Wang TH. Effect of slow abdominal breathing combined with biofeedback on blood pressure and heart rate variability in prehypertension. *J Altern Complem Med* 16(10) (2010): 1039–1045.

Ward NS, Cohen LG. Mechanisms underlying recovery of motor function after stroke. *Arch Neurol* 61(12) (2004): 1844–1848.

Wolpaw JR, McFarland DJ. Control of a two-dimensional movement signal by a noninvasive brain-computer interface in humans. *Proc Natl Acad Sci USA* 101(51) (2004): 17849–17854.

Wolpaw JR, Tennissen AM. Activity-dependent spinal cord plasticity in health and disease. *Annu Rev Neurosci* 24 (2001): 807–843.

Ziemann U, Ilic TV, Pauli C, Meintzschel F, Ruge D. Learning modifies subsequent induction of long-term potentiation-like and long-term depression-like plasticity in human motor cortex. *J Neurosci* 24(7)(2004): 1666–1672.

Zoefel B, Huster RJ, Herrmann CS. Neurofeedback training of the upper alpha frequency band in EEG improves cognitive performance. *NeuroImage* 54 (2011): 1427–1431.

23 | BCI APPLICATIONS FOR THE GENERAL POPULATION

BENJAMIN BLANKERTZ, MICHAEL TANGERMANN, AND KLAUS-ROBERT MÜLLER

The main focus of this book is the use of BCIs to restore communication and control to people with disabling neuromuscular disorders. At the same time, BCIs have a variety of other possible uses beyond serving as a new form of assistive technology. Chapter 22 of this volume addresses BCI use for rehabilitation and other therapeutic purposes. This chapter addresses BCI applications for the general population (i.e., applications that are not specifically intended for people who are disabled). These nonmedical uses fall into three major categories.

The first category includes BCI applications for improving, stabilizing, or otherwise *optimizing* conventional neuromuscular performances. For example, BCI-based monitoring of brain signals that correlate with poor attention might be used to trigger stimuli that encourage attention. The second category includes applications of BCI technology that *enhance* conventional neuromuscular performances *beyond* their normal capacities. For example, BCI-based monitoring of brain signals associated with a difficult visual-detection task might be used to improve the speed or accuracy of detection. The third category includes BCI applications that *broaden* or *enrich* life experience. These include BCI-based internet-browser applications, computer games, relaxation applications, and applications that enable artistic expression such as music or painting. In addition, technology developed for BCIs can also be used for applications that do not fit the BCI definition described in chapter 1, such as neuromarketing (Fisher et al., 2010).

These three kinds of *nonmedical* use of BCI technology are addressed in the following three sections. Each section discusses particular issues specific to that category, reviews applications developed up to the present, and considers possibilities for the future. At the same time it is important to note that the realization of these possibilities will depend in large measure on substantial improvements in BCI convenience, control capacity, and consistency. Particularly important in this regard will be advances in EEG recording methodology (e.g., availability of reliable dry electrodes) and advances in feature extraction and translation algorithms. Obstacles and advances in these critical areas are addressed in chapters 6–8 of this volume.

OPTIMIZING CONVENTIONAL PERFORMANCE

Although the brain signals associated with conventional neuromuscular actions typically exhibit substantial trial-to-trial variability, the actions themselves are usually very stable from one performance to the next (see, e.g., the example of professional piano players in Slobounov et al., 2002). However, the effectiveness of the actions may vary greatly from one performance to the next when the tasks have high memory load or when they require recognition of barely noticeable differences or detection of stimuli that are near threshold. New methods for reducing this variability and thereby ensuring more stable performances could be extremely useful. BCI technology, with its capacity for supporting real-time interactions based on the user's brain signals, could allow the implementation of such methods. For example, a BCI-enhanced vocabulary trainer might present new word pairs only at times when the user is in a mental state suitable for memory encoding (Guderian et al., 2009). (A different but related approach would be based on the prediction of the success of encoding from the evoked responses to presented vocabulary, in the spirit of Karis et al., 1984.) Such BCI-based methods for timing behaviors according to the user's concurrent mental state could improve the reliability of a wide range of psychophysiological experiments and could also find many real-world applications. These methods might improve the productivity, consistency, and safety of industrial operations by avoiding or reducing the deleterious effects of inattention, fatigue, or emotion.

Up to the present, information about mental state has typically been acquired through offline analyses of data garnered from questionnaires, videotaping, or error tabulation (ITU–T Rec. P. 910, 2008; Wältermann et al., 2008). Such methods may help in redesigning behavioral tasks or work environments, but they cannot be used for real-time interactive optimization of performance. In contrast, BCI technology could assess mental state in real time and could thereby optimize the timing of behaviors and/or produce immediate outputs that improve performance. The development of such BCI applications has just begun. This chapter reviews several promising initiatives.

ATTENTION

The neurophysiological substrates of attention are the focus of substantial research efforts, and these have generated increasingly complex and specific conceptual frameworks (e.g., Fan et al., 2007). Reliable and convenient methods for real-time monitoring of attention are particularly relevant for safety-critical applications, in which human performance is often the most variable factor. For example, fatal car accidents are one of the leading causes of death in the United States (Mokdad et al., 2004, 2005; Subramanian, 2007) and the leading cause among

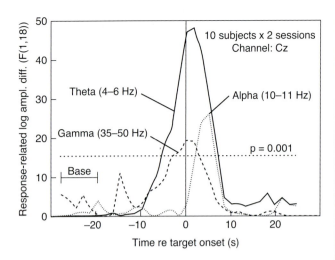

Figure 23.1 *Average time courses from 10 subjects of the hit-versus-error differences (measured as F-statistic) in log amplitudes for the theta (solid), alpha (dotted), and gamma (dashed) frequency bands. The dashed horizontal line is the p = 0.001 significance level for independent comparisons. Consistent hit-versus-error differences in the theta and gamma bands begin about 10 sec before the response, whereas an alpha difference appears only after the response. (From Makeig and Jung, 1996, with permission.)*

children (9–18 years) worldwide (Xu et al., 2010). Two main causes for crashes are visual distractions (Ranney, 2008; Klauer et al., 2010) and decreases in vigilance (Lyznicki et al., 1998; Fletcher et al., 2005). Physiological measures such as eye-blink and heart rate have been used to detect such lapses of attention (e.g., Papadelis et al., 2007). However, EEG-based markers, which are likely to be more directly related to attention, have been used only rarely, due to the practical limitations of standard EEG recording systems. Nevertheless, there is strong evidence that EEG features could be of high value for online monitoring of attention.

In an impressive study by Makeig and Jung (1996), EEG was recorded from central and posterior midline locations Cz and POz while people performed a difficult auditory detection task. They were asked to detect brief (260-msec) 6-dB increases occurring at random times at an average rate of 10/min in a 62-dB white-noise background. The investigators analyzed the correlations between specific EEG frequency bands and the occurrence of errors (i.e., failures to detect the increase). They found that errors were correlated with specific EEG frequency bands on both short (i.e., trial-to-trial) and longer (e.g., minute-to-minute) time scales. Most important in the present context, they found in most subjects that 4–6 Hz theta activity began to increase, and >35 Hz gamma activity began to decrease, about 10 sec prior to errors (i.e., failures to detect) (fig. 23.1). This implies that theta/gamma monitoring might be used online to detect error-prone states and prevent errors by alerting the person or by delaying the task. Another approach worth exploring would be use of the so-called "error-preceding potentials," which are systematic changes in brain activity that foreshadow behavioral errors (Eichele et al., 2010).

A recent study (Müller et al., 2008) evaluated the use of EEG signals to detect errors in a setting similar to that found in many important tasks. It simulated a security surveillance system in which the person needs to maintain close attention to a rather boring task. The objective was to determine whether a BCI might use EEG signals to detect, and hopefully predict, mental states associated with a high probability of errors. Each subject viewed 2000 x-ray images of suitcases and was asked to indicate those that did or did not contain dangerous objects by immediately pressing a key with the left or right index finger, respectively (fig. 23.2). Successive images were presented. Each image was shown for 750 msec, and as soon as the subject responded (1.750 msec on average), the next image was presented. EEG was recorded from 128 channels at 1000 Hz. The monotonous nature of the task and the long duration of the experiment (i.e., ten 200-image blocks over a total of about 120 min) were expected to produce a gradual decrease in attention and a consequential increase in errors in the later blocks.

The time course of error occurrences (mainly misses, but also 6–25% false positives) was smoothed to form a measure of

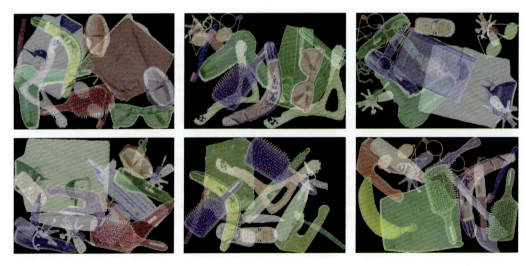

Figure 23.2 *Examples of x-ray images used in the detection task. The upper row shows three suitcases that do not contain a weapon, and the lower row shows three that do (i.e., machine gun, knife, and axe). (From Blankertz et al., 2010.)*

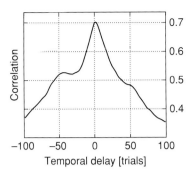

Figure 23.3 *Correlation coefficient between the CII (derived from the EEG) and performance (i.e., error rate) for different time shifts. The highest correlation is at zero time shift, as expected. In addition, and most important, the CII correlates strongly with an error even before the error occurs.*

attention, or concentration, which was called the *error index*. To enhance the analysis, two threshold values of this error index were established for each subject. Values above the higher threshold indicated insufficient concentration, and values below the lower threshold indicated sufficient concentration. The EEG data for periods of high and low error index were compared, and a detailed description of this analysis was provided (Müller et al., 2008). A prominent feature of the results was the finding that decreased alpha (8–12 Hz) activity over the left parieto-occipital scalp region was associated with high error index. Based on the contrast between periods of high- and low-error index, a *Concentration Insufficiency Index* (CII) was derived from EEG data. Figure 23.3 plots the correlation between the error index and the CII as a function of the temporal difference between them. It is clear that the two are highly correlated at zero-time difference. Furthermore, and most important in the current context, the correlation is high even for 50 trials into the future. This implies that the CII derived from the EEG data can provide a method to anticipate an increase in errors and thus to guide interventions to prevent or correct them.

WORKLOAD

Many common and important tasks are complex combinations of multiple subtasks that must be performed simultaneously or in rapid succession. Driving a car exemplifies such a complex task. The driver must control the vehicle, attend to the road, respond quickly and appropriately to a wide variety of possible expected or unexpected obstacles or other events, select or follow a specific set of directions, and may also add optional tasks such as conversing or listening to music. At some point, as the total composite workload increases, performance on the various subtasks will deteriorate, and grievous consequences, such as an accident, may follow. A number of studies have identified EEG correlates of workload in ongoing brain signals (Gevins et al., 1995; Smith et al., 2001; Berka et al., 2007; Holm et al., 2009) and in event-related potentials (Isreal et al., 1980; Donchin, 1987; Kramer et al., 1995; Prinzel et al., 2003; Allison and Polich, 2008).

Offline analyses of such EEG measures of workload obtained during the testing of new vehicles or other products

could be used to ensure that the workloads associated with their operation do not reach dangerous levels. For example, one of the optional accessory systems might be switched off when the workload demanded by critical tasks reached high levels. Such EEG measures might also be used to avoid new product features that elevate workload to unacceptable levels, or, conversely, to validate new features intended to reduce workload (e.g., automatic control of the distance from a vehicle being followed). Furthermore, and most relevant in the current context, such measures might be used in a real-time BCI-based system to ensure that workload never reaches dangerous levels for individual users.

In a recent study performed in collaboration with Daimler AG, Kohlmorgen et al. (2007) developed and tested an EEG measure of workload. They recorded EEG (32 channels located according to the International 10–20 system) from 17 people while they actually drove on a highway at a speed of 100 km/hr. This was their primary task. At certain times, additional secondary and tertiary tasks were superimposed. The secondary task was an auditory reaction task in which one of two buttons mounted on the left and right index fingers had to be pushed about every 7.5 sec in response to a vocal prompt. The tertiary task was either mental calculation or attending to one of two simultaneously presented voice recordings. In an initial calibration phase, an EEG-based workload detector was calibrated for each individual driver. Basically, this workload detector classified spatial patterns of band power in subject-specific frequency bands. Initially, unstable channels and channels appearing to contain muscle or eye-movement artifacts were removed. Then different parameter configurations (frequency bands, sets of channels, spatial filters, hysteresis thresholds) were evaluated, and the configuration that provided the best discrimination of the two workload conditions was selected. The algorithms to accomplish this are presented in Kohlmorgen et al., 2007.

After this calibration, the system could determine the driver's workload in real time (see fig. 23.4). In the test phase of the study, the system turned off the auditory reaction-time task whenever it detected a high workload. In this way, it reduced, or mitigated, the driver's workload.

The results of this study showed that the average reaction time was 100 msec faster during the test phase (i.e., when the additional reaction-time task was turned off by the workload detector) than in the calibration phase (i.e., when the task continued despite a high workload). The improvement in performance during the test phase may be explained by the fact that the workload detector successfully predicted periods of potentially reduced reactivity and exempted drivers from needing to react during increased workload (Kohlmorgen et al., 2007).

These and other similar results (e.g., Sterman and Mann, 1995; Gevins et al., 1995; Horne and Baulk, 2004; Lal and Craig, 2005; Lin et al., 2005; Berka et al., 2007) suggest that such BCI-based methods might improve the stability and overall level of performance in a variety of situations in which high workload is a risk. At the same time, it is important to note that the EEG workload detector was substantially more effective in some subjects than in others. Although product development using these measures might be limited to such

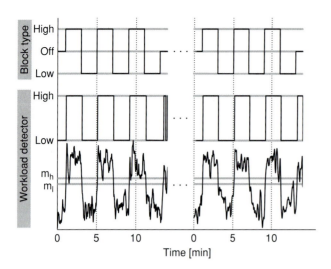

Figure 23.4 *Time course of the classifier output (lower panel) for the best-performing subject and the corresponding binary high/low workload indication used to control the mitigation (middle panel). The true high- and low-workload conditions (auditory) are shown in the upper panel. The close correspondence between the top and middle panels indicates that the classifier accurately detected the workload (95.6% correct). (From Blankertz et al., 2010.)*

modify the task or the emotional state whenever a deleterious emotional state is detected. For example, the task might be delayed or simplified whenever frustration or stress is detected. Alternatively, it may be possible to train people to reduce EEG measures known to be associated with emotional states that impair performance. Important research in this direction investigates the classifiability of emotions in music listening (Lin et al., 2010).

In a pilot study, Blankertz et al. (2009) explored neuronal correlates of emotional reactions related to interaction. Multichannel EEG was recorded from pairs of subjects while they competed in a two-alternative forced-choice task. For specific periods of performance (and unbeknownst to the subjects), the task was biased so as to give one subject or the other an unfair advantage (i.e., by earlier presentation of the stimulus). This bias was designed to induce positive or negative emotional states (e.g., elation, stress, frustration) in the subjects. The behavioral data were consistent across the four subjects of this initial study. For example, when placed at a disadvantage, subjects adapted their strategy (e.g., accepting higher error rates in order to achieve faster reaction times to cope with the competitor), probably reflecting an uncomfortable emotional state. EEG analysis revealed significant within-subject differences between periods of negative and positive emotions in theta-, alpha-, or beta-frequency bands. Within subjects, these differences had widely distributed and spatially coherent topographies (i.e., explainable by one or two dipoles) (see chapters 3 and 6). The relevant frequency bands as well as their spatial foci varied across subjects. Figure 23.5 shows the results from one subject.

The variety of EEG correlates found among the subjects demonstrates the need for adaptive methods in order to successfully enhance task performance by emotional decoding. Studies with a larger number of subjects will show whether some EEG measures correlate with individual attitudes toward a particular emotion provoking situation. In addition, further investigation is needed to establish that the observed changes in the EEG reflect emotions rather than other aspects of task performance (e.g., more forcefully pressing the buttons when annoyed).

individuals, their application in actual products for wider use will presumably require that they be effective for all or almost all potential users.

EMOTION

Emotional states such as anger, frustration, and depression have been shown to affect the event-related potentials (ERPs) elicited by specific stimuli and to be reflected in brain rhythms (Aftanas et al., 2004; Olofsson et al., 2008). Activity recorded over prefrontal cortex appears to be particularly affected by emotional state (Davidson, 2004; Sotres-Bayon and Quirk, 2010). Furthermore, emotional state can affect task performance (Herrington et al., 2005; Gray, 2001; Cohen et al., 2010; Janelle, 2002). Thus, it may be possible to use concurrent EEG analysis to improve or stabilize performance by intervening to

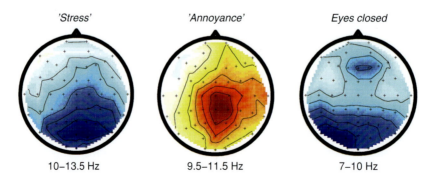

'Stress'   'Annoyance'   Eyes closed

10–13.5 Hz   9.5–11.5 Hz   7–10 Hz

Figure 23.5 *Topographic maps of (upper) alpha-band power for the emotional states "stress" and "annoyance" (minus baseline) in one subject. For comparison, a map of (lower) alpha band power is shown for the condition eyes closed. Note that the eyes closed condition shows modulation in a different frequency band from the affective conditions. The maps differ in their spatial foci.*

ENHANCING CONVENTIONAL PERFORMANCE

Thus far, we have examined some of the ways in which BCIs may help to ensure that people consistently perform specific tasks at the upper levels of their abilities. BCIs might also allow people to *exceed* their normal performance ranges in accuracy or speed. This section discusses several possible approaches to using BCIs to enable such supranormal performance.

OBJECT DETECTION

Several studies (Gerson et al., 2006; Parra et al., 2008; Sajda et al., 2010) have provided impressive illustrations of using EEG decoding to enhance performance in a search and decision-making task. A person is presented with complex images, a few of which contain target objects. The person's task is to detect the targets and to indicate detection by reacting (e.g., pressing a button) as quickly as possible. Despite recent advances in computer vision technology (i.e., technology that allows computers to "see," that is, to extract from images information important to a given task (Ballard and Brown, 1982), humans perform more accurately than real-time object-recognition systems in detecting objects in complex scenes (Bundeskriminalamt, 2007). Furthermore, in humans, brain signals can reflect the detection process *prior* to the actual response of the muscles (i.e., button-pressing) and can do so even in the absence of any requirement for muscles to respond.

Parra et al. (2008) used real-time BCI-based EEG analysis to assist in a detection task in humans. In the first step (a screening or triaging step), the complex images were presented at a very rapid rate (i.e., 10–20 per second). The expectation was that the images containing target objects (i.e., the target images) would evoke P300 responses (see chapter 12), whereas images not containing target objects (i.e., the nontarget images) would not do so. Each image was assigned a priority score indicating to what extent it had evoked a P300-like response. Then, in the second step, the images were ordered according to their scores (i.e., higher scores first) and were presented to the subject at a slow rate to permit careful examination and definitive detection.

This two-step approach was expected to produce performance exceeding the normal range for several reasons. In the triage step the images can be presented at speeds considerably greater than those possible when an actual neuromuscular response is required. Furthermore, a conventional self-paced search is usually much slower because the person responds only after reaching a given certainty threshold. Although the initial rapid image presentation is essentially a coarse-grained approach and is likely to produce some errors, the image prioritization can greatly facilitate the subsequent self-paced examination that makes final decisions.

Parra and his colleagues employed a learning-based approach to discriminate between the EEG responses to target and nontarget images. They recorded 64 EEG channels, extracted sliding 50-msec time windows, and computed a linear discriminant (see chapter 8) from training data that determined the probability that a given image was a target image. They computed 10 discriminative EEG features derived from multiple windows in the first second after image presentation and linearly combined those features to yield results indicating the probability that the image was a target image. The procedure was designed to be robust against slow drifts and fast sample-by-sample fluctuations. With a group of five subjects, these investigators showed that the rapid-presentation triaging step with BCI-based analysis could correctly detect 92% of the target images. These were then given a high priority for subsequent more careful evaluation.

Parra and colleagues coined the term *cortically coupled computer vision* for their BCI-enhanced two-step image detection (Gerson et al., 2006; Parra et al., 2008; Sajda et al., 2010). The term indicates that it integrates traditional computer-vision and BCI technology in order to increase the speed and accuracy of image search.

OTHER POSSIBLE BCI-BASED PERFORMANCE ENHANCEMENTS

Many studies have described EEG features that precede and or even predict the details of spontaneous or stimulus-triggered motor actions, such as hand movement or finger flexion (Blankertz et al., 2006; Waldert et al., 2008). A BCI system able to accurately detect such premovement potentials might be used to produce an action that is faster than is possible by actual muscle contraction. The resulting enhancement in effective reaction time could be particularly valuable in time-critical situations such as the need for a vehicle operator to react quickly to unexpected obstacles or other sudden events.

Another possible BCI-based performance enhancement is suggested by a variety of studies showing that performance errors are associated with particular EEG features (e.g., the error-related negativity) (Falkenstein et al., 2000; Nieuwenhuis et al., 2001; Schalk et al., 2000; Blankertz et al., 2003; Parra et al., 2003; Chavarriaga and Millán, 2010). One promising possibility is that preceding or concurrent brain signals that correlate with successful or unsuccessful performance (e.g., Schubert et al., 2009; Mathewson et al., 2009; Thut et al., 2006; Chen et al., 2008; Fernández et al., 1999; Eichele et al., 2010) might be used in real time to abort or correct errors in neuromuscular performances such as in rapid forced-choice tasks.

BROADENING OR ENRICHING LIFE EXPERIENCE

In this final section, we discuss BCI applications that do not optimize or enhance the performance of conventional neuromuscular tasks but, rather, *broaden* or *enrich* social interactions, creative endeavors, entertainment options, or other life experiences. Although the initial development of these BCI applications is generally intended for people with severe disabilities, they are likely to become appealing to people in general as their convenience and capacities increase.

MEDIA-RELATED ACTIVITIES

People with or without neuromuscular disabilities are interested in a variety of media-related activities: surfing the Internet; assembling photo, video, and music collections and sharing them with family and friends; joining interactive venues such as Internet chat rooms; participating in computer-based painting or music composition; and, of course, consuming audiovisual material for entertainment, education, or employment. These activities can be categorized into exploration, social interaction, self-expression, and consumption. Because an individual's access to such activities usually has a major role in determining his or her quality of life, BCI-based methods for improving this access might greatly improve the lives of people with severe disabilities and perhaps the lives of others as well.

At present BCI applications for media-related activities must accommodate the severe limitations in speed, accuracy, and complexity characteristic of current BCI output commands. These limitations are analogous to, and quite similar to, those that apply to media-related activities on small hand-held mobile devices such as smartphones (Murray-Smith, 2009). As a result, the development of BCI-based media activities can profit from the field of human-computer interaction, which is constantly improving the interaction models for these devices.

Although BCI-based media applications are still in their infancy, several intriguing early examples have been described. These clearly go beyond text-input applications like the original P300-speller grid of Farwell and Donchin (1988) and its successors, Hex-o-Spell (Blankertz et al., 2007; Williamson et al., 2009) and Dasher (Wills and MacKay, 2006).

Figure 23.6 shows an example of the BCI-based browser interface *Nessi* (Bensch et al., 2007). It enables users not only to browse web pages but also to access web-based services and web-based applications in general. It is platform-independent and open source. Its functionality has been demonstrated with a two-class motor-imagery paradigm (Bensch et al., 2007). Two sets of selectable links are each highlighted by one of two different colors. To select a link, the user generates the control command (i.e., the motor imagery that he/she has been instructed to use to represent a given color) to select the set of links that contains the desired link. The chosen set of links is then divided into two smaller sets, each in a different color; selection is repeated in this way until a single link is chosen and accessed.

ARTISTIC EXPRESSION

Kübler et al. (2008) described a BCI-based brain-painting application that uses P300 evoked responses to visual stimuli

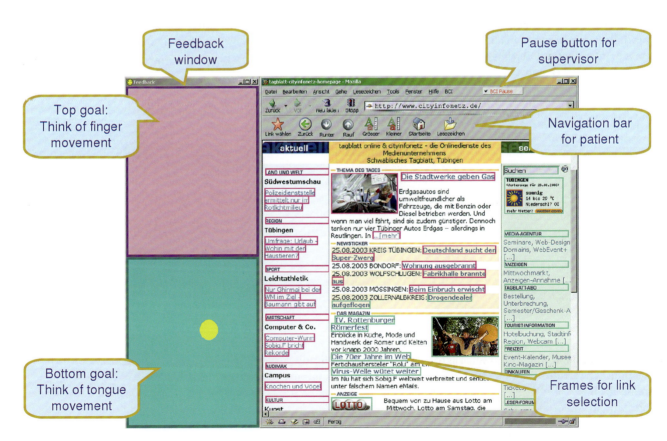

Figure 23.6 Screenshot of the Nessi BCI-based internet browser. On the left, the user observes feedback from the BCI control signals generated by two motor imagery tasks (e.g., imagined finger movement vs. imagined tongue movement). In a series of two-choice imagery-based selections, the user steps down a binary tree to arrive at a single link. (From Bensch et al., 2007.)

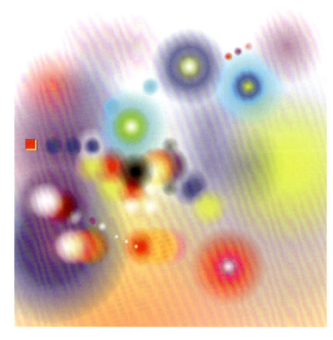

Figure 23.7 *Artistic work generated by BCI-based brain-painting application (Kübler et al., 2008). (Image by courtesy of Adi Hösle.)*

(see chapter 12). By attending to desired items on a matrix of simple painting tools (e.g., colors, shapes, etc.), the user can place shapes on a digital canvas and color them. To date, this application has been used by a number of people with ALS and by an artist without disabilities. Although this application is somewhat restricted by its tool and shape set, it enables artistic expression that does not depend on neuromuscular function. Figure 23.7 shows a sample composition.

GAMES

BCI-controlled gaming applications range widely from strictly medical to completely nonmedical applications. The application can be controlled by the BCI alone, or the BCI can be an additional input that supplements conventional control. Surveys that discuss approaches and requirements of BCI-controlled games on a general level are discussed in Nijholt, 2009, as well as in Allison and Grainmann, 2008. Lécuyer et al. (2008) provides a good overview of several BCI games and virtual-environment applications.

BCI-BASED GAMES

Games can provide strong motivation for practicing, and thereby achieving, better control with a BCI system. Thus, simple BCI-based games can assist naive users in mastering BCI-based communication and control applications. They can be designed to increase the intensity or duration of attention, increase the speed and accuracy of brain-signal control, or improve other important capabilities. The expectation is that these improvements will transfer to the actual communication or control usage of the BCI. For example, Lalor et al. (2005) describe a game intended to improve the concentration needed to operate a BCI that uses steady-state visual evoked potentials

(SSVEPs) (chapter 14). Ramsey et al. (2009) describe a goal-keeper game designed to encourage rapid generation of motor imagery–based BCI commands. These simple BCI games are useful in training for BCI use, but they probably do not have the appeal or immersive properties that would lead people to play them for entertainment alone, apart from their novel method of control compared to standard games (i.e., brain signals rather than muscle-based movements).

Figure 23.8 shows a recently published BCI-based game that requires only two-class control, but requires precise timing and simulates complex physical interactions (Tangermann et al., 2009). This application demonstrates that BCI control signals derived from motor imagery can be precise enough in timing to play a fast and reactive game in real time. Although trade-offs between timing precision and classification precision were necessary for all users, the users found the game to be highly immersive and engaging (Tangermann et al., 2009).

Another notable BCI game is one based on the extremely popular video game "Tetris" (Tetris Holding, www.tetris.com). In this game, variously shaped pieces that are slowly falling down a computer screen can be moved horizontally or rotated in 90-degrees steps by the player so that they fit together exactly upon reaching the bottom. In the BCI version of this game (fig. 23.9), left- or right-hand motor imagery moves the pieces left or right respectively, mental rotation (Ditunno and Mann, 1990) rotates it clockwise, and foot motor imagery makes it fall faster. Although hand and foot motor imagery have been used often in BCI applications, *mental rotation* is a newer BCI paradigm that was first used for BCI control of a robot (Millán et al., 2004). In this BCI version of Tetris, mental rotation was used to rotate pieces and thus was ostensibly quite natural. It was found to be associated with a predominantly right parietal focus (fig. 23.9). This finding is consistent with the neuronal activity that has been reported to be associated with such tasks (Farah, 1989; Ditunno and Mann, 1990; Harris et al., 2000). However, bilateral (Tagaris et al., 1996) and even left hemispheric (Mehta and Newcombe, 1991) dominance has also been reported. Milovojevic et al. (2009) suggest an approach to resolving these seemingly contradictory results.

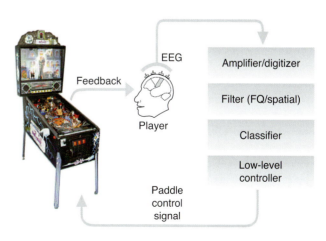

Figure 23.8 *A BCI-based game in which the user controls a pinball machine by motor imagery with left- and right-hand motor imagery.*

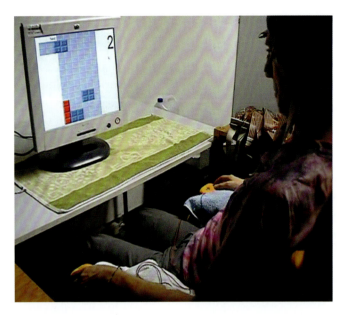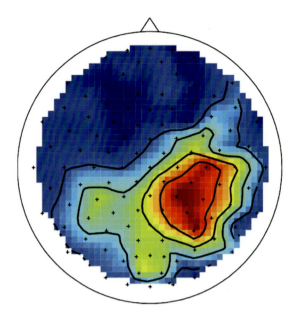

Figure 23.9 BCI-based "Tetris" (Tetris Holding, www.tetris.com) game. (Left) The player uses left- or right-hand motor imagery to move the falling piece right or left, respectively, mental rotation to rotate it clockwise, and foot motor imagery to make it fall faster. (Right) The topographical pattern of desynchronization (i.e., decrease in power) in the 18–24 Hz beta band associated with mental rotation. This desynchronization (red) indicates cortical activation. The right parietal focus is in accord with reports in the literature (e.g., Ditunno and Mann, 1990), but see discussion in the main text regarding contrary findings. (Photograph and topography from an exploratory experiment, by personal communication of the Berlin BCI group.)

BCI-based games, and especially games that can be played *either* with a BCI or through conventional neuromuscular function such as a joystick (i.e., *BCI-capable games*), can also increase social integration for people who are severely disabled by allowing them to cooperate or compete with others, including people without significant disabilities. BCI versions of strategic games such as chess that do not require fast or precisely timed actions enable two people to compete on equal terms, regardless of their respective neuromuscular capabilities. Games that require cooperation (rather than competition), in which two or more players work together to reach a common goal, may provide still greater and more immersive social integration.

In BCI-capable games that reward fast actions or precise timing, such as speed chess or Tetris, the able-bodied player could be slowed down or otherwise impeded (e.g., by adding delays or uncertainty to keyboard inputs) so that the other player could compete on equal terms. Adjustments of this kind might enable people with disabilities to compete on equal terms. They would also allow people without disabilities to experience, and thereby gain greater understanding of, the daunting obstacles constantly faced by people with disabilities.

BCI methods might also be used in otherwise conventional games to optimize the moment-to-moment match between the user's mental state and the demands of the game, and thereby to enhance the user's experience. BCI or BCI-capable versions of both slow strategic games and quick reactive games could also be played remotely over the Internet. Joining a gaming community provides opportunities for social interactions and could allow people with severe disabilities to become active members of communities made up of people with or without disabilities.

In designing a BCI-based game, the limited information-transfer rate of current BCI methods must be taken into account. The greatest challenge is to develop a user interface that accommodates the BCI's limited speed and precision and still provides an attractive, highly immersive gaming experience. The limited control can in part be compensated for by providing rich and timely feedback for each control command issued by the user. This is a fruitful field for cooperation between the BCI research community and the human-computer interface community.

BCI-SUPPLEMENTED GAMES

Whereas a BCI can serve as the sole source of control for a game, it might also provide an *additional* control channel in conventionally controlled games. In the future, as the robustness and convenience of EEG recording devices grow and their costs continue to decline, game players in general may be interested in exploring BCI supplements to standard game-pad, mouse, or keyboard input devices in order to expand and enrich their gaming experiences. The creation and use of such hybrid (i.e., combined BCI/conventional) games should benefit from the development of reliable dry electrodes and algorithms that can reliably separate brain signals from artifacts such as EMG- or eye-movement-related activity (see chapters 6 and 7). At present, the manner in which BCI control and muscle control interact, and the paradigms that enable them to operate concurrently and effectively, remain to be defined.

The development of hybrid games should benefit from the methods developed for real-time monitoring of mental states such as attention and workload described in the first section of this chapter. A game might use this information to adjust the speed or complexity of its ongoing operation to increase the user's immersion and enjoyment. The game experience could be tailored in real time to optimize each gamer's experience.

SUMMARY

As BCI systems become more convenient and affordable, as their information-transfer rates improve, and as their performance becomes more reliable, they are likely to find new applications that go far beyond the assistive-communication and control applications that are the primary focus of current research and development. They may then come to serve people both with and without disabilities—and for a wide variety of purposes.

This chapter discusses three broad categories of actual or conceivable nonmedical uses of BCI technology. First, BCI systems might be used to *optimize* or stabilize performance in conventional neuromuscular tasks. Thus, they might intervene when attention wanes, or they might adjust workload when it reaches a level that is likely to produce errors or otherwise degrade performance.

Second, BCI systems might be used to *enhance* neuromuscular performance beyond that possible conventionally. For example, BCI detection of EEG features specific to target stimuli might increase speed and accuracy in a detection task, BCI recognition of EEG premovement potentials might enable shorter reaction time, or BCI error detection might allow the canceling or correction of a mistake.

Third, BCIs may enable the creation of systems that *broaden* or *enrich* life experiences through media-related activities (e.g., Internet access), new methods of artistic expression, or appealing new computer games that engage the interest and effort of numerous people both with and without disabilities. BCI-based games, or games capable of being operated in either a BCI or conventional fashion, can level the playing field for both able-bodied and disabled users, and can promote social interactions and integration, including those that use the Internet. BCI methods might also be used in otherwise conventional games to optimize the moment-to-moment match between the user's mental state and the demands of the game and thereby to enhance the user's experience.

In summary, in the future, nonmedical BCI applications are likely to affect many kinds of activities for both able-bodied and disabled people, changing and improving the ways in which important and demanding tasks are accomplished, stabilizing and even enhancing task performance, and expanding opportunities for social interactions and entertainment.

REFERENCES

Aftanas, LI, Reva, NV, Varlamov, AA, Pavlov, SV, Makhnev, VP . Analysis of evoked EEG synchronization and desynchronization in conditions of emotional activation in humans: temporal and topographic characteristics. *Neurosci Behav Physiol* 34: 859–867, 2004.

Allison, B, Grainmann, B. Why use a BCI if you're healthy? *IEEE Intell Syst* 23: 76–78, 2008.

Allison, B, Polich, J. Workload assessment of computer gaming using a single-stimulus event-related potential paradigm. *Biol Psychol* 77: 277–283, 2008.

Ballard, DH, Brown, CM. *Computer Vision*. Upper Saddle River, NJ: Prentice Hall, 1982.

Bensch, M, Karim, A, Mellinger, J, Hinterberger, T, Tangermann, M, Bogdan, M, Rosenstiel, W, Birbaumer, N. Nessi: An EEG controlled web browser for severely paralyzed patients. *Comput Intell Neurosci*, 2007.

Berka, C, Levendowski, DJ, Lumicao, MN, Yau, A, Davis, G, Zivkovic, VT, Olmstead, RE, Tremoulet, PD, Craven, PL. EEG correlates of task engagement and mental workload in vigilance, learning, and memory tasks. *Aviat Space Environ Med* 78: B231–244, 2007.

Blankertz, B, Dornhege, G, Lemm, S, Krauledat, M, Curio, G, Müller, KR. The Berlin Brain-Computer Interface: Machine learning based detection of user specific brain states. *J Univ Comput Sci* 12: 581–607, 2006.

Blankertz, B, Dornhege, G, Schäfer, C, Krepki, R, Kohlmorgen, J, Müller, KR, Kunzmann, V, Losch, F, Curio, G. Boosting bit rates and error detection for the classification of fast-paced motor commands based on single-trial EEG analysis. *IEEE Trans Neural Syst Rehabil Eng* 11: 127–131, 2003.

Blankertz, B, Krauledat, M, Dornhege, G, Williamson, J, Murray-Smith, R, Müller, KR. A note on brain actuated spelling with the Berlin Brain-Computer Interface. In: Stephanidis, C (Ed.), *Universal Access in HCI, Part II, HCII 2007, Stephanidis.*Berlin, Heidelberg: Springer, 4555: 759–768, 2007.

Blankertz, B, Müller, KR, Curio, G. Neuronal correlates of emotions in human-machine interaction. In: *BMC Neuroscience 2009*, Eighteenth Annual Computational Neuroscience Meeting: CNS*2009. 10, (Suppl 1): 80.

Blankertz, B, Tangermann, M, Vidaurre, C, Fazli, S, Sannelli, C, Haufe, S, Maeder, C, Ramsey, L, Sturm, I, Curio, G, Müller, KR. The Berlin brain-computer interface: Non-medical uses of BCI technology. *Front Neurosci* 4: 198, 2010.

Bundeskriminalamt. Face recognition as a search tool—"Foto-Fahndung." Technical report, Bundeskriminalamt, 2007.

Chavarriaga, R, Millán, JdR. Learning from EEG error-related potentials in noninvasive brain-computer interfaces. *IEEE Trans Neural Syst Rehabil Eng* 18: 381–388, 2010.

Chen, YN, Mitra, S, Schlaghecken, F. Sub-processes of working memory in the N-back task: An investigation using ERPs. *Clin Neurophysiol* 119: 1546–1559, 2008.

Cohen, N, Henik, A, Mor, N. Can emotion modulate attention? Evidence for reciprocal links in the attentional network test. *Exp Psychol*, 2010. In press.

Davidson, RJ. What does the prefrontal cortex "do" in affect: Perspectives on frontal EEG asymmetry research. *Biol Psychol* 67: 219–233, 2004.

Ditunno, PL, Mann, VA. Right hemisphere specialization for mental rotation in normals and brain damaged subjects. *Cortex* 26: 177–188, 1990.

Donchin, E. The P300 as a metric for mental workload. *Electroencephalogr Clin Neurophysiol Suppl* 39: 338–343, 1987.

Eichele, H, Juvodden, HT, Ullsperger, M, Eichele, T. Mal-adaptation of event-related EEG responses preceding performance errors. *Front Hum Neurosci* 4, 2010.

Falkenstein, M, Hoormann, J, Christ, S, Hohnsbein, J. ERP components on reaction errors and their functional significance: A tutorial. *Biol Psychol* 51: 87–107, 2000.

Fan, J, Byrne, J, Worden, MS, Guise, KG, McCandliss, BD, Fossella, J, Posner, MI. The relation of brain oscillations to attentional networks. *J Neurosci* 27: 6197–6206, 2007.

Farah, MJ. The neural basis of mental imagery. *Trends Neurosci* 12: 395–399, 1989.

Farwell, L, Donchin, E. Talking off the top of your head: Toward a mental prosthesis utilizing event-related brain potentials. *Electroencephalogr Clin Neurophysiol* 70: 510–523, 1988.

Fernández, G, Effern, A, Grunwald, T, Pezer, N, Lehnertz, K, Dümpelmann, M, Van Roost, D, Elger, CE. Real-time tracking of memory formation in the human rhinal cortex and hippocampus. *Science* 285: 1582–1585, 1999.

Fisher, CE, Chin, L, Klitzman, R. Defining neuromarketing: Practices and professional challenges. *Harv Rev Psychiatry* 18: 230–237, 2010.

Fletcher, A, McCulloch, K, Baulk, SD, Dawson, D. Countermeasures to driver fatigue: a review of public awareness campaigns and legal approaches. *Aust N Z J Public Health* 29: 471–476, 2005.

Gerson, A, Parra, L, Sajda, P. Cortically coupled computer vision for rapid image search. *IEEE Trans Neural Syst Rehabil Eng* 14: 174–179, 2006.

Gevins, A, Leong, H, Du, R, Smith, ME, Le, J, DuRousseau, D, Zhang, J, Libove, J. Towards measurement of brain function in operational environments. *Biol Psychol* 40: 169–186, 1995.

Gray, JR. Emotional modulation of cognitive control: approach-withdrawal states double-dissociate spatial from verbal two-back task performance. *J Exp Psychol Gen* 130: 436–452, 2001.

Guderian, S, Schott, BH, Richardson-Klavehn, A, Düzel, E. Medial temporal theta state before an event predicts episodic encoding success in humans. *Proc Natl Acad Sci USA* 106: 5365–5370, 2009.

Harris, IM, Egan, GF, Sonkkila, C, Tochon-Danguy, HJ, Paxinos, G, Watson, JD. Selective right parietal lobe activation during mental rotation: A parametric PET study. *Brain* 123 (Pt 1): 65–73, 2000.

Herrington, JD, Mohanty, A, Koven, NS, Fisher, JE, Stewart, JL, Banich, MT, Webb, AG, Miller, GA, Heller, W. Emotion-modulated performance and activity in left dorsolateral prefrontal cortex. *Emotion* 5: 200–207, 2005.

Holm, A, Lukander, K, Korpela, J, Sallinen, M, Muller, KM. Estimating brain load from the EEG. *ScientificWorldJournal* 9: 639–651, 2009.

Horne, JA, Baulk, SD. Awareness of sleepiness when driving. *Psychophysiology* 41: 161–165, 2004.

Isreal, JB, Wickens, CD, Chesney, GL, Donchin, E. The event-related brain potential as an index of display-monitoring workload. *Hum Factors* 22: 211–224, 1980.

ITU–T Rec. P. 910. Subjective video quality assessment methods for multimedia applications. Geneva: International Telecommunications Union, 2008.

Janelle, CM. Anxiety, arousal and visual attention: a mechanistic account of performance variability. *J Sports Sci* 20: 237–251, 2002.

Karis, D, Fabiani, M, Donchin, E. P300 and memory: Individual differences in the von Restorff effect. *Cog Psychol* 16: 177–216, 1984.

Klauer, SG, Guo, F, Sudweeks, J, Dingus, TA. An analysis of driver inattention using a case-crossover approach on 100-car data: Final report. Technical report, Virginia Tech Transportation Institute, 2010.

Kohlmorgen, J, Dornhege, G, Braun, M, Blankertz, B, Müller, KR, Curio, G, Hagemann, K, Bruns, A, Schrauf, M, Kincses, W. Improving human performance in a real operating environment through real-time mental workload detection. In: Dornhege, G, del R. Millán, J, Hinterberger, T, McFarland, D, Müller, KR, Eds. *Toward Brain-Computer Interfacing*, Cambridge, MA: MIT press, 409–422, 2007.

Kramer, AF, Trejo, LJ, Humphrey, D. Assessment of mental workload with task-irrelevant auditory probes. *Biol Psychol* 40: 83–100, 1995.

\, A, Furdea, A, Halder, S, Hösle, A. Brain painting–BCI meets art. In: Müller-Putz, GR, Brunner, C, Leeb, R, Pfurtscheller, G, Neuper, C, Eds. *Proceedings of the 4th International Brain-Computer Interface Workshop and Training Course 2008*. Graz: Verlag der Technischen Universität Graz, 2008, 361–366.

Lal, SK, Craig, A. Reproducibility of the spectral components of the electroencephalogram during driver fatigue. *Int J Psychology* 55: 137–143, 2005.

Lalor, E, Kelly, S, Finucane, C, Burke, R, Smith, R, Reilly, R, McDarby, G. Steady-state VEP-based brain-computer interface control in an immersive 3D gaming environment. *EURASIP J Appl Signal Processing* 19: 3156, 2005.

Lécuyer, A, Lotte, F, Reilly, RB, Leeb, R, Hirose, M, Slater, M. Brain-computer interfaces, virtual reality, and videogames. *Computer* 41: 66–72, 2008.

Lin, CT, Wu, RC, Jung, TP, Liang, SF, Huang, TY. Estimating driving performance based on EEG spectrum analysis. *EURASIP J Appl Signal Process* 19: 3165–3174, 2005.

Lin, YP, Wang, CH, Jung, TP, Wu, TL, Jeng, SK, Duann, JR, Chen, JH. EEG-based emotion recognition in music listening. *IEEE Trans Biomed Eng* 57: 1798–1806, 2010.

Lyznicki, JM, Doege, TC, Davis, RM, Williams, MA. Sleepiness, driving, and motor vehicle crashes. Council on Scientific Affairs, American Medical Association. *JAMA* 279: 1908–1913, 1998.

Makeig, S, Jung, TP. Tonic, phasic, and transient EEG correlates of auditory awareness in drowsiness. *Cogn Brain Res* 4: 15–25, 1996.

Mathewson, KE, Gratton, G, Fabiani, M, Beck, DM, Ro, T. To see or not to see: Prestimulus alpha phase predicts visual awareness. *J Neurosci* 29: 2725–2732, 2009.

Mehta, Z, Newcombe, F. A role for the left hemisphere in spatial processing. *Cortex* 27: 153–167, 1991.

Milivojevic, B, Hamm, JP, Corballis, MC. Hemispheric dominance for mental rotation: It is a matter of time. *Neuroreport* 20: 1507–1512, 2009.

Millán, J, Renkens, F, No, JM, Gerstner, W. Non-invasive brain-actuated control of a mobile robot by human EEG. *IEEE Trans Biomed Eng* 51: 1026–1033, 2004.

Mokdad, AH, Marks, JS, Stroup, DF, Gerberding, JL. Actual causes of death in the United States, 2000. *JAMA* 291: 1238–1245, 2004.

Mokdad, AH, Marks, JS, Stroup, DF, Gerberding, JL. Correction: Actual causes of death in the United States, 2000. *JAMA* 293: 293–294, 2005.

Müller, KR, Tangermann, M, Dornhege, G, Krauledat, M, Curio, G, Blankertz, B. Machine learning for real-time single-trial EEG-analysis: From brain-computer interfacing to mental state monitoring. *J Neurosci Methods* 167: 82–90, 2008.

Murray-Smith, R. Empowering people rather than connecting them. *Int J Mobile Hum Compur Interact* 1: 18–28, 2009.

Nieuwenhuis, S, Ridderinkhof, K, Blom, J, Band, G, Kok, A. Error-related brain potentials are differentially related to awareness of response errors: Evidence from an antisaccade task. *Psychophysiology* 38: 752–760, 2001.

Nijholt, A. BCI for games: A "state of the art" survey. In: *ICEC '08: Proceedings of the 7th International Conference on Entertainment Computing*. Berlin, Heidelberg: Springer-Verlag, 225–228, 2009.

Olofsson, JK, Nordin, S, Sequeira, H, Polich, J. Affective picture processing: An integrative review of ERP findings. *Biol Psychol* 77: 247–265, 2008.

Papadelis, C, Chen, Z, Kourtidou-Papadeli, C, Bamidis, P, Chouvarda, I, Bekiaris, E, Maglaveras, N. Monitoring sleepiness with on-board electrophysiological recordings for preventing sleep-deprived traffic accidents. *Clin Neurophysiol* 118: 1906–1922, 2007.

Parra, L, Christoforou, C, Gerson, A, Dyrholm, M, Luo, A, Wagner, M, Philiastides, M, Sajda, P. Spatiotemporal linear decoding of brain state. *IEEE Signal Process Mag* 25: 107–115, 2008.

Parra, L, Spence, C, Gerson, A, Sajda, P. Response error correction—a demonstration of improved human-machine performance using real-time EEG monitoring. *IEEE Trans Neural Syst Rehabil Eng* 11: 173–177, 2003.

Prinzel, LJ, Freeman, FG, Scerbo, MW, Mikulka, PJ, Pope, AT. Effects of a psychophysiological system for adaptive automation on performance, workload, and the event-related potential P300 component. *Hum Factors* 45: 601–613, 2003.

Ramsey, L, Tangermann, M, Haufe, S, Blankertz, B. Practicing fast-decision BCI using a "goalkeeper" paradigm. In: *BMC Neuroscience 2009*, Eighteenth Annual Computational Neuroscience Meeting: CNS*2009, 10 (Suppl 1): P69.

Ranney, TA. Driver distraction: A review of the current state-of-knowledge. Technical report, National Highway Traffic Safety Administration, 2008.

Sajda, P, Parra, LC, Christoforou, C, Hanna, B, Bahlmann, C, Wang, J, Pohlmeyer, E, Dmochowski, J, Chang, SF. In a blink of an eye and a switch of a transistor: Cortically-coupled computer vision. *Proc IEEE* 98: 462–478, 2010.

Schalk, G, Wolpaw, JR, McFarland, DJ, Pfurtscheller, G. EEG-based communication: Presence of an error potential. *Clin Neurophysiol* 111: 2138–2144, 2000.

Schubert, R, Haufe, S, Blankenburg, F, Villringer, A, Curio, G. Now you'll feel it—now you won't: EEG rhythms predict the effectiveness of perceptual masking. *J Cogn Neurosci* 21: 2407–2419, 2009.

Slobounov, S, Chiang, H, Johnston, J, Ray, W. Modulated cortical control of individual fingers in experienced musicians: An EEG study. Electroencephalographic study. *Clin Neurophysiol* 113: 2013–2024, 2002.

Smith, ME, Gevins, A, Brown, H, Karnik, A, Du, R, Gevins, AS. Monitoring task loading with multivariate EEG measures during complex forms of human-computer interaction. *Hum Factors* 43: 366–380, 2001.

Sotres-Bayon, F, Quirk, GJ. Prefrontal control of fear: More than just extinction. *Curr Opin Neurobiol* 20: 231–235, 2010.

Sterman, MB, Mann, CA. Concepts and applications of EEG analysis in aviation performance evaluation. *Biol Psychol* 40: 115–130, 1995.

Subramanian, R. Motor vehicle traffic crashes as a leading cause of death in the USA, 2004. NHTSA-Report DOT HS 810 742, NHTSA, 2007.

Tagaris, GA, Kim, SG, Strupp, JP, Andersen, P, Uğurbil, K, Georgopoulos, AP. Quantitative relations between parietal activation and performance in mental rotation. *Neuroreport* 7: 773–776, 1996.

Tangermann, M, Krauledat, M, Grzeska, K, Sagebaum, M, Blankertz, B, Vidaurre, C, Müller, KR. Playing pinball with non-invasive BCI. In: *Advances in Neural Information Processing Systems 21*, Cambridge, MA: MIT Press, 1641–1648, 2009.

Thut, G, Nietzel, A, Brandt, SA, Pascual-Leone, A. Alpha-band electroencephalographic activity over occipital cortex indexes visuospatial attention bias and predicts visual target detection. *J Neurosci* 26: 9494–9502, 2006.

Waldert, S, Preissl, H, Demandt, E, Braun, C, Birbaumer, N, Aertsen, A, Mehring, C. Hand movement direction decoded from MEG and EEG. *J Neurosci* 28: 1000–1008, 2008.

Wältermann, M, Scholz, K, Möller, S, Huo, L, Raake, A, Heute, U. An instrumental measure for end-to-end speech. In: *Proceedings of the 11th International Conference on Spoken Language Processing*, 2008, 61–64.

Williamson, J, Murray-Smith, R, Blankertz, B, Krauledat, M, Müller, KR. Designing for uncertain, asymmetric control: Interaction design for brain-computer interfaces. *Int J Hum Comput Stud* 67: 827–841, 2009.

Wills, S, MacKay, D. DASHER—an efficient writing system for brain-computer interfaces? *IEEE Trans Neural Syst Rehabil Eng* 14: 244–246, 2006.

Xu, J, Kochanek, KD, Murphy, SL, Tejada-Vera, B. Deaths: Final data for 2007. *National Vital Statistics Reports* 58: 1–137, 2010.

24 | ETHICAL ISSUES IN BCI RESEARCH

MARY-JANE SCHNEIDER, JOSEPH J. FINS, AND JONATHAN R. WOLPAW

Scientific and engineering advances often bring with them important ethical issues. As a prominent part of the progress that now promises unprecedented understanding of and access to the brain and its disorders, BCI research in humans raises ethical issues that engage the attention and affect the actions of scientists, engineers, clinicians, and policy makers. Some of these issues are straightforward and can be addressed effectively (although not always easily) by adhering to well-established principles. Others are new and unique. Arising from the practical realities of BCI research or from the fundamental nature of BCIs themselves, they may have no clear solutions at present.

This chapter discusses the ethical issues raised by BCI research in humans. It is organized around the three principles set out in the Belmont Report of 1978 (National Commission for the Protection of Human Subjects, 1978), which is generally considered the founding document of modern human research standards. The three principles are *beneficence, respect for persons*, and *justice*. Stated most simply, *beneficence* requires that the potential benefits of human research (to humanity and perhaps to the research subjects) far outweigh its risks to the subjects. *Respect for persons* requires that informed consent be obtained from the subjects. *Justice* requires that the benefits and burdens of the research be fairly distributed. Each of these principles is complex both in theory and in practice, and together they have generated a large and steadily growing literature (Institute of Medicine, 2005; Ackerman, 2006; Illes, 2006; Leshner, 2007; Beauchamp and Childress, 2009). In this chapter, we focus on those aspects most relevant to current BCI research.

In applying these principles, it is helpful to divide BCI research into two distinct, though potentially overlapping, categories. The first category comprises BCI research aimed at helping people with disabilities to obtain a functional status equal to that of people who are not disabled. In terms of the BCI definition presented in chapter 1 and used throughout this book, this category includes research aimed at restoring or replacing natural CNS output, or at improving natural output to equal that of people who are not disabled. This area has been and continues to be the major focus of BCI research, and it is also the major focus of this chapter. The second category comprises research aimed at the general population. In terms of the chapter 1 definition, this category includes research aimed at enhancing or supplementing natural CNS output or at improving natural output to supranormal levels. Because work of this kind is just beginning, and because the additional ethical issues that it raises remain largely hypothetical at present, its treatment here is relatively brief.

BCI RESEARCH TO HELP PEOPLE WITH DISABILITIES

Restoring communication and control capacities to people with severe neuromuscular disabilities has been and continues to be the major focus of BCI research. The human research essential to this enterprise raises a variety of ethical questions. Some are more or less standard issues that arise in many other areas of biomedical research. Others are unique to BCI research or to the broader field of neurotechnology in general.

BENEFICENCE: DOING GOOD AND NOT DOING HARM

The first prerequisite for assessing the beneficence of any enterprise is a clear definition of beneficence, that is, specification of the precise nature of the *good* that is being pursued. For BCI research aimed at people with disabilities, this definition is clear: research is beneficial if it helps people to regain normal function—to communicate, to move about, to work and play, and so forth. By this definition, the potential benefits of BCI research are not in serious doubt. The chapters in this book provide ample evidence that, even with their current limitations, BCIs can restore basic communication and control capacities to those with the most severe neuromuscular disabilities and can do so with minimal risk. With little or no capacity for independent action, these individuals may be completely dependent on caregivers. A BCI can restore some measure of autonomy and independence, enabling them to maintain social relationships with family and friends, to convey their desires to caregivers, to operate environmental control or entertainment systems, or even to continue gainful employment (e.g., Sellers et al., 2010). Indeed, it has been argued that society has an ethical obligation to enable people who have the capacity to communicate to do so (Fenton and Alpert, 2008; Fins, 2009a). As BCI technology improves, it is likely to become useful to much larger numbers of people with less severe disabilities. In sum, the potential human benefits of BCI technology are clear and provide ample justification for the human research necessary to realize them. At the same time, attention to a number of important factors is essential in order to maximize these benefits.

Many of the risks associated with BCI research are not as obvious as those associated with other new neurotechnologies and therapies, such as deep brain stimulation or other brain-stimulation methods, drugs that manipulate neurotransmitter function, or agents that encourage neuronal regeneration (Farah et al., 2004; Illes and Bird, 2006; Schermer, 2009; Gillett, 2006; Hamilton et al., 2011). Unlike these other methodologies, BCIs do not act directly on the brain; they act only as receptive devices that measure CNS activity. As described in chapter 1, BCIs convert that activity into new outputs that replace, restore, augment, supplement, or improve natural CNS output. Nevertheless, these new BCI-based outputs do come with risks. They might, for example, induce undesirable plasticity in the brain, and invasive BCIs involving surgical implantation introduce attendant dangers of bleeding, tissue reaction, and infection. These and other risks may be substantial, and research studies should be designed and executed so as to minimize them. The following subsections discuss measures intended to maximize the benefits and minimize the risks of BCI research in humans.

THE NEED FOR MULTIDISCIPLINARY EXPERTISE AND COLLABORATION

As illustrated abundantly in many chapters of this book, BCI research is inherently and necessarily multidisciplinary. It involves neuroscience, physics, mechanical and electrical engineering, applied mathematics, computer science, clinical neurology, neurosurgery, rehabilitation, assistive technology, behavioral psychology, human factors engineering. (Indeed, the multidisciplinary nature of BCIs and other neurotechnology is reflected in the necessarily interdisciplinary nature of neuroethics [Fins, 2011].) Contributions from and collaboration among all these different disciplines are needed for BCI research to be successful in its central goal, to restore communication and/or other capacities to those with disabilities. This reality imposes two specific ethical requirements on BCI research studies.

ENSURING QUALITY OF CARE

First and most obviously, the personnel conducting a human (or animal) study should possess adequate expertise in all disciplines relevant to the study. Indeed, this requirement dates back to the Nuremberg Code (1949), which states that the quality of care provided in research settings must equal that provided in clinical settings. For example, if a group of researchers whose primary expertise and interest is in development of signal-processing algorithms seeks to collect EEG data from human subjects, they need to ensure (often through collaboration) that the details of EEG recording (i.e., electrode placements, reference selection, impedance reduction, digitization resolution and rate, artifact detection, etc.) are properly handled. This multidisciplinary requirement may be more difficult to satisfy when the subjects are people with specific disabilities, since clinician involvement is then needed for subject access and selection. It can become still more difficult when BCIs are tested for long-term use by people with disabilities (when expert hardware/software support and skills in handling the often complex interactions with caregivers and family are needed), or when invasive BCIs are studied (when device engineering and neurosurgery also become essential components). Analogous multidisciplinary requirements apply to BCI research groups with primary expertise in engineering, assistive technology, behavioral psychology, and others.

Deficiency in any one of the disciplines relevant to a study may prevent it from yielding substantive results or may even pose additional risks to the research subjects. Thus, for BCI research, as for other neurotechnology research (e.g., Fins et al., 2006), engaging the multidisciplinary expertise needed to ensure that every aspect of a study is well designed and executed is an ethical necessity.

ENSURING ACCESSIBILITY OF RESULTS

The second ethical implication of the multidisciplinary nature of BCI research is that the results of any BCI study should be made easily accessible to other research groups. This is consistent with good science and with the principle of justice articulated in the Belmont Report; such intellectual collegiality promotes progress and should enhance access to new technologies. Furthermore, it is also consistent with the fact that most BCI research is supported by public funds. This implies that the results are not meant to be proprietary but rather to be shared in a way that promotes and benefits a scientific community engaged in collaborative work (Fins, 2010).

From a practical point of view, an open-access approach to methods and results facilitates the growth of the field. Many groups who lack the kinds of expertise or access needed to acquire particular kinds of data are able, by virtue of the expertise they do possess, to use data gathered by others for further analyses that amplify and extend the value of the data. Excellent examples of the value of making BCI data widely available are the several BCI data competitions, in which a relatively small number of groups have provided specific kinds of BCI data for analysis by signal-processing groups throughout the world (Sajda et al., 2003; Blankertz et al., 2004; Blankertz et al., 2006). These essentially collaborative efforts have produced important advances in signal-processing methods. However, despite such encouraging examples, the vast majority of BCI studies to date have not produced fully accessible data. Certainly, even though common data formats do exist (e.g., Schalk and Mellinger, 2010), providing data with sufficient information to make it useful to another research group, and ensuring that subject confidentiality is maintained, may still be a substantial task. Nevertheless, the necessary efforts should be undertaken whenever possible so that BCI data, which often require special circumstances and substantial efforts for their collection, are as productive as possible. Maximizing the yield from such data is especially critical in view of the considerable expense often involved in obtaining them and the generally severe limitations on research funding from NIH and elsewhere.

INVASIVE BCI RESEARCH: MOVING FROM ANIMALS TO HUMANS

The implants used in invasive BCI methods entail risks of tissue damage and reaction, infection, device failure, and long-term functional instability (see chapters 5 and 16). These risks can in large measure be evaluated and reduced through animal studies that optimize electrode designs, develop better implantation procedures, and assess long-term safety and efficacy. The need for such animal studies as an essential prerequisite for human studies was first articulated in the

Nuremberg Code (1949). For invasive BCIs, the necessary studies are conducted mainly in rats and monkeys. Rat studies are suitable for some questions (e.g., tissue compatibility, device durability). However, the substantial differences between rodents and primates (e.g., in infection susceptibility, brain anatomy, and tissue movements) mean that monkey studies are needed to address other key questions (e.g., infection risks, long-term recording stability). Furthermore, because monkeys can be trained to perform complex protocols, monkey studies can in principle address many questions about BCI control capacities. Of course, these animal studies must adhere to established requirements for the care and use of laboratory animals, and must be reviewed and approved by the local Institutional Animal Care and Use Committee (Committee for the Update of the Guide for the Care and Use of Laboratory Animals, 2011).

Although animal studies are generally a necessary prerequisite to invasive BCI studies in humans, the determination of the point at which human studies, with the risks they entail, become justifiable or necessary is a complex problem with a significant ethical component. The most extreme position is that human implantation is not appropriate until all the questions that can possibly be addressed in animals have been addressed and have satisfactory answers, that is, until wholly implantable systems that are safe and perform effectively for many years in monkeys have been developed and validated and have shown that they can provide function that significantly exceeds that possible with noninvasive BCI systems. By this extreme position, only then will human implantations and human studies be justified. However, the actual implementation of this position is highly problematic because of the unique capabilities and complexity of the human brain. It has not been widely adopted, either by researchers or by those charged with regulating human studies.

At present, invasive BCIs are under study both in animals and in humans. Several factors justify these human studies. First, the risks entailed (e.g., of infection, tissue damage, device failure) appear to be very modest, and complications that do occur are generally transient and appear to do no lasting harm (see chapter 16). Second, the studies are generally limited to people in whom the risks are not amplified by concurrent health problems, adverse environmental factors, or the burden of an unrealistic *therapeutic conception* (i.e., an incorrect and overly optimistic concept of the benefits of the device and its ability to restore lost function) (Lidz et al., 2004). That is, the subjects are healthy and medically stable aside from their severe neuromuscular disabilities, they have supportive living environments, and they understand that they are participating in research and that the BCI is not intended to be, and may well not be, a solution to their own communication and control needs. Thus, their participation does not constitute an excessive additional burden. Indeed, they generally welcome the study, primarily as an opportunity to contribute to important research, and only secondarily as something that might conceivably be of benefit to them personally in the future. Third, the major aims of these studies generally include aims that are difficult or even impossible to address in monkeys. Despite the fact that some BCI control applications can theoretically be tested in monkeys, only human testing can readily test applications such as complex communication or elaborate, highly flexible movement control. On the other hand, issues such as the long-term safety, stability, and efficacy of fully implantable system prototypes are best assessed first, and exhaustively, in monkeys prior to comparable human testing.

STUDYING BCI USE BY PEOPLE WITH DISABILITIES

The essential final step in the development of a BCI system is the demonstration that it is usable by and useful to those people for whom it is intended. Although this step can begin with short-term studies in which people with severe disabilities use the BCI under close supervision, it ultimately requires long-term (i.e., >6 months) studies of independent use (generally in the users' homes) in which the day-to-day operation and oversight of the system is handled by the user and the caregivers, with minimal ongoing technical support from the research group. These demanding long-term studies are discussed in detail in chapter 20. Here we address the risks this work may involve. We begin with physical and psychological risks that are largely analogous to those encountered in many other areas of biomedical research. We then address risks that are specific to BCI research, either because of the basic nature of BCIs or because of their current state of development.

Physical Risks

The physical risks associated with noninvasive BCI use are generally minimal. With proper education of the caregivers responsible for supporting BCI use, problems such as skin irritation due to daily electrode application can be prevented or readily addressed should they develop. BCI systems use medical-grade electronic components so that the risks of inadvertent shocks are almost nonexistent. At the same time, both researchers and caregivers need to ensure that hardware and software are checked regularly and properly maintained.

Physical risks will increase when and if invasive BCI systems enter testing in long-term independent home use. Users and caregivers will need to be instructed in how to recognize local or systemic signs of infection or implant malfunction (e.g., erythema, swelling, fever, performance decline), and researchers will need to have in place appropriate oversight procedures as well as protocols for quickly and successfully responding to such problems. At the same time, assuming that preclinical studies have been thorough and successful, these risks should have very low probability and should be able to be addressed effectively if they occur.

Psychological Risks

Like any study of a promising new treatment method, whether a drug or a device, BCI studies in people with severe disabilities run the risk of subject disappointment if the system proves not to be usable or useful. This risk may be mitigated, but not eliminated, by emphasizing the limitations and uncertainties of the study in the informed consent process and throughout the subject's participation.

In order to minimize these psychological risks, researchers should emphasize that subjects who volunteer to participate are performing a service, for the research group certainly, and, more importantly, for humanity in general. It should be carefully explained that benefiting subjects is not the study's primary purpose (even though it might do so). Rather, it is actually the subject's altruism and willingness to volunteer that are providing benefits in new knowledge and, hopefully, in useful new assistive technology. Researchers should emphasize this point when they first invite people to participate, during the informed consent process, and throughout the course of the study. Certainly, some subjects may still choose to participate mainly because they hope to benefit themselves. This is understandable and to be expected, but it is critical that all subjects understand that no personal benefit is promised (particularly in an early trial), and that their participation is mainly a very admirable and highly appreciated contribution to BCI research and development. This understanding will often help to reduce the risk of a therapeutic misconception on the part of the subject, that is, unrealistic expectations that may lead to disappointment (Lidz et al., 2004).

Psychological risks may be particularly significant for subjects who see the BCI as a last resort because conventional assistive devices have failed. In the most extreme situations, particularly prevalent in those with progressive disorders such as ALS, subjects and family members may want to consider the possibility of BCI-based communication in making life decisions, such as whether or not to accept full-time artificial ventilation. In fact, 42% of people with ALS on long-term mechanical ventilation indicated that such ventilation should be stopped if and when they became unable to communicate (Moss et al., 1996). Prospective BCI users and their families may be desperate for a way to prevent the total isolation and dependency they foresee coming. As a result, the researchers may be drawn into extremely complex and highly emotional dilemmas that go far beyond the bounds of scientific research and that may entail major psychological and other risks to the subject and his or her family members. These potential risks should be considered carefully by the research group in designing the study and in defining the subject selection criteria. For example, to reduce risk the experimenters might elect, at least initially, to study only people who have already made the difficult decision to accept mechanical ventilation, or people with stable disabilities for whom other communication and control options exist.

Limiting a study to people with stable disabilities also reduces the risk that disease progression will render the BCI less and less useful to them. If and when this occurs, the research group may feel obligated, or may be asked, to try to modify the BCI so as to restore its effectiveness. Certainly, some provisions for simple modifications can be incorporated into the initial research plan. However, beyond such basic responses, ad hoc modification efforts can often require extra effort that places enormous demands on usually very limited resources. Furthermore, any such effort is essentially new research and may thus require its own approval process. At the same time, the desire to help the subject may be compelling. Studying subjects with stable disabilities is one way to reduce the probability that such dilemmas will arise. Nevertheless, each research group should try to consider in advance how these situations will be handled if they occur.

A study limited to subjects who have already accepted mechanical ventilation must avoid giving the impression that it is coercing the continuation of ventilation. The subject must continue to feel completely free to discontinue ventilation; prior acceptance of a BCI should not in any way constrain this decision.

For BCI systems that have already demonstrated safety and some measure of efficacy, better approaches might be to include possibilities such as the acceptance or rejection of mechanical ventilation in the study protocol and to learn how subjects and their families actually consider (or even use) BCI systems in making such difficult choices. After all, it is important to test these devices in the real-life contexts in which they are likely to both improve and perhaps also complicate the care of people with severe and often progressive disabilities. Studies of this kind should closely involve both local ethics committees and palliative-care specialists who can help ensure that the rights of these individuals, who are both study subjects and patients, are fully protected throughout the life cycle (Fins, 2006).

The Risk of Inappropriate Outputs

Studies in which people use BCIs in their daily lives may also encounter risks associated with this use. For example, through human or system error, a BCI used for environmental control and simple communication with a caregiver might set the room temperature incorrectly or might fail to notify a caregiver of an acute problem, such as a respirator malfunction. Possibilities of this kind make it incumbent on the research group to design and configure the BCI applications so as to minimize the likelihood of such malfunctions and to educate both user and caregiver in avoiding and detecting these malfunctions. Fulfilling this obligation requires careful and imaginative consideration of all possible malfunctions and continued meticulous attention to their prevention and their detection.

The Risk of Invasion of Privacy

One concern often voiced about BCIs is that their users might inadvertently reveal private thoughts and emotions, or even that outside authorities might use BCIs to extract information without consent. Indeed, the P300 evoked potential, which is the basis for one widely used BCI, has been suggested as a method for lie-detection (Levy, 2007). This concern about BCI technology is part of the general concern about the potential abuses of the new brain-imaging technologies (e.g., MRI, fMRI) and other new diagnostic methods (e.g., genetic analysis) (e.g., Farah et al., 2004; Illes and Bird, 2006).

In reality, however, the danger to privacy posed by BCIs, although plausible at first glance, may not become a major problem. As discussed in chapter 1, BCIs provide the brain with new nonmuscular output channels; they enable the user to communicate with and act on the world through brain signals rather than muscles. As such, they generally require the active engagement of the user and are therefore not mind-reading devices. It is important that investigators and ethicists make these points explicitly, lest unjustified fears undermine the legitimate uses of BCIs and limit their availability to populations in need of new assistive communication and control devices (Fins, 2007).

BCIs that use cortical neurons or sensorimotor rhythms require at least as much user involvement and skill development as normal muscular control; and even the P300-based BCI depends on the user attending to the stimuli that are being presented. Thus, BCIs, that is, systems that provide the brain with new outputs, may not constitute substantial new threats to individual privacy. In the future if BCIs incorporate methods such as targeted brain stimulation (e.g., to provide sensory feedback) in order to improve their performance, additional ethical concerns may arise. However, such systems would be more than simply BCIs, and thus are beyond the scope of the present discussion.

On the other hand, the data collection and analyses conducted as part of long-term studies of independent BCI use may introduce invasion-of-privacy risks. For example, if the user employs the BCI to communicate with family, friends, or co-workers and complete data on BCI use are collected, the data will necessarily include these communications. Although these communications may be accessible only to the researchers, their knowledge in itself might constitute an invasion of privacy or be viewed as such by the user or by the user's correspondents. Thus, data collection might be designed to avoid collecting the messages (e.g., by measuring only the number of letters or words spelled and assessing errors by the number of backspaces).

The Problem of Time-Limited Studies

Another particularly difficult ethical issue arises from the nature of most research studies: they are designed, and funded, to cover certain time periods. For a study of long-term BCI use, the period may be lengthy, even several years, but it is not indefinite, if only because the research is generally not funded indefinitely. Although this time limitation presents no problem in subjects for whom the technology is not useful, it may be a problem in subjects for whom the technology proves useful: they may want to continue using it beyond the study period. In the most extreme examples, their continued ability to communicate may depend entirely or largely on continued use of the BCI. Their continued possession of the BCI system itself may not present a problem, since its initial cost was presumably covered by the study budget. However, funding is still needed for supplies (e.g., electrode caps), and, most important, expert personnel are needed to provide technical support. Even if the subject can pay for this support, it may not be available except from the research group, which is usually not designed or empowered to provide such support outside of a research setting. Research groups may manage in one way or another to continue to provide technical support, but this usually cannot be guaranteed in advance. Thus, mention of this uncertainty should be included in the informed consent process.

This issue of continued support is a problem for which there will be no definitive solution until BCI technology becomes more widely available and is routinely supported by service, rather than research, organizations. Until then, funding agencies, review boards, and research groups must address it according to their own best lights and capacities.

When ethicists speak of such dilemmas they speak of the principle of nonabandonment, that is, not walking away from one's professional obligation to those who are in need or vulnerable. Subjects with implanted devices and those requiring special supplies or specific interfaces are highly dependent on the research team, and the members of the team are morally obligated to do all they can not to abandon them when the formal study is completed (Fins, 2009b). To formally recognize this obligation, and to increase the probability that it will be honored, Institutional Review Boards (IRBs) should require that study protocols include provisions for it. These might involve setting aside sufficient resources ahead of time and/or ensuring that the needed long-term services will be covered by conventional health insurance. Without such provisions, subjects may be exceedingly vulnerable in the poststudy phase, and this risk should be minimized to the greatest extent possible.

The Risk of Deleterious CNS Plasticity

As discussed in chapter 1, the brain's neuromuscular skills (e.g., actions such as walking, talking, etc.) are acquired and maintained by initial and continuing plasticity in the many different CNS areas involved. Throughout life, CNS neurons and synapses change continually to master new skills and to preserve those already mastered. BCIs, by providing new output channels (i.e., brain signals rather than muscles), ask the CNS to adapt in new ways so as to use these new outputs effectively. Studies to date provide substantial evidence that such plasticity does occur and that it is important (e.g., see chapter 13). Its occurrence is clearly desirable if it allows BCI use to become as easy as normal muscular control, and thereby enables the disabled user to function more normally in the world. In this case, the person's dependence on technology should be no more troubling than the dependence of a visually impaired person on eyeglasses or a hearing-impaired person on a hearing aid.

At the same time, due to the ubiquitous capacity for plasticity in the CNS and the fact that the CNS must maintain many different skills, BCI use is likely to produce plasticity that is extremely complex and that may affect other aspects of CNS function. The dangers of such associated plasticity are unknown. On the one hand, any new technology (e.g., automobiles, typewriters, video games) that changes how people interact with the world presumably produces extensive CNS plasticity. On the other hand, these other technologies involve only the brain's natural neuromuscular outputs. BCIs are unique in providing new, wholly artificial outputs. Furthermore, the fact that BCI operation is based on the interaction of two adaptive controllers, the user's brain and the BCI (chapter 1), introduces unprecedented possibilities for new plasticity (Wolpe, 2007). Thus, the brain of an individual who becomes accustomed to using a BCI may change in unprecedented ways.

The extent, nature, and functional effects of such additional plasticity are unknown. At present, there is no evidence for deleterious effects, and this theoretical risk is justifiable in view of the substantial human promise of BCI technology. In addition, the limited capabilities and applications of current BCIs suggest that any inadvertent plasticity they produce is likely to be modest. Nevertheless, BCI researchers and others involved in BCI development should be aware of this potential problem, should watch for it, and should be prepared to respond appropriately to its appearance. At the same time, it is important to stress that this risk remains purely theoretical and lacks any supporting evidence whatsoever. Thus, it should not be allowed to inhibit well-designed and carefully executed BCI research that may offer substantial benefits to people with severe disabilities.

The Risk of Uncensored Actions

People often imagine, or even seriously consider, actions that are inappropriate, antisocial, or harmful to themselves or others. These contemplated actions do not normally occur because activity in certain brain areas (e.g., the frontal lobes) ensures that they do not reach the cortical and subcortical motor areas and from them proceed to the spinal and brainstem motoneurons. However, BCI outputs are produced by brain signals, not by motoneurons, and the signals may come from nonmotor brain areas. Thus, it is conceivable that BCI-based actions might sometimes bypass the brain's normal censoring processes, so that BCI users might produce actions (or language) that they would never produce through conventional muscle-based outputs.

Just as the likelihood that BCIs may cause deleterious CNS plasticity, the likelihood that they might produce uncensored actions is unknown at present. There is as yet no evidence for such actions. It might be hoped, or even expected, that the process of skill acquisition involved in learning how to use a BCI would include incorporation of the normal censoring processes. Nevertheless, the possibility of uncensored actions exists, and some precaution against it is practical and appropriate. At present, the proper precaution is summed up in a paraphrase of the first part of Isaac Asimov's First Law of Robotics (Asimov, 1942), specifically: *a BCI should be configured so that it cannot injure a human being.* (This rule is similar to the well-known medical aphorism, *Primum non nocere*, or *First, do no harm*.)

The first, and easiest, human to protect is the user. Thus, a BCI-operated wheelchair should not be able to drive off a cliff, a BCI-operated robotic arm should not be able to strike its user, a BCI-operated orthosis should not be able to force limb joints beyond their normal ranges of motion, and a BCI-operated environmental control system should not be able to raise or lower the room temperature beyond a physiologically acceptable range. Certainly, many of these simple strictures will already be required as precautions against malfunctions of the BCI itself. However, when other improper actions are considered, and especially when harm to other humans is considered, prevention becomes considerably more demanding. For example, should a BCI-operated wheelchair refuse to cross a dangerously busy street, and how would it decide? Or, must a BCI-operated robotic arm that can point a remote control at a television be at the same time unable to point a gun at another person, and how would it make the distinction?

Such questions raise difficult technical, ethical, societal, and legal liability issues comparable to those associated with the development of other computer-based technologies. The degree to which uncensored actions are a BCI risk will become clear only as BCI usage and capabilities increase. At the same time, on a positive note, the limited capabilities of current BCIs mean that their potential for inappropriate actions is commensurably limited and readily addressed by simple safeguards. Furthermore, continued experience with these first BCIs should reveal the extent of the problem and guide efforts to deal with it as more capable BCIs are developed.

RESPECT FOR PERSONS: INFORMED CONSENT

Like any human research study, BCI research requires that the subjects provide informed consent. For the majority of people, even those with severe disabilities, the informed-consent process is usually not a major problem. The process can be satisfactorily executed as long as the subject can understand the information provided and has a reliable means of communication. This communication capacity can be very simple, even a single-switch capacity, as long as it is configured (e.g., with conventional assistive technology) to enable the subject to ask questions and express concerns as necessary. At the same time, it is important to ensure that the prospective subject's autonomy in making the decision to participate is not compromised by compelling (and perhaps unrealistic) expectations (on the part of the subject and/or family members) as to what the BCI will provide (e.g., continued communication capacity) (Haselager et al., 2009). This risk, and measures that may reduce it, were addressed in the section on minimizing psychological risks.

For the small number of subjects without reliable communication, informed consent may in principle be obtained from those surrogates deemed to be legally authorized representatives who have assumed official responsibility for the person according to established procedures (e.g., Buchanan, 1989; Winslade, 2007; Fins 2009a). Whereas this alternative is generally straightforward for studies of noninvasive BCIs, it becomes more complex and difficult for studies of invasive BCIs, given their potential risks. The risk of discomfort or pain is of particular concern for a subject with no reliable means of communication.

One approach to this problem is to plan ahead, which is often possible for people with progressive diseases, such as ALS. This may be accomplished through an advance directive for research (similar to those often completed by prospective research subjects with psychiatric illnesses or in the early stages of dementing diseases). Such a directive would articulate the person's preferences in regard to BCI research participation and/or would name an individual to make these decisions if and when the person loses the ability to communicate. Just as people in the early stages of ALS often decide whether or not they will accept mechanical ventilation when it becomes necessary for their survival, they might decide whether they will participate in a specific BCI study. They may even plan ahead by beginning BCI usage immediately.

Of course, such prospective solutions are not possible for people who have lost communication ability due to disorders that began suddenly and without warning, such as brainstem stroke. While the BCI experience to date with people who lack all communication ability has not been encouraging (e.g., Birbaumer, 2006; Hill et al., 2006), further careful study is essential. The notable achievements of individuals such as Judy

Mozersky (Mozersky, 1996) and Jean-Dominique Bauby (Bauby, 1997) encourage such efforts.

One distinctive aspect of the informed-consent process for studies of long-term independent BCI use is that it may involve more than just the prospective BCI user. The subject's principal caregivers usually have essential roles in such studies, and thus their informed consents are also needed. Furthermore, the assessment of the perceptions of caregivers, family members, and others as to the impact of the BCI on the subject's quality of life and on their interactions with the subject may be a key part of the study; and their informed consents are required for this purpose.

JUSTICE: RESPONDING TO APPEALS, REPORTING RESEARCH RESULTS, AND FACILITATING WIDESPREAD DISSEMINATION

The principle of *justice* stipulates that the benefits and burdens of the research be fairly distributed. It may be difficult to assess the *benefit* aspect of this statement, especially in early trials when the nature and likelihood of the benefits are as yet largely unknown. The *burden* aspect of the statement is easier to address. Other sections of this chapter have indicated how selection of study participants can avoid inclusion of people whose participation would be likely to constitute an undue burden. This might frequently be the case for people in the throes of deciding whether or not to accept ventilation, people with unstable medical conditions, and people in difficult living environments or with unreliable caregivers.

In selecting subjects for a study, researchers are generally severely limited by practical factors such as whether a person lives close enough to be accessible for initial evaluation and for ongoing technical support. Nevertheless, researchers may contribute in several ways to helping larger number of prospective BCI users, and to ensuring that the benefits of the research are widely available.

RESPONDING TO APPEALS FROM PROSPECTIVE USERS

BCI research and development draw substantial media attention. As a result, research groups are frequently approached by a family member or friend of a severely disabled person who is seeking, often desperately, for a way to provide this person with the ability to communicate. If the researchers are conducting a study of long-term independent BCI use, and if this person meets the inclusion criteria, such an appeal may be timely and easily handled by recruiting the subject into the study. However, this fortuitous coincidence is rarely the case. Most groups are not involved in such clinical studies, and, for those who are, the study populations are limited, must satisfy strict inclusion criteria, and are generally confined to people located relatively nearby. Certainly, if the researchers know of another BCI group conducting a study for which the person is a good candidate, a referral is appropriate. But this is unlikely given the relatively small number and sizes of BCI clinical studies.

How then, do researchers respond to such requests from people in dire need? However appealing it may seem, one response to be avoided in most cases is to try to provide and maintain a BCI system for the person outside of a formal and properly approved research protocol. First, such efforts are likely to fail, since research groups will generally lack the funding, personnel, and/or the full range of expertise needed to establish and sustain them. Second, such efforts are inherently improper, in that they constitute neither research nor clinical practice. They are not research because they are not conducted under a fully defined and IRB-approved protocol, and they are not routine clinical care because the technology they are providing has not been formally demonstrated to be effective and has not been approved for use by the relevant regulatory body (e.g., the FDA in the United States). Although the FDA Humanitarian Device Exemption (see chapter 21) may offer researchers an alternative option in special circumstances, its use can be problematic (Fins et al., 2011), and it does not produce generalizable results, which are better pursued through the standard route of an investigational device exemption (often as part of a premarket approval [PMA] process) and a well-designed and IRB-approved clinical trial (chapter 21). It is this latter route that will ultimately best serve the people in need of BCI technology. In sum, providing a research-grade BCI system simply as an ad hoc response to an individual appeal is generally neither ethical, effective, nor consistent with regulatory expectations and prevailing law.

Obviously, the ultimate solution to such appeals is the widespread dissemination and support of powerful and practical BCI systems (chapter 21). Unfortunately, such dissemination remains in the as yet indefinite future. In the meantime, it is in the best interests of prospective BCI users, and the field in general, for BCI usage to remain almost entirely under the auspices of established research protocols.

Nevertheless, research groups can, in the interim, still respond in a substantive and often helpful way to many of the appeals for help that they receive. With many such appeals, a brief conversation will reveal that BCI technology has little or nothing to offer the person, and, if this is true, it should be communicated to the inquirer. Most important, whether or not this is the case, the research group can usually give substantive help by providing information about the growing range of powerful conventional (i.e., muscle-based) assistive communication devices (e.g., eye-tracking systems) and about organizations (hospitals, clinics, foundations) in the person's vicinity that can perform comprehensive assistive technology (AT) evaluations and provide access to appropriate devices.

In the authors' experience, which now includes over 200 such appeals, most people are largely or totally unaware of such conventional technology or of the entities that can provide guidance and access to it. BCI research groups should make themselves familiar with this referral information and should be prepared to provide it as appropriate to those who inquire. Simply by doing this, they can often furnish invaluable help to those who appeal to them.

Furthermore, as discussed at length in chapter 11, BCI-based AT is best understood and disseminated as an important new extension of the spectrum of conventional muscle-based AT devices. Thus, by putting prospective users in touch with AT clinics and other institutions, BCI researchers can facilitate their eventual access to BCI-based AT. Such actions serve the Belmont principle of justice.

REPORTING RESEARCH RESULTS

As in other productive research fields, the focus in BCI research should be on producing peer-reviewed primary articles in high-quality scientific and engineering journals. In addition, researchers should recognize that the intense and often distorted media attention that BCIs attract, although an advantage in some respects, is also a potential disadvantage, because it engenders unrealistic expectations in the public and skepticism in other scientists.

Thus, it is extremely important for BCI researchers to be resolutely realistic and tempered in their interactions with the popular and scientific media (Illes et al., 2010). This does not preclude responsible engagement with the media; it simply calls for prudence and the avoidance of hyperbolic and unrealistic claims or speculations about new devices and their capabilities. Although this approach may sometimes reduce a scientist's media prominence, it should ultimately redound to the credit of both the scientist and the entire research field.

For similar reasons, researchers should adhere as nearly as possible to the *Ingelfinger rule*, the principle that peer-reviewed publication must precede any other detailed dissemination of research results. Although studies are frequently first reported in meeting presentations and abstracts, and may reach the scientific and popular media in that way, their first full description and documentation should be in a peer-reviewed format (Relman, 1981).

FACILITATING WIDESPREAD DISSEMINATION

Like many new technologies, BCIs are expensive to produce and maintain. Although the initial cost of noninvasive BCIs is likely to drop as development continues, the cost of technical support is likely to remain substantial. Furthermore, invasive BCIs, because they require surgery, are generally much more costly. Thus, ensuring that BCIs are widely available to those who need them, whatever their financial resources, is a considerable problem, and it is considered in some detail in chapter 21. Although this is not only (or even mainly) a research problem, BCI researchers may still help in several ways to realize effective solutions; and, in doing so, they can further serve the principle of justice.

Researchers can contribute to BCI dissemination by considering expense in designing them, by incorporating goals such as minimizing the necessary technical support into their research studies, and by developing BCI applications that reduce the need for constant caregiver oversight or even enable the user to resume gainful employment. These efforts can substantially reduce the cost and increase the personal and economic appeal of BCIs, and thus they should be considered important aspects of the development of clinically practical BCI systems.

The widespread dissemination and support of BCIs for people with disabilities depend ultimately on the participation and success of commercial enterprises. The complex factors that will determine whether and how commercial involvement occurs are considered in chapter 21. These factors go well beyond scientific and technical issues. Nevertheless, BCI researchers can help in ensuring that BCIs reach those who most need them by considering carefully where and how they become involved in efforts to develop commercially viable BCIs. Thus, they might choose to participate only in commercial initiatives that include a serious intent and a well-structured plan to produce BCI systems for the primary target population, people with substantial disabilities. Certainly, such initiatives might include and benefit from other goals, such as BCI-based video games. Nevertheless, by choosing to participate in commercial initiatives that include BCI-based assistive technology as a major component of their product line, BCI researchers can promote the dissemination of BCI technology to those who need it most and can thereby observe the principle of justice. At the same time, researchers who are involved in commercial ventures should guard against real or apparent conflicts of interest (e.g., Fins and Schiff, 2010) and should disclose and justify this involvement in the informed-consent process, in their interactions with regulatory bodies, and in their presentations and publications.

BCI RESEARCH FOR THE GENERAL POPULATION

BCI research began primarily as a response to the needs of people with severe disabilities, and these needs continue to be its major focus. At the same time, researchers are turning also to developing BCIs to be used by the general population for a wide variety of purposes. Companies are developing and marketing BCI-based computer games and BCIs for artistic expression, and researchers are exploring BCI-based methods for facilitating tasks such as object detection (chapter 23). In terms of the BCI definition articulated in chapter 1, these efforts seek to use BCIs to enhance or supplement natural CNS output or to improve natural output to supranormal levels.

Like research developing BCIs for clinical purposes, the research aimed at BCIs for nonclinical purposes is governed by the Belmont principles of beneficence, respect for persons (i.e., informed consent), and justice. The issues surrounding the principle of informed consent are less complex for people without disabilities. Communication limitations and uncertainties about mental status are not present, and prospective subjects are not unduly influenced or coerced by an acute need for the communication capabilities that the BCI might be able to provide. On the other hand, if and when BCIs are able to enhance the performance of particular groups (e.g., airline pilots) the issue of coercion may arise, and it could be potentially severe for BCIs that require implanted sensors (Moreno, 2006; Foster, 2006).

The application of the principle of beneficence is more difficult in this wider area, first because beneficence is harder to define, and second because the range of possible nonclinical uses is as yet unknown. Whereas the beneficence of BCI research intended to help people with severe disabilities is clear, the beneficence of BCI research intended to enhance, supplement, or improve the CNS output of people without disabilities depends on the purposes to which the new capabilities are to be applied and on the value that human research committees or society in general places on these purposes.

BCI research to improve the performances of airline pilots or surgeons would presumably be considered highly beneficial, much more so than BCI research to improve video-game or basketball performance. In reality, however, BCIs that improved performance in any one of these areas would almost certainly be applicable in the others as well. Indeed, it would probably be difficult to imagine any BCI that enhanced, supplemented, or improved CNS output that could not be put to a purpose that most would consider worthwhile. The fact that the same BCIs could also serve less desirable or even undesirable purposes is not an ethical issue specific to BCIs or to BCI research. It is an issue that applies to most effective new technologies. As such, it may be addressed by established societal norms and legal codes, or it may require their further development. The need to extend or modify established norms to prevent misuse is a frequent and unavoidable consequence of scientific and technological progress. The possibility that BCIs will be misused need not discourage or impede research, particularly in view of the substantial human benefits this work may provide.

The specific risks of BCI research for people who are not disabled are in general less complex than those of BCI research for people with disabilities, since the psychological risks of BCI failure, the complications of personal and familial situations, and the issues raised by disease progression and study termination are much less severe or are entirely absent. Certainly, the physical risks and the risks of BCI malfunction or incorrect outputs are comparable and require comparable precautions. The risks of infection, damage, and device failure associated with invasive BCIs are likely to be addressed and minimized in clinical studies before these BCIs are ever used by the general population. BCI implantations in people who are not disabled appear to be unlikely in the near future. Indeed, they should be undertaken only after all difficulties and dangers have been resolved and after their superiority over noninvasive alternatives has been convincingly demonstrated.

The largely undefined risks of unexpected and possibly deleterious CNS plasticity and of uncensored actions exist also in this kind of BCI research. Some information on the nature and extent of these risks is likely to come from studies of BCIs for people with disabilities. In the context of BCIs to be used by the general population for many different purposes, these risks are potentially greater and could have significant societal implications. BCIs that are fully integrated into people's daily lives are likely to have individual and societal effects that are unpredictable and perhaps even unforeseeable at present. However, they are in this regard essentially no different from other new technologies that extend the capabilities of CNS outputs, such as the printing press, the automobile, or the Internet.

Finally, in regard to the principle of justice, BCIs that supplement or enhance natural CNS outputs raise the danger of further stratifying society by providing those with greater access to new technology with still more advantages. Although this is a risk associated with many new technologies, it should be noted that the Belmont Report opposed the use of psycho-

surgery for enhancement (National Commission for the Protection of Human Subjects of Biomedical and Behavioral Research, 1977; Fins, 2003). This consideration provides further reason to defer BCI implants in people without disabilities until the physical risks have been essentially eliminated, the unique benefits have been established, and the societal issues are better understood.

SUMMARY

The recent advent of a broad spectrum of new technologies and therapies that promise unprecedented understanding of and access to the brain and its disorders has raised a host of practical and theoretical ethical issues. This chapter focuses on those issues most important to BCI research and development. It is organized around the three principles set out in the Belmont Report of 1978: *beneficence*, *respect for persons*, and *justice*. Beneficence requires that the benefits of the research (to humanity and perhaps to the research subjects) far outweigh its risks to the subjects. Respect for persons requires that the subjects provide informed consent. Justice requires that the benefits and burdens of the research be fairly distributed.

BCI research for people with severe disabilities, which has already demonstrated substantial human benefits, is clearly ethically justified. At the same time, the inherently multidisciplinary nature of BCI research means that groups engaged in it are ethically obligated to ensure that they have adequate expertise in every discipline relevant to the proposed study and that their research results are available for further analysis by other researchers.

The development of invasive BCI methods involves both animal and human research. In accordance with ethical research principles, human studies should be limited primarily to issues that can be resolved only in humans, whereas other issues (e.g., realization of safe and effective long-term implant methods) should be addressed first in animals. Furthermore, invasive BCI research requires a reasonable expectation that it will yield capacities not possible with noninvasive BCI methods.

Studies of BCI use by people with disabilities should be designed and executed to ensure: that subjects and their families understand that they are doing a service by participating and may very well not benefit themselves; that the psychological and physical risks of BCI failure or malfunction are minimized; that the risks of inappropriate BCI outputs are minimized; that procedures to prevent invasion of privacy are in place; and that the possibility that the subject may want to use the BCI beyond the term of the study or that disease progression may degrade BCI usefulness is considered and addressed as effectively as possible.

BCIs pose several theoretical risks. One is that long-term BCI use will induce deleterious CNS plasticity. The second is that BCI-based actions may circumvent the normal censoring processes to which muscle-based actions are subjected. Although there is as yet no evidence for the reality of these risks, BCI researchers should consider them in study design and remain vigilant for their occurrence.

In defining subject criteria and in obtaining informed consent from subjects with severe disabilities, it is important to take into account: their communication limitations due to their disabilities; the possibility that the severity or expected progression of their disabilities may tend to coerce their participation; and the possible need to obtain consent also from caregivers and/or family members.

BCI research groups frequently receive appeals for help on behalf of people with severe disabilities. Researchers are not usually able to provide and maintain BCIs in response to such appeals, and they should not do so outside of a formally approved research protocol. Nevertheless, they may still give substantial help simply by educating people about the wide range of available conventional assistive technologies and guiding them to facilities that provide and maintain these technologies.

High-quality peer-reviewed publications should be the primary goal of BCI studies; and BCI researchers should be consistently realistic in their interactions with the popular and scientific media.

BCI researchers can help to facilitate the realization and widespread dissemination of clinically useful BCI systems by incorporating clinically relevant practical aims into their studies and by focusing their involvement with commercial enterprises on those that include among their aims a serious intent to produce systems useful to people with severe neuromuscular disabilities.

Research aimed at BCIs for the general population is also subject to the principles enunciated in the Belmont Report (1978). Although some issues specific to people with severe disabilities are less important for this much larger population, the determination of benevolence is more complicated, and the possibilities for misuse may raise societal and legal questions that go far beyond science and engineering. At the same time, the knowledge gained through BCI research for people with disabilities, particularly regarding risks such as inadvertent CNS plasticity or uncensored actions, should help guide development of BCIs for general use.

REFERENCES

Ackerman, S. Hard Science, Hard Choices: Facts, Ethics, and Policies Guiding Brain Science Today. New York: Dana Press, 2006.

Asimov, I. Runaround. In: Astounding Science Fiction. March, 1942.

Bauby, J.-D. The Diving Bell and the Butterfly, translated by J. Leggatt. New York: Vintage International, 1997.

Beauchamp, T. L., and Childress, J. F., Principles of Biomedical Ethics, 6th ed. New York: Oxford University Press, 2009.

Birbaumer, N. Editorial: Brain-computer interface research: coming of age. Clinical Neurophysiology 117:479–483, 2006.

Blankertz, B., Müller, K-R., Curio, G., Vaughan, T. M., Schalk, G., Wolpaw, J. R., Schlögl, A., Neuper, C., Pfurtscheller, G., Hinterberger, T., Schröder, M., and Birbaumer, N. The BCI competition 2003: Progress and perspectives in detection and discrimination of EEG single trials. IEEE Transactions on Biomedical Engineering, 51, 1044–1051, 2004.

Blankertz, B., Müller, K.-R., Krusienski, D., Schalk, G., Wolpaw, J. R., Schlögl, A., Pfurtscheller, G., Millán, J., Schroder, M., and Birbaumer, N. The BCI competition III: Validating alternative approaches to actual BCI problems. IEEE Transactions on Neural Systems and Rehabilitation Engineering, 14, 153–159, 2006.

Buchanan, A. E. Deciding for Others: The Ethics of Surrogate Decision Making. Cambridge: Cambridge University Press, 1989.

Committee for the Update of the Guide for the Care and Use of Laboratory Animals. Guide for the Care and Use of Laboratory Animals, 8th ed. Washington, DC: The National Academies Press, 2011.

Farah, M. J., Illes, J., Cook-Deegan, R., Gardner, H., Kandel, E., King, P., Parens, E., Sahakian, B., Wolpe, P.R. Neurocognitive enhancement: what can we do and what should we do? Nature Reviews Neuroscience 5: 421–425, 2004.

Fenton, A., and Alpert, S. Extending our view on using BCIs for locked-in syndrome. Neuroethics 1:119–132, 2008.

Fins, J. J. From psychosurgery to neuromodulation and palliation: History's lessons for the ethical conduct and regulation of neuropsychiatric research. Neurosurgery Clinics of North America 14:303–319, 2003.

Fins, J. J. A Palliative Ethic of Care: Clinical Wisdom at Life's End. Sudbury, MA: Jones and Bartlett, 2006.

Fins, J. J. A review of Mind Wars: Brain Research and National Defense by Jonathan D. Moreno. New York: Dana Press, 2006. Journal of the American Medical Association 297:1382–1383, 2007.

Fins, J. J. Being conscious of their burden: severe brain injury and the two cultures challenge. In Disorders of Consciousness, Ann. N.Y. Acad. Sci. 1157:131–147, 2009a.

Fins, J. J. Deep brain stimulation, deontology and duty: The moral obligation of non-abandonment at the neural interface. Journal of Neural Engineering 6:50201. Epub Sept 1, 2009b.

Fins, J. J. Deep brain stimulation, free markets and the scientific commons: Is it time to revisit the Bayh-Dole Act of 1980? Neuromodulation 13:153–159, 2010.

Fins, J. J. Neuroethics and the lure of technology. In Handbook of Neuroethics. Illes, J. and Sahakian, B. J, (Eds.) New York: Oxford University Press. In Press.

Fins, J. J., Mayberg, H. S., Nuttin, B., Kubu, C. S., Galert, T., Strum, V., Stoppenbrink, K., Merkel, R., and Schlaepfer, T. Neuropsychiatric deep brain stimulation research and the misuse of the Humanitarian Device Exemption. Health Affairs 30:302–311, 2011.

Fins, J. J., Rezai, A. R., Greenberg, B. D. Psychosurgery: Avoiding an ethical redux while advancing a therapeutic future. Neurosurgery 59:713–716, 2006.

Fins, J. J., and Schiff, N. D. Conflicts of interest in deep brain stimulation research and the ethics of transparency. Journal of Clinical Ethics 21:125–132, 2010.

Foster, K. R., 2006. Engineering the Brain. In J. Illes, Neuroethics: Defining the Issues in Theory Practice, and Policy. Illes, J. (Ed.) New York: Oxford University Press, 185–199.

Gillett, G. Cyborgs and moral identity. Journal of Medical Ethics 32:79–83, 2006.

Hamilton, R., Messing, S., Chatterjee, A. Rethinking the thinking cap. Neurology 76:187–193, 2011.

Haselager, P., Vlek, R., Hill, J., and Nijboer, F. A note on ethical aspects of BCI. Neural Networks 22:1352–1357, 2009.

Hill, N. J., Lal, T. N., Schröder, M., Hinterberger, T., Wilhelm, B., Nijboer, F., Mochty, U., Widmer, G., Elger, C., Scholkopf, B., Kübler, A., and Birbaumer, N. Classifying EEG and ECoG signals without subject training for fast BCI implementation: Comparison of nonparalyzed and completely paralyzed subjects, IEEE Transactions in Neural Systems and Rehabilitation Engineering, 14:183–186, 2006.

Illes, J. Neuroethics: Defining the Issues in Theory, Practice, and Policy. New York: Oxford University Press, 2006.

Illes J., Bird S. J. Neuroethics: A modern context for ethics in neuroscience. Trends in Neurosciences 29:511–517, 2006.

Illes, J., Moser, M. A., McCormick, J. B., Racine, E., Blakeslee, S., Caplan, A., Hayden, E. C., Ingram, J., Lohwater, T., McKnight, P., Nicholson, C., Phillips, A., Sauvé, K. D., Snell, E., and Weiss, S. NeuroTalk: Improving the communication of neuroscience. Nature Reviews Neuroscience 11: 61, 2010.

Institute of Medicine Responsible Research: A Systems Approach to Protecting Research Participants. Washington, DC: IOM, 2005.

Leshner A. I. Ethical issues in taking neuroscience research from bench to bedside, In Glannon W. (Ed.), Defining Right and Wrong in Brain Science New York: Dana Press, 2007.

Levy, N. Neuroethics: Challenges for the 21st Century, Cambridge: Cambridge University Press, 2007.

Lidz, C. W., Appelbaum, P. S., Grisso, T., Renaud, M. Therapeutic misconception and the appreciation of risks in clinical trials. Social Science & Medicine 58:1689–1697, 2004.

Moreno, J. D. Mind Wars: Brain Research and National Defense. New York: Dana Press, 2006.

Moss, A. H., Oppenheimer, E. A., Casey, P., and Carroll, P. A. Patients with amyotrophic lateral sclerosis receiving long-term mechanical ventilation: Advance care planning and outcomes, Chest 110:249–255, 1996.

Mozersky, J. Locked In: A Young Woman's Battle with Stroke, Ottawa: Golden Dog Press, 1996.

National Commission for the Protection of Human Subjects of Biomedical and Behavioral Research. Use of psychosurgery in practice and research: Report and recommendations of National Commission for the Protection of Human Subjects of Biomedical and Behavioral Research. Federal Register 42:26318–26332, 1977.

National Commission for the Protection of Human Subjects The Belmont Report: Ethical Principles and Guidelines for the Protection of Human Subjects of Research, Washington, DC: Government Printing Office, 1978.

Nuremberg Code. Trials of War Criminals before the Nuremberg Military Tribunals under Control Council Law No. 10. Vol. 2:181–182. Washington, DC: U.S. Government Printing Office, 1949.

Relman, A. S. The Ingelfinger rule. New England Journal of Medicine 305: 824–826, 1981.

Sajda, P., Gerson, A., Müller, K.-R., Blankertz, B., and Parra, L. A data analysis competition to evaluate machine learning algorithms for use in brain-computer interfaces. IEEE Transactions on Neural Systems and Rehabilitation Engineering, 11:184–185, 2003.

Schalk, G., and Mellinger, J. A Practical Guide to Brain-Computer Interfacing with BCI2000. Berlin: Springer, 2010.

Sellers, E. W., Vaughan, T. M., and Wolpaw, J. R. A brain-computer interface for long-term independent home use. Amyotrophic Lateral Sclerosis 11:449–455, 2010.

Winslade, W. J. Severe brain injury: Recognizing the limits of treatment and exploring the frontiers of research. Cambridge Quarterly of Healthcare Ethics 16:161–168, 2007.

Wolpe, P. R. Medicine and society: Ethical and social challenges of brain-computer interfaces. Virtual Mentor: American Medical Association Journal of Ethics 9:128–131, 2007.

PART VI. | CONCLUSION

25 | THE FUTURE OF BCIs: MEETING THE EXPECTATIONS

JONATHAN R. WOLPAW AND ELIZABETH WINTER WOLPAW

This book began with the holiday greeting that Herbert Jasper sent to Hans Berger 74 years ago (fig. 1.1). The BCI that Jasper drew was pure fantasy at the time and remained so for many more years. Now, however, fantasy has become reality. Starting about 25 years ago, scientists around the world began to develop capabilities comparable to those imagined in Jasper's drawing. From early demonstrations of electroencephalography (EEG)-based spelling and single-neuron-based device control, they have moved on to apply EEG, intracortical, electrocorticographic (ECoG), and other brain signals to increasingly complex control of cursors, robotic arms, prostheses, wheelchairs, and other devices. Jasper and Berger would presumably be pleased, though probably not surprised, to learn that BCIs are possible and even useful. Their continued development is the focus of a rapidly growing research and development enterprise that generates tremendous excitement in scientists, engineers, clinicians, and the general public. This excitement reflects the promise of BCIs, which is indeed rich.

THE PROMISE

By the definition used throughout this book, BCIs are systems that use brain signals to replace, restore, enhance, supplement, or improve the brain's natural outputs (fig. 1.3). Replacement and restoration of natural outputs are intended mainly for people with severe disabilities. They have been, and continue to be, the primary focus of BCI research. Such BCIs might eventually prove sufficiently effective to be used routinely to replace or restore useful function to many people disabled by neuromuscular disorders. With advances in technology and training, these BCIs might support communication that is as fast as normal typing or talking, might reanimate paralyzed limbs to produce normal movements, and might restore bladder, bowel, and other autonomic functions. They might, in short, enable the realization of a revolutionary new class of assistive technology.

BCIs might also enhance or supplement natural motor outputs for pilots, surgeons, soldiers, air-traffic controllers, and other highly skilled professionals. They might furnish artists, athletes, video-gamers, and others with new opportunities and challenges. Thus, they might constitute a major new technology that would be widely used by large segments of the general population and would fundamentally change important aspects of daily life.

BCIs might also be used to improve the recovery of people with strokes, head trauma, and other disorders by furnishing powerful new methods for inducing and guiding CNS plasticity so as to restore useful function beyond that possible with other methods. They could thereby be a potentially major addition to the armamentarium of rehabilitation therapies. As CNS regeneration methods are discovered and as they advance, BCIs, through their capacity to induce adaptive plasticity, may play an important role in guiding functional regrowth of neuronal connections. Because they could help very large numbers of people, these kinds of therapeutic BCI applications would greatly increase the clinical significance of BCI technology.

These visions of the future understandably inspire the excitement and energy, and attract the resources, now centered on BCI research and development. Nevertheless, and despite the remarkable achievements of the past 20 years and the growing interest and activity in the field, this future is not assured. The future of BCI technology will depend on many factors. It is not yet known whether the inherent limitations of outputs produced directly from brain signals will limit the success of BCI technology, and researchers have no control over these limitations. Nevertheless, we can certainly control the choices of the problems we address and the strategies we use to address them. Focused and effective attention to several crucial issues is needed for the inspiring future envisioned to actually occur.

THE MOST IMPORTANT PROBLEMS

In our view, problems must be solved in three crucial areas in order to achieve truly practical and effective BCIs. These areas are: *signal acquisition hardware*, *validation and dissemination*, and *reliability*. We will look at the needs in each of these areas and consider how they may best be addressed.

SIGNAL ACQUISITION HARDWARE

Both noninvasive and invasive BCI systems rely on the sensors and associated hardware that acquire brain signals. Substantial improvements in this hardware are critical to the future success of BCIs. Some of the needed improvements are straightforward and achievable with current technology, whereas others hinge on further bioengineering advances.

NON-INVASIVE BCIs

For EEG-based BCIs, the hardware needs are well known to anyone who uses EEG for BCI or other long-term purposes outside of protected laboratory or clinical environments. Electrodes and amplifiers for BCI use should ideally:

- not require skin abrasion or conductive gel (i.e., so-called *dry electrodes*)

- be small and fully portable

- have comfortable, convenient, unobtrusive, and cosmetically acceptable mountings

- be easy to set up, initialize, and monitor

- function for many hours without maintenance

- perform well in all environments without significant artifacts

- operate by telemetry instead of using extensive wiring

- interface easily and reliably with BCI applications

For many of these requirements, the path to achievement is reasonably clear, and the work simply needs to be done. However, with or without dry electrodes, it may be particularly difficult to satisfy the need for robust performance in all environments. Robust performance should therefore be a major objective of continuing research.

For functional near-infrared (fNIR)-based BCIs, the desirable hardware improvements are largely analogous to those needed for EEG-based BCIs. However, the overall capability of fNIR-based BCIs is less well defined at present and may be severely limited by the inherent slowness of BOLD signals (see chapters 4 and 18). On the other hand, if this technology proves able to monitor more rapid metabolic processes (chapter 4), this limitation might disappear or become considerably less significant.

BCIs based on functional magnetic resonance imaging (fMRI) or magnetoencephalography (MEG) have prospects quite different from those of BCIs based on EEG or fNIR. Because of the expense, bulk, and environmental requirements of their hardware, these methods will, at least for the foreseeable future, remain confined to research laboratories. Major (as yet unforeseen) innovations would be needed to render them more practical. Nevertheless, as described in chapter 4, such methods might be extremely useful in helping to locate optimal sites for placement of invasive BCI sensors such as microelectrode arrays.

IMPLANTED (INVASIVE) BCIs

Implanted (invasive) BCIs present a more complex picture. The overall goal is to realize wholly implantable systems that:

- are safe

- remain intact, functional, and reliable for decades

- record stable signals for many years

- convey the recorded signals by telemetry

- can be recharged in situ by wireless energy transfer or other methods (or have batteries that last for many years)

- have external elements that are robust, comfortable, convenient, and unobtrusive

- interface easily and effectively with high-performance applications

Although some of the improvements needed to achieve these goals for implantable BCI interfaces are straightforward and attainable, others are more challenging.

The development of advanced-technology sensors, such as the Utah array, the Michigan electrode, and micro-ECoG arrays, has extended the functioning lifespan of implanted sensors, improved their recording stability and fidelity, and attenuated the tissue damage associated with their insertion and continued presence. Despite these great strides, sensors that fully satisfy the needs listed here remain to be achieved. Although the electrode arrays now being used function effectively in the short term, and sometimes also in the long term, significant long-term tissue reaction occurs, and there is instability in the neuronal populations that are recorded. To a considerable degree, further work can be expected to clarify and resolve these issues.

Nevertheless, microelectrode arrays, no matter how finely machined and miniaturized, are foreign bodies inserted into the delicate and dynamic biological environment of brain tissue. As such, they induce a host of effects, from simple mechanical damage to complex electrophysiological, biochemical, and immunological events (chapter 5). A variety of novel approaches to reducing these effects or their functional impact have been proposed and some are currently under investigation. At present, it is not clear which approaches will be successful, or how successful they will be. It is possible that major as yet undefined innovations in sensor technology will be needed for invasive BCIs to realize their full promise. Innovation for BCI implants will certainly benefit from research and development of brain sensors and stimulators that are used for other clinical purposes. Up to the present, development of sensors for any of these purposes has progressed primarily through animal studies, and this will undoubtedly be the case for the future. This is not only required for safety, but it is also prudent, since initial human studies of new technology run the risk that an early failure with significant adverse consequences could inhibit further research for a long time.

Finally, for several of the potentially most useful BCI applications, it is likely that additional implanted devices will be needed to stimulate specific CNS or peripheral structures. For example, implanted stimulators will be needed to support BCI-based restoration of bladder or bowel function or BCI-based restoration of limb movements through activation of individual muscles. Such implants do exist at present, but further improvements in their capabilities, convenience, and reliability are desirable, and they will need to be effectively interfaced with BCI outputs.

VALIDATION AND DISSEMINATION

COMPARING DIFFERENT SIGNALS AND METHODS

BCI researchers are exploring a wide variety of promising non-invasive and invasive brain signals and methodologies. Up to the present, the primary goal has been simply to show that a given BCI design works. However, as the field progresses and as BCIs begin to enter actual clinical use, two other questions become important. The first question is how good a given BCI can get (e.g., how reliable, how fast, how many degrees of freedom it can provide, etc.). The second question is which BCI designs are best for which purposes.

The first question implies that each promising design should be optimized and that, furthermore, the ultimate limits on users' capabilities with the design should be defined. This will require well-structured methods for reaching and defining the upper limits of performance. It will be important to develop protocols that push the performance limits of both the user and the signal-analysis methods, as well as the performance limits of the two together.

The second question is which designs are best for which kinds of applications. This will be a more difficult question to answer. It will require some measure of consensus among research groups in regard to which applications should be used for comparing designs and how performance on them should be measured. At some point in the not too distant future, this question will require reasonably formal attention. The most obvious pertinent example is the question of whether the performance possible with intracortical signals is markedly superior to that possible with ECoG signals, or even EEG signals. As noted in chapter 1, the data to date (e.g., see chapters 13, 15, and 16) do not give a clear answer. Presumably, for many prospective users, invasive BCI designs will need to be markedly superior to be considered preferable to noninvasive designs. As the various designs move toward clinical use, it will become increasingly important to reach some agreement on how they should be compared.

THE VALUE OF A CLINICAL FOCUS

BCI research benefits in several ways from the fact that its primary purpose is to replace or restore useful function for people with severe disabilities. First, this purpose attracts substantial funding from government and private entities interested in advancing health and helping people with disabilities. Second, it promotes a careful focus on actual brain signals and avoidance of the artifacts that commonly occur (e.g., cranial electromyographic [EMG] activity). It also sets relatively modest and achievable goals. Indeed, the modest level of functionality of current BCIs is of value mainly to people who have lost almost all normal neuromuscular function.

At the same time, the development of BCIs for people with disabilities requires as its final step convincing validation of real-life value in terms of efficacy, practicality, and impact on quality of life. As described in chapter 20, this is a demanding enterprise. It requires committed multidisciplinary teams with the time and resources needed for prolonged studies of real-life use under complex and often difficult circumstances. Nevertheless, validation studies are an essential step if BCIs are to realize their promise. The results of these studies can also encourage and guide the development of BCI applications for the general population. The validation of BCIs designed to improve rehabilitation after strokes or in other disorders will be similarly demanding and will require carefully controlled comparisons with the results obtained by conventional methods alone.

THE PROBLEM OF DISSEMINATION

With their current capabilities, which make them useful mainly for people with the most severe disabilities, BCIs are essentially an *orphan technology*. As discussed in chapter 21, an orphan technology is one that is proven in the laboratory (and perhaps in field tests as well) but that does not provide adequate incentive for commercial interests to produce it and to promote its widespread dissemination. Convincing demonstrations that BCIs can improve motor rehabilitation could markedly expand the potential user population. However, the efficacy of BCI usage for such therapeutic purposes remains uncertain at present (see chapter 22 in this volume). In any case, if and when further research improves the functionality of BCIs and makes them commercially attractive, their dissemination will require viable business models that provide not only financial incentive for the commercial company but also adequate reimbursement to the clinical and technical personnel who will deploy and support the BCIs.

The best achievable scenario might be one in which BCIs designed to help people with severe disabilities develop synergistically with BCIs for use by the general population (chapter 23). Development of the former would provide essential scientific knowledge, technical capabilities, and clinical experience, while development of the latter would provide the commercial incentive, simplifications, and robustness essential for large-scale dissemination.

RELIABILITY

The third and probably most difficult problem is that of BCI reliability. Although the future of BCI technology certainly depends on improvements in signal acquisition, as well as on convincing validation studies and viable dissemination models, the difficulties and uncertainties of these problems pale next to those associated with the problem of BCI reliability. This problem is critical to the success of BCI technology and is likely to have the greatest impact on its future.

The magnitude of the problem is perhaps revealed best by the efforts to achieve BCI-based control of multidimensional movements. The results of these efforts have been well described in impressive reports in high-profile articles that have received extensive coverage in the scientific and general media. Nevertheless, they have been successful only up to a point.

First, they are all laboratory demonstrations and have not proven themselves in real-world environments. Second, even with the data collected under highly controlled, optimal conditions in simplified environments with continual expert oversight, BCI performance varies markedly and unpredictably from trial to trial, minute to minute, day to day, and individual to individual. Although stretches of good performance certainly occur (enough to provide statistically significant data for publication and impressive videos), and although performance does tend to improve with practice, it never approximates normal muscle-based motor control; and, most important, it never achieves, even in protected laboratory environments, the reliability essential for actual practical use.

In all hands, no matter the signal type, the signal-processing method, the task learned, or the application for which it is used, BCI reliability, particularly for applications such as movement control, remains poor. BCIs suitable for translation into real-life usefulness must be as reliable as natural muscle-based actions. Without a qualitative upgrade of as yet unknown nature, the real-life usefulness of BCIs will, at best, remain confined to only the most basic communication functions for those with the most severe disabilities; they will not provide control useful to many people for many purposes in their daily lives. It is reliability, more than maximum speed or degrees of freedom, that is most likely to determine the future of BCI technology.

How can this knotty problem be solved? Paths to probable solutions may be identified by recognizing and engaging three fundamental issues. The first is the central role of *adaptive interactions* in enabling and maintaining successful BCI operation. The second is the need for BCI systems that recognize and imitate as far as possible the *distributed* functioning of the normal CNS. The third is the need to take into account the complexity of nervous system function by looking beyond the brain signals currently used for BCI control and the kinds of feedback now provided, that is, by incorporating additional brain signals and providing additional sensory inputs.

ADAPTATION

The need for continuing interactive adaptation of both the BCI and the CNS was introduced in chapter 1 and has been discussed in several other chapters. This final chapter returns to it because of its critical importance to the ultimate success of BCIs in providing control that is both precise and reliable, which is the only kind of control of any significant value in real life.

BCIs provide the CNS with the opportunity to acquire new skills in which brain signals take the place of the spinal motoneurons that produce conventional muscle-based skills. The neuromuscular skills that are the natural function of the CNS depend for their initial acquisition and long-term maintenance on continual activity-dependent plasticity in many places in the CNS, from the cortex to the spinal cord (chapter 1). This plasticity, which generally requires intensive practice over months and even years, allows babies to learn to walk and talk, children to master reading, writing, and arithmetic, and adults to acquire specialized athletic, artistic, and intellectual skills. The acquisition and maintenance of reliable BCI-based

skills, such as multidimensional movement control, will presumably require comparable activity-dependent plasticity. Studies with both noninvasive and invasive BCIs provide ample evidence (e.g., chapters 13, 15, and 16) that the new skills learned during BCI practice involve their own CNS adaptations, certainly in the brain area producing the relevant signals, and probably in multiple connecting areas as well.

As noted in chapter 1, BCI operation depends on the effective interaction of two adaptive controllers, the CNS and the BCI. The BCI must adapt to ensure that its outputs correspond to the user's intentions. That is, it must adapt so that it focuses on the brain signal features that encode the user's intent. At the same time, the BCI should also encourage and facilitate CNS plasticity that improves the precision and reliability with which the user's intent is encoded in the brain signals. Thus, the BCI and CNS must work together to acquire and maintain an effective and completely reliable partnership under all circumstances.

Although BCIs are typically adapted initially to the user's brain signals, the importance of *ongoing* adaptation, especially for complex applications such as movement control, is less widely appreciated. Furthermore, only the simplest methods have been used: the BCI periodically parameterizes its translation algorithm to make the best use of the brain signals as they have been in the past, and it expects the CNS to adapt to that algorithm going forward. Whereas this basic operant-conditioning design can be effective, the persistent unreliability of current BCIs indicates that it is not sufficient. Managing the ongoing mutual adaptations of CNS and BCI so as to maximize and stabilize the encoding of the user's intent and the BCI's recognition of that intent depends on the development of algorithms that enable and optimize such adaptation. It will also depend on finding answers to several key questions. Which brain areas are best able to adapt? Which brain signals are most amenable to adaptation (e.g., mu/beta/gamma rhythms in EEG or ECoG; local field potentials; multi- or single-neuron activity)? What are the most effective training protocols? What are the time scales of adaptation (i.e., from seconds to hours to weeks to years)?

The work needed to address these unknowns has just begun, and it is certain to be difficult and labor-intensive. One need only consider the prolonged practice required to acquire other life skills. Complex BCI-based skills may also require lengthy training in which the benefits become evident only very gradually. Furthermore, the optimal solutions to the key issues affecting adaptation are likely to differ from one BCI application to another, and from one user to another.

Engaging and managing CNS adaptation involve fundamental neuroscientific questions and may yield important insights into CNS function in general. By learning which signals and which areas can or cannot adapt most effectively, and which protocols can induce effective and stable adaptation, and, eventually, by exploring the functional and structural mechanisms of effective adaptations, BCI research is likely to illuminate the properties of natural CNS function and to lead to better understanding of how the CNS produces its natural neuromuscular outputs. Indeed, because it provides unique models for elucidating nervous system function, BCI research has value for neuroscience in general, independent of the practical applications that are the primary focus of most current efforts.

The central importance of CNS adaptation has a further implication. It implies that the most critical (but hopefully not intractable) problems in BCI development may be neurobiological rather than technical. The principles governing how the CNS acquires, improves, and maintains its natural muscle-based functions may be the best source of guidance for designing effective BCI systems. In accord with this view, we consider briefly how BCI-based function might improve its reliability by more closely imitating normal muscle-based function.

DISTRIBUTION OF CONTROL

CNS control of motor actions is normally distributed across multiple areas. Although cortical areas may control the goal and the overall outline of an action, many of the details, particularly the high-speed sensorimotor interactions during the course of performance, are often handled mainly at subcortical levels. For example, spinal reflex pathways produce the earliest responses to sudden load increases or postural instabilities; the cortex learns of these perturbations only later and may or may not produce additional corrective responses. Furthermore, the distribution of control depends on the requirements of the task. Playing the piano entails cortical control of individual finger movements, but grasping an object may not. For the latter, high-speed control of finger muscle contractions may be delegated largely to spinal and subcortical pathways that can respond very quickly to sensory inputs reflecting the physical properties of the object (i.e., shape, hardness, weight).

BCI performance is also likely to benefit from distribution of control. In BCI design, the comparable distribution would be between the BCI's output commands (i.e., the user's intent) and the application device that receives the commands and turns them into action. Chapter 1 describes two possible extremes of this distribution. In *goal selection*, the BCI simply specifies the goal to be achieved, and the application device then handles the production of the action that achieves the goal. In *process control*, the BCI controls every detail of the action. Figure 1.6 illustrates these two alternatives. The optimal solution for a particular BCI will probably vary from application to application and may often be a combination involving both goal selection and process control. For example, consider BCI control of a robotic hand. If the task is playing the piano, the BCI will need to specify individual finger movements. However, if the task is grasping a bottle, the BCI can simply specify that the goal is to grasp the bottle, and the application and its software can then execute the action using feedback from pressure sensors in the robotic hand to control individual fingers so as to maintain effective grasp. In this latter scenario, the BCI's task is much simpler (both in degrees of freedom and required speed) than it would be if it controlled all aspects of the task; and the achievement of consistent high-quality performance is thus likely to be considerably easier and more reliable. The distribution of control in this scenario allows the cortex to operate more as it does during normal neuromuscular performances, in which many details,

particularly those requiring high-speed responses, are often delegated to subcortical areas.

In sum, the achievement of reliable, high-quality BCI performance may be substantially facilitated by incorporating into the application itself as much control as is consistent with the action to be produced. Ideally, if applications such as robotic arms are to be capable of many different kinds of actions, the distribution of control between the BCI and the application should adapt to suit each action, just as the distribution of control within the CNS normally adapts to suit each neuromuscular action.

SIGNALS FROM MULTIPLE AREAS AND ADDITIONAL SENSORY INPUTS

The neuromuscular outputs of the normal CNS reflect the collaborative contributions of many brain areas from the cortex to the spinal cord. For example, the direct corticospinal-tract connections to spinal motoneurons represent only one of many influences that reach motoneurons and control their activity. The differing contributions of various cortical areas and subcortical centers, and their interconnections, are considered in chapter 2. For the present discussion, the most relevant observation is that, despite the fact that the activity in these many brain areas can vary substantially from trial to trial, neuromuscular actions are nevertheless impressively stable and reliable even under widely varying conditions.

This observation suggests that BCI performance might be improved and stabilized by using signals from multiple brain areas and by including features that reflect relationships between areas (e.g., coherences). By enabling the CNS to operate more as it does in producing muscle-based skills (i.e., through cooperation among different areas), this strategy might ultimately reduce the unreliability typical of current BCIs. Work has begun in this area and more is needed. It is complex and demanding because there are so many possible combinations of features from different areas and so many different ways in which their relationships could be measured.

Using signals from multiple areas might also help eliminate another obstacle to fully practical BCIs. Current BCIs are mainly *synchronous*; that is, the BCI rather than the user determines when output is produced (chapter 10). Ideally, BCIs should be *asynchronous* (i.e., *self-paced*), so that the BCI is always available and the user's brain signals alone control when BCI output is produced. BCIs that record signals from multiple areas are more likely to be sensitive to the relevant current context, including both the environment and the user's state and activities. Thus, such BCIs may be better able to recognize when their output is or is not appropriate.

Up to the present BCI applications have provided mainly visual feedback, which is relatively slow and often imprecise. In contrast, conventional muscle-based skills generally rely on numerous sensory inputs that differ in modality (e.g., proprioceptive, cutaneous, visual, auditory) and/or in site of origin (e.g., distal or proximal limbs, trunk). BCIs that control tasks involving high-speed complex movements (e.g., limb movement) are likely to need forms of sensory feedback that are faster and more precise than vision. As noted in chapter 5, efforts to provide such feedback via stimulators in sensorimotor cortex, thalamus, or elsewhere have begun. At this point, the optimal peripheral or central sites and the most effective kinds of stimulation are largely unknown. The choices will presumably vary with the BCI type, the application, and the etiology of the user's disability (e.g., peripheral inputs will often not be effective in people with spinal cord injuries). The selection of sites and stimuli should also benefit from improved understanding of the normal roles of these sites and the kinds of inputs they produce or receive during natural muscle-based control.

SUMMARY

BCI development has a bright future, with many energetic and effective researchers in laboratories all over the world realizing BCI systems that only a few years ago seemed in the realm of science fiction. These BCI systems use many different brain signals, recording methods, and signal-processing approaches. They can control a variety of external devices, from cursors and avatars on computer screens, to televisions and wheelchairs, to robotic arms and neuroprostheses. People with and without disabilities have tested these devices, and a few are already using them for important purposes in their daily lives. With improved signal-acquisition hardware, convincing clinical validation, effective dissemination models, and, probably most important of all, with increased reliability, BCIs are poised to become a major new technology for people with disabilities—and possibly for the general population as well. BCI research and development will continue to be a consummately multidisciplinary effort, and the years ahead should be exciting indeed.

INDEX

Page numbers followed by *f* or *t* indicate figures or tables, respectively

393

discrete decoding, 281
discrete wavelet transform (DWT), 136–37
discriminant models, in signal processing, 148, 149*f*
dissemination, of BCI applications, 10–11, 389
dorsal visual streams, 23
dry electrodes, 106
in EEG, 167
DSP chips. *See* digital signal processing chips
DWT. *See* discrete wavelet transform

eBCIs. *See* extraparenchymal BCIs
echo planar imaging (EPI), 309
ECoG. *See* electrocorticography
EEG. *See* electroencephalography
EEG reference electrode selection, 110
efferent fibers, 20
electric circuits, 47–49
current sources, 47–48, 47*f*
fluid flow rate, 47*f*
impedance in, 48
linear supposition in, 48–49, 49*f*
Ohm's Law, 47
in tissues, volume conduction in, 49–50
voltage sources, 47–48
electric fields, in brain
action potential sources in, 53
dipole current sources, 52–53, 53*f*
ECoG and, 53–54
EEG recording, 54, 57–58
experimental coarse-graining, 52
intraskull recordings, 54
LFPs and, 45–46, 53
low frequencies, 46
macrocolumns, 55*f*
mesoscopic source strength for, 55–56
microsource functions, 55
monopole current sources, 52
multiple cortical sources, 54–55
quasistatic, 46
recordings of, 51–54
by scale, 51–52, 52*f*
scalp-recorded potentials, 56–57
spatial resolution comparisons, 54, 54*t*
static membrane charges in, 46
theoretical coarse-graining, 52
volume conduction in, 46
electrocorticography (ECoG), 251–61
arrays for, 252*f*
artifact vulnerability in, 253
bandwidth of, 253, 254*f*
BCI recording, 8, 8*f*, 81, 256–59
beta rhythms in, 253, 254*f*
BOLD signals, 254
clinical implementation of, 261*f*
controls, 257–58, 258*f*
for disabled people, 252
electric field recording, 53–54
electrodes in, 168–69, 251, 259
feature detection by, 253–56
gamma rhythms in, 253–54
generators of, 46
hardware for, 168–69
history of development of, 251
in human studies, 259–60
item selection in, 258
LFPs, 251
limitations of, 259
LMP and, 255
mesoscale fields, 45
for motor function, 257
mu rhythms in, 253, 254*f*

online applications, 257–58
power demands of, 260
protocol design for, 256–57
recording devices, 260, 260*f*
recording domains, 252*f*
research applications for, 259–61
research studies for, 251
sampling rates in, 256
sensors for, 168–69
sensory input in, 256
signal amplitude for, 253, 253*f*
signal modalities for, 261
signal origin for, 256, 256*f*
spatial resolution in, 252, 259
SSVEPs and, 255
success rates from, 258
surgical implantation and, 260
thalamocortical oscillations in, 255, 261
time domain with, 254–55
tracking tasks, 255*f*
wireless, 260
electrodes
active, 106, 167
closely spaced, 113–15
cone, 273
DBS, 278
dry, 106, 167
in ECoG, 168–69, 251, 259
in EEG, 81, 105–6, 167–68
impedance, 167
inactive, 112
in intracortical recording, 169
Michigan, 273
multisite, 273
neurotropic, 84
placement of, 167–68
in P300 BCIs, 216*f*
recording, 56, 168*f*
reference, 56–57, 111–14, 112*f*
sensors, 167–69, 168*f*
signal characteristics for, 167–68
Utah arrays, 37, 85–86, 85*f*
wet, 106
electrode signal conditioning, 37–38
electrode tissue interface, 87–88
electroencephalography (EEG), 105–9
active electrodes in, 106
for ADHD, 352–53
artifacts and, 108–9
AVE in, 115–17. *See also* common average reference
bipolarity of, 106–7
CAR in, 115–17. *See also* average reference
closely space electrodes, 113–15
coherence in, 59
components of, 106*f*
contact impedance guidelines, 105–6
cortical generation of, 54
for CSF, 118
cursor controls, with BCIs, 81, 133, 179, 233, 307
dry electrodes in, 106
dura imaging approach to, 60
for electric fields, in brain, 54, 57–58
electrodes, 81, 105–6, 167–68
Engineer's Nyquist criterion, 107, 117–18
EPs in, 59–60
ERPs in, 60
feedback with, 352–60
FFTs in, 59
filters and, 109
forward problem for, 57–58
generators of, 46
hardware for, 167–68
for head models, 51

high-resolution methods, 58–61, 119–20
inactive electrodes, 112
inverse problem for, 58
Laplacian in, 60
linked-ears reference in, 115
linked-mastoid reference in, 115
macroscale fields, 45
mathematical transformations of, 58–59
montages for, 107, 108*f*
motor function recovery with, 353
after neural injury, 353
phase-locking in, 107
phase synchronization for, 59
for P300 BCI, 218
quantitative, 58–61
random references in, 115
reference electrodes in, 111–14, 112*f*
REST in, 117
sampling rates for, 107–8
for seizures, 352
sensitivity comparisons, 110–11, 111*f*
sensors, 166–68, 166*f*
signal sources, 110*f*
SMRs in, 236
source dynamics in, 61–62
spatial sampling of, 117–19
SSVEPs, 60
surface Laplacian in, 60, 120
system gains with, 105
VEP in, 112, 114*f*
volume conduction in, 61–62
wet electrodes in, 106
electromyographic (EMG) activity, 231
eloquent cortex, 15. *See also* cerebral cortex
EMG activity. *See* electromyographic activity
emotional reactions, BCIs and, 366, 366*f*
Engineer's Nyquist criterion, 107, 117–18
enhancement applications, in BCIs, 4
environmental interference, in signal processing, 132–33
EPI. *See* echo planar imaging
epilepsy, BCIs for, 321
EPs. *See* evoked potentials
ERD. *See* event-related desynchronization
ERPs. *See* event-related potentials
error-blind protocols, 193
error-detection protocols, 193, 364, 364*f*
ERS. *See* event-related synchronization
Ethernet, 175
ethics, BCI research and, 373–82
in accessibility of results, 374
appeals and, 379–80
beneficence and, 373–74
CNS plasticity and, 377–78
in general population, 380–81
inappropriate outputs and, 376
in informed consent, 378–79
invasion of privacy risks, 376–77
for invasive research, 374–80
justice principles in, 373, 379
multidisciplinary expertise and, 374
for people with disabilities, 375–80
physical risks and, 375
psychological risks and, 375–76
quality of care and, 374
respect for persons, 373, 378–79
for results reports, 380
for time-limited studies, 377
uncensored actions and, risks with, 378
European Union, BCI approval process in, 341
Evarts, Edward, 15

event-related desynchronization (ERD), 227–28, 228*f*
grand average patterns, 229*f*
event-related potentials (ERPs), 215
definition of, 223
in EEG, 60
event-related synchronization (ERS), 227, 228*f*
grand average patterns, 229*f*
evoked potentials (EPs). *See also* steady-state visually evoked potentials; visual evoked potentials
ASSEP, 245
in EEG, 59–60, 241
f-VEP, 241
excitatory synapses, 55
experimental coarse-graining, 52
extraparenchymal BCIs (eBCIs), 265–67
iBCIs and, 266–67
extrinsic noise, in neural recordings, 90

failure modes and effects analysis (FMEA), 339
fast decoding, 295–96
fast Fourier transforms (FFTs)
in EEG, 59
in feature extraction, 134–35, 135*f*
FDA. *See* Food and Drug Administration
feature extraction, in signal processing, 123–24, 129–39
application of, 133–38
AR modeling in, 135–36
band power, 134, 134*f*
block processing in, 133–34
coherence in, 137
conditioning, 138–39
data decimation in, 129–30
environmental interference in, 132–33
feature smoothing in, 139
FFT in, 134–35, 135*f*
frequency features, 134–36, 137*f*
frequency-range prefiltering, 129
ICA and, 139
integration in, 134
log-normal transforms, 138
Mahalanobis distance in, 137–38, 138*f*
method selection in, 133
normalization of, 129–30, 138
PCA and, 139
peak-picking in, 134
phase locking value in, 137
signal conditioning, 129–33
spatial filtering in, 130–32, 131*f*
template matching in, 134
temporal features for, 134
wavelets in, 136–37
feature smoothing, 139
feature vectors, in signal processing, 147
feature weights, in social processing, 147
federal grants, 347–48
SBIR, 347
STTR, 347
feedback, as therapeutic tool. *See also* augmented sensory feedback; biofeedback; motor function recovery, with BCI-based feedback; sensory feedback; somatosensory feedback, in motor control
with ADHD, 352–53
applications for, 351–52
BOLD responses and, 358*f*
connectivity analysis for, 358–59
with EEG, 352–60
for emotion processing, 357–58
with fMRI, 357–60
in hospital settings, 357

nerve fibers, 20
Nessi interface, 368, 368f
neural populations, 82, 270
neural recording
  electrodes for, 56
  with implantable microelectrodes,
    87–90
  of intracortical microelectrode arrays,
    90–97
  lumped-element functional models
    for, 89
  noise factors in, 89–90
  selectivity in, 88
  sensitivity in, 88
  of spikes, 36–38
  stability of, 88–89
  in supplementary motor cortex, 29f
neuroimaging. See also
  electrocorticography;
  electroencephalography; functional
  magnetic resonance imaging;
  functional near-infrared
  spectroscopy; functional
  transcranial Doppler;
  magnetoencephalography; positron
  emission tomography
  for blood flow, 66
  hardware for, 70
  resolution in, 65–67, 66f
  task design for, 74
neurons, 94–95
  in nonlinear signal processing models,
    153, 154f
neuronal spikes, 279–81
  Bayesian models in, 280
  bins in, 279
  nonstationarities in, 280
neurotropic electrodes, 84
noise, in neural recordings, 89–90
noise reduction, 37–38
nonlinear models, in signal processing,
    153–54
  continuous output in, 154
  kernel methods, 153
  neurons in, 153
nonstationarities, 149–50, 150f, 280
normalization, 129–30, 138
notch filters, 109
Nyquist Limit, 107, 125
Nyquist-Shannon sampling theorem, 125

object detection, with BCIs, 367
occipital lobe, 17
Oddball Paradigm, 215–16
  time course in, 216f
offline evaluations, for BCI, 159–60
Ohm's Law, 47
  action potentials and, 53
  tissues, volume conduction in, 49–50
oligodendrocytes, 95
open-loop decoding, 280–81
OpenViBE software, 178
operating protocols, BCI, 189–94
  application command to, 191–92
  asynchronous directed-output, 193
  directed-output, 193
  error-blind, 193
  error-detection, 193
  feature extraction in, 191
  goal selection, 9–10, 9f, 192
  initiation of, 189
  intentional control, 189
  no intentional control, 189
  preparameterized, 191
  process control, 9–10, 9f, 192

self-paced, 190–91
self-parameterized, 191
  SMRs in, 191
synchronous, 189–91, 190f
  for system testing, 193
  translation errors in, 192–93
  translation process in, 191
  for user training, 193
optodes, 302
orphan products, 342, 344, 348–49
output latency, 183–84, 184f
outputs. See artificial outputs, of BCIs;
  natural outputs, of CNS

pain management, 359
parameterization, 155–56
paraplegia, 319
parietal cortex
  action decoding and, 292–98
  action planning by, 290–96, 291f
  anatomy of, 289, 290f
  BCI signals in, 289–98
  external stimuli for, 291
  eye movements and, 290–91
  grasping activity in, 292, 293f
  PRR, 296–97
  reaching movements and, 290–91
parietal lobe, 16–17
parietal reach region (PRR), 296–97
participant recruitment, 327–28
passive BCI, 5–6
PCA. See principal component analysis
PCI. See peripheral component
  interconnect
peak-picking, in signal processing, 134
Penfield, Wilder, 15, 15f
people with disabilities. See also assistive
  technology; classical locked-in
  syndrome; incomplete locked-in
  syndrome; residual motor function,
  AT for; total locked-in syndrome
  ethics and, 375–80
peripheral component interconnect
    (PCI), 175
peripheral nervous system (PNS), 3
PET. See positron emission tomography
phase locking value, 137
  in SMRs, 230
phase synchronization, 59
photon banana, 70
physical risks, 375
pick-up coil, 109
planar gradiometer, 110
plasticity, CNS, 377–78
  artificial outputs, 6
  definition of, 351
  ethics in BCI research and, 377f
  importance for BCIs, 6–8
plug-and-play assistive technology,
    198, 209
PNS. See peripheral nervous system
Poisson process, 140
population coding, 265, 270
positron emission tomography (PET),
    66, 68f
  temporal resolution in, 68–69
posterior parietal cortex (PPC), 17, 23
  as associational, 23
  coding in, for motor control, 29
  directional tuning in, 25
  dorsal visual streams, 23
  motor control, 25
  ventral visual streams, 23
PPC. See posterior parietal cortex
Predictive speller, use with BCI, 207, 223

prefrontal cortex, 23–24
  motor control and, 25
  spatial working memory and, 24
prehension behaviors, 30–31
  primary motor cortex and, 31
premotor cortex, 22
  action decoding and, 292–98
  action planning by, 290–96, 291f
  anatomy of, 289, 290f
  BCI signals in, 289–98
  coding in, for motor control, 29
  external stimuli for, 291
  eye movements and, 290–91
  grasping activity in, 292, 293f
  motor control and, 24–25, 30
  PRR, 296–97
  rate modulation of movement by,
    25, 26f
  reaching movements and, 290–91
preparameterized protocols, 191
primary motor cortex, 20–22, 24–25.
    See also intraparenchymal BCIs;
    motor control
  action potential in, 15–16
  directional tuning in, 27, 27f
  electrical stimulation of, 15
  eloquent cortex in, 15
  encoding in, of motor control, 27–28
  firing rate profiles, 25f
  kinematic information in, 27
  lesions in, 31
  in macaque monkeys, 21f, 22f
  motor homunculus in, 15, 15f
  population vectors, 27–28
  prehension behaviors and, 31
  research studies on, 28
  SMA, 29–30
  subdivision of, 22
principal component analysis (PCA), 38,
    131–32
  for feature extraction, 139
  in fNIRS, 303–4
probes. See Michigan electrode;
  subcellular edge electrode probes
process control protocols, 9–10, 9f, 192,
    197, 203–4
proprioception
  in somatosensory cortex, 22
  somatosensory feedback and, 31–32
prosthesis control, 208
protocols. See specific protocols
PRR. See parietal reach region
psychological risks, 375–76
P300 BCIs, 215–24
  alternative electrode montages, 220
  alternative stimuli in, 220–21
  amplitude in, 217–18, 221
  auditory stimuli in, 222
  clinical evaluation of, 326f
  context-updating model, 217
  EEG recording, 218
  electrode locations, 216f
  e-mail applications for, 330f
  FLD in, 220
  function of, 217
  gaze direction in, 221–22
  ICA for, 220
  improvement of, 222–23
  independent home use of, 223
  latency in, 216–17
  matrix formats in, 221
  mental prosthesis, 218
  offline data analysis, 219
  origin of, 217
  signal-processing methods, 220
  stability function in, 217–18

stimulus presentation parameters in,
    220–21
  studies, 218–20
  support vector machines, 220
  SWLDA in, 220
P300 ERPs, 215–17
  Oddball Paradigm and, 215–16
pulse sequences, 73
pyramidal cells, 18

QoL assessments. See quality of life
  assessments
quality of life (QoL) assessments,
    332–33
quantization, in signal processing, 125
quasistatic electric fields, 46
quasistatic magnetic fields, 46

radiofrequency transmitters, 72
rate-coding hypothesis, 35
RC filters. See resistor and capacitor
  filters
reach decoding, 292–94, 297f
reaching movements
  delayed-cascade tasks, 290
  delayed-reach tasks, 290–91
  grasping, 292, 293f
  neural activity for, 290–91
readiness potential, 245
receiver antennae, 72
reconstruction computers, 73
recording. See neural recording
recording electrodes, 56
reference electrodes, 56–57
  in EEG, 111–14, 112f
  strategy summaries, 117
  true testing for, 113
  VEPs with, 113–14
reference electrode standardization
  technique (REST), 117
regression models, in signal
  processing, 148
regulatory considerations, for BCIs,
    339–41
reimbursement considerations, for BCIs,
    344–46
  coding for, 345
  coverage and, 344–45
  global marketing and, 346
  insurers and, 346
  payment and, 345
  reasonable proof and, 345–46
  strategy elements, 344
reliability, of BCIs, 389–92
  for iBCIs, 267
remote controls, BCIs for, with
  televisions, 378
Remote data transfer, in BCI, 330–31
repetition time (TR), 309–10
residual motor function, AT for,
    199–200
  manual scans in, 200
  user options in, 200
resistor and capacitor (RC) filters, 172
resolution, in neuroimaging, 65–67, 66f
  for EEG, 58–61, 119–20
  in PET, 68–69
  temporal, 65
resonance frequency, 72
REST. See reference electrode
  standardization technique
reversion rights, 348
robotics, 207
  motor function recovery with, 355–56